MANUAL OF CLINICAL PROBLEMS IN ADULT AMBULATORY CARE

WITH ANNOTATED KEY REFERENCES

MANUAL OF CLINICAL PROBLEMS IN ADULT AMBULATORY CARE

WITH ANNOTATED KEY REFERENCES

EDITED BY

LAURIE DORNBRAND, M.D.
Robert Wood Johnson Foundation Clinical Scholar and Fellow
in Internal Medicine, Division of General Medicine, University of North
Carolina at Chapel Hill School of Medicine, Chapel Hill

AXALLA J. HOOLE, M.D.
Associate Professor of Medicine and Administrative and Social Medicine,
Division of General Medicine, University of North Carolina at Chapel
Hill School of Medicine; Associate Attending Physician, Department
of Medicine, North Carolina Memorial Hospital, Chapel Hill

ROBERT H. FLETCHER, M.D., M.Sc.
Director, Robert Wood Johnson Clinical Scholars Program and Professor
of Medicine, University of North Carolina at Chapel Hill School
of Medicine; Co-Chief, Division of General Medicine, North Carolina
Memorial Hospital, Chapel Hill

C. GLENN PICKARD, JR., M.D.
Professor of Medicine and Social and Administrative Medicine,
University of North Carolina at Chapel Hill School of Medicine;
Associate Attending Physician, Division of General Medicine, North
Carolina Memorial Hospital, Chapel Hill

LITTLE, BROWN AND COMPANY   BOSTON/TORONTO

CONTENTS

CONTRIBUTING AUTHORS

RICHARD M. ADERHOLD, M.D.
Director, Adult and Addiction Services, Wilson-Greene Mental Health Center, Wilson, North Carolina

MARIO C. BATTIGELLI, M.D.
Professor of Medicine, Division of Pulmonary Diseases, University of North Carolina at Chapel Hill School of Medicine; Attending Physician, Department of Medicine, North Carolina Memorial Hospital, Chapel Hill

PAUL BECK, M.D.
Professor and Director, Program on Aging, University of North Carolina at Chapel Hill School of Medicine, Chapel Hill; Director, Medical Teaching Service, Wake County Medical Center, Raleigh, North Carolina

RAYMOND F. BIANCHI, M.D.
Clinical Assistant Professor of Medicine, University of North Carolina at Chapel Hill School of Medicine, Chapel Hill; Attending Physician, Department of Medicine, Charlotte Memorial Hospital, Charlotte, North Carolina

EUGENE M. BOZYMSKI, M.D.
Professor of Medicine, Division of Digestive Diseases and Nutrition, University of North Carolina at Chapel Hill School of Medicine; Attending Physician and Chief, Diagnostic and Treatment Center, North Carolina Memorial Hospital, Chapel Hill

JAMES P. BROWDER, M.D.
Clinical Assistant Professor of Surgery, Division of Otolaryngology, University of North Carolina at Chapel Hill School of Medicine; Attending Physician, Department of Surgery, North Carolina Memorial Hospital, Chapel Hill

JAMES A. BRYAN II, M.D.
Professor of Medicine, Division of General Medicine, University of North Carolina at Chapel Hill School of Medicine; Attending Physician, Department of Medicine, North Carolina Memorial Hospital, Chapel Hill

ERNEST BURKES, JR., M.D.
Professor of Oral Diagnosis, University of North Carolina at Chapel Hill School of Dentistry, Chapel Hill, North Carolina

ROBERT M. CALIFF, M.D.
Assistant Professor of Medicine, Division of Cardiology, Duke University School of Medicine; Staff Physician and Director, Cardiac Care Unit; Duke University Medical Center, Durham, North Carolina

DAVID R. CLEMMONS, M.D.
Assistant Professor of Medicine, Division of Endocrinology and Metabolism, University of North Carolina at Chapel Hill School of Medicine; Assistant Attending Physician, Department of Medicine, North Carolina Memorial Hospital, Chapel Hill

ROMULO E. COLINDRES, M.D.
Professor of Medicine, Division of Nephrology, University of North Carolina at Chapel Hill School of Medicine; Attending Physician, Department of Medicine, North Carolina Memorial Hospital, Chapel Hill

PETER CURTIS, M.R.C.P., F.F.C.A.P.
Associate Professor, Department of Family Medicine, University of North Carolina at Chapel Hill School of Medicine; Attending Physician, Family Practice, North Carolina Memorial Hospital, Chapel Hill

MARION DANIS, M.D.
Assistant Professor, Department of Medicine, University of North Carolina at Chapel Hill School of Medicine; Attending Physician, Department of Medicine, North Carolina Memorial Hospital, Chapel Hill

RICHARD A. DAVIDSON, M.D.
Associate Professor of Medicine, Division of General Medicine, Department of Medicine, University of Florida College of Medicine, Gainesville, Florida

ROBERT S. DITTUS, M.D.
Assistant Professor of Medicine, Department of Medicine, Indiana University School
of Medicine; Assistant Attending Physician, Wishard Memorial Hospital and Indiana
University Hospital, Indianapolis

JAMES F. DONOHUE, M.D.
Associate Professor of Medicine, Division of Pulmonary Diseases, University of North
Carolina at Chapel Hill School of Medicine; Attending Surgeon and Director,
Pulmonary Outpatient Clinic, North Carolina Memorial Hospital, Chapel Hill

LAURIE DORNBRAND, M.D.
Robert Wood Johnson Foundation Clinical Scholar and Fellow in Internal Medicine,
Division of General Medicine, University of North Carolina at Chapel Hill School of
Medicine; Physician, On Lok Senior Health Services, San Francisco

DOUGLAS A. DROSSMAN, M.D.
Associate Professor of Medicine and Psychiatry, University of North Carolina at
Chapel Hill School of Medicine; Attending Physician, Division of Diseases and
Nutrition, North Carolina Memorial Hospital, Chapel Hill

BRUCE B. DUNCAN, M.D.
Adjunct Assistant Professor of Epidemiology, University of North Carolina at Chapel
Hill School of Public Health, Chapel Hill, North Carolina

ROBERT W. ECKEL, M.D.
Clinical Instructor, Department of Neurology, Georgetown University School of
Medicine, Washington, D.C.; Staff Neurologist, Kaiser-Georgetown Health Plaza,
Washington, D.C.

LAMAR E. EKBLADH, M.D.
Private Practice, Obstetrics, Williamsburg Community Hospital, Williamsburg,
Virginia

JEFFERY J. FAHS, M.D.
Resident in Neurology, University of Arizona Health Sciences Center, Tucson,
Arizona

MARY L. FIELD, R.N., M.S.N., F.N.P.
Assistant Professor, Department of Primary Care, University of North Carolina at
Chapel Hill School of Nursing; Family Nurse Practitioner and Coordinator, Health
Maintenance Clinic, North Carolina Memorial Hospital, Chapel Hill

WILLIAM F. FINN, M.D.
Associate Professor of Medicine, University of North Carolina at Chapel Hill School
of Medicine; Associate Attending Physician, Department of Medicine, North Carolina
Memorial Hospital, Chapel Hill

ROBERT H. FLETCHER, M.D., M.Sc.
Director, Robert Wood Johnson Clinical Scholars Program, Professor of Medicine
and Co-Chief, Division of General Medicine, University of North Carolina at Chapel
Hill School of Medicine; Attending Physician, North Carolina Memorial Hospital,
Chapel Hill

SUZANNE W. FLETCHER, M.D.
Professor of Medicine, Division of General Medicine, University of North Carolina at
Chapel Hill School of Medicine; Attending Physician and Co-Chief, Division of
Medicine, North Carolina Memorial Hospital, Chapel Hill

TERRY L. FRY, M.D.
Assistant Professor of Surgery, Division of Otolaryngology, University of North
Carolina at Chapel Hill School of Medicine; Attending Physician, Department of
Surgery, North Carolina Memorial Hospital; Chapel Hill

JORGE T. GONZALEZ, M.D.
Assistant Professor of Medicine, University of North Carolina at Chapel Hill School
of Medicine; Senior Attending Physician and Director of Medicine, Outpatient
Department, New Hanover Memorial Hospital, Wilmington, North Carolina

WILLIAM H. GOODSON III, M.D.
Associate Professor of Surgery, University of California, San Francisco, School of
Medicine; University of California Medical Center, San Francisco

MAC A. GREGANTI, M.D.
Associate Professor, Division of General Medicine, University of North Carolina at Chapel Hill School of Medicine; Attending Physician, Department of Medicine, North Carolina Memorial Hospital, Chapel Hill

JOHN T. GWYNNE, M.D.
Associate Professor of Medicine, Division of Endrocrinology, University of North Carolina at Chapel Hill School of Medicine; Attending Physician, Department of Medicine, North Carolina Memorial Hospital, Chapel Hill

NORTIN M. HADLER, M.D.
Associate Professor of Medicine and Microbiology, Division of Rheumatology and Immunology, Department of Medicine, University of North Carolina at Chapel Hill School of Medicine; Attending Physician, North Carolina Memorial Hospital, Chapel Hill

JOHN J. HAGGERTY, M.D.
Associate Professor of Psychiatry and Clinical Assistant Professor of Family Medicine, University of North Carolina at Chapel Hill School of Medicine; Attending Psychiatrist, Division of Consultation and Liasion Psychiatry, North Carolina Memorial Hospital, Chapel Hill

ALAN K. HALPERIN, M.D.
Associate Professor of Medicine, Division of General Medicine, Department of Medicine, The University of New Mexico School of Medicine; Director, General Medicine Clinics, Veterans Administration Medical Center, Albuquerque

LINN HATLEY, M.D.
Clinical Assistant Professor of Obstetrics and Gynecology, Division of General Gynecology, University of North Carolina at Chapel Hill School of Medicine; Private Practice, Obstetrics and Gynecology, Durham, North Carolina

WILLIAM D. HEIZER, M.D.
Professor of Medicine, Division of Gastroenterology, University of North Carolina at Chapel Hill School of Medicine; Director, Nutrition Support Services, North Carolina Memorial Hospital, Chapel Hill

MICHAEL C. HINDMAN, M.D.
Assistant Professor of Medicine, Division of Cardiology, Duke University School of Medicine; Director of Preventative Cardiology Program, Duke University Medical Center and Veterans Administration Hospital, Durham, North Carolina

J. PACK HINDSLEY, JR., M.D.
Private Practice, Urology; Staff Physician, Beaufort County Hospital, Washington, North Carolina

MARK A. HLATKY, M.D.
Associate in Medicine, Duke University School of Medicine; Physician, Division of Cardiology, Duke University Medical Center, Durham, North Carolina

AXALLA J. HOOLE, M.D.
Associate Professor of Medicine and Administrative and Social Medicine, Division of General Medicine, University of North Carolina at Chapel Hill School of Medicine; Associate Attending Physician, Department of Medicine, North Carolina Memorial Hospital, Chapel Hill

KATHERINE A. HUFFMAN, M.D.
Clinical Assistant Professor, Division of Nephrology, University of North Carolina at Chapel Hill School of Medicine; Attending Physician, North Carolina Memorial Hospital, Chapel Hill

STEPHEN B. HULLEY, M.D., M.P.H.
Professor of Epidemiology, University of California, School of Medicine, San Francisco

ERIC W. JENSEN, M.D.
Associate Professor of Psychiatry, University of North Carolina at Chapel Hill School of Medicine; Attending Physician, Department of Psychiatry, North Carolina Memorial Hospital, Chapel Hill

JOHN S. KIZER, M.D.
Associate Professor of Medicine and Pharmacology, University of North Carolina at Chapel Hill School of Medicine; Attending Physician, North Carolina Memorial Hospital, Chapel Hill

THOMAS KOTTKE, M.D.
Assistant Professor of Medicine and Public Health, University of Minnesota Medical School—Minneapolis; Director of Cardiac Rehabilitation, Department of Medicine, University of Minnesota Hospitals and Clinics, Minneapolis

TIMOTHY W. LANE, M.D.
Assistant Professor of Medicine, Division of Infectious Diseases, University of North Carolina at Chapel Hill School of Medicine; Internal Medicine Teaching Program, Moses H. Cone Memorial Hospital, Greensboro, North Carolina

ROBERT S. LAWRENCE, M.D.
Charles S. Davidson Associate Professor of Medicine, Harvard Medical School, Boston; Director, Department of Medicine, The Cambridge Hospital, Cambridge, Massachusetts

SIDNEY L. LEVINSON, M.D.
Clinical Assistant Professor of Medicine, Division of Gastroenterology, University of North Carolina at Chapel Hill School of Medicine; Attending Physician, Department of Medicine, North Carolina Memorial Hospital, Chapel Hill

MATTHEW H. LIANG, M.D., M.P.H.
Assistant Professor of Medicine, Harvard Medical School; Assistant Physician, Department of Rheumatology and Immunology, Brigham and Women's Hospital, Boston

MACK LIPKIN, M.D.
Visiting Professor of Clinical Medicine, University of North Carolina at Chapel Hill School of Medicine; President, Zlinkoff Foundation, New York

BERNARD LO, M.D.
Assistant Professor of Medicine, University of California, San Francisco, School of Medicine, San Francisco

WILLIAM D. MATTERN, M.D.
Professor of Medicine, University of North Carolina at Chapel Hill School of Medicine; Medical Director, Dialysis Program, North Carolina Memorial Hospital, Chapel Hill

CHERYL F. MCCARTNEY, M.D.
Assistant Professor of Psychiatry, University of North Carolina at Chapel Hill School of Medicine; Attending Psychiatrist Division of Consultation and Liaison Psychiatry, Chapel Hill

JACK D. MCCUE, M.D.
Associate Professor of Medicine, Chief, Section on General Medicine and Geriatrics, The Bowman Gray School of Medicine of Wake Forest University, Winston-Salem, North Carolina

JOHN C. MERRITT, M.D.
Professor Ophthalmology, University of North Carolina at Chapel Hill School of Medicine; Attending Surgeon, Glaucoma and Pediatric Clinics, North Carolina Memorial Hospital, Chapel Hill

PHILLIP A. MOORING, M.S.
Supervisor of Substance Abuse Services, Wilson-Greene Mental Health Center, Wilson, North Carolina

C. RICHARD MORRIS, M.D.
Associate Professor of Pediatrics, Division of Nephrology, University of North Carolina at Chapel Hill School of Medicine; Attending Physician, Department of Pediatrics, North Carolina Memorial Hospital, Chapel Hill

C. THOMAS NUZUM, M.D.
Associate Professor of Medicine, Division of Digestive Diseases and Nutrition, University of North Carolina at Chapel Hill School of Medicine; Attending Physician, North Carolina Memorial Hospital, Chapel Hill

MICHAEL Y. PARKER, M.D.
Private Practice; Staff Physician, Rex Hospital, Raleigh Community Hospital, and Wake County Memorial Hospital, Raleigh, North Carolina

C. GLENN PICKARD, JR., M.D.
Professor of Medicine and Social and Administrative Medicine, University of North Carolina at Chapel Hill School of Medicine; Associate Attending Physician, Division of General Medicine, North Carolina Memorial Hospital, Chapel Hill

DUNCAN S. POSTMA, M.D.
Assistant Professor of Surgery, Division of Otolaryngology University of North Carolina at Chapel Hill School of Medicine; Attending Physician, North Carolina Memorial Hospital, Chapel Hill

SHELDON M. RETCHIN, M.D.
Assistant Professor of Medicine, Division of General Medicine University of North Carolina at Chapel Hill School of Medicine; Attending Physician, Director, Medicine Clinics, North Carolina Memorial Hospital, Chapel Hill

CELESTE ROBB-NICHOLSON, M.D.
Fellow in Rheumatology, Harvard School of Medicine; Brigham and Women's Hospital, Boston, Massachusetts

JOHN F. ROGERS, M.D.
Assistant Professor of Medicine, Division of Clinical Pharmacology, Department of Medicine, The Johns Hopkins University School of Medicine; Director, Clinical Pharmacology Unit, Good Samaritan Hospital, Baltimore

C. STEWART ROGERS, M.D.
Assistant Professor of Medicine, Division of General Medicine, University of North Carolina at Chapel Hill School of Medicine; Internal Medicine Teaching Service, Moses H. Cone Memorial Hospital, Greensboro, North Carolina

DESMOND K. RUNYAN, M.D.
Assistant Professor of Social and Administrative Medicine University of North Carolina at Chapel Hill School of Medicine; Attending Physician, Department of Pediatrics, North Carolina Memorial Hospital, Chapel Hill

R. BALFOUR SARTOR, M.D.
Assistant Professor of Medicine, Division of Gastroenterology, University of North Carolina at Chapel Hill School of Medicine; Attending Physician, Department of Medicine, North Carolina Memorial Hospital, Chapel Hill

SUZANNE V. SAUTER, M.D.
Assistant Professor of Medicine, Director Rehabilitation Program Office, University of North Carolina at Chapel Hill School of Medicine; Attending Physician, North Carolina Memorial Hospital, Chapel Hill

REBECCA A. SILLIMAN, M.D.
Assistant Professor of Medicine, Division of General Medicine, Department of Medicine, Brown University Program in Medicine; Assistant Attending Physician, Roger Williams General Hospital, Providence, Rhode Island

ROSS J. SIMPSON, JR., M.D.
Assistant Professor of Medicine, Division of Cardiology, University of North Carolina at Chapel Hill School of Medicine; Attending Physician, North Carolina Memorial Hospital, Chapel Hill

DAVID S. SISCOVICK, M.D., M.P.H.
Assistant Professor of Medicine and Clinical Assistant Professor of Epidemiology, University of North Carolina at Chapel Hill School of Medicine; Attending Physician, Department of Medicine, North Carolina Memorial Hospital, Chapel Hill

PHILIP D. SLOANE, M.D.
Assistant Professor, Department of Family Medicine, University of North Carolina at Chapel Hill School of Medicine; Attending Physician, North Carolina Memorial Hospital, Chapel Hill

HUNTER R. STOKES, M.D.
Clinical Associate Professor of Ophthalmology, University of South Carolina School of Medicine, Columbia; Chairman, Section of Ophthamalogy, McLeod Regional Medical Center, Florence, South Carolina

GREGORY STRAYHORN, M.D.
Assistant Professor of Family Medicine, University of North Carolina at Chapel
Hill School of Medicine; Attending Physician, North Carolina Memorial Hospital,
Chapel Hill

PETER C. UNGARO, M.D.
Associate Professor of Medicine, University of North Carolina at Chapel Hill School
of Medicine; Senior Attending Physician, Department of Medicine, New Hanover
Memorial Hospital, Wilmington, North Carolina

ROBERT D. UTIGER, M.D.
Professor of Medicine, Division of Endocrinology, University of North Carolina at
Chapel Hill School of Medicine; Attending Physician, North Carolina Memorial
Hospital, Chapel Hill

EDWARD H. WAGNER, M.D.
Director, Center for Health Studies, Group Health Cooperative of Puget Sound,
Seattle, Washington.

LAURENCE O. WATKINS, M.D.
Assistant Professor of Medicine, Medical College of Georgia School of Medicine;
Attending Physician and Director, Noninvasive Cardiac Laboratory Eugene Talmadge
Memorial Hospital, Augusta, Georgia

ROBERT A. WAUGH, M.D.
Associate Professor of Medicine, Duke University School of Medicine; Associate
Physician, Cardiac Center, Duke University Medical Center, Durham, North Carolina

ANDREAS T. WIELGOSZ, M.D., F.R.C.P.
Associate Professor of Medicine, University of Ottawa School of Medicine;
Cardiologist, University of Ottawa Heart Institute, Ottawa, Ontario, Canada

MARK E. WILLIAMS, M.D.
Assistant Professor of Medicine, Division of General Medicine, University of North
Carolina at Chapel Hill School of Medicine; Attending Physician, North Carolina
Memorial Hospital, Chapel Hill

PARK W. WILLIS IV, M.D.
Assistant Professor of Medicine, Department of Medicine, University of North
Carolina at Chapel Hill School of Medicine; Attending Physician, Cardiology
Division, North Carolina Memorial Hospital, Chapel Hill

Clinicians often perceive a gap between the information available in the traditional medical literature and the day-to-day concerns of patient care. In *Manual of Clinical Problems in Adult Ambulatory Care* we have endeavored to bridge the gap and thereby meet the needs of clinicians—whether they be internists, family physicians, nurse practitioners, or subspecialists—who provide general care.

Most of the problems reviewed in the Manual were selected because they are among the ones frequently recorded in surveys of ambulatory medical care. Others—for example, bereavement, problem patients, and exercise—were added because they seemed to be encountered often, even though they may not be recorded as medical problems. For each topic, the discussion is directed toward questions that must be answered by clinicians. In this way we have attempted to make the text comprehensive, although not all-inclusive. Even though dermatologic complaints are very common, we had insufficient space to cover them, adequately; there are excellent references available in this field.

Each chapter is accompanied by an annotated bibliography of articles and books that are particularly influential, well done, or provocative. In many cases, the literature fell short and answers to clinical questions were not available from published research. We hope some readers will be stimulated to pursue answers themselves through clinical research.

In organizing the chapters, we found it difficult to choose between a diagnosis-oriented and a problem-oriented approach. We have elected to use both, depending on the level of resolution with which medical conditions are ordinarily encountered in practice. Thus, we have chapters on diagnostic entities such as mitral valve prolapse, parkinsonism, and asthma. Other chapters are about medical problems such as lymphadenopathy, proteinuria, and shoulder pain. The reader may find it necessary to refer to the index, rather than the table of contents, to find where a given problem is located.

We have aimed throughout to present information in a way that is immediately useful to physicians in office and clinic. We hope the reader will find the Manual a practical but scholarly companion during the complex task of caring for patients in ambulatory care settings.

L.D.
A.J.H.
R.H.F.
C.G.P., Jr.

ACKNOWLEDGEMENTS

We are grateful to the contributing authors for their scholarship and for the graciousness with which they adapted their individual styles to conform to a single book of relatively uniform style and format. Regardless of the level of formal affiliation with us, all became involved in an active and productive collaboration that proved to be very satisfying. We also wish to thank our colleagues who reviewed many of the chapters and made valuable suggestions for change.

All typescripts were edited in the offices of The Division of General Medicine and Clinical Epidemiology, and The Robert Wood Johnson Clinical Scholars Program at Chapel Hill. We are deeply indebted to the staff in these offices: Heidi McMurray, Shelley Chalmers, Ruth Long, and Theresa Brooks. Their effort, good will, and high standards made the editors' responsibilities seem lighter.

Finally, we are indebted to the housestaff of the Department of Medicine. Efforts to answer their questions prompted us to undertake this project.

L.D.
A.J.H.
R.H.F.
C.G.P., Jr.

I. CONSTITUTIONAL SYMPTOMS

1. DIZZINESS

James P. Browder

Patients who complain of "dizziness" present a major diagnostic problem. Most will prove to have a benign, self-limited illness often attributed to tension or anxiety. However, this "diagnosis" is made in part by ruling out other diseases, many of which are quite serious and in some cases life-threatening.

In taking the initial history, the essential first step is to decide whether or not the dizzy patient has vertigo, because the presence of vertigo greatly limits the possible diagnoses.

Vertigo

In general, most patients with vertigo, as opposed to other kinds of dizziness, will complain of a sensation of movement in space when by other means (their visual and proprioceptive-exteroceptive systems) they do not appear to be moving. Vertigo is thus described as a hallucination of movement. Very often this sensation will be accompanied by nausea, with or without vomiting. In many patients there will be associated otologic complaints such as hearing loss, tinnitus, or a feeling of "fullness" in the ear.

Vertigo is characteristically episodic; dizziness that is described as "continuous" is almost certainly not vertigo. Typically, each episode of vertigo is sudden in onset and relatively short in duration. Attacks last from a few seconds to several hours at the most, although a residual "queasy feeling" may last for several days. Head movement almost always aggravates vertigo, whereas in other forms of dizziness it has little or no effect. Finally, the intensity of vertigo is usually more dramatic and severe than in other forms of dizziness.

If the patient is experiencing vertigo when seen for evaluation or if the vertigo can be induced by one of several maneuvers described below, then one should be able to demonstrate nystagmus when testing the extraocular movements. Failure to demonstrate nystagmus in a patient who has acute, severe vertigo at the time is most unusual and should cause one to question whether the symptom is really vertigo.

Most patients with vertigo can be shown to have one of the entities discussed below, and a definite diagnosis, prognosis, and plan of treatment can be established.

Middle Ear Disease

If there is an associated complaint related to the ear, such as earache or hearing loss, primary middle ear pathology should be considered. Acute otitis media, for example, can produce a mild labyrinthitis with vertigo, tinnitus, and hearing loss (primarily conductive).

Vertigo can be an ominous sign when associated with chronic otitis media and/or cholesteatoma, because the symptom suggests extension into the labyrinthine structures. The presence of foul-smelling pus or, if cholesteatoma, squamous debris in the external auditory canal would suggest these diagnoses.

Otitis Externa

Otitis externa can present as otorrhea and vertigo.

Meniere's Disease

Meniere's disease should be considered if vertigo is associated with a fluctuating hearing loss, "roaring" tinnitus, and occasionally a feeling of fullness in the ear. All of these symptoms occur together in episodes that may last for several hours and can be severely incapacitating. Recurrences occur at intervals of a few days to several months. Examination of the ear shows no abnormalities. All patients with suspected Meniere's disease and/or other conditions presenting with vertigo and hearing loss require referral to an otolaryngologist to establish the definitive diagnosis.

Positional Vertigo

Patients with a strong positional component to their vertigo form another distinct group. Hearing symptoms are not present, and vertigo is not provoked unless the patient changes head position. Symptoms are usually mild and of short duration. Two types occur: one classically comes on at night, when the patient turns over in bed, and is called *benign positional vertigo* (BPV); the other occurs when the patient is standing and tilts the head back and is called *paroxysmal positional vertigo* (PPV). Paroxysmal positional vertigo can be elicited by rapidly taking the patient from a sitting to a supine position while the head is forcibly turned to one side (the Dix-Hallpike maneuver). This maneuver should be performed with caution or not at all in older patients, who may be susceptible to vertebral artery compression and stroke. The classical response indicating PPV consists of rotatory nystagmus with a latent period prior to onset, fatigue in the intensity of the nystagmus if the maneuver is repeated, and the associated feeling of vertigo.

Both types of positional vertigo are self-limited and will resolve within several months of onset. In the classic examples no additional evaluation is indicated; less clear-cut instances of positional vertigo should have a more thorough evaluation, including audiometry and electronystagmogram (ENG), usually by a specialist.

Vestibular Apoplexy

Two fairly common causes of severe vertigo without hearing loss, headache, or other symptoms are vestibular neuronitis and viral labyrinthitis. Vestibular neuronitis is the term usually given to an acute attack of severe vertigo that may recur, but does so in a milder form. Neurologic, ear, nose, and throat examination, and audometric evaluation are entirely normal, although caloric testing shows a unilateral loss of vestibular function. Viral labyrinthitis is a similar illness preceded by a viral syndrome. These names presume more about the disease than is actually known; therefore a less specific name, "vestibular apoplexy," is preferable. In either case, the diagnosis is one of exclusion and requires audiometric testing to rule out occult cochlear involvement. Treatment is symptomatic, and both illnesses are self-limited.

Cervical Vertigo

Cervical vertigo is uncommon and must be mentioned primarily because of its medicolegal implications. Some individuals develop vertigo induced by neck motion following a "whiplash" injury to the neck. The diagnosis of cervical vertigo can be made conclusively only by ENG, so referral to a specialist is necessary if the diagnosis is suspected.

Other Causes

Other, less common, causes of vertigo include perilymph fistula, otosclerosis, epilepsy, multiple sclerosis, polyarteritis nodosa, and cerebrovascular accidents.

Unsteadiness

The majority of patients complaining of dizziness but not having vertigo are usually better described as having "unsteadiness," and they will usually readily agree that this is an accurate description of their complaint. Others will offer a variety of vague descriptions. Rarely is this group of patients confused with those having vertigo.

In contrast to patients complaining of vertigo, patients with unsteadiness represent a heterogeneous group with diagnoses ranging from gastrointestinal bleeding or aortic stenosis to mild, self-limited adverse reactions to drugs or tension/anxiety states. In nearly all cases, the underlying cause will be evident from the initial complete history and physical examination. Among the most common causes of unsteadiness are drugs (particularly antihypertensive and psychotropic drugs, as well as many over-the-counter drugs, such as the antihistamines), any of the causes of classic syncope when the syndrome is not fully expressed (e.g., postural hypotension and arrhythmias), and psychiatric conditions (e.g., depression, chronic anxiety, and anxiety attacks, particularly with hyperventilation). Other medical conditions causing unsteadiness are less common: anemia, neurologic disease, such as cerebrovascular accidents and autonomic peripheral neuropathy, and valvular heart disease. Not infrequently older patients complain of dizziness but in fact have a gait disturbance from deterioration of one or more of several systems—ophthalmalogic, vestibular, or neurologic (proprioception). Failing eyesight is frequently found in isolation or in combination with other processes. Vestibular deterioration is unusual as an isolated event.

Laboratory assessment of the unsteady patient should include a measure of hema tocrit or hemoglobin at the minimum because anemia is a cause of unsteadiness. The pursuit of other studies should depend on some clue, such as an arrhythmia that might require a Holter monitor.

Treatment

Vertigo
Management of vertigo is almost always directed at controlling symptoms. Patients should remain quietly in bed, making no attempt to read or watch television. Light usually exacerbates nystagmus (and vertigo). Most patients quickly learn on their own that bed rest is helpful, and such advice is rarely needed. Mild sedatives, such as diazepam (Valium), 5 mg orally three times a day, are sometimes prescribed. A variety of antihistamine-like drugs have been recommended, such as dimenhydrinate (Dramamine) and meclizine hydrochloride (Antivert, Bonine). These often seem useful, although their specific efficacy beyond the sedative and placebo effects has not been established.

Unsteadiness
Therapy for unsteadiness depends on the underlying disease. Treatment of the group of patients with unsteadiness attributed to tension or anxiety presents a common dilemma. Reassurance is often therapeutic but may well not suffice. Alleviation of stress, where possible, is always a primary goal, and many patients in this group are insistent that tranquilizers or mild sedatives be prescribed. Personal philosophy and beliefs guide the practitioner in this area. Diazepam, 5 mg orally three times a day, for 1- to 2-week periods may prove very beneficial in many cases. Antihistamine-like drugs are often used, but they are unlikely to have any specific effect on unsteadiness.

Wolfson RJ (Ed.). Vertigo *Otolaryngol* Clin *North Am* 6(1), Feb. 1973.
  A state of the art review of the treatment of vertigo with articles devoted to Meniere's disease, vestibular neuronitis, positional vertigo, acoustic tumors, and central vertigo.
Spector M. *Dizziness and Vertigo: Diagnosis and Treatment.* New York: Grune & Stratton, 1967.
  A systematic presentation of the anatomy, physiology, diagnosis, and treatment of dizziness and vertigo. Clinical syndromes of both otologic and nonotologic origins are discussed.
Gay AJ, et al. *Eye Movement Disorders.* St. Louis: Mosby, 1974.
  A comprehensive but very readable presentation of ophthalmokinetic pathology, emphasizing clinical diagnosis based on a thorough understanding of the underlying pathophysiology. Essential reading for anyone wishing to understand electronystagmography interpretation.

2. FATIGUE
Mack Lipkin

The complaint of fatigue is a challenge to clinicians because possible causes range from the trivial to the lethal. Fatigue is a common complaint and often the first symptom of physical or mental illness, unhealthy life-styles, unhappy experiences, or any combination of these. It may be presented in varied language: "I can't get out of bed in the morning," "I have no pep," "I'm tired out all the time," or "I just don't feel good."

Fatigue can be both an effect of many disorders and itself a cause of further morbidity. For example, hepatitis and infectious mononucleosis are accompanied by both lassitude and depression, which in turn can lead to problems in work, social life, and nutrition, resulting in more depression and fatigue. This interweaving of cause and effect, along with imprecise language, has made it impossible to find reliable data about the frequency of various causes of fatigue in ambulatory practice. According to several surveys, physical disorders are found in anywhere from 3 to 39% of patients who present to internists and family practitioners with a primary complaint of fatigue. Such figures reflect the variability of medical practice and are not helpful in dealing with individual patients. In the absence of hard data to dictate a standardized workup the problem may be considered in terms of three etiologic categories: "organic" disease, unhealthy life-styles and habits, and depression. A meticulous history is likely to yield the critical clues to assessment and management.

"Organic" Disease

Fatigue may precede or follow the more specific symptoms of many diseases, or it may be associated with frequently used medications, especially diuretics and antihypertensives. It is common during the active phase of most illnesses and may persist for days months, or years. As the first and only symptom of insidious disease, fatigue is more frequently seen with diabetes mellitus, hypothyroidism, diuretic-associated electrolyte imbalance, neoplasms such as lymphoma and carcinoma of the cecum, slowly progressing renal or heart failure, early dementia, and chronic anemia, especially pernicious anemia. Chronic fatigue deserves a full review of systems to reassure both doctor and patient about possible "organic" disease. Laboratory studies and elimination of possibly offending drugs should be ordered as deemed appropriate. The search is best done at the beginning of treatment to forestall the patient's fear that the doctor is not being conscientious.

Clinical experience suggests that several findings make "organic" disease as the primary etiology less probable but do not rule it out. These include (1) fatigue present for several months without other symptoms and signs, (2) fatigue chiefly or only in the morning, especially if it disappears with activity, distraction, or exercise, (3) evidence of depression (although depression accompanies many diseases), (4) evidence of life patterns conducive to tiredness, and (5) normal temperature, when actually taken and recorded three times a day.

Life-style Problems

Fatigue associated with unhealthy life-styles and habits is probably the most common type seen in ambulatory practice. What we know about this cause of fatigue is based mainly on clinical observations; there have been few rigorous studies of the relationship between life-style and symptoms. Inquiry to elicit such problems should explore the following areas.

Occupational History

A detailed description of the patient's work may uncover such factors as problems with associates and supervisors, limited future prospects, monotony, or chronic dissatisfaction, all of which may contribute to chronic fatigue or even exhaustion. "Overwork" is a common complaint and often misleading; most people enjoy hard work if it is satisfying. Those who are unhappy in their jobs or who work compulsively are more likely to complain to physicians. The elderly usually decrease work effort gradually as their energy and endurance fade; those who insist on maintaining their former patterns may complain of fatigue.

Domestic Environment

Evaluation of the domestic environment should include compatibility with spouse or other companions, degree of mutual support, financial problems, sexual satisfaction and troubles with children or other relatives.

Exercise Patterns

Inadequate exercise over a long period of time may lead to decreased vigor and ready fatigability. Patients with depression, anxiety, and tension often report temporary relief with exercise, whereas those whose fatigue stems from active disease often feel worse after exercise.

Eating Habits

People who do not eat properly often feel tired. This includes both those who grossly overeat and those who substitute coffee and carbohydrates for meals.

Rest and Recreation

Imbalance in work, play, and rest, patterns of recreation, and the range of hobbies and interests can result in fatigue.

Drug Use

The excessive use of substances with stimulant or depressive effects, including alcohol, caffeine, and tobacco as well as amphetamines, sedative-hypnotics, and minor tranquilizers, may also result in cyclical patterns of activity and fatigue.

Treatment

When problems in any of the above areas are elicited, simply pointing them out to the patient may be a useful first step in dealing with the associated physical symptoms. Changes in diet, exercise, and recreation patterns may be suggested. Some problems at work and home may be amenable to counseling from the primary physician; others require more specialized intervention.

Depression

Depressive reactions are seen in many forms and degrees of severity. The term *depression* is applied, often quite vaguely, to a miscellany of clinical conditions ranging from an endogenous disorder to a situational reaction, normal or excessive, to unfortunate life events.

Regardless of the type of depression, it is commonly accompanied by morning fatigue, whether or not the patient slept well. Although many depressed patients blame poor sleep for their fatigue, the two are probably not cause and effect but associated manifestations of the underlying mechanism. The patient who describes feeling abysmally tired in the morning, but less fatigued a few hours later, is almost always a depressed person. In contrast, people with chronic disease seldom show such diurnal rhythm and, unlike depressed patients, generally feel somewhat better after resting.

The suspicion of depression should lead to a search for further evidence such as a history of previous depression, dysphoric mood, sleep disturbance, loss of an important person, disappointment, or failure. Obsessive-compulsive patients are prone to recurring depressions. The elderly, especially the physically ill, are notoriously subject to depressions, and the presentation is often deceptive, masked by physical complaints.

Once again a careful drug history is essential. Depression may be a side effect of a number of commonly prescribed drugs, including reserpine, alpha-methyldopa, propanolol, benzodiazepines, chlorpromazine, and birth control pills. Improper use of prescribed sedatives, tranquilizers, or amphetamines may result in cycles in which symptoms are temporarily relieved, followed by a let-down feeling, which causes more drug use and results in more fatigue and/or depression.

In any case, the diagnosis of depression should always be made on positive evidence, not solely on an inability to find an "organic" cause. Positive evidence, properly elicited, often offers clues to appropriate management. Further information on treatment of depression is contained in Chapter 113.

The cause of a patient's complaint of fatigue may stem from any illness in the books or from patterns of living not conducive to well-being. Persistent fatigue is a warning that the problem may be serious and warrants careful investigation. About 90% of the time a meticulous history will yield adequate clues to both diagnosis and effective management. Additional examination and the clinical course should clarify the remainder.

Lipkin M. *The Care of Patients: Concepts and Tactics.* New York: Oxford University Press, 1974. Etiology: pp. 36–49, 88–97; Diagnosis: pp. 107–135, 156–160; Treatment: pp. 163–164, 171–182, 211–214, 220–230.
Useful background material.

Engel GL. Differential Diagnosis of Nervousness and Fatigue. In CM MacBryde and RS Blacklow (Eds.), *Signs and Symptoms: Applied Pathologic Physiology and Clinical Interpretation* (5th ed.). Philadelphia: Lippincott, 1970. Pp. 641–646.
Comprehensive review of nervousness and fatigue as encountered in a university medical center more often than in ambulatory practice. Scholarly and well written.

Halberstam MF. Fatigue. In HF Conn and RB Conn (Eds.), *Current Diagnosis Six.* Philadelphia: Saunders, 1980. Pp. 50–53.
   Engaging written discussion by a good internist-cardiologist.

Plutzky M. Identifying the depressed patient. *Primary Care* 7(4):585, Dec. 1980.
   A useful, simple summary of "depression" as encountered in primary care practice.

Blumenthal MD. Depressive illness in old age: Getting behind the mask. *Geriatrics* 35:34, 1980.
   A realistic and practical summary of the problem.

Morrison JD. Fatigue as a presenting complaint in family practice. *J Fam Pract* 10(5):795, 1980.
   Review of 176 patients with isolated diagnosis of fatigue. One of the few attempts at a quantitative study of fatigue.

Barsky AJ. Hidden reasons some patients visit doctors. *Ann. Intern Med* 94:492, 1981.
   Sensible discussion of psychological problems in ambulatory practice.

Postoperative fatigue (editorial). *Lancet* 1:84, 1979.
   Good article pointing to multifaceted etiology. Little is known about this common troublesome occurrence.

Simanson E, Weiser PC (Eds.). *Psychological Aspects and Physiological Correlates of Work and Fatigue.* Springfield, Ill.: Thomas, 1979. Pp. 285–335.
   An excellent summary of some "biopsychosocial" factors.

3. OBESITY

Bruce B. Duncan

Obesity is an excess of body fat. Because body fat is extremely difficult to measure, however, obesity is in practice defined in terms of relative weight for height. Insurance companies' data on mortality rates analyzed in 1959 have been translated into tables of "desirable body weight" (DBW), that is, the weight apparently associated with minimum mortality for a given height and frame size. More recent studies, however, show DBW to be about 10% above these 1959 figures, and as used in this chapter DBW includes that 10% upward adjustment.

Large prospective studies demonstrate that the risk of death is only marginally related to weight in the broad range between 20% below and 20% above DBW, but increases in a curvilinear fashion beyond these bounds. It has been estimated that being 30 to 50% over DBW has a greater impact on mortality than smoking one or more packs of cigarettes a day.

The overall increase in mortality related to obesity results predominantly from ischemic heart disease, as obesity exerts a major effect on the cardiac risk factors of hypertension, hyperglycemia, and hypercholesterolemia. It also increases mortality from diabetes, cerebrovascular disease, cancer, and some diseases of the digestive tract (e.g., cirrhosis, cholelithiasis). Clinical experience, supported in most cases by epidemiologic studies, suggests that obesity is associated with, and probably causes, increased morbidity from a variety of other conditions. Among these are osteoarthritis of the weight-bearing joints, dermatologic and pulmonary disorders, poor reproductive and sexual function, increased accident proneness, and perioperative complications. In addition, the obese suffer increased psychopathology and psychosocial disability, at least in part because our society reveres slimness.

Diagnostic Evaluation

Degree of Obesity

The degree of obesity should be assessed by comparison of the patient's weight with the appropriate DBW. Tables of desirable body weight can be readily found in textbooks, but those in books published prior to 1983 are based on 1959 data and should be adjusted upward by 10%. When tables are not available, DBW can be estimated as follows: starting from 100 pounds for women and 110 pounds for men, 5 pounds are

dded or subtracted for each inch of the patient's height above or below 5 feet. Ten
ercent is added for individuals with an average frame, 20% for those with a large
rame.

On initial evaluation, one must determine if obesity is primary or secondary.

Secondary Obesity

Secondary obesity is rare. Endocrine causes such as hypothyroidism and Cushing's syn-
rome can usually be excluded by physical examination. Excess skinfold thickness of
atty consistency cannot be explained by hypothyroidism, while a normotensive patient
vithout cushingoid features almost certainly does not have Cushing's syndrome. Other
econdary causes include a variety of rare congenital syndromes, which almost always
roduce associated physical findings and are usually present in childhood. Drugs that
an cause obesity include insulin, phenothiazines, corticosteroids, tricyclic antidepres-
ants, and cyproheptadine.

Primary Obesity

Primary obesity results from caloric intake in excess of caloric expenditure. This sim-
le statement belies a very complicated matter, however. Evidence indicates that more
han sloth and gluttony underlies obesity. Some studies suggest a genetic predisposi-
ion. Many studies document that individuals differ widely in their ability to utilize
ietary energy. Variability in thermogenesis, or the body's tendency to produce heat
uring the processes of daily living, may explain much of this difference.

Childhood-onset obesity is widely held to be more resistant to therapy than adult-
nset obesity, perhaps due to fat cell hyperplasia occurring during the early years.

Treatment

Conventional Dietary Therapy

Conventional dietary therapy is aimed at decreasing caloric intake with or without
ncreased caloric expenditure. The standard dietary approach has been the balanced
eduction of all three caloric constituents (protein, fats, and carbohydrates). One simple
pproach to this is the following:

. Calculate total calories necessary to maintain DBW by multiplying DBW in kilo-
    grams times energy expenditure per kilogram, estimated at 30 kcal/kg for sedentary
    activity, 35 to 40 kcal/kg for moderate activity, and 45 kcal/kg for strenuous activity.
. Calculate a hypocaloric intake using the same formula, but assuming energy expen-
    diture to be 20 to 25 kcal/kg of DBW.
. Translate calories obtained into a dietary plan of at least three meals per day, using
    the hypocaloric diet for weight reduction and stressing that the maintenance caloric
    intake should not be exceeded after DBW is achieved. Patients should be encouraged
    to become familiar with the caloric contents of common foods and to participate in
    diet-planning. Commercially available booklets of calorie counts may help patients
    to identify unsuspected high-calorie items they have been consuming, such as potato
    chips. A dietician may facilitate this whole process.

Unfortunately, the balanced reduction diet is, by itself, of limited effectiveness, par-
icularly in patients who are substantially overweight. In the short term, only 25% of
atients lose more than 20 pounds and less than 5% more than 40 pounds. More long-
erm studies have shown that over a period of a few years virtually all patients return
o near their original weight. Dismay at these facts has led to newer dietary ap-
roaches, such as the addition of behavioral modification techniques. Community and
ommercial weight loss programs such as TOPS and Weight Watchers provide an or-
anized, relatively inexpensive group approach. With behavioral techniques, initial
veight losses comparable to or greater than those with a balanced reduction diet alone
an be expected. Unfortunately, long-term follow-up studies of behaviorally oriented
veight reduction programs have failed to show maintenance of weight loss.

Exercise

Exercise is an important adjunct to dietary therapy. It increases dietary-induced ther-
nogenesis, directly consumes some (albeit a small amount) of calories, and provides a
ense of well-being important for change of behavior. However, it is no substitute for

dietary management. Simple calculations reveal just how few calories are expended even in vigorous exercise. An expenditure of 3500 kcal is needed to consume 1 pound of body fat. A 70-kg person running at 6 mph expends 500 kcal per hour and therefore by running one such mile per day, would lose only 1 pound every 6 weeks. The concept of local exercise or heat, upon which gadgets for spot reduction and passive exercise are based, has been shown not to produce local fat reduction.

Drugs

Drugs are another frequent adjunct to weight reduction diets. Except for a few bulk agents and low-calorie packaged liquid diets, all of the over-the-counter slimming drugs are appetite suppressants consisting of phenylpropanolamine with or without caffeine. Numerous placebo-controlled trials demonstrate, over a 12-week period, minimal (1–4 kg) weight loss with these agents or their more toxic prescription counterparts. No study has demonstrated effective retention of weight loss once the drug is discontinued. These drugs have side effects, and many have addictive potential; none is recommended. Other commonly used drugs include human chorionic gonadotropin, diuretics, digitalis, and pharmacologic doses of thyroid hormone. They are neither effective nor sufficiently safe for treatment of obesity. The effect of replacement levels of thyroid hormone used as an adjunct to dieting has not been sufficiently studied to recommend its use.

Radical Therapy

Because simple approaches to weight reduction are often not effective, many individuals have turned to more radical and unconventional ones.

Diets

Patients not infrequently inquire about various diets. Most of these are fad diets that arise from an enthusiastically written book based on nothing more than eclectic theory and glowing case reports. Fad diets usually fall into one of several categories. The low carbohydrate diet is exemplified by the Drinking Man's Diet, the Air Force Diet, the Scarsdale Diet, and the Stillman Diet. It induces an exhaustion of glycogen stores leading to a salt and water diuresis of 2 to 4 kg in the first few days, which produces enthusiasm in the absence of reduction in fat stores. The high carbohydrate–high fiber diet, such as the rice diet, produces weight loss on the basis of early satiety from bulk. The high fat and low carbohydrate diet (e.g., Dr. Atkin's diet), in addition to initiating a diuresis, produces anorexia, probably on the basis of ketosis.

Much study has been conducted recently on two other types of radical diets: the protein-sparing modified fast (PSMF) and its near equivalent, the very low calorie diet (VLCD). Fasting results in dramatic weight losses, attributable in part to the anorexia it induces. However, the marked negative nitrogen balance produced by fasting has led to its abandonment in favor of diets that introduce small quantities of protein of high biologic value, with (VLCD) or without (PSMF) small quantities of carbohydrate. The total energy content of these diets is less than 800 kcal per day. The Cambridge Diet is a commercially popular version of the VLCD. In published series, very low calorie, high biologic value protein diets have been remarkably successful.

Reports of cardiac arrhythmias and sudden death resulting from the use of "liquid protein diets" have made many hesitate to employ these diets, particularly in the liquid form. However, the protein source in nearly all cases was not one of high biologic value but rather digested collagen. In contradistinction, in one series of over 3000 obese patients treated with a VLCD, many with cardiac disease, only 1 patient had an unexpected death. If the safety of these diets can be established, and if their reported success is also found in routine practice, they will answer for many obese patients the question of how to lose weight. However, they will not answer the equally important problem of how to maintain weight loss.

In giving advice concerning a fad diet, the clinician should consider

1. Whether the diet appears to provide the minimum balance of amino acids, vitamins, and minerals
2. Whether it provides an excess of undesirable foodstuffs, such as cholesterol and animal fat
3. Whether its side effects (e.g., orthostatic hypotension or hypokalemia from rapid diuresis)

uresis) are likely to be a risk for a given patient and, if so, whether adequate supervision is provided
4. Whether the patient's obesity is of sufficient degree to provide medical justification for a radical (and perhaps serious) departure from balanced eating habits
5. Whether the dieting approach will lead to a permanent change in the patient's eating habits

Obesity is a chronic disease. A fad diet, by definition, engenders enthusiasm and zeal, which, unless accompanied by behavioral change, cannot result in sustained reduction in weight.

Surgery
At present, surgery is the only therapy for morbid obesity that appears to provide long-term weight loss. Jejunoileal bypass, the first such procedure, has fallen into disfavor because of excessive long-term side effects, including liver failure and cirrhosis, metabolic bone disease, arthritis, renal calculi, and persistent diarrhea and flatulence. Currently, gastric surgery is preferred. Long-term complication and success rates of the gastric procedures are difficult to assess because the operations are constantly changing. Mortality in experienced hands is 1 to 2%, and morbidity, which is usually of no long-term consequence, about 25%. In one large series, patients lost an average of 44 kg after 2 years and successfully maintained this loss in 5-year follow-ups.
A 1978 National Institutes of Health (NIH) consensus development conference produced guidelines for the selection of patients for surgery. The patient should (1) be either 100 pounds overweight or 180% or more of DBW, (2) have serious health or psychosocial problems, and (3) have failed a suitable nonsurgical therapy.

Choosing Treatment
Given the difficulty of therapy and the likelihood of relapse, the decision of how aggressively to treat obesity must be individualized. One must consider, among other things, patient age, motivation, resources, degree of obesity, and presence of current or likelihood of future obesity-related illness. Because the risk associated with obesity is synergistic with other cardiac risk factors (e.g., cigarette smoking, hypertension) and because obesity may be less amenable to change, the patient may benefit more from strict attention to changing the other cardiovascular risk factors than from further attempts at weight reduction.

Van Itallie TB. Obesity: Adverse effects on health and longevity. *Am J Clin Nutr*32:2723–2733, 1979.
In-depth discussion of morbidity and mortality associated with obesity.
Bray GA. Obesity in America, an overview of the second Fogarty International Center Conference on Obesity. *Int J Obes* 3:363–375, 1979.
Summary of an NIH convened conference of experts. Contains, among other things, a body mass index nomogram and weight for height tables without frame size.
Genuth SM, et al. Weight reduction in obesity by outpatient semistarvation. *JAMA* 230:987–991, 1984.
Largest outpatient series documenting mean weight loss of 38 kg with a very low calorie, high biologic value, liquid protein regimen.
Howard AN. The historical development, efficacy and safety of very-low-calorie diets. *Int J Obes* 5:195–208, 1981.
Summary article in an issue of the International Journal of Obesity dedicated predominantly to VLCDs. Of note is the apparent safety of VLCDs in small case series, the ready efficacy in weight reduction of palatable VLCDs, and the very poor weight maintenance after VLCD termination.
Volkmar FB, et al. High attrition rates in commercial weight reduction programs. *Arch Intern Med* 141:426–428, 1981.
Suggests that the commonly held belief that commercial programs may offer benefit over traditional dietary counseling may be due, in part, to inadequate study of the former.
Wing RR, Jeffery RW. Outpatient treatments of obesity: A comparison of methodology and clinical results. *Int J Obes* 3:261–279, 1979.
Cites behavior therapy for best maintenance of weight loss, but mean follow-up only 23 weeks. Does not include PSMF data.

Joffe, SN Progress reports: Surgical management of morbid obesity. *Gut* 2:242–254, 1981.
   A non-surgeon's review of surgical approaches.
Stunkard AJ, Penick SB. Behavior modification in the treatment of obesity: The problem of maintaining weight loss. *Arch Gen Psychiatry* 36:801–806, 1979.
   Analysis of long-term follow-up of series of patients undergoing behavioral therapy reveals poor retention of weight loss over 10-month to 5-year periods.
Franklin BA, Rubenfire M. Losing weight through exercise. *JAMA* 244:377–379, 1980.
   Concise but somewhat superficial overview of the role of various forms of exercise, emphasizing the futility of "effortless weight reduction" and "spot reduction."
Douglas JG, Munro JF. The role of drugs in the treatment of obesity. *Drugs* 21:362–373, 1981.
   Broad summary of controlled trials of anti-obesity drugs, lacking only emphasis on long-term failure of drug therapy.
Massachusetts General Hospital Dietary Department, Boston. *Diet Manual.* Boston: Little, Brown, 1976.
   A brief but comprehensive aid in calculating diet for many needs. Included is a more sophisticated approach to calculation of caloric goals and food exchange lists with an explanation of their use.
Frank A, et al. Fatalities on the liquid protein diet: An analysis of possible causes. *Int J Obes* 5:243–248, 1981.
   Up-to-date analysis summarizing deaths and noting the possible etiologic factors of potassium, other electrolyte, or micronutrient deficiency; prolonged QT interval; inadequate quantity or poor quality protein; inadequate medical supervision; and post-diet binge eating. Authors conclude that no properly managed patient died as a direct result of the liquid protein diet.

4. WEIGHT LOSS
William D. Heizer

Body weight may fluctuate as much as 1 kg from day to day as a result of short-term imbalances in the intake and output of energy and water. Over long periods of time, however, the weight of most healthy adults remains remarkably constant.

Because body weight is so well maintained in the normal state, an unintentional loss of more than 5% of the usual weight should be investigated, although it does not necessarily indicate a serious physical problem.

Weight loss is a presenting complaint in about 4% of outpatients. Approximately half of these have not actually lost a significant amount of weight, and other explanations for the visit must be sought. On the other hand, approximately half of the outpatients who have lost a significant amount of weight do not mention that as a presenting complaint. Therefore, evidence of weight loss should be sought routinely in the history and physical examination and by comparison with previous weights.

Causes
The list of conditions that cause weight loss is lengthy, and the prevalence of various causes of weight loss has not been investigated extensively. In a recent study of patients enrolled at a Veterans Administration medical center who had involuntarily lost 5% or more of their usual body weight in 6 months, no cause for the weight loss was found in 26% despite extensive diagnostic evaluation and prolonged follow-up. Cancer and gastrointestinal diseases were found in 19 and 14% of the patients, respectively. Depression, congestive heart failure, alcoholism, and chronic obstructive pulmonary disease each accounted for between 5 and 10%. A variety of other disorders, including diabetes, thyrotoxicosis, infection, sarcoidosis, rheumatoid arthritis, drug-induced gastrointestinal symptoms, and neurologic diseases, each accounted for less than 5% of the total group of patients.

Documentation of Weight Loss

The surest evidence of weight loss is comparison of the current weight with previously recorded values. In the absence of such documentation, a history of weight loss may be corroborated if the patient recalls the amount of measured but unrecorded weights at one or more times in the previous years; if there has been a recent change in clothing size, especially the belt size; or if friends or relatives think the patient has lost weight. Pathologic weight loss also should be considered in the obese patient who is having unusual success on a weight reduction program.

Occasionally, loss of body tissue is accompanied by a nearly equal gain in extracellular fluid. People who see the patient infrequently are most likely to note the loss of soft tissue mass that has occurred in the patient's face and limbs. When patients with edema or ascites are weighed, some estimate of the quantity of extracellular fluid present should be recorded so that subsequent weights can be interpreted correctly.

Mechanism of Weight Loss

The history should attempt to uncover the mechanism of weight loss.

Decreased Intake

Decreased food intake is the most frequent cause of weight loss. Reasons include the following:

1. The thought, sight, and/or odor of food is not appealing (malignancy, gallbladder disease, drugs, depression).
2. The sensation of taste is abnormal (hepatitis, drugs, zinc deficiency).
3. Mechanical problems or pain limit chewing or swallowing (neurologic, dental, oral mucosal or esophageal abnormalities).
4. The intake of food is curtailed due to abdominal pain (intestinal ischemia, partial small bowel obstruction, inflammatory bowel disease, abdominal malignancy), diarrhea (infectious enteritis, inflammatory bowel disease, occasionally lactase deficiency, rarely irritable bowel syndrome), or nausea or vomiting.
5. Lethargy or weakness (neurologic and muscular diseases, drug abuse).
6. Overzealous adherence to diets prescribed, often unnecessarily, for gastrointestinal disease or allergy.
7. Learned aversion to foods that were given following a nauseating stimulus such as cancer chemotherapy.
8. Anorexia nervosa or bulimia: These increasingly prevalent syndromes most often occur among young, relatively affluent, white women who lose weight as a result of decreased intake and, in many instances, self-induced vomiting, purgation, or excessive exercise as well. The disorder often first appears shortly after separation from previous social support (e.g., leaving home, death of parent). Although they rarely acknowledge it, patients often view food intake and body weight as the only thing in their life over which they have control, and fear of losing that control may be intense.

Increased Metabolic Rate

Increased metabolic rate (energy expenditure) can contribute to weight loss in many disease states. For example, resting energy expenditure is increased 10 to 13% for each degree centigrade of temperature above normal. The presence of inflammation, burns, bone fractures, and, in some instances, cancer causes an increase in resting energy expenditure. Weight loss from this cause is usually modest, however, as energy utilization in disease seldom, if ever, exceeds twice the normal resting energy expenditure, even in the severely burned patient. On the other hand, hyperthyroidism, by increasing resting energy expenditure and activity, can cause profound weight loss.

Significant weight loss due only to an increase in physical activity is rare because of the relatively small amount of energy expended in even strenuous activities (about 500 calories for a 70-kg person running 6 miles) and the large number of calories in body fat, 3500 calories per pound. A 70-kg person would lose approximately 1 pound per week with an increase in activity equivalent to running 6 miles every day.

Calorie Loss

Malabsorption (especially pancreatic insufficiency) and uncontrolled diabetes mellitus are well-known causes of weight loss in the face of normal or even supranormal intake.

Diagnosing the Cause of Weight Loss

In attempting to determine whether changes in food intake or activity might account for weight loss, it is helpful to ask the patient to describe a typical recent day—time of arising, meals, snacks, activities, time of going to bed.

In a majority of instances in which a physical cause for weight loss will be found, the cause will be obvious after the history, physical examination, and minimal investigation are completed. For example, when 91 male veterans were studied for involuntary weight loss, in 55 of the 59 with physical causes, the cause was clinically evident on the initial evaluation. The likelihood of a physical cause was increased in the presence of nausea or vomiting, recent change in cough, and a variety of physical findings such as cachexia, abdominal mass, adenopathy, or thyromegaly; it was decreased among patients who did not smoke heavily or who had no decrease in activities due to fatigue.

The types of laboratory studies done should obviously be guided by the results of the history and physical examination. Studies should include chest x-ray, at least three stools for occult blood, urinalysis, complete blood count with differential count, glucose, and liver function tests. With the addition of an upper gastrointestinal series and small bowel follow-through, most patients with a physical cause for weight loss will have that cause detected.

When the history strongly suggests that food intake has not decreased and initial laboratory studies do not indicate diabetes, then hyperthyroidism and malabsorption should be considered. However, in the absence of signs and symptoms of hyperthyroidism, thyroid function tests are most helpful in older patients, in whom signs of hyperthyroidism may be less apparent. Screening tests for malabsorption should include a Sudan stain of the stool fat and tests for serum carotene and folic acid. These tests are only valid when the patient has been eating an adequate diet for several days. The definitive test for malabsorption is a quantitative determination of fat absorption by means of a 72-hour stool collection or possibly a breath test where available. The only definitive method for making or excluding the diagnosis of celiac sprue is a jejunal biopsy.

If the cause for a patient's weight loss is not apparent on history and physical examination and the tests mentioned are normal, the best management might then be watchful waiting, with further investigation primarily dictated by continuing weight loss or development of new symptoms. Follow-up visits should also be used to explore any possible psychological causes for weight loss, including depression, drug abuse, and anorexia nervosa. Depression is probably the leading psychological cause for weight loss seen in the outpatient setting and can be recognized by appetite and sleep disturbance, anhedonia (low energy, poor motivation, decreased libido), feelings of sadness, agitation or psychomotor retardation, and poor concentration or memory (see Chap. 113). A diagnosis of depression or other psychosocial problems does not, of course, rule out the simultaneous presence of a physical cause for weight loss, because both may be present independently or they may be related (e.g., depression appearing as an early manifestation of malignancy).

Complications

Weight loss, as described below, regardless of cause, results in weakness, depressed cellular immunity, skin breakdown, increased susceptibility to infection, emotional changes, and delayed wound healing. In addition to patient dysfunction and discomfort, malnutrition may delay therapeutic and diagnostic procedures and will make therapeutic measures, especially surgery, more hazardous.

The presence and severity of these manifestations depend on the degree of malnutrition and probably on how rapidly it develops. There are no measures of nutrition status suitable for clinical use that are specific and sensitive.

Serious malnutrition may be defined as the presence of weight loss of 7% or more, albumin less than 3.4 gm/dl, and anergy in the absence of a valid non-nutritional explanation for these findings. A more quantitative estimate of the risk of malnutrition, at least for surgical patients, is called the Prognostic Nutritional Index (PNI), the percent likelihood of mortality or serious morbidity following surgery. The PNI is calculated as follows:

$$PNI(\%) = 158 - 16.6(ALB) - 0.78(TSF) - 0.2(TFN) - 5.8(DH)$$

where ALB = serum albumin (gm/dl); TSF = triceps skinfold thickness (mm); TFN = serum transferrin (mg/dl); and DH = cutaneous delayed hypersensitivity to any of three recall antigens, which are graded as 0, nonreactive, 1, < 5 mm induration, 2, > 5 mm induration.

Although nutrition repletion may lower the PNI, it has not been rigorously established that this will decrease postoperative morbidity and mortality. Nevertheless, a PNI greater than 40 to 50% suggests that the patient will likely benefit from special nutritional support before and after surgery.

Treatment

Obviously, it is preferable to prevent rather than treat serious nutritional deficiency, and prevention should begin early. Usually, the first effort should be to increase oral intake. This may include

1. More frequent feeding of foods with high-calorie density
2. Avoiding restrictive diets of unproven benefit
3. Avoiding drugs that suppress appetite or hinder gastrointestinal function whenever possible
4. Avoiding accidental or unnecessary restriction of intake in association with investigative procedures
5. Using commercial dietary supplements.

A number of liquid diets are commercially available for use as supplements or meal replacement. Their disadvantage is that few, if any, patients find them as palatable as ordinary food. Their advantages are that they are liquid, nutritionally complete, and require little or no preparation. Many are lactose free. Most of the formulas have a calorie density of 1 cal/ml. A few with greater calorie densities may be especially useful for patients with early satiety.

A decision to use special means of nutritional support—tube feeding or intravenous nutrition—should be based on an assessment of the patient's intake of energy and protein currently and in the near future, expenditure of energy and protein that is increased by catabolic illness, and current energy and protein stores. The number of these risk factors present and the intensity of each should be considered in determining the need for intensive nutritional support.

Marton KI, Sox HC Jr, Krupp JR. Involuntary weight loss: Diagnostic and prognostic significance. *Ann Intern Med* 95:568–574, 1981.
  The only recent prospective study to establish the prevalence of various causes of weight loss. The patients studied were those enrolled at a Veteran's Administration medical center between 1975 and 1978 and being evaluated for weight loss.
Grande F, Keys A. Body Weight, Body Composition, and Calorie Status. In RS Goodhard and ME Shils (Eds.), *Modern Nutrition in Health and Disease.*Philadelphia: Lea & Febiger, 1980. P. 3.
  A general discussion of normal body weight, body composition, and the relationship between changes in body composition and changes in calorie balance.
Hodges RE, Adelman RD. Evaluation of the Nutrition Status of Patient. In RE Hodges (Ed.), *Nutrition and Medical Practice*. Philadelphia: Saunders, 1980. P. 1.
  Discussion of traditional nutritional assessment of children and adults, including the elderly, concentrating on the history, physical examination, and anthropometric measurements.
Grant JP, Custer PB, Thurlow J. Current techniques of nutritional assessment. *Surg Clin North Am* 61:437–463, 1981.
  Perhaps the best summary of current, clinically available methods of nutritional assessment, including history, physical examination, body composition analysis, anthropometric measurements, and biochemical measurements.
Bain ST, Spaulding WB. The importance of coding presenting symptoms. *Can Med Assoc J* 97:953–959, 1967.
  A study of the chief or presenting symptoms for 500 consecutive new outpatients attending a Toronto General Hospital clinic.
Foster DW. *Alterations in Body Weight*. In Isselbacher KJ et al. (Eds.), *Principles of*

Internal Medicine (9th ed). New York: McGraw Hill, 1980. Pp. 213–214.
Brief summary of the detection and causes of weight loss.

Floch MH. Weight Loss and Nutritional Assessment. In MH Floch, *Nutrition and Diet Therapy in Gastrointestinal Disease.*New York: Plenum, 1981. P. 101.
Categorizes diseases that often cause weight loss and reviews methods for assessing nutritional status.

Drossman DA, Ontjes DA, Heizer WD. Anorexia nervosa. *Gastroenterology* 77:1115–1131, 1979.
Review of the psychosocial, endocrine, medical, and nutritional features of anorexia nervosa and current management of the condition.

Shil ME, Bloch AS, Chernoff R. *Liquid Formulas for Oral and Tube Feeding.* Order from Nutrition Support Kitchen, Box 279, Memorial Sloan-Kettering Cancer Center, 1275 York Avenue, New York, New York 10021.
Tables listing the composition of a large number of commercially available liquid diets and supplements. An excellent starting point but incomplete because of the number of new products being marketed.

II. EYE PROBLEMS

5. OCULAR FOREIGN BODIES

Hunter R. Stokes

Foreign bodies in and around the eye are usually quite painful and can cause significant permanent loss of vision if not properly managed. They may be embedded in the skin of the lid, sometimes penetrating the lid onto or into the conjunctiva, or embedded in the cornea, either superficially or deeply.

Lid and periocular orbital foreign bodies are usually from shattered particles in a work-related accident (nails, wood) or from explosions (gunshot, fireworks). The immediate danger is related to the depth of penetration and the resultant damage to the eyeball. Penetrating lid injuries by large foreign bodies (nails, sticks) are very painful. Immediate removal is indicated but is best done by an ophthalmologist, because the distal end of the foreign body may have penetrated the globe. Retained foreign bodies from projectiles (shotguns, BB guns) may be in the soft tissue of the lid, in the orbit, or within the eyeball. It is important to know the exact location of the foreign body, but routine x-ray studies are usually of little value. For transport of patients with retained foreign bodies, the primary consideration is protection from further damage by preventing any movement (e.g., rubbing) of the foreign body, especially if a portion of the object protrudes from the eye or eyelids. A simple paper cup, either flat-bottomed or pointed, can be taped over the eye. This allows the foreign body to remain in place and puts no pressure on the eye.

Evaluation

Foreign bodies in the cul-de-sacs and under the upper lid can occur without any noticeable trauma, such as a gust of wind while walking or dust from an automobile air conditioner duct. Common foreign bodies causing trauma include work-related particles (from drilling, sanding) and, especially in children, sand or dirt. In these situations, there are typical complaints. First, there is the obvious foreign body sensation—"trash in my eye." Second, the foreign body seems to "move around in the eye." Actually, the foreign body is almost always lodged in the substance of the conjunctiva under the upper lid and is not moving; but, with each blink, a different area of the cornea is irritated, giving the impression that the foreign body is moving.

If the foreign body is in the inferior cul-de-sac, it can be seen by having the patient look up while the lower lid is pulled down. Foreign bodies in the superior cul-de-sac can sometimes be seen with elevation of the upper lid while the patient looks down. Most of these foreign bodies will, however, be lodged in the conjunctiva on the under surface of the upper lid and can only be seen by eversion of the lid. The presence of such a foreign body is suggested by abrasions of the superior cornea in a multiple linear pattern (vertical) usually confined to one quadrant, which can be seen by fluorescein stain.

Eversion of the upper lid is essential in locating foreign bodies under the upper lid. The proper method is (1) have the patient look down with both eyes open and (2) grasp the lashes of the upper lid and lift up while depressing the midportion of the upper lid laterally with a blunt instrument. As long as the patient continues to look down, the upper lid will remain relaxed and everted so that a careful examination can be performed. As soon as the patient looks up or, as often occurs with children, an attempt is made to squeeze the eye shut, the lid will return to its usual position.

The best "instrument" for a lid eversion is a double-tipped cotton swab (Q-tip) with one end moistened with a local anesthetic, such as proparacaine (Ophthetic or Ophthaine) or tetracaine (Pontocaine). The dry end is used to press the lid in the eversion maneuver and the damp end is available to sweep across the conjunctival under-surface of the lid to remove any foreign body that may be found. A small sulcus just under the upper lid margin must be carefully examined. Small foreign bodies can be lodged in this indentation and are easily overlooked.

If no foreign body is found with lid eversion but there is a strong suspicion that a foreign body should have been found, one of two things can be assumed: the foreign body is still there and not found, or it has been washed out, but the eye still hurts. The instillation of fluorescein may reveal a "spot" of dye concentration that may indicate a relatively transparent foreign body (sand, insect wing, fiberglass particle), which can usually be wiped away with the cotton swab. Even if no foreign body is found with this method, it is a good idea to sweep completely across the conjunctival surface underneath the upper lid with the moist cotton swab to wipe away a missed foreign body. If still no foreign body is seen, it may have become dislodged by tears and is no longer in the eye. This is a diagnosis of exclusion.

Often a patient will report that glass may be in the eye, such as from a broken light bulb or windshield. Obvious glass may be found in the cul-de-sac. But, if the patient continues to complain of a sensation of a foreign body for days after and no foreign body is seen, a thin sliver of glass may have been imbedded in the conjunctiva and is intermittently presenting itself at the surface to create a scratchy sensation. These patients should be referred to an ophthalmologist for evaluation under a slit lamp.

Treatment

Conjunctival Foreign Bodies

Conjunctival foreign bodies that are on the surface of the conjunctiva or that have superficially penetrated the conjunctiva of the eyeball (bulbar conjunctiva) can usually be wiped off with the cotton swab or lifted off with a toothless forcep after the eye is anesthetized. If there is any difficulty in removing the foreign body, if it appears to be deeply embedded, or if there is severe pain when the foreign body is touched, then attempts at removal should be discontinued and the patient immediately referred to an ophthalmologist.

Sometimes, when a conjunctival foreign body is removed, an underlying laceration of the conjunctiva is discovered. In cooperative patients, two damp cotton swabs can be used to spread the wound edges and explore the wound. This is important, as it may reveal an additional subconjunctival foreign body or laceration of sclera, which may need to be referred for treatment. For children or others in whom this maneuver is not possible, it is important enough to identify deep, penetrating trauma to admit them to the hospital for evaluation under general anesthesia.

Corneal Foreign Bodies

Corneal foreign bodies are common and are easily embedded, so that removal with a cotton swab may not be possible. Removal cannot be attempted without anesthetizing the cornea with a topical anesthetic. Irrigation of the cornea with sterile water or sterile saline, directing the flow toward the foreign body, will dislodge many foreign objects. If this fails, wiping with a damp cotton swab is indicated. Next, a spud or 25-gauge needle can be used if the head can be held still and the physician has excellent near vision. The cornea is only 1 mm thick, and the slightest unpredicted movement of the head can cause more damage by the spud or the needle than the foreign body. An excellent light source and some form of magnification (examiner loop) are necessary. If the spud or needle effort is not immediately successful, efforts to remove a foreign body should be discontinued and referral made for removal under a slit lamp. Also, if the removal of the foreign body is immediately followed by a shallowing of the anterior chamber or an obvious leakage of fluid, perforation of the cornea must be suspected and the patient immediately referred to an ophthalmologist.

Although many corneal foreign bodies are metallic, the use of a magnet for removal is not recommended. Many metallic foreign bodies are nonmagnetic or weakly magnetic. Also, even if the foreign body is magnetic, it may be only partially removed by the magnet.

Iron foreign bodies (quite common from drilling or hammering steel) cause rust in the underlying corneal tissue within only 2 to 4 hours. A metallic foreign body present for 8 hours may have a complete rust ring formed around or beneath it. The foreign body may be relatively easily removed with a needle tip or spud but not the cotton swab, while the rust ring remains. Patients with a rust ring should be referred to an ophthalmologist for removal with a hand drill under the magnification of a slit lamp.

If a metallic corneal foreign body has been imbedded for 2 to 4 days before medical attention is sought, the necrosis of tissue underlying the rust ring may permit removal of the foreign body and the entire ring rather easily. However, while this makes removal of the foreign body easier, there is a greater risk of infection leading to corneal ulceration and subsequent scar formation. These patients should also be referred to an ophthalmologist.

After a foreign body has been removed from the cornea, the management is the same as the management of a corneal abrasion with several further considerations. Topical anesthetics should never by dispensed or prescribed; corneal defects will heal slowly, or not at all, with frequent instillation of topical anesthetics. Except for small abrasions (less than 3 mm long), a long-acting cycloplegic, such as scopolamine (¼% Isopto Hyoscine), should be instilled to relieve severe pain, which may last for several days. This pain is from ciliary spasm, which is a reflex reaction to stimulation of corneal nerve endings exposed by the abrasion. Cycloplegics paralyze the ciliary body muscle, relieving the spasm.

Because few, if any, foreign bodies are sterile when they are embedded in the cornea, antibiotic coverage is essential (see Chap. 7). If no haze is present around the site of the foreign body, a pressure bandage should be applied for 24 hours after an antibiotic is instilled. After 24 hours, antibiotics should be used every 3 hours, four times a day, until the epithelium is healed. As for abrasions, if there is still fluorescein staining after 72 hours, referral to an ophthalmologist is indicated. The pressure patch for 24 hours encourages rapid healing of the corneal wound, but it should not be applied if there is any hint of infection, such as haze in the surrounding cornea or marked injection of adjacent conjunctiva. After instillation of the cycloplegic, topical antibiotics should be started immediately and used frequently, every 2 to 3 hours for the first 24 to 48 hours.

Topical steroids should be avoided in the management of corneal defects after foreign body removal. Steroids inhibit wound healing, encourage fungal infections (a real consideration when the foreign body is vegetable matter, such as wood or pine needles), and in susceptible patients, may increase intraocular pressure to levels high enough to cause damage to the optic nerve.

The prognosis is good for most corneal foreign bodies because treatment is usually instituted in time to avoid damage to vision and complications. Many primary care physicians who initially see patients with corneal foreign bodies choose to remove only superficial foreign bodies and refer all others to an ophthalmologist. Also, they elect to refer all patients for follow-up care after the foreign body is removed. All foreign bodies located in the central cornea should at least be referred for follow-up slit lamp examination. Even a faint scar, if located centrally, in or near the visual axis, can lead to a permanent reduction in vision.

Havener WH. *Synopsis of Ophthalmology* (2nd ed.). St. Louis: Mosby, 1963.
   There is an excellent discussion in this book of a variety of situations related to foreign bodies and also an excellent demonstration of eversion of the lids with photographs.
Gardiner, PA. "Accidents and First Aid"—ABC of Ophthalmology Series. Br Med J 2:1347, 1978.
   This series covers a variety of ocular problems, and the particular one on injuries is certainly complementary to this discussion of corneal foreign bodies.

6. CORNEAL ABRASION
Hunter R. Stokes

Corneal abrasion is a rather common and quite painful eye condition. Any superficial contact with the anterior surface of the eyeball may remove a portion of the epithelial surface of the cornea. In addition, extensive exposure of the cornea to ultraviolet light (sunlamp, welder's arc) can also produce abrasions. Most corneal abrasions, especially smaller ones, can be managed by primary care or emergency room physicians.

Diagnosis

A diagnosis of corneal abrasion should be suspected when trauma to the eye leads to pain or sensation of a foreign body. The diagnosis can usually be made using oblique illumination of the cornea with a penlight, which discloses an irregular area of the usually smooth, glistening surface of the cornea. Direct or slightly tangential illumination may cause a shadow on the surface of the iris that moves in the opposite direction to the movement of the light. Following fluorescein instillation into the inferior cul-de-sac, any area of abrasion will be outlined by absorbed dye and will be more visible. Cobalt blue filter (a small filter that can be attached to the tip of a penlight) will further illuminate the fluorescein. Fluorescein strips (dampened with water or sterile saline, or lightly touched to the moist lower lid conjunctival surface if the eye is tearing) should be used instead of fluorescein solution, which is an excellent culture medium for *Pseudomonas*.

Differential Diagnosis

The most important problem that may be confused with an abrasion is herpes simplex keratitis. One should look for (1) a prior history of herpes keratitis, (2) coexisting fever blister, (3) recent upper respiratory infection, (4) no history (or vague history) of corneal trauma, (5) a dendritic (branching) corneal stain pattern, and (6) reduced corneal sensitivity (this is impossible to test if a topical anesthetic has been instilled or used to dampen the fluorescein strip).

Winter, with its associated increase in viral infections, and the early weeks of hot weather in the summer are the times when herpes keratitis is most frequently seen. The persistence of pain and a linear stain in a patient with no good history of ocular trauma and no foreign body under the upper lid dictates referral to an ophthalmologist, because the dendritic pattern may be very difficult to appreciate without a slit lamp. If the history and symptoms suggest a corneal abrasion, even when none is seen using fluorescein, it is appropriate to treat the eye as an abrasion for 24 hours. If symptoms persist, referral to an ophthalmologist is necessary.

Uncomplicated corneal abrasions almost always heal without scarring, and vision returns to normal; however, herpetic corneal lesions always leave a scar, and delayed management can lead to significant permanent loss of vision.

Treatment

The first step in the management of corneal abrasion is to make certain that there is no retained foreign body either on or in the cornea or under the upper lid. The instillation of a topical anesthetic may be necessary to examine the eye adequately, especially with ultraviolet burns, but should *never* be prescribed or dispensed for use by the patient.

Dispensing topical anesthetics is absolutely contraindicated for several reasons. First, additional damage may be done as the anesthetized cornea is further exposed to trauma as the natural blink reflex is diminished. Second, the anesthetic delays re-epithelialization and precludes adequate healing. Third, the patient may use the leftover portion for the next "scratched eye," which may instead be a corneal ulcer, a penetrating foreign body, or some other serious, potentially blinding eye problem.

Topical steroids and topical medications containing steroids should never be used in treating corneal abrasions. Not only can the steroid enhance the growth of a herpes lesion of the cornea, but it also encourages the growth of fungal lesions and can cause an elevation of intraocular pressure. The most important reason for not using topical steroids, however, is that they inhibit corneal wound healing.

Very small, uncomplicated corneal abrasions will often heal spontaneously within 12 to 24 hours. However, if an abrasion is large enough to be visible to the naked eye of the physician examiner, it should be treated with antibiotic drops and a pressure patch.

Antibiotic or sulfonamide solution, not ointment, should be instilled before patching. There is evidence that ointment may lead to delayed healing and a higher incidence of recurrent erosion because ointment particles may be trapped under the healing epithelium. A firm pressure patch is placed over the injured eye unless the other eye does not have good vision. Bilateral abrasions (as in ultraviolet burns) may require bilateral patches or patching of the more seriously injured eye. Healing is improved by applying the patch with pressure sufficient to keep the eyelids from rubbing over the abrasion. This is accomplished by applying tape strips, usually three to five parallel strips of 1-

inch tape, with the superior ends pointing to the central forehead and the inferior ends toward the lateral cheek on the injured side. After 24 hours, the patch should be removed and an antibiotic or sulfonamide drops used four times a day for 24 to 48 hours. If the abrasion is larger, a moderately long-acting cycloplegic such as ¼% scopolamine (Isopto Hyoscine) should be used because it reduces ciliary spasm (a major cause of pain) and dilates the pupil for approximately 72 hours. With all corneal abrasions, however, pain is rather severe, and analgesia (codeine or meperidine [Demerol]) may be needed. If there is still pain or any stain after 48 hours, referral to an ophthalmologist is indicated.

Complications

An uncomplicated epithelial abrasion heals without scarring and without vision loss. A corneal abrasion, however, can become infected and develop into a superficial ulcer that leads to slower healing and a permanent scar. Any haze of the cornea around an abrasion dictates immediate referral to an ophthalmologist.

If the abrasion does not heal in 48 to 72 hours, then a transparent embedded foreign body or a missed foreign body under the upper lid should be suspected. These patients should be referred for slit lamp examination.

In up to 10% of corneal abrasions, recurrent epithelial erosions result from failure of epithelium to adhere to the underlying basement membrane. The patient may note immediate pain on awakening or on rubbing the previously injured eye. This can occur weeks or months after the injury. A lubricating ointment (e.g., Lacri-Lube) at bedtime or when drying of the cornea may be anticipated (such as during airline travel or exposure to direct air from an automobile heating/air conditioning unit) may be sufficient treatment. Referral to an ophthalmologist is indicated for recurrences. Ultimately, removal of the epithelium may be necessary to allow a better rehealing process.

Referral

Large or deep abrasions, suspected herpes lesions, and abrasions with haze (possible ulcer) should be referred to an ophthalmologist at the time of injury. Many primary care and emergency room physicians treat corneal abrasions initially and refer the patient to an ophthalmologist for follow-up the next day. Recurrent erosion, continuing pain, or positive fluorescein stain after 48 hours should also be referred.

Vaughn D, Asbury T. *General Ophthalmology* (9th ed.). Los Altos, Calif.: Lane Medical Publications, 1980.
  This excellent general textbook in ophthalmology is valuable to both the family physician and the ophthalmologist. There are several sections on trauma, including corneal abrasions (p. 38), and the related subjects—herpes keratitis (pp. 96–98) and recurrent erosion (pp. 106, 109)—are also covered well.
Adrieni J, et al. *Symposium on Ocular Pharmacology and Therapeutics.* St. Louis: Mosby, 1970.
  This is the seventh symposium that was presented and represents the transactions of the New Orleans Academy of Ophthalmology. It includes some excellent discussion on a variety of subjects. Outstanding arguments are presented against using ophthalmic ointments (p. 96); the discussion focuses on the treatment of the conjunctiva, but it is at least as appropriate for the cornea.
Eiferman RA. Recurrent corneal epithelial erosions. *Perspect Ophthalmol* 4:3–7, 1981.
  This is an excellent discussion with photographs.
Baum JL, Silbert AM. Aspects of corneal wound healing in health and disease. *Trans Ophthalmol Soc UK* 98:348–351, 1978.
  Outstanding discussion of healing in corneal abrasion. The potential for recurrent erosion is described, and the contraindication of ointment with evidence of healing by sliding of epithelial cells and adhesions of epithelium to the basement membrane is demonstrated.
Kenyon KR. Recurrent corneal erosion: Pathogenesis and therapy. *Int Ophthalmol Clin* 19:169–196, 1979.
  Excellent review of clinical condition (symptoms and signs) and therapy. Also photomicrographs showing histopathology with electron-microscopic photographs.

Duane TD. *Light and Photometry. Biomedical Foundations of Ophthalmology.* Philadelphia: Harper & Row, 1983. Vol. 2, Chap. 15, pp. 17–18.
This is an excellent basic scientific explanation for the damage done to the cornea by ultraviolet light.
Petroutsos G, et al. Corticosteroids and corneal epithelial wound healing. *Br J Ophthalmol* 66:705–708, 1982.
This discussion regards the retardation of corneal wound healing by topical ocular steroids. The other problems with topical ocular steroids are also mentioned and referenced.

7. CONJUNCTIVITIS
Hunter R. Stokes

The conjunctiva is a thin, transparent tissue that covers the posterior surface of the lids (palpebral conjunctiva) and the anterior surface of the sclera (bulbar conjunctiva). Inflammation and/or infection of the conjunctiva is the most common eye disease in the western hemisphere. Trachoma, a form of chlamydial conjunctivitis that is rare in the United States, is the most common infectious disease in the world.

The common causes of conjunctivitis include bacteria, chlamydia, viruses, and allergies. Other, less common types—fungal, chemical, and idiopathic—are important but uncommon and rarely need to be considered by the primary care practitioner.

The diagnosis of conjunctivitis can usually be made from the history and physical examination. In general, bacterial conjunctivitis is associated with mucopurulent discharge, smooth, inflamed conjunctiva with red dots (papillae), and no preauricular lymphadenopathy. Viral conjunctivitis is associated with a watery discharge, follicles (hypertrophied translucent lymph tissue surrounded by blood vessels), and enlarged preauricular lymph nodes. Allergic conjunctivitis is associated with chemosis and mucoid discharge. In studies comparing laboratory analysis with clinical diagnosis of bacterial, viral, and allergic conjunctivitis, correlations range from poor to 75%. Most authorities agree, however, that in primary care practices smears and cultures are impractical and are not indicated unless management proves difficult or an unusual or virulent organism, such as *Neisseria gonorrhoeae,* is suspected.

Bacterial Conjunctivitis
Bacterial conjunctivitis, the most common type of conjunctivitis, is most often caused by *Pneumococcus, Hemophilus influenzae,* and *Staphylococcus aureus.* It has a rather sudden onset, beginning usually in one eye, to be followed in the other eye in 2 to 5 days. There is severe irritation with a foreign body sensation and a purulent exudate. The reaction is more prominent in the palpebral conjunctiva than in the bulbar conjunctiva, with mild injection of the conjunctival vessels. Usually there is lid edema. In the chronic bacterial conjunctivitis caused by *S. aureus,* there may be an associated blepharitis (infection of the lid margins, often described as granulated eyelids from swelling of the lid margins and crusting of the lashes) and a stye (external hordeolum).

Conjunctival secretions in bacterial conjunctivitis are infectious for 24 to 48 hours after therapy begins. Family members must take care when applying medication to the eyes of infected patients.

Treatment
Acute bacterial conjunctivitis is self-limited and usually clears in 2 weeks without treatment. With treatment, dramatic clearing occurs in 48 to 72 hours. A variety of topical antibiotics (chloramphenicol, neomycin, gentamicin, polymyxin, bacitracin, to-

bramycin, and sulfonamides) are very popular, cost approximately the same, and are equally effective. Neomycin is the most frequently used and most frequently associated with allergic reactions. In such cases, the purulence and exudate of infection clears, but is shortly replaced by severe itching and burning of the eyes, red swollen lids, and a dry, almost scaly appearance to the skin of the lid. The drug should be stopped and cold compresses applied.

Referral
Recurrent or chronic conjunctivitis should be referred to an ophthalmologist. In chronic bacterial conjunctivitis, a combination of steroid/sulfonamide (e.g., Blephamide, Vasocidin) or steroid/antibiotic (e.g., Maxitrol, NeoDECADRON) has been demonstrated to be more effective than either alone. However, the steroid-containing compound should be prescribed only by an ophthalmologist.

Viral Conjunctivitis
Many viruses can cause conjunctivitis, but the two most often encountered are adenoviruses: adenopharyngeal conjunctivitis (APC) and epidemic keratoconjunctivitis (EKC). Swimming pool conjunctivitis is commonly caused by the APC virus and occasionally by the EKC virus. Both are rather common in children, and neither is eliminated by proper chlorination. These characteristics are especially associated with APC. The infectivity of EKC is dramatic, and it is often the explanation for a summer outbreak of severe pink eye. Precautions must be taken with hands, ophthalmic solutions, and bathroom linen. Hand towels used by those with EKC must be washed in hot water to reduce the chance of spread. Physicians must be careful because hand to eye, as well as tonometer contamination, has been implicated in epidemics.

Clinical Manifestations
In APC, there is fever of 100 to 104°F, a severe pharyngitis, and bilateral follicular conjunctivitis with marked watery discharge. The eyes are quite red, and large preauricular nodes are usually present. Because of multiple, small subepithelial corneal ulcers (infiltrates), vision is often reduced.

In EKC, the infection usually begins in one eye with marked conjunctival injection and tearing. There is pain and blurred vision associated with corneal infiltrates (which may persist for months after the infection clears), follicles as in APC, and marked chemosis. A huge preauricular node is not unusual.

Herpes simplex conjunctivitis is associated with a fever blister on the lip or upper face, typical vesicular lesions on the skin of the eyelids, and/or dendritic corneal herpes lesions. The conjunctivitis is typically unilateral with follicles.

Treatment
There is no specific therapy for viral conjunctivitis. However, a topical antibiotic is usually prescribed for 10 to 14 days to prevent secondary bacterial infection. Symptomatic treatment is indicated for the fever and sore throat of APC, and topical lubricants (e.g., methylcellulose) may relieve eye redness. Referral to an ophthalmologist is indicated for management of EKC cases with painful corneal involvement.

The possibility of herpetic infection should discourage primary care practitioners from prescribing steroid medications in any conjunctival infections. Even though herpetic infection is not always associated with a typical corneal ulcer, topical steroid preparations can dramatically enhance proliferation of herpes simplex, resulting in permanent vision loss from a corneal scar.

Allergic Conjunctivitis
There are several forms of allergic conjunctivitis. The common finding is a history of allergy.

Hay Fever Conjunctivitis
Hay fever conjunctivitis is a mild but frightening condition. The patient suddenly notes itching, tearing, and "fullness" of one or both eyes and finds redness of the conjunctiva with associated marked chemosis. The eye seems to "sink" into the conjunctiva, and the conjunctiva may protrude beyond the lid margins when the eyelids are closed. There is almost always a history of an immediate past confrontation with a known

allergen (e.g., pollen, grass). Treatment includes cold compresses, vasoconstrictors for 24 to 48 hours (Albalon-A Liquifilm or Vasocon-A Ophthalmic Solution), and systemic antihistamines for 24 hours, and the condition clears as rapidly as it appears.

Vernal Keratoconjunctivitis

Vernal keratoconjunctivitis occurs more often in males than females. It occurs annually in the spring or early summer, usually in warm climates, is bilateral, and causes severe itching with watery discharge and severe papillary conjunctivitis. The papillae on the conjunctiva of the lids (upper more frequently than lower) are so large that they are described as "cobblestone." Each huge papilla has a flat surface and a tuft of capillaries that are readily visible. Particularly in young blacks, the lesions may be prominent at the limbus (the junction of the conjunctiva and cornea) where the papillae form a gelatinous mounded lesion, which is more prominent from 10 AM to 2 PM and from 5 to 7 PM.

This condition is recurrent for 5 to 10 years but is eventually self-limited. However, patients are quite uncomfortable. Cold compresses help. Topical steroids relieve the symptoms, but the chronicity of the condition often leads to prolonged steroid use.

The primary care practitioner will be happy to refer patients with vernal conjunctivitis to an ophthalmologist. Although the diagnosis is easy, the patient is miserable, the condition recurrent, and the management disappointing.

Wilson LA, et al. Treatment of external eye infections: A double-masked trial of tobramycin and gentamycin. *Ocular Ther Surg*, pp. 364–367, Nov./Dec. 1982.
  This discusses the relative values of two of the more recent antibiotics. It also includes an excellent clinical description of many cases of bacterial conjunctivitis.
Eiferman RA. A primer of conjunctivitis. *Primary Care* 6(3):561–586, Sept. 1979.
  An overview of the treatment of conjunctivitis.
Stenson S, et al. Studies in acute conjunctivitis. *Arch Ophthalmol* 100:1275–1277, 1982.
  An analysis of 700 cases of conjunctivitis comparing laboratory and clinical findings.
Leibowitz H, et al. Human conjunctivitis. *Arch Ophthalmol* 94:1747–1749 and 1752–1756, 1976.
  A report divided into two parts. The first found poor correlation between laboratory and clinical findings. The second examined treatment and found steroid/antibiotic preparations were better than antibiotics alone and both were better than placebos in relieving symptoms.

8. CHALAZION AND HORDEOLUM
Hunter R. Stokes

Almost all localized swollen masses of the eyelids are either chalazia or hordeola. The two are often confused and to some extent are managed similarly. However, the history, anatomic position of the swelling, and degree of inflammation are usually sufficiently different to distinguish between them and allow specific therapy.

Chalazion

A chalazion is a chronic, granulomatous inflammation of a meibomian gland, a sebaceous gland located in the tarsal plate. Chalazia occur at any age. They are always located deep within the lid tissue adjacent to the inner (conjunctival) surface. A small, nontender nodule ("English pea") is palpable within the lid, and there is a corresponding area of redness and elevation on the everted lid.

Treatment

Small, chronic chalazia can be left alone. If they are large enough to cause an obvious cosmetic swelling or to create pressure on the eyeball (which can actually blur vision by creating astigmatism), then surgical excision by an ophthalmologist is indicated. Chalazia can become infected, leading to painful swelling. This complication is managed with warm compresses, applied for 15 minutes four times a day, and topical sulfonamides or antibiotics, either ophthalmic solution or ointment, four times a day.

Hordeolum

A hordeolum (stye) is essentially a localized, superficial abscess, usually caused by *Staphylococcus aureus,* of one of the sweat or sebaceous glands of the eyelids. It presents as a red, swollen, and quite tender mass, which most commonly points to the skin surface of the lid (external hordeolum). Less often an internal hordeolum occurs; it is usually larger than an external one and points toward the inner conjunctival surface.

Treatment
Warm compresses for 15 minutes four times a day, followed by topical medication (same as for an infected chalazion), are usually sufficient. Drainage can be expected to begin in 24 to 48 hours. If drainage does not start after 48 hours of treatment, then incision and drainage at the area of pointing, either internal or external, may be necessary. The procedure can be done by a nonspecialist. However, sometimes a large hordeolum (usually internal) can progress to localized cellulitis that involves the entire lid and threatens cavernous sinus thrombosis. With the first hint of cellulitis, systemic antibiotics to treat *S. aureus* should be added to local therapy. Systemic antibiotics are not necessary for simple, localized hordeola.

Occasionally, patients have recurrent hordeola. They are usually in one eye and are caused by a chronic staphylococcal infection. Systemic antibiotics may help; usually referral to an ophthalmologist is indicated for lid cleansing.

Abramson, IA Jr. *Color Atlas of Anterior Segment Eye Disease.* New York: McGraw-Hill, 1964.
This color atlas includes excellent photographs of chalazia and hordeola.

9. CATARACTS
Hunter R. Stokes

The human lens is colorless, biconvex, and transparent. Clouding of the lens creates a cataract, which is both the most common cause of severe visual impairment in the United States and the most common cause of correctable severe visual disability. Well over 90% of all cataracts are considered to be due to the normal aging process of the human lens and not to any secondary disease. Cataracts are usually bilateral; however, the degree of opacification and rate of progression may differ from one eye to the other. Cataracts are a function of human aging and are present to some degree in at least 70% of patients over 70 years of age, but they occur more frequently in diabetics and are also associated with hypoparathyroidism, myotonic dystrophy, and atopic dermatitis.

Less commonly, cataracts are traumatic, congenital, or associated with the use of a number of drugs. Congenital cataracts and cataracts from rubella in the first trimester of pregnancy are usually visible at birth and present as a white pupillary reflex when fundoscopy is attempted. Traumatic cataracts can be caused by blunt, nonpenetrating trauma to the eye as well as by perforating injuries to the globe with direct injury and/or laceration of the lens. Systemic corticosteroids and topical echothiophate iodide (used for glaucoma treatment) have been found to be associated with an increased incidence of cataract formation.

Diagnosis
The diagnosis of cataract is made by detecting an opacity in the lens. An opacity can usually be seen by directing a penlight into the pupil or by looking through the

ophthalmoscope. Opacities of the lens can best be seen with the ophthalmoscope set at approximately +10 and with the examiner approximately 12 inches from the patient's face. The examination can be facilitated by dilating the pupil with two drops of 10% Neo-Synephrine Hydrochloride (Ophthalmic) solution. The risk that this procedure will cause acute angle-closure glaucoma is small. These opacities may be located in the anterior portion of the lens, the center (nucleus), or posteriorly. The level of the opacity as well as the degree of opacification determines how vision is affected, but these details are best studied by an ophthalmologist with a slit lamp. Usually the patient complains of reduced vision; however, some patients may actually report an improvement in either distance or near vision, even discarding glasses for some visual functions ("second sight"). This occurs because the shape as well as the transparency of the lens is altered during the cataract formation. This change in shape can result in myopia, which changes the refractive error and may allow farsighted patients to perform close work without glasses for months or years.

As soon as a patient is suspected of having a cataract, referral to an ophthalmologist is indicated. This does not mean that the patient will immediately have cataract surgery. A thorough ophthalmologic examination to detect possible associated eye conditions (glaucoma, retinal disorders, retinal holes and/or detachment) must be performed. Often a change in the patient's glasses, suggested by careful refraction, will improve visual acuity so that the patient can continue to function visually without surgery. Occasionally, dilating drops may also improve vision and preclude immediate surgery. It is rare that referral is delayed long enough for a cataract to become hypermature and threaten the health of an eye. After the initial visit, semiannual or annual examinations by the ophthalmologist are continued until surgery is ultimately indicated.

Treatment

The only specific management of cataracts is surgical removal of the lens (cataract extraction). Cataract extraction is indicated when the level of visual impairment reduces the ability of the patient to perform daily activities.

In recent years, development in instrumentation, sutures, and microscopes has revolutionized cataract surgery, allowing earlier ambulation and improved visual results. Now most cataract surgery is done under local anesthesia, and the average hospital stay has been reduced to 3 days. Patients are usually out of bed in several hours and discharged on the first postoperative day. In early 1983, Medicare began to reimburse outpatient surgery, and soon the number of cataracts done as outpatient surgery will approach 50%.

Several types of operations are available for cataract extraction, including intracapsular extraction, extracapsular extraction, and phacoemulsification. In intracapsular extraction the entire lens is removed using a cryoextractor ("freezing" the lens for removal). In extracapsular extraction, the anterior capsule is opened, the contents of the lens (nucleus and cortex) removed, and the posterior capsule left in place. This was the procedure of choice in the United States before 1955, and it has been enjoying a major resurgence in popularity in this country in the late 1970s and early 1980s. Phacoemulsification is a special form of extracapsular extraction. It is now the method of choice in younger patients and is preferred for all patients by some ophthalmic surgeons. An instrument is inserted into the eye, the nucleus is emulsified, and then the nucleus as well as the cortex is aspirated. Operative and postoperative pain is minimal with all techniques unless complications occur.

After the first postoperative week, the eye is usually patched only at night. Topical medicines are ordinarily used for 1 month. Most sutures are removed at 6 to 8 weeks, and the healing process is sufficiently complete for the patient to see (with new correction eyeglasses, contact lens, or intraocular lens) by 3 months after surgery.

Management After Cataract Extraction

Surgical aphakia (surgical absence of the lens) is corrected by an artificial lens. This lens may be in the form of spectacles, a contact lens, or an intraocular lens.

Spectacle Correction

Spectacle correction in aphakia requires the least surgery (no need to implant an intraocular lens) and the least patient effort (no contact lens to insert). However, there are significant disadvantages to spectacle aphakia lenses. They magnify (by about

33%), distort, and cause a loss of peripheral vision. Because of the magnification, the patient who has had only one eye operated on for cataracts cannot rely on spectacle correction if the other eye still has useful vision, because the difference in image size is intolerable. For these patients, the option is to wear contact lenses or to have an intraocular lens implantation.

Contact Lenses
Contact lenses reduce the problem of magnification and distortion. Moreover, peripheral vision is retained. Both hard and soft contact lenses are available. However, many elderly patients are unable to handle contact lenses because of arthritis, tremor, or anxiety; others have insufficient tears.

Hard contact lenses are less expensive, are more durable, provide consistently clearer vision, can be altered to provide a slight power change, and can be fitted to many eyes with marked astigmatism. Also, the tinting of the hard lenses makes them easier to find and their relative inflexibility makes them easier to handle; both of these are significant advantages in elderly patients with impaired vision.

Some soft contact lenses are inserted daily, while others may be inserted by an ophthalmologist and left in place for weeks or months. Not all eyes can be fitted with this "permanent" contact lens, and if fitted, the patient must return at least bimonthly to be examined in order to ascertain that the contact lens is not damaging to the eye. Soft lenses are more likely to be lost. The average postoperative cataract patient may require up to three soft contact lenses in the first year (Medicare only pays for the first one). Also, many soft lenses that may be worn for weeks or months (extended wear contacts) cause superficial vascularization, which can later preclude further contact lens wear or require topical steroid treatment with all of its potential problems.

Intraocular Lenses
Intraocular lenses are now implanted in some patients by more than three-quarters of all ophthalmologists in the United States. Usually the intraocular lens is implanted at the time of the cataract extraction, but it can be implanted later (secondary implant). Recent improvements in lens design and availability make this a safer and more satisfactory method of correction of aphakia than ever before. It is estimated that, in 1983, 70–80% of all patients undergoing cataract operations in the United States received an intraocular lens implant. All patients are not candidates for implants and the decision regarding the type of correction for aphakia must be made jointly by the operating surgeon and the patient.

Prognosis
With modern techniques of cataract extraction, 95% of patients can expect an improvement in vision and about 90% will have vision correctable to 20/40 or better. The most serious intraoperative and postoperative complications are infection and hemorrhage. Because most cataract operations are performed in elderly patients, other problems, such as macular degeneration and retinal vascular disorders, may reduce the final visual acuity, even though the surgical procedure and healing are without complication. Elderly patients whose vision is reduced significantly by cataracts should be encouraged to have surgery, but should be cautioned about visual expectations. Both the patients and their families are often disappointed when the elderly aphakic patient cannot "read the phone book"; this level of vision may not have been achievable because of other ocular problems.

Sloane AE, Kaufman JH. More on Cataract Surgery. In RJ Brockhurst et al. (Eds.), *Controversy in Ophthalmology*. Philadelphia: Saunders, 1977. P. 62.
  This includes an objective discussion of the differences between intracapsular cataract surgery and the extracapsular method of phacoemulsification.
Wong WW. Indications for cataract surgery: Psycholinguistic considerations. *Arch Ophthalmol* 96:526–528, 1978.
  An excellent philosophical discussion on when cataract surgery should be performed, and the conclusion is that successful cataract extraction should permit the patient to function better visually than before the surgery. This same issue has a good editorial (related to this subject and this article) on page 247.

10. GLAUCOMA
John C. Merritt

The glaucomas are characterized by increased ocular tensions to levels capable of producing optic nerve damage. Most glaucomas cause blindness by producing ischemic changes within the optic nerve tissue, resulting in visual field loss.

The glaucomas may be subdivided according to their mechanism of development into primary (chronic) open-angle glaucoma, primary angle-closure glaucoma, and the secondary glaucomas. This chapter will be limited to the most common glaucoma, primary open-angle glaucoma (POAG), which accounts for over 90% of all cases of glaucoma. The primary angle-closure glaucomas, diagnosed in less than 2% of glaucoma patients, result from appositional closure of functional trabecular meshwork by the peripheral iris. These are treated with iridectomies, by means of either surgery or laser, to eradicate the pupillary block component that maintains the elevated ocular tension. In secondary glaucoma, increase in intraocular pressure is induced by another ocular disease.

Natural History
Elevation in ocular pressure (ocular hypertension) is the first clinically detectable abnormality in most patients who develop POAG. Years later, the increased pressure may lead to optic nerve damage, resulting in the characteristic physical findings commonly termed primary open-angle glaucoma. The period of time between the onset of ocular hypertension and the first signs of glaucoma is not known. Similarly, the risk factors that may affect this progression are unclear. Most patients with ocular hypertension do not proceed to glaucoma during their lifetime.

Frequency
The overall prevalence of POAG in one or both eyes is estimated to be about 3%, based on a survey of 2675 residents in Framingham, Massachusetts in 1973 to 1975. The prevalence of POAG increased with age, to 7.2% for the persons 75 to 85 years old. This study has not been repeated elsewhere, and the results may not be representative of other American communities, particularly among blacks, who appear to be more susceptible to POAG than whites.

At present, no risk factors for POAG have been established. Data collected in 11 states where blindness is uniformly reported suggested that glaucoma blinded three to eight times more nonwhites than whites, although numerous biases could explain these observations. Increased systolic blood pressure is known to induce a concomitant increased ocular tension, but the relationship of POAG to essential hypertension has not been investigated. Similarly, diabetes has not been shown to be a major risk factor, although some data suggest that diabetics might be at increased risk. The Framingham Eye Study found no associations with education, variable blood sugar, systemic blood pressure, height, vital capacity, serum phospholipids, and hand strength.

Diagnosis

Ocular Hypertension
Ocular hypertension can be detected by a variety of instruments. Those practical for non-ophthalmologists include the following:

The Schiotz tonometer is the traditional instrument; it is widely used and relatively inexpensive (about $200). Unfortunately, it is often unreliable, especially in severe myopia, and not infrequently causes corneal abrasions.

The applanation tonometer is safer and more accurate than the Schiotz, but more expensive (about $800). Both tests can be performed by non-physicians.

As with systemic hypertension, there is no sharp delineation between normal and abnormal ocular tension. As a general rule, pressures are considered normal (as long as optic nerves appear normal) below 25 mm Hg and are regarded with some suspicion in the 25 to 30 mm Hg range. Pressures greater than 31 mm Hg are more likely abnormal; when found, visual fields and optic nerves must be examined closely to iden-

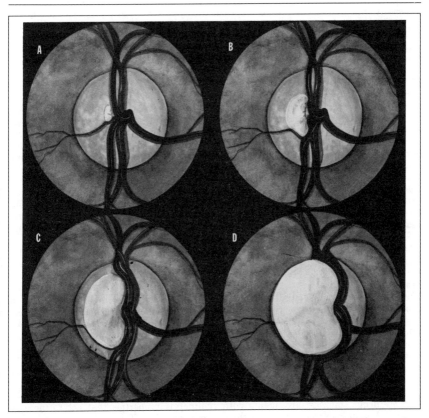

Fig. 10-1. Optic nerve cupping in glaucoma. A. Cup-disk ratio 0.1. Probably normal. B. Cup-disk ratio 0.4. Gray zone. C. Cup-disk ratio 0.8. Pressure-dependent changes of optic nerve. D. Cup-disk ratio 0.9+. Pressure-dependent changes of optic nerve.

tify any pressure-dependent field loss consistent with glaucoma. Pressures normally increase with age and ordinarily display a 2- to 5-mm Hg diurnal variation. Although POAG is characterized by increased ocular tensions, low-tension glaucomas are known to exist. These occur in people with optic nerve damage and visual field loss identical to those of POAG, but with no documented increases in ocular tension during 24 hours of testing.

Screening for glaucoma does not meet the strict criteria for inclusion in a periodic health examination because the effectiveness of early treatment has not been established by clinical trials. However, there are good reasons to support annual screening by primary care physicians in patients after age 40. Patient visits to primary care physicians are more frequent than to eye specialists, measurement of ocular tension is simple and inexpensive, and glaucoma is detected in 35 to 40% of patients referred to ophthalmologists by general physicians.

Glaucoma
The clinical signs in established POAG, in addition to ocular hypertension and open chamber angles (verified by contact lens gonioscopy), are optic nerve changes and visual field loss.

The visible changes in the optic disk that are characteristic of glaucoma include increased cupping and pallor. The cup-disk ratio is estimated in the vertical dimension (Fig. 10-1). The two eyes are usually comparable. Cup-disk ratios less than 0.3 are usually normal; between 0.3 and 0.6 is a gray zone. Cup-disk ratios greater than 0.6, especially if asymmetry is present between the eyes, are usually indicative of POAG. Increased pallor of the optic disk, a manifestation of optic atrophy, may be more difficult for non-ophthalmologists to recognize than the cup-disk ratio. The two eyes are often affected by glaucoma to a different degree. At times, glaucoma is recognized in the more severely affected eye by a "Marcus Gunn pupil" in which, because of afferent pupillary defects, there is a paradoxical dilatation of the pupil when light is shone into it.

Field defects, including isolated scotoma in Bjerrum's area (near the blind spot), arcuate scotomas, paracentral scotomas, and nasal step, are early indications of POAG and are detected by quantitative perimetry. In advanced glaucoma, peripheral field loss continues until there is generalized constriction of field, usually leaving only a temporal field of vision. Other ways of evaluating visual field loss (e.g., confrontation field with moving finger) are not sufficiently precise and would only succeed in detecting extremely large defects, as in far-advanced glaucoma.

Surveillance for Glaucoma

Once the existence of ocular hypertension is established, glaucoma should be ruled out by an ophthalmologist. Following that, patients are kept under observation for early glaucomatous changes by means of yearly examinations in which reproducible quantitative perimetry is done and the optic nerves are examined by ophthalmoscopy. In addition, optic nerve changes may be documented with serial photography and/or fluorescein angiography to detect the earliest possible evidences of optic nerve damage.

Treatment

Because the early pressure-dependent field defects are known to be reversible with lowered ocular tension, the risk-benefit ratio strongly favors no medical or surgical therapies for ocular hypertension alone. The treatment of glaucoma includes outflow-altering and inflow-altering topical drugs, and systemic carbonic anhydrase inhibitors, along with numerous surgical and laser procedures. These treatments are usually initiated by ophthalmologists but become part of the medical regimen that is dealt with by other physicians.

Outflow Drugs

Outflow drugs (miotics) are agents with cholinergic properties that act to increase aqueous humor movement through the anterior chamber. Topical pilocarpine hydrochloride is supplied in solutions of ½ to 4%, commonly given as one drop four times a day. Patients are instructed to occlude lower puncta, located on the eyelid near the inner canthus, so that systemic absorption is minimized. Adverse effects are often reported. The most frequently encountered side effects are miosis from accommodative spasms; induced myopia; blurred vision in elderly subjects with lens opacities; brow aches, headaches, and conjunctival hyperemia; retinal detachments in white patients without lenses with peripheral retinal holes; and cholinergic toxicity (often reported after multiple topical applications to break primary angle closure attacks). Longer-acting miotics (cholinesterase inhibitors) may alter serum cholinesterase levels so that prolonged apnea and respiratory failure result from succinylcholine anesthesia.

Inflow Drugs

The epinephrine compounds lower ocular tension predominantly through decreased aqueous humor production. Most epinephrine compounds in clinically used strengths (¼–2%) do not significantly alter pupil size in POAG subjects, since many are frequently taking miotics. Propine, a derivative of epinephrine that freely enters the anterior chamber, dilates pupils during the early period, though the mydriatic duration is unknown. Side effects from epinephrine compounds include conjunctival hyperemia with prolonged usage; brow aches, which occur with higher concentrations (2%); allergic reactions; rarely, induced arrhythmia in elderly subjects with known cardiac disease; and cystoid macula edema in white aphakic patients. Infrequently systemic hypertension is produced in elderly subjects.

Timolol maleate, a beta-adrenergic blocker, induces ocular hypotension by decreasing aqueous production. Innumerable studies have indicated that timolol (¼ and ½%) lowers ocular tension in chronic open-angle glaucomas. Most common ocular side effects are conjunctivitis, blepharitis, and keratitis with corneal hypothesia; systemic effects can occur (see Chap. 31).

Carbonic Anhydrase Inhibitors
Carbonic anhydrase inhibitors, such as acetazolamide, are agents that induce ocular hypotension by inhibition of the enzyme carbonic anhydrase within the ciliary epithelium and by inducing metabolic acidosis, both resulting in decreased aqueous production. Common clinically used dosages for the glaucomas vary from 125 mg three times a day to 250 mg four times a day orally. Numerous adverse effects have been reported for these drugs: loss of appetite, lethargy and depression, weakness, tinnitus, hypokalemia and metabolic acidosis in elderly patients, loss of libido, altered taste, kidney stone formation, Stevens-Johnson–like syndromes, and aggravation of diabetes mellitus. These complications are not uncommon, and 33% of patients placed on systemic carbonic anhydrase inhibitor therapy become compliance failures within 1 year. There is no evidence that long-term acetazolamide in dosages of 250 mg four times a day produces more ocular hypotension than 125 mg four times a day. Ophthalmologists often conclude that by judiciously adding these systemic agents (in maximum dosages) to topical therapies maximum medical therapies are being employed for the glaucoma.

Surgery
Surgery has traditionally been reserved for patients who are "medical failures." This failure in POAG has classically been defined as the progressive loss of visual field (not progressive increase in ocular tensions) while taking the maximum tolerated medications. The fistulizing operations are approximately 75 to 85% successful in whites, while blacks have both a higher complication and higher failure rate. Recently, laser trabeculoplasties have virtually replaced these filtering operations; however, longer-term results and complications have not been reported.

Kahn HA, et al. The Framingham Eye Study: Part I. Outline and major prevalence findings. *Am J Epidemiol* 106:17–32, 1977.
   Because this was a study of a predominantly white population, its findings do not describe the incidence or prevalence of open-angle glaucoma or other glaucomas within the American population.
Kahn HA, Moorhead HB. *Statistics on Blindness in the Model Reporting Area 1969–1970.* DHEW Publications No. (NIH), 1973, pp. 73–417.
   Suggests a 3½- to 8-times higher incidence of blindness in blacks than in whites, but numerous biases exist in data collection and interpretation.
Klein BE, Klein RI. Intraocular pressure and cardiovascular risk variables. *Arch Ophthalmol* 99:837–839, 1981.
   A recent mass screening study to identify a direct correlation between systemic blood pressure and intraocular pressure and to document that these mean systolic blood pressures and mean ocular tensions were higher in American blacks than in whites.
Kahn HA, et al. The Framingham Eye Study: Part II. Association of ophthalmic pathology with single variables previously measured in the Framingham Heart Study. *Am J Epidemiol* 106:33–41, 1977.
   This retrospective attempt failed to identify any association of ophthalmic pathology documented with single variables listed in the Framingham Heart Study.
Kaback MB, Burde RM, Becker B. Relative afferent pupillary defect in glaucoma. *Am J Ophthalmol* 81:462–468, 1976.
   Early paper documenting the presence of relative afferent pupillary defects in asymmetric open-angle glaucoma.
Armaly MF. The visual field defect and ocular pressure level in open angle glaucoma. *Invest Ophthalmol* 8:105–124, 1969.
   Classic paper demonstrating that lowering ocular tension reverses visual field defects in early open-angle glaucoma; hence, the definition of pressure-dependent visual field defects is derived.
Heilmann K. On the reversibility of visual field defects in glaucomas. *Trans Am Acad Ophthalmol Otolaryngol* 78:304–308, 1974.
   European study documenting similar reversibility of visual field defects in the glaucomas.
Merritt JC. Filtering procedures in American Blacks. *Ophthalmic Surg* 11:91–94, 1980.
   Description of failed glaucoma operations in American blacks.

11. VISUAL IMPAIRMENT
Hunter R. Stokes

The measurement of visual acuity is the most important and revealing test of ocular function. It is appropriate for primary care physicians to check vision in their offices. Careful measurement of the visual acuity should be recorded in all cases of ocular and facial trauma. These data may later prove to be extremely valuable.

Patients whose visual acuity must be measured for the purpose of jobs, legal blindness and disability determinations, military induction, and medicolegal cases should be referred to an ophthalmologist. Often these requests for vision examination require documentation of distance and near vision with and without correction, visual field measurement, and sometimes a refraction. While legal blindness is usually described as vision of 20/200 or less, other factors, such as the field of vision and the degree of ocular motility (including the presence or absence of diplopia), are often a part of the formula necessary to make the final determination.

The most common causes of visual impairment include hereditary defects in people under age 20, diabetic retinopathy in those 21 to 60, and macular degeneration in those over 60.

Even though cataracts are a very common cause of visual impairment (most patients over the age of 70 have at least some degree of cataract formation), it is not considered a major cause of blindness in the United States because most cataracts are operated on before blindness occurs.

Vision Testing

Distance Vision
The major component of the office visual acuity examination is testing distance vision. A hallway is sufficient for testing if the proper distance (20 feet) and lighting are available. In addition to the the usual Snellen chart, charts should be available for children and the illiterate (E chart). The examiner should measure vision in patients with acuity less than 20/200 by recording finger counting (CF) at various distances (e.g., CF 1 foot, CF 66 inches), hand movements (HM), light perception (LP), or total blindness (no light perception [NLP]). Improvement of vision by a pinhole is objective evidence of myopia.

Near Vision
The measurement of near vision is not as important as the measurement of distance acuity and need not be measured by primary care physicians. Children and young adults usually have good vision, and refractive errors (especially myopia) affect distance vision more than near vision. After age 40, all patients begin to develop presbyopia and cannot see "up close" as well as before.

Color Vision
Six percent of males have some degree of color blindness or at least a red/green deficiency. Rarely is color blindness associated with other ocular problems. The only limitations for color-deficient people are certain color-related jobs (interior design, clothing sales, and airplane piloting) and appointments to the military academies. Poor color vision is not considered a disability.

Intraocular Pressure Measurements
Two percent of Americans over age 40 have chronic open-angle glaucoma, a disease that leads to blindness if not diagnosed and treated. Glaucoma usually produces no symptoms and can only be detected by the measurement of intraocular pressure. This test should be performed by primary care physicians. (See Chap. 10.)

Special Problems

Diabetes Mellitus
Patients with diabetes mellitus are at increased risk for ocular problems. Transient myopia with reduction in distance visual acuity is induced by hyperglycemia. Cata-

racts occur earlier than in nondiabetics and with twice the incidence; moreover, the complication rate with cataract surgery is four to five times greater. Chronic simple glaucoma occurs three times more often, and other forms of glaucoma occur more frequently and with greater severity in diabetes. The retinopathy of diabetes mellitus is the fastest rising cause of severe visual impairment and occurs as a function of the duration of the disease.

All diabetics should have a careful examination of the fundus for neovascularities and microaneurysms, and all those noted to have retinopathy should be referred immediately to an opthalmologist for a complete evaluation. Otherwise, all insulin-dependent diabetics should be referred to an ophthalmologist after they have had the disease for 10 years and thereafter should be seen at least annually. The ophthalmologic examination usually includes an intravenous fluorescein angiogram to study the dynamics of the retinal circulation. This examination should identify those patients who may benefit from laser treatment. During the past decade, lasers have reduced the number of diabetics who eventually become blind from proliferative retinopathy.

Floaters

Patients who complain of a "skim over the eyes" are often having visual disturbances from an uncorrected or undercorrected refractive error. However, the presence of floaters is a common complaint among patients over the age of 35 and is often associated with detachment of the vitreous base; this is not a serious problem and is infrequently associated with detachment of the retina or an intraocular hemorrhage. This differentiation can only be made by an ophthalmologist.

Eye Evaluation in Trauma

Careful measurement of visual acuity should be recorded in all cases of ocular and facial trauma. Besides establishing visual acuity at the time of the accident, this data will prove to be extremely valuable in assessing progression of the injury and in determining treatment.

Fonda G. *Management of the Patient with Subnormal Vision* (2nd ed.). St. Louis: Mosby, 1970. Pp. 3–5.
  Excellent reference on the causes of poor vision by age groups.
Faye EE. *Clinical Low Vision* (1st ed.). Boston: Little, Brown, 1976.
  Discussion of patients with diabetes (pp. 283–288).

III. EAR PROBLEMS

12. DEAFNESS AND TINNITUS

James P. Browder

Hearing loss and tinnitus often occur together. They are common complaints, particularly among older people. Most sensorineural hearing loss (SNHL, "nerve deafness") is accompanied by some sort of tinnitus, described variously as "ringing," "whistling," or "crickets in my ear." Conductive hearing loss (CHL) is less often associated with significant tinnitus, although it may unmask a faint, high-pitched ringing that can be detected by most people in very quiet surroundings.

The major questions to be answered when confronted with the complaints of deafness and tinnitus are: Is the condition treatable, and is it a manifestation of an underlying, serious disease? Most deafness is easily treatable, whereas tinnitus is not. Rarely does deafness or tinnitus signal a life-threatening condition, such as an acoustic tumor, although neither complaint can be dismissed as trivial.

Causes of Deafness

Conductive Hearing Loss

The most common cause of hearing loss is CHL secondary to a middle ear effusion resulting from eustachian tube malfunction. This may follow an upper respiratory infection or allergy or, less commonly, nasopharyngeal tumor, cleft palate, or trauma. Otosclerosis also commonly causes CHL, sometimes accompanied by a sensorineural component ("cochlear" otosclerosis). Otosclerosis is more often found in women than in men, with a peak incidence in the third decade of life. Less common causes of CHL in adults are cholesteatoma, fixation of the ossicles secondary to repeated middle ear infections, and traumatic ossicular dislocation. Rarely, middle ear tumors, such as a glomus tympanicum, can cause CHL.

Sensorineural Hearing Loss

High-frequency SNHL, usually associated with a loss of speech discrimination function, is often seen among older people, especially among those with a history of noise exposure. Less common causes of SNHL include Meniere's disease, metabolic disorders such as hyperlipidemia, and, rarely, ototoxic drug exposure, acoustic tumors, congenital deafness, childhood viral illness (e.g., mumps), and trauma.

Presbycusis

Presbycusis is the SNHL often associated with tinnitus that occurs to some degree in almost all elderly patients. Repeated exposure to noise and/or impaired blood supply to the cochlea and its nerve supply are most often cited as the cause. Patients note upper frequency hearing loss with or without a loss of speech discrimination; those with loss of speech discrimination have the most difficulty. They are bothered by high-pitched sounds (particularly children's and females' voices) and loud sounds. Often patients are brought in by family, but the patients may not feel that their hearing has deteriorated. The diagnosis is made by exclusion. Simple instructions to the family will frequently improve communication. Speakers should face the patients to provide visual clues and speak softly and distinctly. Because loud voices or noises are disturbing, families and particularly children should be quiet when around these patients.

Evaluation

History

The history should elicit the duration of symptoms, their laterality, their course, associated symptoms (such as vertigo, pain, or discharge from the ear), a family history, and a drug history (particularly for streptomycin or other aminoglycoside antibiotics).

Examination

The presence of a membrane perforation or other tympanic membrane pathology, or the finding of a discharge in the canal, suggests the presence of middle ear and mastoid pathology; however, a normal tympanic membrane and external auditory canal do not

39

rule out significant pathology. When there is debris in the canal, it may be difficult to differentiate an acute external otitis from an acutely exacerbated chronic middle ear condition. The postauricular region should also be inspected for signs of mastoid disease, and facial nerve function should be tested because it can be affected by destructive mastoiditis.

Assessment of Hearing

An assessment of hearing without an audiometer is approximate at best. The "ticking watch" test yields limited information because of the very narrow range of high-frequency sound that most watches produce. It is better and simpler to use the whispered voice. With a finger occluding the opposite ear, a person with normal hearing should be able to respond to a simple question, such as "How old are you," directed to the test ear at a level at which the examiner can just barely hear it.

Tuning forks are of limited value. The optimum frequency for testing with the fork is 512 Hz, although 256 Hz and 1024 Hz can be used. The 128-Hz fork, which is used for testing vibratory sensation, is not adequate for testing hearing. The Rinne test, which compares air-to-bone conduction, is used to distinguish CHL from SNHL. The Weber test confirms the results of the Rinne test. Tuning forks are useful in cooperative subjects with relatively uncomplicated pathology, such as a unilateral simple SNHL or CHL. More complex clinical problems are best diagnosed by audiometry and/or tympanometry, which should be obtained by referral to an otolaryngologist and audiologist or a hearing and speech center.

Acute Deafness

Trauma

In acute traumatic hearing loss there is usually a straightforward history of trauma. Care should be exercised in examining the ear in the presence of a possible temporal bone fracture to avoid contamination of the central nervous system. There is almost always some tympanic membrane (TM) abnormality. A normal otologic examination when deafness follows trauma usually represents a chronic hearing loss incidentally discovered or, less frequently, a functional hearing loss. All patients with hearing loss following trauma should be referred to an otolaryngologist for documentation and therapy.

Acute Otitis Media/Mastoiditis

Except in children, this disorder rarely represents a strictly acute process; rather it is an exacerbation of preexisting chronic disease. The hallmarks are pain, with or without drainage, and hearing loss. A TM abnormality is almost always present. Postauricular swelling points to a subperiosteal abscess erupting from diseased mastoid air cells. If there is no fever or other systemic symptoms and no clear history for chronic ear disease, treatment with antibiotic/steroid drops is satisfactory, particularly if it is difficult to distinguish otitis media from external otitis. If otitis media is obviously the problem, oral antibiotics are needed (See Chap. 14). Fever, elevated white count, and periauricular inflammation mandate parenteral antibiotics after a culture has been taken. Patients with diabetes, particularly the elderly, also require parenteral antibiotics and close observation because of the possibility of "malignant" external otitis (osteomyelitis of the temporal bone).

Labyrinthitis, manifested by vertigo, is an infrequent but serious complication of an acute middle ear infection. Hearing may be lost, and there is a high risk that infection will spread to the meninges.

Serous Otitis Media

Hearing loss associated with an upper respiratory infection (URI) suggests either acute otitis media or acute serous effusion. A retracted, amber membrane is the hallmark of serous otitis. Bubbles behind the TM are a favorable prognostic sign. This condition is safely treated by decongestants alone, unless the URI itself mandates antibacterial therapy. It may be several days before the patient has significant improvement in symptoms. Myringotomy is not indicated in acute serous otitis media, except for the relief of pain; however, myringotomy and placement of a grommet are effective in chronic middle ear effusion.

Serous otitis media in the absence of a URI or that persists longer than 10 days despite adequate therapy should suggest nasopharyngeal carcinoma. A careful inspection of the nasopharynx by an otolaryngologist is necessary to diagnose this disease.

Functional

Acute deafness, particularly in teenagers with no history of trauma or previous ear disease and a normal otoscopic examination, suggests a functional cause. Audiometric testing is the only reliable way to confirm this diagnosis.

"Idiopathic"

Patients with sudden hearing loss with no clearly identifiable cause should be referred to an otologist immediately. They are treated with steroids and carbon dioxide inhalation, but responsiveness seems to decrease if treatment is delayed a few days; however, effective response to treatment is controversial.

Subacute/Chronic Deafness

For patients presenting with a 2-week or longer history of hearing loss, it is useful to distinguish between those having a normal TM and those demonstrating TM pathology. The causes of subacute/chronic hearing loss with a normal tympanic membrane are shown in Table 12-1.

TM pathology with long-standing hearing loss usually indicates chronic middle ear and mastoid infection. Even if the TM is intact, fixation of the ossicles, which can be surgically corrected, may have come about as a result of an old infection. If foul-smelling pus and dirty, gray debris are found in the ear canal, a cholesteatoma should be strongly suspected and the patient referred to an otolaryngologist for definitive therapy. Vertigo, fever, severe ear pain, or meningeal or other CNS findings in association with a draining ear point to a violation of the bony barrier separating the middle ear from the labyrinth; this condition is a surgical emergency.

Otosclerosis can occasionally present with a blush near the oval window seen through the translucent TM (Schwartze's sign). Audiometric testing can confirm the diagnosis. Tumors of the external auditory canal and middle ear are not common but can present with deafness. Otoscopy usually reveals obvious pathology, although in the case of a glomus tympanicum it may show no more than a localized area of erythema behind the TM.

Wax Impaction

Wax impaction, with or without external otitis, can cause deafness.

Tinnitus

All cases of atypical tinnitus in which the cause is not immediately apparent should be referred to an otolaryngologist for audiometric evaluation and a thorough head and neck examination.

Table 12-1. Causes of subacute/chronic hearing loss with normal tympanic membrane

Etiology	Finding
Otosclerosis	Schwartze's sign (occasional)
Familial	Progressive in young adults
Metabolic (hyperlipidemia)	Abnormalities in blood chemistries
Congenital	Other congenital abnormalities
Viral (mumps, measles)	Nonprogressive in children
Noise-induced	High frequency loss
Drug-induced (salicylates, aminoglycosides)	Tinnitus
Presbycusis	Diagnosed by exclusion
Central	Rare

"Garden Variety" Tinnitus

A high-pitched ringing sound localized to one ear and of varying degrees of intensity and duration is an exceedingly common occurrence in the general population. It may be associated with ototoxic drug exposure, especially aspirin. Occasionally, tinnitus of this nature can be so disturbing that a physician is consulted. Unfortunately, no effective treatment exists except for discontinuing any ototoxic drugs. Because the symptom is most disturbing at night, a soft, monotonous noise, such as a fan or radio, may help mask the tinnitus. Some patients with mild SNHL and tinnitus may benefit from a hearing aid used not so much to amplify what is heard as to provide a source of external background noise to mask the tinnitus. In every case where a patient's primary complaint is tinnitus, an audiogram should be obtained, since tinnitus may signal the onset of progressive deafness.

Roaring Tinnitus

Roaring tinnitus, especially if linked with hearing loss and/or vertigo, suggests Meniere's syndrome.

Pulsatile Tinnitus

Pulsatile tinnitus may accompany a middle ear effusion or may represent a transmitted sound from a cardiac murmur or cervical bruit. If the tinnitus can be shown to be in synchrony with the heartbeat, careful auscultation of the heart, cervical vessels, eye and the mastoid and parietal areas of the skull may reveal a bruit signalling a cardiovascular anomaly, an aneurysm or fistula, or an arteriovenous malformation. Pulsatile tinnitus can also be caused by glomus tumors.

Fluttering tinnitus

Fluttering tinnitus may be caused by intermittent spasm of the tensor tympani muscle or even the presence of an insect in the external auditory canal. Tympanometry is helpful in documenting the former condition. Tensor tympani spasm is normally associated with an acute eye irritation, by a reflex phenomenon, or it may be a manifestation of acute anxiety.

Clicking Tinnitus

Clicking tinnitus is the hallmark of palatal myoclonus. This is a disorder of uncertain etiology that responds to mild sedation. The diagnosis is confirmed by observing a rapid, rhythmic twitching of the ipsilateral palate while the tinnitus is present.

Crunching Tinnitus

Crunching tinnitus in association with chewing may represent temperomandibular joint arthritis or a foreign body, such as a hair, in the external auditory canal that rubs against the TM.

Hearing Aids

Determining whether or not a patient with deafness will benefit from hearing amplification is largely a matter of judgment, based on specific audiometric findings plus a trial of an appropriate device. Two major difficulties are encountered in fitting a patient for a hearing aid. First, the patient does not have sufficient speech discrimination function to understand what is amplified. A patient who is able to comprehend less than half of what is said, even though amplified, will find a hearing aid more a source of frustration than benefit. Second, the patient does not have a sufficiently wide dynamic range. With SNHL, the discomfort threshold from loud sounds is often lowered. Hearing aids are limited in their ability to amplify sounds so that they are loud enough to be heard but not so loud that they cause pain.

Legal restrictions on the sale of hearing aids vary from state to state. Regardless of the law, good practice requires that the patient be tested by a licensed audiologist working in association with an otolaryngologist, that the patient be permitted to rent the device at a moderate fee for a trial in the home and at work of at least 1 month, that appropriate servicing of the aid is available in case of malfunction, and that a limited warranty on the device of at least 1 year is offered.

Glasscock ME (Ed.). Sensorineural deafness. *Otolaryngol Clin North Am* 11(1), Feb 1978.

Over 25 articles by an international panel covering in depth such topics as noise-induced hearing loss, sudden hearing loss, cochlear otospongiosis (otosclerosis), hearing aids, and cochlear implants.

Page JM (Ed.). Audiology. *Otolaryngol Clin North Am* 11(3), Oct. 1978.
    A complete discussion in a number of articles of contemporary audiometric evaluation including testing for central auditory dysfunction, brain stem–evoked response audiometry, impedance testing (tympanometry), and evaluation for hearing aids.

Arenberg IK (Ed.). Meniere's disease. *Otolaryngol Clin North Am* 13(4), Nov. 1980.
    A thorough presentation of both the known and the problematic concerning the pathophysiology, diagnosis/staging, and treatment of Meniere's disease.

13. OTITIS EXTERNA
Marion Danis

Otitis externa is the general term referring to any inflammatory process involving the skin covering the auricle and lining the external auditory canal. Any pathologic process that occurs elsewhere on the skin can occur on the skin of the external ear, and the same principles of treatment apply. The many causes of external otitis can be classified as follows: infectious, allergic (eczematoid), neurogenic, and a small group of other causes (e.g., seborrheic, psoriatic). Diffuse infectious otitis externa is the most common entity.

Frequency
Otitis externa is a very common condition in ambulatory practice. It is five times more common in swimmers than nonswimmers and occurs with greater frequency in hot, humid climates because of the macerating effect of water on the epithelium of the external auditory canal. It occurs in patients of all ages.

Clinical Presentation
Ear pain is the presenting complaint in approximately 85% of patients and varies in severity from slight discomfort that is difficult to distinguish from itching to excruciating aching or throbbing. The severity of pain has been thought to occur because the skin of the external ear is attached directly to the periosteum and perichondrium so that edema of the dermis compresses nerve fibers against the cartilage or bone. Any movement of the auricle, such as chewing, can be painful. Itching is present in two-thirds of cases and often precedes the pain. If the condition becomes chronic, itching is often the chief complaint. Conductive hearing loss may occur from occlusion of the lumen of the external auditory canal by edema, secretions, or other material such as desquamated keratin, cerumen, or debris.

    Physical findings classically include erythema and edema of the skin of the auditory canal, a greenish-tinged discharge, and pain on manipulating the auricle. Involvement of both ears occurs almost 20% of the time.

Differential Diagnosis

Localized Furuncle
Localized infectious external otitis presents as a discrete furuncle involving the skin of the canal and is usually readily distinguishable from diffuse external otitis. Occasionally there will be so much swelling that the canal is obliterated and visualization of the furuncle is difficult. However, with careful, gentle examination, the furuncle will almost always be seen. Spontaneous rupture of the furuncle may result in drainage of purulent material into the canal. The source of the drainage is usually identifiable.

Otitis Media
When the lumen of the external auditory canal is obliterated by pus and debris, it becomes difficult to differentiate external otitis from otitis media, particularly if the

Table 13-1. Clinical features of acute diffuse otitis externa and acute otitis media

Feature	Otitis externa	Otitis media
Pain	Aggravated by moving jaw	Aggravated by swallowing
Tenderness	Prominent	Absent
Systemic symptoms	Usually absent	Fever, rhinitis, sore throat
Hearing loss	Conductive type	Conductive type
Swelling of ear canal	Prominent	Absent
Discharge	Not profuse; may be more malodorous	Occurs with tympanic perforation
Tympanic membrane	Inflamed but intact; no middle ear fluid	May be perforated; fluid in middle ear

latter is chronic otitis media with perforation and drainage. Table 13–1 presents some clinical features that are useful in making the distinction. (See also Laboratory Diagnosis, below).

Other Infectious Causes
Fungal infections of the external ear are not common and should be suspected only in a grossly abnormal ear canal under special environmental conditions (extremely moist, hot climate) or when the external ear has been a site of chronic bacterial infection, a foreign body, or necrotic tumor. Fungal infections may be due to saprophytic (opportunistic) organisms such as *Aspergillus* (which may produce a black exudate), *Mucor*, *Actinomyces*, and *Candida* or pathogenic fungi such as species of *Trichophyton* or *Microsporum*. Mycobacterial infections of the ear need only be considered when chronic granulomatous and ulcerative lesions occur in the ear canal. *Mycoplasma* causes a bullous myringitis. Herpes simplex and herpes zoster can affect the external ear and present with typical vesicles.

Noninfectious Inflammatory Reactions
Inflammation of the skin of the external ear can be produced by contact with many agents, either because of irritation, as in irritant contact dermatitis, or because of an immune-mediated reaction, as in allergic contact dermatitis. Common irritants include strong acids, alkali, and metallic salts, all of which are caustic enough to cause reaction upon first exposure, and less noxious agents such as hearing aid inserts, soaps, and solvents, which may require more prolonged exposure to cause irritation. Allergic contact dermatitis is most commonly caused by poison ivy and certain ingredients of hair sprays and cosmetics, as well as nickel and rubber compounds. Patients with inflammation of the external ear should be asked about any exposure to hair sprays, shampoos, dyes, earrings, or local medications (particularly those containing neomycin) and use of foreign objects in the ear such as hairpins, matches, earplugs, or headphones. Seborrhea and psoriasis should be considered, and characteristic lesions on the skin elsewhere, particularly on the scalp, should be noted.

Once these other conditions are ruled out, neurodermatitis may be considered. In early cases, erythema, edema, vesiculations, and crusting may occur, leading to dry, thickened, lichenified skin that is difficult to distinguish morphologically from other causes. The ear is a favorite site of itching and scratching, which is probably important in the pathogenesis of neurodermatitis.

Laboratory Diagnosis
Because bacteriologic culture results usually will not alter the management of otitis externa, this procedure is not routinely necessary. Cultures may be warranted in rare instances where differentiation of otitis externa from otitis media is unusually difficult; the different spectrum of organisms seen in the two conditions may help to distinguish between them.

The normal bacteriologic flora of the external auditory canal consists of *Staphylococcus epidermidis* (or *Staphyloccocus aureus* in approximately 15% of normal individuals) and *Corynebacterium* species. Organisms seen in diffuse otitis externa, listed in descending order of prevalence, are *Pseudomonas* species, *S. aureus*, *Proteus*, *Escherichia coli*, and other, less common organisms. The organisms causing otitis externa tend to be those causing skin infections, whereas the organisms that cause otitis media are organisms usually seen in respiratory tract infections, such as pneumococci, *Hemophilus influenzae*, and group A beta-streptococcus.

If fungal infection is suspected, the diagnosis may be supported by observation of fungal hyphae on a 10% potassium hydroxide slide preparation of scrapings and confirmed by culture on Sabouraud's medium.

Treatment

If the ear canal is not occluded, diffuse otitis externa should be treated with an appropriate otic solution applied to both ears three times a day for 1 week. Combined antibiotic/steroid preparations (e.g., Cortisporin Otic Solution) have been used for many years with success. Recent controlled trials have shown equally good results using a simpler solution containing propanediol diacetate (VōSoL Otic Solution), which is both antifungal and antibacterial.

If the canal is at all occluded, a simple gauze wick should be inserted in the external canal. The wick should be kept moist with the solution, thus insuring continuous application to the inflamed tissue and preventing the drops from simply rolling out of the canal into the external ear. Recently the use of a stiff, expandable wick (Weck cell ear wick or commercially available as Otowick) has been advocated because it can be inserted into the inflamed canal more easily and with less pain. Cleaning the ear canal is often very difficult and is not necessary.

Pain medication should be prescribed for the first 24 to 48 hours. Topical analgesics are ineffective and not indicated.

A more localized external otitis ought to be treated like any other localized staphylococcal infection on the skin. Warm compresses and observation, followed by incision and drainage, will usually suffice. Inflammation of the surrounding tissue, fever, and lymphadenopathy are indications for antibiotics. Penicillin or a penicillinase-resistant drug such as dicloxacillin is usually used. External otitis caused by fungal infection usually can be treated with propanediol diacetate (VōSoL Otic Solution).

Prevention of otitis externa can be accomplished in individuals who have repeated attacks by aural administration of propanediol diacetate (VōSoL Otic Solution), aluminum acetate (Burow's solution), or acetic acid daily and particularly after swimming.

Complications

The most serious complication of otitis externa is a spreading *Pseudomonas* infection, which rarely occurs except in diabetic patients. Any diabetic patient with otitis externa needs to be observed carefully. Some authorities have recommended beginning the elderly, diabetic, or immunocompromised patient on an oral antibiotic, selected on the basis of the culture and sensitivity of the aural discharge. If there is any progression of the disease, as indicated by persistence of granulation tissue or development of cranial neuropathies, then intravenous antibiotics must be given, and an otolaryngologist should be consulted about possible surgical intervention.

Aside from this cautionary note, diffuse otitis externa is a benign disease that may well resolve with little intervention.

Senturia BH, Marcus MD, Lucente FE. *Diseases of the External Ear* (2nd ed.). New York: Grune & Stratton, 1980.
   This is the most recent and complete reference on diseases of the external ear, and it includes an excellent discussion of various causes of external otitis.
Cassini N, et al. Diffuse otitis externa: Clinical and microbiologic findings in the course of a multicenter study on a new otic solution. *Ann Otol Rhinol Laryngol* 86 (Suppl. 39):1–16, 1977.
   This article provides a good review of the literature on the epidemiology, pathogenesis, and bacteriology of diffuse otitis externa, and it also provides the results of a trial

comparing two antibiotic/corticosteroid formulations. Both formulations had a clinical efficacy rate of 97%.

Wright DN, Dineen M. Infectious otitis externa. *Arch Otolaryngol* 95:241, 1972.

An animal model of otitis externa is used to explore etiologic factors of this disease. It was found that prolonged water exposure caused a shift in bacterial flora from gram-positive to gram-negative and precipitated disease. Removal of the ear canal lipids alone did not result in disease, but did predispose to disease if the canal was subsequently contaminated.

Hoadley AW, Knight DE. External otitis in swimmers and non-swimmers. *Arch Environ Health* 30:445, 1975.

The incidence of otitis externa is five times greater in swimmers than in nonswimmers.

Jenkins BH. Treatment of otitis externa and swimmer's ear. *JAMA* 175:148–150, 1961.

In an uncontrolled trial, 200 patients were treated with cleaning of the ear canal "where necessary" and with VōSoL Otic drops (propanediol diacetate, acetic acid, benzethonium chloride, and propylene glycol) for 8 days. Symptoms were resolved by the fourth to sixth day, and results were excellent in all cases.

Taylor JS. Otitis externa: Treatment using a new expandable wick. *Eye Ear Nose Throat Monthly* 53:33, 1974.

A stiff, expandable Weck cell ear wick (Weck cell sponge) is used to deliver medication to the edematous auditory canal, and much less pain is incurred in its use.

Lambert IF. A comparison of the treatment of otitis externa with "Otosporin" and aluminum acetate: A report from a services practice in Cyprus. *J R Coll Gen Pract* 31:291, 1981.

An extremely useful article that characterizes the presentation of otitis externa in a general practice and compares the results of treatment with either aluminum acetate or an antibiotic/steroid combination (Otosporin). This randomized trial shows no difference in outcome with the two treatments.

Freedman R. Versus placebo in treatment of acute otitis externa. *Ear Nose Throat J* 57:198–204, 1978.

A very useful report in which 91 patients had cleaning of the external ear and half subsequently received Coly-Mycin S Otic (colistin sulfate, neomycin sulfate, hydrocortisone acetate, and acetic acid). There was greater resolution of symptoms in the treated group at 7 days, but by 21 days there was no difference, with equal resolution in both groups.

Chandler JR. Malignant external otitis: Further considerations. *Ann Otolaryngol* 86:417, 1977.

Malignant external otitis is a Pseudomonas *infection occurring in diabetics that spreads to the soft tissues beneath the temporal bone, which, when untreated, leads to facial nerve palsy, mastoiditis, sepsis, osteomyelitis, sigmoid sinus thrombosis, and death. Medical therapy with intravenous carbenicillin and gentamicin is recommended and surgery is withheld unless there is no improvement.*

14. OTITIS MEDIA
Desmond K. Runyan

Although less common in adults than in children, acute otitis media remains a painful problem that may be followed by complications, including mastoiditis, bacterial meningitis, and other central nervous system infections. The clinical diagnosis is sometimes difficult to make, even for experienced physicians, and many aspects of the treatment are controversial.

Otitis media occurs most frequently in the first 2 years of life and declines slowly in incidence after that time, probably because of longer eustachian tubes, better antibody response in the upper respiratory tract, and specific antibodies resulting from prior infections. Factors that are associated with a higher risk for the disease include cleft palate, Down's syndrome, nasopalatine lymphoid hyperplasia, allergic rhinitis, and native American or Eskimo origin. The highest attack rates occur in the winter months during viral epidemics.

The offending infectious agent in otitis media is almost always bacterial. An antecedent viral infection may predispose the patient to the disease, but primary viral infection of the middle ear has rarely been documented. *Pneumococcus* is the most frequent bacterial pathogen in both adults and children and is found in 24 to 44% of middle ear cultures during acute otitis. *Hemophilus influenzae* is the second most common bacteria isolated; it is the presumed pathogen for about one-fourth of all middle ear infections. Conventional wisdom held that *H. influenzae* had a declining role with advancing patient age and was rarely recovered in patients over age 8. However, there are now a number of reports of *H. influenzae* disease in older children and adults. In one series of adolescents, *H. influenzae* was present in one-third of middle ear cultures. About 10% of *H. influenzae* isolates are type B, which is more often associated with ampicillin resistance and central nervous sytem infection; the remainder are usually nontypable. Other known pathogens of the middle ear include group A streptococcus, *Branhamella catarrhalis, Staphlococcus aureus, Escherichia coli,* and *Pseudomonas.*

Diagnosis

The clinical presentation of acute otitis media is usually quite specific in adults: ear pain, otorrhea, hearing loss, and/or vertigo. Fever is common but not universal. Conjunctivitis, rhinitis, and pharyngitis occur if there is a concomitant upper respiratory infection. Adenopathy of the posterior auricular and posterior cervical nodes is often observed.

Differential Diagnosis

Otorrhea may make it difficult to differentiate otitis media with perforation from otitis externa. The former typically has a history of antecedent viral infection and of intense pain followed by acute relief at the time of perforation. Otitis externa often follows exposure to water, and there is severe tenderness on movement of the outer ear (see Chap. 13). The ear canal can often be cleansed well enough to visualize the tympanic membrane when the diagnosis is otitis media, while the swollen canal may be too tender to clean in otitis externa. Techniques for cleaning the ear include swabbing the canal with cotton twisted onto a probe or wooden stick, use of a cerumen spoon or loop, and irrigation with half-strength white vinegar or Burow's solution. If the ear canal cannot be cleaned adequately to see the tympanic membrane and other surfaces, treatment may be begun using the history, with or without an audiogram, to guide the diagnosis. In the absence of complete external canal occlusion, a hearing examination in otitis externa should be normal. Other entities in the differential diagnosis of earache include mumps, dental abscess, ear canal furuncle, ear canal foreign body or trauma, and tonsillitis.

Clinical Diagnosis

The diagnosis of acute otitis media is made on clinical grounds alone. The standard operating head otoscope can be used to facilitate cerumen removal in order to visualize the tympanic membrane. A sealed otoscope with the capability of pneumatic otoscopy is the most appropriate instrument to use in making the diagnosis.

The tympanic membrane should be observed for contour, color, translucence, and mobility. The classic description of otitis media is a red, opaque, bulging tympanic membrane that has "lost" its bony landmarks. Distortion of the luster or "light reflex" of the anterior inferior portion of the tympanic membrane has been suggested as a useful indicator of the presence or absence of otitis media, but this sign is frequently inaccurate. In contrast, the mobility of the tympanic membrane during pneumatic otoscopy has been shown to be both sensitive and specific for otitis media. The normal tympanic membrane should move briskly as small amounts of air are introduced into the sealed otoscope head. Pus accumulated behind the drum impedes normal membrane motility.

Impedance tympanometry is a sensitive and reliable method of detecting middle ear effusion in children. The tympanometer measures the resonance of the ear canal for a fixed sound as the air pressure is systematically varied; it is now being widely used in clinical practice to confirm the presence of middle ear fluid.

Bacteriologic Diagnosis
Definitive bacteriologic diagnosis is usually not necessary for treatment of otitis media. Under some conditions it may be appropriate to perform a tap of the middle ear, using a 20-gauge spinal needle and a tuberculin syringe, to identify a specific organism. Culture of the middle ear is most helpful for immunosuppressed patients with otitis or when otitis develops during antibiotic therapy. Nasopharyngeal cultures do not accurately reflect middle ear flora and so have no clinical utility in routine practice or for either of the above situations.

Treatment

Currently, it is standard practice to prescribe an antibiotic for acute otitis media. However, existing data suggest that the acute clinical course of otitis is affected minimally by the addition of antibiotics. The usual clinical course is nearly complete resolution of pain and fever in less than 48 hours. In one study, the duration of pain and fever among patients with otitis did not differ markedly for patients treated with antibiotics than for those treated with only antihistamines. On the other hand, it is clear that there has been a marked decline in suppurative complications of otitis media, coincident with the introduction of routine use of antimicrobials. Perforation is now rarely seen, perhaps a result of early use of antibiotics. Therefore, while definitive evidence of effectiveness is lacking, physicians should continue to use antimicrobials known to cover the organisms usually responsible for otitis.

Antibiotics
One of four antibiotics is conventionally used. Ampicillin (250–500 mg qid) or amoxicillin (250–500 mg tid) will cover all of the usual organisms including *H. influenzae,* and they are therefore the drugs of choice. Penicillin (200–500 mg qid) is used, with or without the addition of sulfonamide (4 gm to start, then 1 gm qid), to cover *H. influenzae.* Erythromycin (250–1000 mg qid) or tetracycline (200–500 mg qid) is used for penicillin-sensitive patients. Trimethoprim/sulfamethoxazole (1–2 tablets bid) is not currently considered an appropriate first-line drug, but it is frequently prescribed in the event of treatment failure and for patients unlikely to comply with a three- or four-times-a-day regimen. Failure of trimethoprim/sulfamethoxazol to eliminate pneumococcal isolates is not uncommon. The usual course of therapy is 10 days.

The increased incidence of ampicillin-resistant *H. influenzae* among hospital isolates has prompted increasing use of alternative regimens that include sulfonamides, chloramphenicol, and the cephalosporins. The marrow suppression risks of chloramphenicol, and to a much lesser extent of the sulfonamide combinations, argue against routine use of either of these drugs in uncomplicated disease, particularly in view of the low complication rate of otitis in adults. Cefaclor, the most appropriate of the cephalosporins, is quite expensive and recent reports suggest that the recurrence rate is higher than with the other regimens.

Adjunctive Therapies
Antihistamines and oral decongestants have long been advocated as adjuncts to the medical management of acute otitis. Animal studies in the 1960s and 1970s supported their theoretic utility. However, there are now a large number of clinical trials that demonstrate that these medications are of no use. In a few studies, the addition of these drugs appeared to delay clearance of middle ear fluid. They have no place in the routine management of uncomplicated otitis media. Decongestants delivered by nasal spray have not been shown to be useful, but the number of studies is small.

Pain Relief
Topical analgesics for the ear (e.g., Auralgan) appear to be ineffective. The squamous epithelium of the ear canal inhibits adequate absorption. Oral analgesics, including aspirin and acetaminophen, are effective for mild-to-moderate pain. Narcotic preparations may be necessary for a few patients during the first 24 to 48 hours.

Complications

Complications of otitis media include central nervous system infection, mastoiditis, and cholesteatoma. The relationship between acute otitis media and serous otitis is less clear. Middle ear effusion frequently persists after acute infection, but serous otitis is also diagnosed in the absence of a history of acute infection when a patient presents for evaluation of a conductive hearing loss. Mastoiditis is thought to accompany almost all cases of otitis, and simple management of the otitis is adequate to treat the mastoid infection. Untreated mastoid infection can become a surgical emergency with osteitis and thrombosis of the proximate venous sinuses. The chronically infected middle ear may develop a cholesteatoma, which is a mass of desquamated epithelial cells with or without cholesterol crystals. This mass can lead to eventual destruction of middle ear structures and result in a conductive hearing loss.

Serous Otitis

Serous otitis is diagnosed when a middle ear is not acutely inflamed but appears to contain middle ear fluid, seen as decreased translucence, a horizontal fluid level (when the patient is upright), bubbles behind the eardrum, and often retraction of the eardrum. Synonyms include "glue ear" and "secretory otitis." The causes and natural history of serous otitis are unclear, but subacute infection, allergy, barotrauma, eustachian tube dysfunction, and persistent fluid following acute otitis are all believed to play a role. It has recently been established that effusion may persist after an acute infection for as long as 10 weeks. Some investigators have found a variety of bacterial pathogens in middle ear fluid despite the lack of clinical evidence of acute inflammation. The long-term consequences of serous otitis are not known, but at least in children, persistent effusion is associated with conductive hearing loss and delayed acquisition of speech.

Treatment of serous otitis remains controversial. Antihistamine and decongestants have long been advocated as logical and appropriate; however, recent clinical trials have demonstrated their lack of effectiveness. The discovery of bacteria in some middle ear fluid at tympanostomy tube placement has prompted antimicrobial treatment in some centers. Other options include corticosteroids, surgical drainage with or without tympanostomy tube placement, and mechanical efforts at middle ear inflation (i.e., gum-chewing or holding one's nose while inflating the nasopharynx). Because of lack of data regarding treatment, a conservative medical approach, including antibiotic treatment, mechanical efforts, and watchful waiting, is most prudent for the first 2 to 4 weeks. Consultation with an otolaryngologist should follow if the middle ear effusion persists in an otherwise healthy adult because of the remote possibility of nasopharyngeal cancer.

Cantekin E, Mandel E, Bluestone C, et al. Lack of efficacy of a decongestant-antihistamine combination for otitis media with effusion in children: Results of a double blind randomized trial. *N Engl J Med* 308:297, 1983.
A study that is conclusive in its dismissal of antihistamine adjunctive therapy.

Greunfast K. A review of the efficacy of systemically administered decongestants in the prevention and treatment of otitis media. *Otolaryngol Head Neck Surg* 89:432–439, 1981.
A summary of the pharmacology of these drugs and the clinical and animal studies supporting their use.

Henderson F, et al. A longitudinal study of respiratory viruses and bacteria in the etiology of acute otitis with effusion. *N Engl J Med* 306:1377–1383, 1982.
A longitudinal study of the incidence and microbiology of otitis in a known population of children. The best work of its kind to date.

Paradise J. Otitis media in infants and children. *Pediatrics* 65:917–943, 1980.
Probably the most extensive and authoritative review of the otitis media problem ever published. This article should be the basis of any further reading on otitis.

Schwartz R. Bacteriology of otitis media: A review. *Otolaryngol Head Neck Surg* 89:444–450, 1981.
A review of clinical techniques for ear cultures, and a discussion of the microbiologic findings of more than 2800 ear cultures.

15. EARWAX
Michael Y. Parker and Terry L. Fry

Earwax (cerumen) is created by the secretions of the sebaceous glands located in the skin that lines the outer, cartilaginous half of the ear canal. The quantity and consistency of the wax varies with the individual. Swimming or showering can result in water being absorbed by otherwise dry cerumen, causing expansion and displacement of wax into the deeper portions of the ear canal. Cerumen has a protective, antibacterial effect by helping to maintain an acid pH in the ear canal and serving as a barrier to infection. However, when excessive or impacted secretions result in a hearing deficit or obscure the tympanic membrane during an otoscopic examination, cerumen removal becomes necessary.

Cerumen Removal
The use of cotton swabs can be effective in removing cerumen from widely patent, nontortuous, non–hair-bearing ear canals, but in other situations they may serve only to impact the wax more deeply within the medial, bony half of the ear canal, which normally should not contain cerumen. Several safe and simple methods, used singly or in combination, are effective in removing cerumen. These include instrumentation, irrigation, suction, and chemical softeners.

Instrumentation
Firm cerumen may be removed with a smooth cerumen spoon or wire loop. Preferably this should be performed under direct vision, through an operator-held otoscope. The examiner's hand should be stabilized against the patient's head to avoid inadvertent trauma with patient movement.

Irrigation
Irrigation should be done with a liquid warmed to body temperature to avoid caloric stimulation that can result in vertigo. A solution of 1.5% acetic acid is preferable to tap water because the low pH retards the overgrowth of *Pseudomonas* in the wet ear canal. Such an irrigating solution may be readily approximated by diluting 1 part commercially available white vinegar (5% acetic acid) with 2 parts water. Adding to this solution an equal volume of hydrogen peroxide or 1 : 750 benzalkonium chloride (Zephiran Chloride) supplies a detergent effect, which aids in separating the wax from the ear canal.

Irrigation should be done under gentle pressure with the tip of an ear bulb syringe held carefully at the entrance of the ear canal while the pinna is retracted superiorly and posteriorly (in the adult) or posteriorly (in the child). The fluid should be directed toward the superior aspect of the ear canal because a direct blast against the cerumen mass will only cause it to become more deeply impacted. In experienced hands, the Water Pik is also an effective irrigating device. However, if improperly used, the turbulence it creates may cause trauma.

Irrigation is relatively contraindicated in any individual with a known tympanic membrane perforation because of the possibility that it may cause middle ear infection or trauma to the round window. However, these complications are very unusual when diluted vinegar is used as an irrigant, even when an ear with an unrecognized perforation is inadvertently irrigated.

Suction
Soft, semifluid cerumen can often be removed most efficaciously under direct vision with a blunt-tipped 14-gauge needle attached to wall or portable suction, equivalent to approximately 10 cm of water pressure. By compressing the connecting tubing, suction can be terminated immediately if necessary. Excessive suction can cause a caloric stimulation and result in vertigo.

Chemical Softeners
Some cerumen impactions may resist all of the above techniques but may respond to softening agents instilled in the ear canal over a 7- to 14-day period. In cases of dense, hard, inspissated cerumen, these agents will not usually be effective when used alone and must be followed by suction, wire loop, or irrigation for final removal. Softening agents are also the method of choice when a thin layer of cerumen persists against the tympanic membrane after the bulk of the impaction has been removed. The most commonly used softening agents are Debrox, Cerumenex, and acetic acid (1.5%) in combination with water, peroxide, or an emulsifying agent such as benzalkonium chloride. Stool softeners are sometimes suggested for this purpose but are not indicated for cerumen softening because they may cause a severe inflammatory reaction in the ear canal.

Debrox Drops (carbamide peroxide 6.5% in anhydrous glycerol) act as a peroxide by releasing oxygen and thereby debriding and cleansing the ear canal. These drops offer a safe and effective means for softening minimal to moderate amounts of cerumen; 3 to 5 drops are instilled in the affected ear(s) twice a day, and results are seen in several days.

Cerumenex Drops (10% triethanolamine polypeptide oleate condensate in propylene glycol with chlorbutanol 0.5%) emulsify cerumen while maintaining an acid pH. Action is usually complete in 15 to 30 minutes. Cerumenex is appropriate for office rather than outpatient use. At least 1% of patients using these drops will develop a hypersensitivity reaction, with a local dermatitis ranging from mild erythema to a severe eczematoid reaction involving any areas originally contacted by the drops. Even in those patients not hypersensitive to Cerumenex, local reaction may occur if the drops are accidentally applied to the periaural area.

Hydrogen peroxide is a safe and effective agent for loosening the attachment of cerumen to the underlying ear canal. An alternative is sterile Zephiran Chloride. Mixing either of these solutions in a 1:1 ratio with diluted white vinegar maintains an acid pH, so there is little chance the patient will develop an infection from solution remaining in the ear canal after cleaning is finished. Applications once or twice a day are usually effective in 4 to 14 days.

Chronic Care
Many patients ask, "If I can't use cotton swabs or stick anything in my ears, how can I keep them clean?" In responding to this question, the clinician should explain the protective role of cerumen, stressing that its presence does not indicate that the ear is "dirty." Patients with increased cerumen production can use diluted white vinegar warmed to body temperature as an irrigant one to two times per week for an effective, safe, and economical means of cerumen removal.

Caruso VG, Meyerhoff WC. Trauma and Infections of the External Ear. In M Paparella and D Shumrick (Eds.), *Otolaryngology* (2nd ed.). Philadelphia: Saunders, 1980. Pp. 1345–1346.
A good discussion of cerumen and its function in the ear canal.
Senturia BH, Marcus MD, Lucente FE. *Diseases of the External Ear.* New York: Grune & Stratton, 1981. Pp. 26–30.
Discusses role of bacteria in the pathogenesis of otitis externa, supporting the use of solutions with acid pH.

IV. UPPER RESPIRATORY PROBLEMS

16. THE COMMON COLD
Gregory Strayhorn

The common cold is a benign, self-limited viral infection of the upper respiratory tract. It is the leading cause of visits to doctors' offices and days lost from work in the United States.

Causal Agents
The rhinovirus, with more than 100 antigenic serotypes, is responsible for 25 to 38% of colds. The corona virus, parainfluenza virus, respiratory syncytial virus, influenza virus, adenovirus, and enteroviruses cause another 10 to 40% of infections. *Mycoplasma pneumoniae* and other unidentified agents are also responsible for similar infections of the upper respiratory tract.

Seasonal Patterns
Adults average two to four colds per year. The incidence rises in early fall, peaks in winter, and declines in early to late spring and parallels the times when schools are open. There is evidence that exposure to a cold environment per se does not increase susceptibility to respiratory infection. Children appear to be the main reservoir of respiratory viruses. Adults with children in the home have a higher incidence of colds, and women are affected more frequently than men, probably because of greater contact with children.

Transmission
The rhinovirus reproduces primarily in the nose and is shed in nasal secretions. Transmission generally occurs by hand contact with the infectious agent and self-inoculation of the lacrimal sacs and nasal mucosa. Contact with contaminated objects or the skin of infected individuals is sufficient to spread the infection. Transmission via infectious droplets of respiratory secretions transported in air from sneezing and coughing is suspected but not experimentally substantiated. The length of contact with the donor, the severity of the donor's symptoms, and the amount of virus shed in nasal secretions are directly related to transmission of the virus and occurrence of infection.

Clinical infection usually develops 2 days after exposure, with a range of 1 to 6 days.

Diagnosis
Differentiation of the common cold from other infections of the upper respiratory tract is based on the usually mild clinical manifestations of this illness and the absence of pronounced constitutional symptoms.

Symptoms
The usual symptoms include sneezing, congestion, stuffy nose, and a watery nasal discharge, which may become thick and yellowish. A sore or "scratchy" throat generally accompanies nasal symptoms, and pain may be referred to the ear. A nonproductive cough and, less frequently, hoarseness often begin on the first or second day. Less common complaints of malaise, headache, muscle aches, chilliness, and burning eyes can precede the usual symptoms. If present, fever seldom exceeds 102°F. Secondary symptoms include impaired taste and smell and pressure in the sinuses and ears. All symptoms generally reach their maximum severity by the second or third day and subside within 4 to 7 days; however, cough may persist several days to 1 week after the cessation of other symptoms, and the cough is generally prolonged and more severe in smokers.

Physical Findings
Physical findings include mildly swollen and erythematous nasal and pharyngeal mucosa with no exudate. There is usually nasal passage occlusion, postnasal discharge, and enlarged posterior pharyngeal lymphoid tissue. Cervical lymph nodes can be slightly enlarged and/or tender. Eustachian tube obstruction secondary to mucosal edema can lead to tympanic membrane dysfunction with mild transient hearing impairment.

Complications

Complications of the common cold are usually localized to specific sites and include sinusitis, otitis media, pharyngitis, cervical adenitis, laryngitis, tracheobronchitis, bronchiolitis, and pneumonia. Serious bronchial infections are more likely to occur in patients with chronic obstructive pulmonary disease, asthma, or cystic fibrosis. Clinical presentations are more severe; fever above 102°F, moderate to severe respiratory distress, tonsilar and pharyngeal edema and/or exudate accompanied by moderate to severe pain should alert the clinician to consider bacterial complication or a specific viral syndrome. The influenza virsuses may cause mild upper respiratory symptoms but typically include systemic manifestations of fever, malaise, muscle aches, and less commonly, nausea and vomiting. Lower respiratory tract disease may be caused by respiratory syncytial virus, parainfluenza, and occasionally corona virus. Recurrent cold symptoms may be caused by corona virus infection. Viral pharyngitis presentations are discussed in Chapter 18.

Treatment

The usual spontaneous resolution of the common cold makes treatment unnecessary beyond that for symptom relief.

Nasal Symptoms

In a clinical trial, oral pseudoephedrine separately or in combination with an antihistamine relieved symptoms of sneezing and nasal obstruction significantly more effectively than placebo; symptom relief was not enhanced by antihistamines. Pseudoephedrine is usually given in an oral dosage of 60 mg every 6 hours. The most common side effect is insomnia.

Phenylpropanolamine is the decongestant most frequently found in over-the-counter cold preparations. The usual adult dosage is 25 mg to 50 mg orally four times a day. It can cause severe elevation in blood pressure in hypertensive patients. The drug also causes significant blood pressure elevation in healthy volunteers, under controlled conditions. Therefore, it should be used with caution in patients with hypertension and not at all in those with moderate to severe hypertension. It is contraindicated in patients taking monoamine oxidase inhibitors.

Clinical trials to assess the efficacy of antihistamines alone in relieving nasal symptoms have yielded mixed results. A recent trial with chlorpheniramine found it to be significantly more effective than placebo. The dosage of chlorpheniramine ranges from 4 to 8 mg orally every 6 hours. Its use is commonly associated with drowsiness, and it should not be used in situations that require alertness.

Topically applied sympathomimetic drugs, used to shrink swollen nasal mucous membranes, are effective for short periods. Frequent and prolonged use is discouraged because of rebound persistent congestion. The longer-acting xylometazoline hydrochloride (Otrivin), 0.05% spray or drops, has a duration of action up to 8 hours and may decrease the frequency of rebound congestion when used appropriately in a dosage of 2 to 3 sprays or drops every 8 to 10 hours as needed. The judicious use of topical decongestants may be indicated in patients who cannot tolerate the side effects of oral preparations. It has been proposed that topical decongestants may aid in preventing eustachian tube and sinus obstruction and subsequent otitis media and sinusitis; there is no substantial evidence for or against this assertion.

Application of ointments with petroleum base protects the skin of the nares from the irritation of frequent nose blowing and wiping.

Expectorants (e.g., guaifenesin, potassium iodide) are frequently recommended to decrease the viscosity of mucus secretions in the respiratory tract but are ineffective when evaluated by controlled clinical trials. A clinical trial that evaluated the effect of hot and cold liquids on nasal mucus viscosity found that hot chicken soup eaten by sips or straw significantly decreased the viscosity below baseline and was superior to hot water. Cold liquids had the opposite effect.

Cough

Dextromethorphan hydrobromide is recommended for mild to moderate coughs in oral dosages of 10 to 20 mg every 4 hours or 30 mg every 6 to 8 hours. Clinical trials have shown that it has antitussive properties that are equivalent to low doses of codeine.

The drug is not available singly but is included in many over-the-counter cold preparations; however, the amount received using these products' recommended dose is often subtherapeutic. The dose of dextromethorphan can best be adjusted using a simple preparation, such as guaifenesin/dextromethorphan. For more severe coughs, codeine, 30 mg every 6 hours, is recommended. Side effects and the potential for narcotic abuse should be considered.

Sore Throat
Mild sore throat is relieved temporarily with lozenges, sprays, or gargles that contain topical anesthetics such as benzocaine or phenol. Antiseptic mouthwashes are usually not beneficial. Gargles with warm salted water (1 teaspoon in 1 quart of water) are probably as effective. Analgesics are indicated for moderate to severe sore throats.

Fever, Chilliness, and Muscle Aches
Analgesics and antipyretics are recommended for discomfort and fever. In a clinical trial, aspirin reduced the frequency and severity of many cold symptoms but not significantly when compared to placebo. However, the aspirin group shed significantly more viral particles in nasal secretions, which may increase the rate of cold transmission, particularly if patients increase their human contact because their systemic symptoms have improved. To relieve myalgia, chilliness, and fever, aspirin or acetaminophen is given in dosages of 350 to 650 mg every 4 to 6 hours. Patients with fever and/or moderate constitutional symptoms are advised to rest at home and to maintain a moderate fluid intake.

Combination Cold Preparations
A wide variety of over-the-counter combination cold preparations are available. These preparations are more convenient (although often much more expensive) than the equivalent compounds taken separately. In a review of 200 available antitussive and cold preparations, it was found that greater than 75% had subtherapeutic doses of active ingredients or contained no clinically acceptable compounds. Therefore, recommendations about their use must be selective.

Antibiotics
Antibiotics are not indicated for the treatment of common colds in otherwise healthy people. A clinical trial of tetracycline found it to be ineffective in reducing morbidity. However, antibiotics are indicated for specific secondary bacterial infections and are also recommended for patients with chronic obstructive pulmonary disease, who are at a greater risk of developing bacterial infections of the lower respiratory tract.

Prevention
Given the common cold's usual mode of transmission, frequent hand-washing, disposable tissues, and limited human contact during the peak of nasal discharge should help prevent the spread of colds. The multiple viral etiologies and the numerous antigenic serotypes of the rhinovirus make it impractical to develop a vaccine for immunologic protection against the common cold.

Although vitamin C has been advocated for prevention of the common cold, the evidence does not support its use for this purpose or for treatment. A review of clinical trials conducted between 1942 and 1974 to evaluate the efficacy of ascorbic acid to prevent cold symptoms questioned the validity of results in 57% of the studies because of major methodologic flaws. The remaining 43% showed minor differences between the treatment and placebo groups. Subsequent studies have failed to demonstrate efficacy.

Gwaltney, JM. The Common Cold. In GL Mandell, RG Douglas, and JE Bennett (Eds.), *Principles and Practice of Infectious Diseases.* New York: Wiley, 1979.
   A comprehensive discussion of the pathogenesis, causes, epidemiology, transmission, clinical presentation, diagnosis, and treatment of the common cold.
D'Alessio, DJ, et al. Transmission of experimental rhinovirus colds in volunteer married couples. *J Infect Dis* 33(1):28–36, 1976.
   An experimental study that delineates the epidemiology of person-to-person transmission of rhinovirus infections.

Gwaltney, JM, Moskalski, PB, and Hendley, JO. Hand to hand transmission of rhino-virus colds. *Ann Intern Med* 88:463–467, 1978.
An experimental study that finds hand-to-hand transmission of the rhinovirus to be significantly more effective than small and large aerosol particle transmission.

Bye, CE. Effects of pseudoephedrine and triprolidine, alone and in combination, on symptoms of the common cold. *Br Med J,* July 1980, pp. 189–190.
A clinical trial that finds pseudoephedrine effectively relieves the symptoms of the common cold. Its effectiveness was not enhanced by the inclusion of an antihistamine.

Howard, JC. Effectiveness of antihistamines in the symptomatic management of the common cold. *JAMA* 242:214–217, 1979.
This clinical trial finds chlorpheniramine to be more efficacious than placebo in treating nasal symptoms.

Howie, JGR, Clark, GA. Double-blind trial of early demethylchlortetracycline in minor respiratory illness in general practice. *Lancet,* Nov. 1970, pp. 1099–1102.
A randomized double-blind study involving 829 healthy volunteers that did not find a tetracycline beneficial in reducing morbidity of the common cold.

Saketkhoo, K, Januszkiewicz, A, Sackner, MA. Effects of drinking hot water, cold water, and chicken soup on nasal mucus velocity and nasal airflow resistance. *Chest* 74:408–410, 1978.
A small, randomized control study that finds hot chicken soup superior to other liquids in decreasing nasal mucus viscosity.

Stanley, ED. Increased virus shedding with aspirin treatment of rhinovirus infection. *JAMA* 231(12):1248–1251; 1975.
Increased rhinovirus shedding was a secondary finding in volunteers who were randomized to aspirin and placebo to assess the efficacy of aspirin in preventing cold symptoms.

Chalmers, TC. Effects of ascorbic acid on the common cold: An Evaluation of the evidence. *Am J Med* 58:532–535, 1975.
The author evaluates the methodology used to assess the efficacy of ascorbic acid in preventing and treating the common cold.

Tyrrell, DAJ, et al. A trial of ascorbic acid in the treatment of the common cold. *Br J Prev Soc Med* 31:189–191, 1977.
Ten grams of ascorbic acid per day during the first 60 hours of active colds did not significantly reduce morbidity in otherwise healthy volunteers who participated in this randomized, double-blind study.

Federal Register 41:38,352, Sept. 9, 1976.
A comprehensive review, by a panel of medical experts, of all clinical and scientific evidence of the therapeutic and harmful effects of available cold remedies.

17. SINUSITIS
Suzanne W. Fletcher

Sinusitis is acute or chronic inflammation of the mucosal lining of the paranasal sinuses. The diagnosis of sinusitis is common in ambulatory care, accounting for about 1% of office visits in the United States. It is estimated that approximately 25% of people develop sinusitis sometime during their life. However, the diagnosis and management of sinusitis are far from clear.

Sinusitis is somewhat arbitrarily subdivided into acute sinusitis, with symptoms up to 3 weeks; subacute sinusitis, with symptoms from 3 weeks to 3 months; and chronic sinusitis, with symptoms over 3 months. Most of this discussion will be about acute sinusitis.

Sinus inflammation can result from many causes, including infection, allergy, polyps, or even tumors. However, most studies have demonstrated that sinus mucosal abnormalities seen radiographically are almost always associated with an infection, especially in acute sinusitis.

Figure 17-1 shows three of the four pairs of sinuses. The maxillary sinuses are most

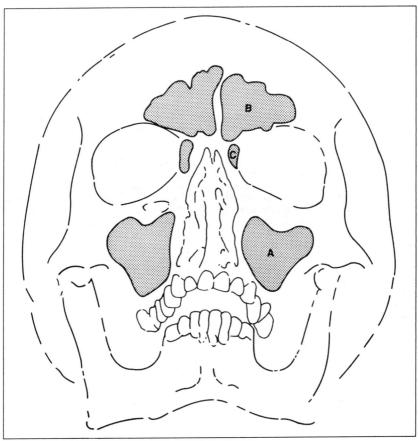

Fig. 17-1. The three pairs of sinuses seen on a Water's view: (A) maxillary, (B) frontal, and (C) ethmoid. The sphenoid sinuses, not shown, are best seen on a lateral view.

frequently involved in adults with acute sinusitis. Because they are also most accessible, the majority of studies have been carried out on maxillary sinuses, so most of what is known about "sinusitis" is really about maxillary sinusitis. Frontal sinusitis is next most frequent in adults, while ethmoid sinusitis is most common in children. Isolated sphenoid sinusitis is rare.

Diagnosis

Symptoms and Signs
The classic "textbook" picture of sinusitis is aching pain, usually over the involved sinus, with congestion, foul nasal discharge, fever, and malaise, often following a recent upper respiratory infection. The pain is made worse by bending over and increases in intensity by late morning ("banker's headache"). On examination, there may be tenderness over the involved sinus, edematous nasal mucosa, and discharge.

The problem with this description is that many of these "classic" symptoms and signs do not correlate well with sinusitis and, more importantly, do not differentiate between sinusitis (for which antibiotics are indicated) and other common problems of the upper respiratory tract, such as rhinitis and upper respiratory infections (for which antibiotics usually are not indicated).

Several symptoms are found more commonly in patients with radiographically proven sinusitis than in those suspected of sinusitis who do not have it on x-ray (Table 17-1). However, these symptoms only partially differentiate between sinusitis and other upper respiratory problems; none alone is highly sensitive or specific. Studies of the sensitivity, specificity, and predictive value of combinations of symptoms and signs have not been reported. To diagnose sinusitis by history alone, therefore, is very difficult.

On examination, sinus tenderness does not differentiate sinusitis from rhinitis, but mucopurulent secretion in the nose suggests sinusitis. Using a nasal speculum, examination of the lateral wall of the nose may show pus draining from the inferior (maxillary sinus drainage) or middle meatus (maxillary and frontal sinus drainage). Pus draining from the superior meatus (ethmoid sinus drainage) is not likely to be seen.

Transillumination

Transillumination of maxillary and frontal sinuses can help establish the diagnosis of sinusitis. An attachment to the otoscope made specifically for this purpose is the best source of light. The easiest technique to examine the maxillary sinuses is to place a transilluminator over the lower orbital rim of the patient, in a completely darkened room, and look for a glow on the hard palate of the opened mouth. No transmission of light indicates increased likelihood of infected sinuses. In one study, 24 of 24 sinuses that showed no transillumination were infected on sinus aspiration, whereas in 15 cases in which transillumination results were clearly normal, aspiration demonstrated no infection in all but 1 case. Transillumination was less helpful when findings were equivocal: of 26 sinuses in which transillumination was dull or decreased, 7 were infected on aspiration and 19 were not.

Frontal sinuses can also be transilluminated by placing the light against the floor of the frontal sinus at the superior medial edge of the orbit. A glow should be transmitted through the anterior wall of the sinus. When interpreting this test, remember that approximately 5% of people have not developed one or both frontal sinuses.

Laboratory Tests

Laboratory tests for sinusitis include culture of nasal swabs and x-rays. Several studies have shown that the results of cultures from the nasal mucosa do not correlate well with cultures of sinus mucosa. Also, cultures of nasal swabs tend to be costly. Therefore, they should not be used for evaluating uncomplicated cases of suspected acute sinusitis.

Table 17-1. Symptoms and signs of acute maxillary sinusitis and their relation to radiologic findings

Symptoms and Signs	Radiologic Finding (%)	
	Normal (60 patients)	Abnormal (60 patients)
URI preceding complaints	67	90
Hyposmia	40	75
Pain on mastication	8	30
Fever >38°C	2	28
Mucopurulent secretion in nasal passages	18	50
Pus in middle or inferior meatus	3	30
Speech indicates "fullness of the sinuses"	5	25
General malaise	42	60
Cough (bronchitis)	42	75

Source: From A. Axelsson and U. Runze, Symptoms and signs of acute maxillary sinusitis. *ORL J Otorhinolaryngol Relat Spec* 38:298–308, 1976.

X-rays of sinuses are the "gold standard" for the diagnosis of sinusitis in clinical practice. Comparisons of radiographic results with culture results of maxillary sinuses have shown good correlation. In one study, 34 of 34 radiographically normal sinuses were normal on aspiration, and 30 of 31 sinuses with opaque sinuses, air fluid levels, or mucosa more than 8 mm thick were infected. The problem is cost. A full series of sinus films can cost the patient (or an insurance company) as much as $75. In some places a single view can be ordered, and when this is possible, the Water's view is usually the most helpful: the head is tilted to prevent the temporal bone from overlapping the maxillary sinuses, and therefore the maxillary, frontal, and ethmoid sinuses are well seen (see Fig. 17-1). Because of expense, and inconvenience for patients not near x-ray facilities, x-rays should not be a routine part of the evaluation of every patient presenting with possible sinusitis.

At the present time, transillumination appears to be a simple and inexpensive first step in diagnosing uncomplicated acute maxillary sinusitis, and physicians should learn this procedure. Radiographic evaluation is reasonable for patients who are at high risk (e.g., patients on immunosuppressive drugs or with diabetes), who have suspected sinusitis in the other paranasal sinuses, who have suspected chronic sinusitis, and/or whose illnesses do not resolve as expected.

Treatment

The most common bacterial causes of sinusitis are *Hemophilus influenzae, Streptococcus pneumoniae,* and various anaerobes. Less commonly, infections with *Neisseria* species, beta-hemolytic streptoccoccus, *Staphylococcus aureus, Pseudomonas aeruginosa,* and *Escherichia coli* are reported. Viruses account for 10 to 15% of sinusitis cases, and rhinovirus is most commonly recovered. Fungal infections are a rare cause of sinusitis in healthy persons and when they occur are usually caused by aspergilli.

With the above picture it is not surprising that antibiotics to which the most common organisms are sensitive have been shown to be effective in treating sinusitis by rigorous studies, including randomized, controlled trials. Ampicillin (500 mg q6h), amoxicillin (250 mg or 500 mg tid), doxycycline (200 mg initially followed by 100 mg qd), and trimethoprim/sulfamethoxazole (2 tablets bid) all have been shown to work, without striking differences. The choice among them should be made according to convenience and cost. There is evidence that frequently sinus x-rays are still abnormal and symptoms are still present after 7 to 10 days, so a 14-day course is probably best.

Topical sympathomimetic amine decongestants (e.g., Otrivin) are usually added. The typical dosage is several drops in each nostril every 8 hours. The pediatric strength reputedly protects against rebound congestion sometimes seen with adult-strength decongestants. Prescribing analgesics for symptomatic relief of pain is appropriate, and heat and steam inhalation (standing in a shower or near a steaming kettle) is often advised. None of these recommendations has been subjected to rigorous evaluation, but they sound reasonable and are not expensive.

When to Refer

Clinicians who are not ear, nose, and throat (ENT) specialists are likely to want help from otolaryngologists on individual patients with sinusitis when the patient appears toxic, is immunocompromised, or has findings of a complication of sinusitis. In addition, the following general categories of patients deserve referrals.

Acute Frontal Sinusitis

Because the frontal sinuses drain poorly and because of the possibility of serious complications (e.g., osteomyelitis or intracranial extension leading to meningitis, subdural abscess, cavernous sinus thrombosis, frontal lobe abscess), some ENT specialists advise that acute frontal sinusitis be considered an emergency and that an otolaryngologist be consulted immediately. The otolaryngologist may want to hospitalize the patient for intravenous antibiotic therapy, close observation, and surgical drainage procedures.

Lack of Improvement After a Full Course of Therapy

Patients who do not improve after 2 weeks of therapy should be evaluated for unusual organisms (e.g., anaerobes, fungi) or for other conditions affecting the sinuses. Most of these patients should be referred for ENT evaluation.

Chronic Sinusitis
Patients with chronic or recurring sinusitis may require surgical drainage procedures.

Axelsson A, Runze U. Symptoms and signs of acute maxillary sinusitis. *ORL J Oto-rhinolaryngol Relat Spec* 38:298–308, 1976.
Analyzes symptoms and signs of acute maxillary sinusitis and correlates these with radiographic results. One of the few studies critically evaluating the clinical presentations of sinusitis.
Evans FO, et al. Sinusitis of the maxillary antrum. *N Engl J Med* 293:735–739, 1975.
Transillumination and x-ray results correlated well with examination of maxillary antrum aspirates. Nasal swab cultures did not.
Axelsson A, et al. Treatment of acute maxillary sinusitis. *Acta Otolaryngol (Stockh)* 91:313–318, 1981.
Hamory BH, et al. Etiology and antimicrobial therapy of acute maxillary sinusitis. *J Infect Dis* 139:197–202, 1979.
Redstone PM, Bergstrom L, Dans PE. The diagnosis and treatment of acute maxillary sinusitis. *Colo Med,* November 1980, pp. 407–414.
Studies of the effect of treatment regimens.
Coleman JA, et al. Sinus disease. *J Fla Med Assoc* 65:728–731, 1978.
Good overview.
Lew D, et al. Sphenoid sinusitis: A review of 30 cases. *N Engl J Med* 309:1149–1154, 1983.
Review of a rare type of sinusitis in adults.

18. SORE THROAT
Gregory Strayhorn

Sore throat is the fourth most common presenting complaint in medical practice. However, it is estimated that only about one in four patients with sore throat seeks medical care for it, suggesting that most episodes of pharyngitis are self-limited.

Viruses are responsible for about half of all episodes of sore throat; these infections are self-limited, are not specifically treatable, and require only palliation. An important minority of sore throats, 15 to 30%, are caused by group A beta-hemolytic streptococci; these occur mainly in young people and should be recognized and treated to prevent rheumatic fever and perhaps infrequent local suppurative complications. Other causes of bacterial pharyngitis are much less common but are both potentially dangerous and treatable: gonococcus, hemophilus, diphtheria, and mixed and anaerobic infections. *Mycoplasma pneumoniae* can cause upper respiratory infection. As many as one-quarter to one-half of all episodes of pharyngitis are of unknown cause, even after extensive laboratory investigation.

Specific Syndromes

Streptococcal Pharyngitis
The group A beta-hemolytic streptococci (GABHS) are the main cause of bacterial pharyngitis. Streptococcal pharyngitis is most prevalent during ages 6 to 12, is associated with crowding and close personal contact, and occurs generally during winter and early spring. Outbreaks of group G streptococcal pharyngitis have been reported among college students; the presentation and clinical course are similar to those of group A streptococcal pharyngitis.

The classic illness includes severe pharyngeal pain, dysphagia, temperature elevation to 104°F, exudate covering the tonsils and posterior pharynx, and enlarged, tender cervical lymph nodes. Lethargy, headaches, myalgias, and anorexia are also common. Improvement in symptoms occurs between the third and fourth day, and a gradual decrease in fever by the fourth to sixth day. Most occurrences of streptococcal pharyngitis are not classic and 40% of patients have imperceptible disease or symptoms indistinguishable from those of the common cold.

Local complications of GABHS infections are rare and include peritonsillar and retropharyngeal abscess, otitis media, and septicemia.

Late, nonsuppurative complications—rheumatic fever and glomerulonephritis—occur 2 to 3 weeks after the onset of pharyngitis. The incidence of acute rheumatic fever is estimated to be 2 cases per 100,000 annually; the attack rate is about 0.12% in untreated streptococcal infections. The attack rate of glomerulonephritis among patients with nephrogenic strains of streptococci ranges from 0 to 28%.

Viral Pharyngitis

Viral pharyngitis is caused by many different viruses and often resembles bacterial pharyngitis. Three specific syndromes are sufficiently characteristic to allow a clinical diagnosis.

With adenovirus infection (pharyngoconjunctival fever), conjunctivitis and pharyngitis occur together in approximately 90% of cases. The clinical presentation also includes fever of 103 to 104°F, malaise, myalgias, chills, and erythema and exudate on tonsils. Pharyngeal pain is mild. Fever lasts for 5 to 6 days. Infections occur primarily during the summer months and are associated with swimming in adenovirus-contaminated water.

Coxsackievirus causes an acute pharyngitis (herpangina) with small vesicles on the tonsillar pillars, soft palate, and uvula. The walls of the vesicles are fragile and rupture, leaving a small, shallow, grayish ulcer with an erythematous halo. Temperature elevation to 105°F may occur, along with anorexia and abdominal pain mimicking appendicitis. The illness clears within 3 to 6 days.

Infectious mononucleosis is discussed in Chapter 119.

Gonococcal Pharyngitis

The prevalence of gonococcal pharyngeal infections is 5 to 28% among homosexual men, 3 to 17% in women seen in venereal disease clinics, and 0.2 to 1.4% in heterosexual men; it is more prevalent among patients who practice fellatio. The majority of gonococcal pharyngeal infections are asymptomatic. Pharyngeal pain is the most frequent clinical symptom. Clinical findings are not distinguishable from those of pharyngitis from other causes and are generally less prominent. Untreated, gonococcal pharyngitis can persist up to 1 to 4 months.

Hemophilus *Epiglottitis*

Hemophilus influenzae type b can cause acute epiglottitis, a potentially life-threatening illness. Up to 12% of cases occur in adults. This illness can present with sore throat that rapidly progresses, within hours, to inflammation and edema of the epiglottis and supraglottic structures, difficulty swallowing, pooling of saliva, and a soft, muffled voice. Intermittent or constant stridor indicates a compromised airway. The epiglottis is bright red and swollen. Roentgenogram of the lateral neck shows distortion of the supraglottic structures. With appropriate treatment, symptoms resolve in 2 to 6 days.

Vincent's Angina

Vincent's angina is an anaerobic and spirochetal infection of the pharynx characterized by inflammation and exudate in the pharyngotonsillar area and foul odor of the breath. The appearance resembles streptococcal pharyngitis.

Peritonsillar Infections

Peritonsillitis and peritonsillar abscesses are caused by mixed anaerobic bacteria, streptococci, and *Staphlococcus aureus*. The infections are characterized by severe pharyngeal pain, dysphagia, and fever. Unilateral inflammation and swelling of the peritonsillar area with medial displacement of the tonsil occur. Bilateral involvement may cause partial pharnygeal obstruction.

Diphtheria

Outbreaks of diphtheria are uncommon, but have occurred among groups with poor sanitation, high rates of alcoholism, and inadequate immunization status. The early clinical picture consists of malaise, fever of 100 to 101°F, and mild pharyngeal discomfort. Pulse rate is usually more rapid than expected with the degree of fever. One to three days after the onset of symptoms, a light to dark gray pseudomembrane, which is firmly adherent to the underlying tissue, covers the tonsillar area. The exudate may obstruct the upper respiratory tract and necessitate surgical intervention. Marked swelling and tenderness of the cervical nodes can cause a "bullneck" appearance.

Evaluation

The evaluation of pharyngitis usually involves efforts to detect streptococcal pharyngitis. Clinical diagnosis is inaccurate because many other syndromes commonly resemble streptococcal pharyngitis. The probability of streptococcal infection is increased during winter and early spring, during an epidemic, and in the presence of fever, pus on the tonsils, and cervical adenopathy.

The most accurate means of diagnosing streptococcal pharyngitis is by culture on sheeps' blood agar. Results can be available within 1 day. False negative results occur in 10% of people with streptococci in their throats. Positive results may not represent disease because about one-half of people with positive throat cultures are "carriers," without evidence of invasion (e.g., rise in antistreptococcal antibody titres). Antibodies develop late in the course of infection; thus, antibody screening is not useful for early detection.

Because of the expense and administrative effort involved in culturing all people with sore throats and treating only those with positive cultures, other strategies have been recommended. In one cost-effectiveness analysis, it was shown that the best strategy depends on the prevalence of positive throat culture (either in the community or by the estimated likelihood for an individual patient, given the clinical findings). The recommendations were, according to pretreatment probability of positive throat culture, greater than 20%, treat all patients; 5 to 20%, treat only patients with group A streptococci–positive throat cultures; and less than 5%, treat no one.

These considerations apply mainly to people under age 30. Above that age, sore throat is less often seen in physicians' offices, and rheumatic fever is unusual.

Viral pharyngitis is often diagnosed by exclusion; sometimes it is based on characteristic clinical presentations, the season, and community epidemics. Diagnosis by serologic studies is generally not cost-effective and not routinely available.

Less common causes of bacterial pharyngitis are suspected in high-risk patients (e.g., homosexuals, people with low immunization rates) and sometimes by clinical findings. The diagnosis is confirmed by specific laboratory procedures. *Neisseria gonorrhea* is diagnosed by a throat culture using Thayer-Martin selective medium. Epiglottitis, peritonsillitis, or peritonsillar abscess is diagnosed from clinical findings. Pharyngeal and blood cultures are required in epiglottitis to isolate the type *H. influenzae* and to select the appropriate antibiotic. Vincent's angina is confirmed by presence of fusobacteria and spirochetes on a crystal violet–stained smear. If diphtheria is suspected, a throat culture using Loeffler's medium should be obtained promptly.

Treatment

Streptococcus

The primary reason for prompt diagnosis and treatment of GABHS infection is prevention of acute rheumatic fever (ARF); treatment does not alter clinical symptoms or the risk of glomerulonephritis. To prevent rheumatic fever, treatment need not be extremely prompt; the reduction in ARF is 98% in the first 8 days of infection, 67% on the 14th day, 42% on the 21st day, and 8% on the 27th day.

Treatment of culture-proven GABHS pharyngitis should include a 10-day course of oral penicillin V, 250 mg every 6 hours; compliance ranges from 50 to 80%. Benzathine penicillin G, 1.2 million units, is recommended when compliance is a potential problem. Erythromycin, 250 mg per day orally for 10 days, is recommended for patients who are allergic to penicillin.

Treatment of peritonsillitis and peritonsillar abscess is the same as that for streptococcal pharyngitis. Patients with severe dysphagia and pharyngeal obstruction require parenteral penicillin. Rarely, incision and drainage are necessary.

Vincent's Angina
Vincent's angina is treated with oral penicillin in dosages recommended for streptococcal pharyngitis.

Hemophilus *Epiglottitis*
Hemophilus epiglottitis is managed by careful observation (usually in a hospital) for signs of airway obstruction, maintenance of an adequate airway, and appropriate antibiotics. Ampicillin, 200 mg/kg per day intravenously in four divided doses, is recommended. For ampicillin-resistant strains of *H. influenzae,* chloramphenicol, 100 mg/kg per day in four divided doses, is recommended.

Gonococcal Pharyngitis
Gonococcal pharyngitis is treated with aqueous penicillin, 4.8 million units intramuscularly, and probenecid, 1 gm orally; tetracycline, 500 mg orally four times a day for 5 days; or sulfamethoxazole/trimethoprim (400/80 mg per tablet), 2 tablets orally three times a day for 7 days or 9 tablets taken once a day for 5 days. Ampicillin, amoxicillin, and spectinomycin are not recommended because of high failure rates. Post-treatment cultures should be obtained to assess treatment success. Tetracycline is recommended for post-treatment failure with penicillin.

Diphtheria
Diphtheria is treated mainly with antitoxin, given immediately if strong clinical evidence is present because neutralization of the toxin is ineffective once it enters cells. Antibiotics are given to reduce the microbial load and eradicate the carrier state, but they do not alter the effect of the toxin. Erythromycin is recommended in an oral dosage of 0.5 to 1.0 gm every 6 hours or 1 to 4 gm per day intravenously in four divided doses.

Palliation
Palliation of sore throat is described in Chapter 18.

Gwaltney JM. Pharyngitis. In GL Mandell, RG Douglas, and JE Bennett (Eds.), *Principles and Practice of Infectious Diseases.* New York: Wiley, 1979.
  An overview of the pathogenesis, etiology, epidemiology, diagnosis, and treatment of pharyngitis.
Joseph P. Gaining ground on gonorrhea: Update on Dx and Rx. Mod Med, March 1981, pp. 28–40.
  A fine presentation of the diagnosis and treatment of N. gonorrhea infections.
McCue JD. Group G streptococcal pharyngitis. *JAMA* 248:1333–1336, 1982.
  A retrospective study of the clinical and treatment characteristics of an outbreak of group G streptococcal pharyngitis among college students.
Monto AS, Ullman BM. Acute respiratory illness in an American community: The Tecumseh Study. *JAMA* 227:164–169, 1974.
  An epidemiologic study of acute respiratory illness in an entire community that included surveillance of all residents regardless of whether they sought medical attention.
Pantell RH. Pharyngitis: Diagnosis and management. *Pediatr Rev* 3(2):35–39, 1981.
  A review of the diagnosis and treatment of streptococcal pharyngitis, with a theoretic cost-benefit analysis.
Peter G, Smith AL. Group A streptococcal infections of the skin and pharynx. *N Engl J Med* 297:365–369, 1977.
  A comprehensive review of the epidemiology, diagnosis, treatment, and prevention of complications of streptococcal pharyngeal infections.
Rammelkamp CH, Monson TP. Strep infections: Time is not on your side. *Res Staff Phys,* July 1971, pp. 44–51.
  A concise discussion of the clinical presentation, diagnosis, and treatment of streptococcal pharyngitis, with a focus on time between infection and treatment as it relates to the prevention of acute rheumatic fever.
Sanchez RM. Etiology and Differential Diagnosis of Pharyngotonsillitis. In PK Peter-

son, et al. (Eds.), *The Management of Infectious Diseases in Clinical Practice*. New York: Academic, 1982.

The author reviews the major causes of pharyngitis with emphasis on clinical presentation, diagnosis, and treatment.

Tompkins RK, Burnes DC, Cable WE. An analysis of the cost-effectiveness of pharyngitis management and acute rheumatic fever prevention. *Ann Intern Med* 86:481–492, 1977.

Decision analysis is used to determine the most cost-effective clinical approach to preventing primary acute rheumatic fever by oral or benzathine penicillin treatment.

Komaroff AL. A management strategy for sore throat. *JAMA* 239:1429–1432, 1978.

A review, with particular attention to the questions facing clinicians caring for patients with sore throat.

19. HOARSENESS
Duncan S. Postma and James P. Browder

Hoarseness is an abnormality of voice production characterized by breathiness or harshness of the voice. It results from a lack of smooth approximation of the vocal cords, either from intralaryngeal pathology or a lack of normal vocal cord mobility. Hoarseness rarely presents as a functional disorder and is usually associated with a demonstrable laryngeal abnormality. If persistent, the symptom demands definitive diagnosis because lesions such as laryngeal carcinoma require early and specific treatment.

Causes

Primary Intralaryngeal Causes

Primary intralaryngeal conditions are the most common causes of hoarseness. Viral laryngitis is characterized by the acute onset of hoarseness without dyspnea and is usually accompanied by rhinopharyngitis. The syndrome is more common in the winter months. Bacterial laryngitis is less common but can be life-threatening, as in the case of acute epiglottitis (supraglottitis), caused by *Hemophilus influenzae*. Acute epiglottitis typically produces a "muffled" voice rather than true hoarseness.

Chronic exposure to tobacco smoke, even passively, can produce irritative laryngitis with edema of the laryngeal mucosa, particularly along the free edge of the vocal cord where vibration is most intense. This trauma, plus exposure to the carcinogens in tobacco smoke, can lead to dysplasia of the laryngeal mucosa, in situ cancer, and eventually frankly invasive epidermoid carcinoma.

Voice abuse is also a common cause of vocal cord lesions. They occur in children who are habitual "screamers," cheerleaders, workers in noisy environments, singers, teachers, and lawyers. Lesions of the vocal cords include nodules ("singer's nodes"), polyps (more closely linked to smoking), and contact ulcers. The ulcers usually present as hoarseness with upper neck or pharyngeal pain, which is exacerbated by speaking or singing.

Malignant tumors are less common but should be considered in anyone with hoarseness, particularly those who smoke or abuse alcohol. The incidence is highest in the sixth and seventh decades of life, and they affect men more frequently than women.

Other, less common intralaryngeal causes of hoarseness are foreign body ingestion, benign tumors, traumatic granulomas from intubation, granulomatous diseases, myxedema, and esophageal reflux.

Secondary Intralaryngeal Causes

Weakness of the intrinsic laryngeal muscles, because of myasthenia gravis or a bulbar palsy (usually associated with significant dysphagia), can cause hoarseness. Cricoarytenoid joint arthritis or fixation can also cause hoarseness and has been documented in association with rheumatoid arthritis, gout, systemic lupus erythematosus, intubation trauma, and accidental injury.

Laryngeal Nerve Damage

Laryngeal nerve damage is an infrequent cause of hoarseness. Because the left recurrent nerve has a longer course than the right, it is affected almost ten times more often. The superior laryngeal nerves are less often paralyzed than the recurrent laryngeal nerves, and their paralysis is probably less often recognized, since the effects are more subtle. The most frequently identified causes of recurrent laryngeal nerve palsy are surgical procedures of the thyroid, neck, or chest and malignancies of the thyroid, esophageal, pulmonary, or other tissues that either directly invade or compress the nerve. Other causes include diabetic or viral neuropathy. In many cases, the cause is never identified.

Functional Hoarseness

Functional hoarseness refers to changes in voice quality not attributable to any detectable organic pathology. Dysphonia plicae ventricularis ("false cord hoarseness") results from using the false instead of the true vocal cords for phonation. It often follows laryngitis and persists after the infection has resolved. Spastic dysphonia, a jerky, poorly coordinated voice with variations in pitch and intensity, may be the result of disease in the central nervous system. Aphonia (complete absence of the voice) is rarely conscious malingering, although secondary gain from the illness may play a major role in its occurrence.

Diagnosis

History

The history should focus on five important areas:

1. What was the nature of the onset of the hoarseness, and how long has it been present? An acute onset, without antecedent trauma or history of foreign body ingestion, suggests an infectious or inflammatory cause. A more chronic course is consistent with voice abuse, irritation from smoking, or neoplasia. Hoarseness that develops only late in the course of a day suggests a neuromuscular disorder (e.g., myasthenia gravis or a partially compensated recurrent laryngeal nerve palsy).

2. Is the hoarseness constant or intermittent? Constant hoarseness suggests a persisting structural change in the larynx such as those secondary to tumor, trauma, or a poorly compensated cord palsy. Functional aphonia is usually constant, although the patient can produce a normal cough on demand, demonstrating physiologic closure of the glottis. Dysphonia plicae ventricularis presents as a constantly harsh voice ("stage whisper"), but also is associated with a normal cough. Intermittent hoarseness usually implies a benign or temporary condition, and its cause may be voice fatigue, "postnasal drip," or idiopathic.

3. What are the associated regional symptoms? Sore throat, ear pain, and dysphagia with hoarseness of more than 2 weeks' duration strongly suggest malignancy. Dyspnea can also signal a cancer or, less often, bilateral vocal cord palsies. Pain can also be a prominent symptom with a contact ulcer or arthritis. A more acute course suggests infection or a foreign body; dyspnea and drooling with a muffled voice strongly suggest acute epiglottitis. Aspiration may accompany a tracheoesophageal fistula (either congenital or associated with trauma or tumor erosion) or, more commonly, unilateral vocal cord palsy, in which case the voice usually has an "especially breathy" or "raspy" quality. Reflux of acid gastric contents may result in hoarseness secondary to an irritative laryngitis, which is typically worse in the mornings.

4. What are the associated systemic symptoms? For example, is there weight loss (malignancy); cough, hemoptysis, or chest pain (intrathoracic etiology); fever (infection); or generalized weakness without weight loss (neuromuscular disorder)?

5. What are possible etiologic or contributing factors? For example, is there a history of voice abuse or trauma, including surgery and cigarette or alcohol abuse?

Physical Examination

Emphasis should be placed on the oral cavity, oropharynx, and neck.

An indirect (mirror) examination of the larynx is usually indicated in patients complaining of hoarseness. It is mandatory in three situations: (1) if hoarseness has persisted for more than 2 weeks; (2) in patients at high risk for laryngeal cancer, i.e., older people and anyone who is a heavy smoker and/or drinker; and (3) in patients with the associated symptoms of dyspnea, pain, aspiration, or dysphagia. Indirect laryngoscopy is not usually indicated in a clear-cut situation of recent voice abuse or with the typical clinical presentation of laryngitis. Prompt evaluation is necessary if hoarseness of acute onset is associated with severe sore throat, dysphagia, or dyspnea. These are the symptoms of acute epiglottitis, which is a medical emergency because it can produce early acute airway obstruction secondary to edema of the supraglottic tissues. If acute epiglottitis is suspected, care must be taken in examining the patient, lest laryngospasm and asphyxiation be induced.

The definitive diagnosis of a mucosal lesion of the larynx can often be made by indirect examination alone. Smoker's laryngitis usually appears as edematous and erythematous vocal cords, often with polypoid changes. Vocal cord nodules typically appear as bilaterally opposing "knots" at the junction of the anterior and middle thirds of the vocal cords. Polyps occur in the same location as nodules but appear as erythematous, smooth, mobile lesions, usually larger than the typical nodule. Contact ulcers appear like any ulcer; they are found at the junction of the middle and posterior thirds of the vocal cords at the tip of the vocal process of the arytenoid cartilage.

Malignancies, when advanced, present as angry, exophytic mass lesions or ulcerations, typical of epidermoid cancer. However, early cancer of the vocal cord may be subtle, presenting as a small, white plaque or an erythematous nodule. A mass or ulcer involving a vocal cord that is immobile for no apparent cause is an ominous sign and may represent occultly invasive cancer.

With laryngeal paralysis, the affected vocal cord is usually in the paramedian position (slightly lateral to the midline). With a unilateral recurrent nerve palsy, the paralysis may not be obvious for several reasons: the paralyzed cord may adduct slightly because of the action of muscles that are innervated either bilaterally or by another nerve; also, the nonparalyzed cord may cross the midline to make contact with the paralyzed cord as a compensatory maneuver, giving the impression of a normal glottis. A superior laryngeal nerve or a combined paralysis is more unusual, and the findings may be subtle. Usually the cord is slightly bowed and flaccid; with speaking, it is seen to be at a lower level than its partner.

With functional hoarseness, there are no laryngeal abnormalities on indirect inspection. Dysphonia plicae ventricularis, however, usually can be identified by demonstrating close approximation of the false cords during phonation, which obscures the true cords.

Treatment

The treatment of viral laryngitis is supportive; increased household humidity, cough suppressants, and analgesics are usually sufficient therapy. "Laryngitis" that does not improve in 7 to 10 days may indicate more significant pathology, and treatment should not be continued without a thorough diagnostic evaluation.

Early vocal cord nodules, polyps, or contact ulcers often respond favorably to strict voice rest. Ideally, this means no use of the voice at all, although in practice minimal use of the voice is usually the best one can hope to achieve. Whispering should be discouraged, since it causes nearly as much vocal strain as yelling. If the patient must speak, a soft, breathy voice is least traumatic. If hoarseness persists for longer than 2 weeks, referral to a speech pathologist or otolaryngologist is indicated.

All patients with laryngeal mass lesions persisting longer than 2 or 3 weeks should be referred to an otolaryngologist for laryngoscopy and possible biopsy. Recurrent laryngeal nerve palsy is evaluated by a careful node examination, posteroanterior and lateral chest x-ray with special lordotic views, and barium swallow if needed. With minimal symptoms and no identifiable etiology, hoarseness can be managed by waiting for 9 to 12 months. Teflon augmentation of a unilaterally paralyzed vocal cord is often very helpful and is a relatively uncomplicated procedure.

Deweese DD, Saunders WH. *Textbook of Otolaryngology.* St. Louis: Mosby, 1982. Pp. 84–128.

   A general overview of the anatomy and physiology of the larynx with a discussion of lesions associated with hoarseness.

Friedman J. Hoarseness. In CD Blueston and SE Stool (Eds.), *Pediatric Otolaryngology.* Philadelphia: Saunders, 1983. Pp. 1181–1189.

A good discussion of the clinical approach to hoarseness, with particular emphasis on the pediatric age group.
Schwartz L, Noyek AM, Naiberg D. Persistent hoarseness. *NY State J Med* 66(20):2658–2662, 1966.
A good review of 1000 cases of persistent hoarseness from the most common causes.

20. RHINITIS
Robert H. Fletcher

Rhinitis is a general term for a variety of unpleasant nasal symptoms that tend to occur together: obstruction, discharge, and sometimes itching and sneezing. These symptoms can result from one of several specific syndromes, which have characteristic presentations, causes, and responses to treatment. These include allergic rhinitis, vasomotor rhinitis, nasal polyps, rhinitis medicamentosa, and miscellaneous endocrine and anatomic conditions. Not uncommonly, more than one of these syndromes occur together, or symptoms are not typical of any one syndrome so that a specific diagnosis cannot be made.

The diagnostic process consists mainly of matching the patient's symptoms, clinical course, and response to treatment (and to a lesser extent, physical findings) to one of the syndromes described below.

Allergic Rhinitis
Large inhaled particles (> 25 μm) are deposited in the upper airway, mainly in the nose. If these particles are allergenic, they can cause an immunoglobulin E (IgE) response in susceptible individuals. When antigen and antibody bind to mast cells in the respiratory epithelium, histamine and other chemical mediators of inflammation are released, which cause nasal obstruction and discharge, itching of the nose and palate, and sneezing. (If particles are small enough to be deposited lower in the airway, bronchospasm can also occur.) A similar reaction in the conjunctivae causes itching, tearing, redness, and swelling.

Allergic rhinitis occurs in two patterns, seasonal and perennial, depending on the occurrence of the responsible antigen. Seasonal rhinitis occurs at the times of year when specific allergens, which vary from region to region, are present in the environment. In general, in temperate climates the allergens are tree pollens in the early spring, grass pollen later, ragweed in late summer, and mold spores in the fall; winter is a time of few symptoms. Seasonal rhinitis is often associated with allergic conjunctivitis. About 10% of adults in the general population suffer from seasonal rhinitis. Symptoms most often begin in children and young adults but can occur at any age. Many patients "outgrow" the condition after several years.

Perennial rhinitis occurs in response to allergens present throughout the year, often in house dust, a complex mixture of particles including fragments of mites and cockroaches, house pet dander, feathers, and synthetic fibers. Perennial rhinitis is less likely to be associated with eye symptoms than seasonal rhinitis. The disease mainly affects children and young adults. In most cases it lasts several years, but sometimes it continues for much longer.

Diagnosis
The diagnosis of allergic rhinitis is made primarily by the presense of typical symptoms. The nasal mucosa is pale and swollen. Nasal secretions are thin and watery. Eosinophils ($> 5\%$) can often be seen on a Wright's stain of nasal secretions; peripheral eosinophilia is uncommon. The diagnosis of allergic rhinitis is also confirmed by response to topical corticosteroids.

The responsible allergens can often be identified by an in-depth history, but this may require a great deal of time. Positive skin tests identify people with specific IgE who are at high risk for allergic rhinitis and other atopic conditions. But skin tests are nonspecific; the majority of people with positive reactions do not have clinically important symptoms. Skin tests are more helpful in seasonal than in perennial rhinitis. In vitro tests for specific IgE are available (radioallergosorbent tests [RAST]) but are expensive and little better than skin tests in identifying people with clinical disease. Reproducing symptoms by nasal challenge with suspected antigens is the standard of accuracy; however, the end point is difficult to interpret, and the test is time-consuming.

Treatment
Choice of treatment, from the wide variety of available agents, depends on the duration of symptoms, severity of disease, convenience, cost, and individual preference. It is reasonable to aim for reduction in symptoms to tolerable levels, not their elimination.

In seasonal rhinitis, considerable relief can be obtained by avoiding exposure to the offending antigens—by staying indoors, running air conditioners, changing air filters, and even leaving the area during peak seasons. For perennial rhinitis, similar but less dramatic results can be achieved by avoiding house pets and feather pillows and by keeping a "dust-free" house.

Antihistamines reduce itching, sneezing, and rhinorrhea but not congestion; drowsiness is their main side effect. Antihistamines are often combined with an oral symphathomimetic, ephedrine, which has a weak effect on nasal congestion. Sympathomimetic nasal sprays and drops dramatically relieve congestion but not irritation and discharge. They cannot be used for chronic symptoms (e.g., > 1–2 weeks) because of tolerance and rebound congestion (see Rhinitis Medicamentosa, below).

Topical corticosteroids are remarkably effective for allergic rhinitis; several randomized, controlled trials have established that the majority of patients achieve substantial relief. Nasal preparations are available containing decadron (Turbinaire), beclomethasone dipropionate (Vancenase, Beconase), and flunisolide (Nasalide). The last two are preferable because they are more active topically and less systemically absorbed. The typical dosage is 1 puff four times a day (or 2 puffs bid), but the dosage can be reduced gradually if symptoms remain under control. The onset of action is usually in a few days and sometimes a few weeks. When there is marked intranasal swelling, a brief course of systemic corticosteroids is sometimes used first to allow the topical preparations to reach the mucosa. Complications are infrequent and not severe: fragility of the nasal mucosa with minor bleeding, transient irritation, and rarely mucosal ulcerations or *Candida* infections. Atrophy of the mucosa, anticipated on theoretic grounds, has not been reported.

Intranasal cromolyn sodium, a mast-cell stabilizer, is sometimes used to prevent attacks of allergic rhinitis. Most patients with seasonal rhinitis, and some with perennial rhinitis, respond—but only partially.

Immunotherapy, with injections of extracts containing the offending antigens, is ordinarily undertaken only in seasonal rhinitis that cannot be controlled by other means. The treatment is time-consuming and expensive, requiring weekly to monthly visits for years. Randomized, controlled trials have shown that the majority of patients with seasonal rhinitis respond with a meaningful reduction in symptoms. Immunotherapy has not been shown to be efficacious for perennial rhinitis, although it is sometimes tried. Immunotherapy is ordinarily prescribed by an allergist and can then be carried out by a nonspecialist.

Vasomotor Rhinitis
At least half of all patients with rhinitis have vasomotor rhinitis. The mechanism of vasomotor rhinitis is apparently an abnormality of autonomic control of the nasal mucosa. Infection and allergy do not play a role but may coexist. The underlying cause is unknown.

Patients with vasomotor rhinitis are troubled by nasal congestion and sometimes watery nasal discharge, which can be profuse. They may have facial discomfort, located around the bridge of the nose and the frontal sinuses, from pressure on the mucosa. The discomfort is sometimes described as a headache and confused with sinusitis. Symptoms are aggravated by a variety of nonspecific irritants: heat, cold, smoke, fumes, dust, and changes in the weather. There are no sneezing paroxysms, nasal itching, or eye symptoms.

The diagnosis is made in the presence of typical symptoms and by excluding other causes of rhinitis. There is no specific test.

Treatment of vasomotor rhinitis is palliative and not very effective. Patients are instructed to avoid nonspecific irritants. Drugs that are effective for allergic rhinitis have little if any effect on the symptoms of vasomotor rhinitis, and their effect has not been established by clinical trials. Some relief of symptoms may be obtained with oral decongestants. The condition is often lifelong, although the symptoms may vary in severity over time.

Nasal Polyps

Polyps can arise in the nasal mucosa in association with allergic rhinitis, sinusitis, or aspirin hypersensitivity. They are usually multiple and result in nasal obstruction and discharge. Fleshy, pale masses can be seen projecting into the nasal cavity.

Polyps can be treated by surgical excision or topical corticosteroids. The surgery is an outpatient procedure, performed by an otolaryngologist, and is both safe and effective. However, polyps tend to recur, and so polypectomy must be repeated, often every 1 to 2 years. Topical corticosteroids are used for patients who must have frequent surgical polypectomies or whose symptoms persist after surgery because of generalized mucosal disease. About 80% of patients improve. Because of shrinkage of swollen nasal mucosa, symptoms diminish within a few days. Weeks to months later, polyps decrease in size as well.

Rhinitis Medicamentosa

Application of sympathomimetic drugs to the nasal mucosa, either by spray or drops, ordinarily causes dramatic relief from nasal congestion, followed in several hours by reactive hyperemia and return of symptoms. Patients may mistake rebound congestion for inadequate control of the original disease and increase use of the drug. Because tachyphylaxis occurs, rebound congestion may be responsible for a larger and larger part of nasal symptoms until, within a few weeks, most of the symptoms are secondary to medication. The problem is less likely if patients use weak preparations, follow prescribed dosage schedules, and use the drugs for no more than 1 to 2 weeks. The problem is fully reversible within several days after medication is withdrawn; a short course of corticosteroids may be helpful in accomplishing withdrawal.

Other drugs associated with nasal congestion include oral contraceptives, various antihypertensive medications (sympathetic blockers), and aspirin (the triad of aspirin sensitivity, asthma, and nasal polyposis).

Miscellaneous Causes of Rhinitis

Pregnant women frequently notice slight nasal congestion, but rarely complain of it. Hypothyroidism is reported to cause a stuffy nose, but this is an uncommon association and may not be specific for the disease. Deviated nasal septum and nasal tumors are anatomic causes of nasal obstruction, usually unilateral.

Intranasal corticosteroid aerosols for noninfectious rhinitis. *Med Lett Drugs Ther* 23:101–102, 1981.
   A review of intranasal corticosteroid aerosols for allergic rhinitis: their efficacy, adverse effects, and cost.
Mygind N. *Nasal Allergy.* Oxford: Blackwell, 1978.
   A comprehensive and well-written monograph.
Blair H, Herbert RL. Treatment of seasonal allergic rhinitis with 2% sodium cromoglycate (BP) solution. *Clin Allergy* 3:283–288, 1973.
   A randomized, double-blind, placebo-controlled trial. By both patients' and clinicians' assessments, the sodium cromoglycate was more effective than placebo.
Mercke U, Wihl JA. Clinical evaluation of an oral combined antihistaminic sympathomimetic preparation. *Acta Allergol* 28:108–117, 1973.
   A randomized, placebo-controlled, crossover trial using patients' symptoms as the outcome. The active combination was significantly better than placebo by all studied parameters: sneezing, irritation, obstruction, and secretion.
Van Metre TE, et al. A comparative study of the effectiveness of the Rinkel method and the current standard method of immunotherapy for ragweed pollen hay fever. *J Allergy Clin Immunol* 66:500–511, 1980.
   Compared to placebo, the standard method of ragweed immunotherapy reduced symp-

toms substantially during the pollen season. A randomized, controlled, double-blind trial.

Mullarkey MF. A clinical approach to rhinitis. *Med Clin North Am* 65:977–986, 1981.
A succinct review.

Toohill RJ, et al. Rhinitis medicamentosa. *Laryngoscope* 91:1614–1621, 1981.
Reports experience with 130 patients in an otolaryngologic practice.

Bickmore JT. Vasomotor rhinitis: An update. *Laryngoscope* 91:1600–1605, 1981.
Compares vasomotor rhinitis to nasal allergy and nasal polyposis.

Small P, et al. Beclomethasone dipropionate in the management of rhinitis—a review. *Ann Allergy* 49:127–130, 1982.
A compact, clinically oriented review.

Arbesman C, et al. Multi-center, double-blind, placebo-controlled trial of fluocortin butyl in perennial rhinitis. *J Allergy Clin Immunol* 71:597–603, 1983.
Describes experience with 306 patients with allergic rhinitis, nonallergic rhinitis, or both, treated with a new topical corticosteroid.

21. MOUTH LESIONS

Ernest Burkes, Jr.

The clinical appearance of disease in the mouth is extremely variable. A differential diagnosis can be developed by grouping lesions into ulcerative lesions, white lesions, red lesions, and exophytic lesions.

Singular Ulcers

Trauma

Trauma is a common cause of oral ulcerations. Healing time is determined by the amount of tissue damage, location, and in many instances pathogenic organisms, tooth fragments, foreign matter, and so on, embedded into the tissue. Recognition of the causative agent and its removal by debridement will usually be sufficient treatment. If trauma occurs on the ventral surface of the tongue in the elderly, a chronic, long-standing ulceration may result. This ulcer has a central depression and raised margins, resembling cancer. Healing commonly occurs following biopsy. Squamous cell carcinoma in the mouth can appear as an ulcer, located in areas where trauma is chronic. To cover this possibility, mouth ulcers should always be re-examined after local factors have been removed.

Aphthous Ulcers

Aphthous ulcers, commonly called canker sores, are singular oval ulcers, 2 to 8 mm in diameter, with regular, broad, red borders, occurring on mobile, nonkeratinized mucosa. From 20 to 50% of people suffer from aphthous ulcers. There is strong evidence that aphthous ulcers result from a cell-mediated or type IV delayed hypersensitivity reaction. These ulcers are painful and last from 1 to 2 weeks. They heal without scar formation and recur at irregular intervals apparently associated with diverse events such as trauma, psychological stress, gastrointestinal upsets, and menstruation. Recommended treatment is application of a topical anesthetic to the surface followed by local debridement with hydrogen peroxide on a cotton swab, a rinse of tetracycline, and then coverage with a topical steroid such as Kenalog in Orabase. The tetracycline reduces the number of potentially infective bacteria and has been shown, in controlled studies, to reduce the duration of pain and lesions.

Squamous Cell Carcinoma

Squamous cell carcinoma in the oral cavity is frequently an ulcerative condition seen in the floor of the mouth and ventral tongue, more commonly in older individuals and in those who use tobacco and alcohol heavily. Because of this possibility, any ulcer lasting longer than 2 weeks should be biopsied.

Periadenitis Mucosae Necrotica Recurrens

Periadenitis mucosae necrotica recurrens, an uncommon condition, may be confused with recurrent aphthous ulceration. However, the ulcers are generally larger and more severe, and they frequently last for several months, healing with scar formation. Treatment is similar to that for recurrent aphthous ulcers.

Syphilitic Lesions

Syphilitic lesions, both primary and secondary, may appear as ulcers (chancres), usually on the lips or tongue.

Tuberculosis and Fungal Infections

Tuberculosis and fungal infections may appear as solitary, deep, firm ulcerations, usually on the tongue and in the presence of systemic infections.

Multiple Ulcers

Multiple ulcers are generally indicative of systemic conditions and viral diseases.

Herpes Simplex Type I

Herpes simplex type I, frequently called "cold sores," is the most common cause of multiple ulcers. The initial herpesvirus infection, called primary herpetic gingivostomatitis, is usually seen during childhood as a febrile illness accompanied by ulcers in the mouth and on the lips. Herpetic ulcers recur almost exclusively on the vermillion border of the lips, attached gingiva, and hard palate. They begin as small vesicles, which break, enlarge, and coalesce, producing large ulcers with irregular borders. These lesions are painful and last from 1 to 2 weeks. Herpetic ulcers tend to recur in the same location each time, because the virus resides within the ganglion that supplies innervation to the area. Multiplication of the virus is stimulated by trauma, wind and sun exposure, and fever. The diagnosis is usually evident from appearance; when necessary, a biopsy, which shows a ballooning degeneration of the nuclei and multinucleation, is diagnostic. Various treatments are advocated, none of which is of established value. New antiviral medications and lysine may prove to be effective. Persons examining these lesions may contract the virus on the fingers (herpes Whitlow), and if steroids are given early, the disease may spread.

Lichen Planus

Lichen planus is a common condition that can present in the mouth as multiple diffuse ulcers or as white, lacy lines. The ulcerative lesions vary in size and extent and often are bilateral and superficial, with angular margins. Ulcerations may be confined to the attached gingiva and resemble a severe gingivitis. Lichen planus is characteristically seen in anxious individuals who report irregular exacerbations and remissions. Lichenoid reactions occur with numerous medications. The treatment of choice, topical steroid application in water-soluble or Orabase vehicles, is very effective.

Benign Mucous Membrane Pemphigoid

Benign mucous membrane pemphigoid (BMMP), also a common ulcerative condition, must be differentiated from lichen planus because the eye lesions of BMMP can lead to blindness. BMMP severely affects the attached gingiva, leaving it red, atrophic, and desquamative. The lesions vary in intensity and occasionally leave scars. Topical corticosteroids in water-soluble vehicles have been recommended, as well as systemic corticosteroids.

Pemphigus Vulgaris

Pemphigus vulgaris is an uncommon but potentially fatal disease, which may begin with ulcers in the mouth. Diffuse ulceration, rimmed by epithelium that can be easily separated and removed in large sheets, is characteristic. A biopsy showing intraepithelial separation is diagnostic. Topical and systemic steroids are the most effective medications.

Erythema Multiforme
Erythema multiforme (Stephens-Johnson syndrome) presents as an abrupt onset of hemorrhagic ulcers of the lips and oral mucosa. Although it is thought to be an allergic manifestation, in many cases no specific cause is found.

Acute Necrotizing Ulcerative Gingivitis
Acute necrotizing ulcerative gingivitis ("trench mouth") is characterized by ulcers occurring only on the gingiva adjacent to and between teeth. It is a fusospirochetal infection, seen in young adults with poor oral hygiene, poor diet, and stress. Typically, these patients complain about bad breath, bad taste, and pain. Antibiotics like penicillin reduce the acute manifestations; however, thorough cleaning and preventive maintenance (e.g., brushing and floss, saline rinses, and calculus removal by a dentist) must be accomplished, or recurrence is common and may lead to tooth loss.

White Lesions

Chronic Trauma
Chronic trauma causes oral mucous membranes to become keratinized. Removal of the irritant should result in reversal of the lesions. Since the attached gingiva is normally keratinized, white lesions on the attached gingiva are generally less dangerous than in other areas. Because white lesions may be premalignant or malignant, especially in patients who use tobacco or alcohol, any lesion that cannot be scraped off or reversed in 2 weeks should be biopsied.

Squamous Cell Carcinoma
Squamous cell carcinoma may be a localized white lesion present in one or more areas in the mouth. Piled up or speckled areas are especially suspicious.

Chronic Hyperplastic Candidosis
Chronic hyperplastic candidosis is a common condition that produces white lesions sometimes appearing similar to carcinoma. It is caused by overgrowth of *Candida albicans* and may occur in healthy individuals or in patients with systemic diseases. The lesions occur throughout the mouth but most frequently at the corners. They scrape off with difficulty. Biopsy shows hyphae invading and causing hyperplasia of the epithelium. The condition is treated successfully with topical antifungal agents, such as nystatin, and by correction of associated systemic conditions.

Wart-like Lesions
A "wart" is a localized, rough-surfaced, usually singular, white lesion ranging from 1 to 5 mm in size, caused by a virus. Condyloma accuminatum must be considered if multiple, larger wart-like lesions are present. Differentiation between verruca vulgaris and a papilloma is made histologically. These three lesions are similar in clinical appearance, and excisional biopsy is the treatment of choice.

Geographic Tongue
Geographic tongue occurs in 1% of the population. It can present as red patches outlined by a white raised border. These lesions change constantly, offer no threat to the patient, and require no treatment.

Nicotine Stomatitis
Nicotine stomatitis occurs in patients who use tobacco heavily. Typically the lesions from snuff occur at the mandibular mucobuccal fold ("snuff dipper's pouch"), while those from cigarettes are mostly on the palate. The oral mucosa may also be diffusely white with areas of white plaque. Because both these conditions are associated with oral cancer, any area of ulceration or focal areas of thickening that persist for 2 weeks should be biopsied to rule out cancer.

Lichen Planus
The most common form of lichen planus occurs as diffuse interlacing white lines in the buccal mucosa bilaterally. It may be an incidental finding or may cause the patient extensive irritation. Its relationship to carcinoma is controversial.

Red Lesions

Vascular Lesions
Many localized red lesions are vascular. Hemangiomas in the oral mucosa, when blanched, will often reveal deep feeder vessels. Vascular lesions are treated surgically, or by cryosurgery, when bleeding or cosmetic appearance is a problem.

Mucoceles
Mucoceles are red or bluish and are common in the lower lip. They ordinarily persist and cause intermittent swelling and drainage unless they are removed surgically.

Premalignant and Malignant Epithelial Tumors
Premalignant and malignant epithelial tumors may begin as localized or diffuse red patches. A velvety surface with areas of ulceration and small white plaques especially suggests malignant change. A history of tobacco and alcohol use is common when this lesion is found in the floor of the mouth or soft palate.

Candidiasis
Candidiasis is commonly a diffuse, red granular surface lesion scattered through the mouth.
    Shallow, diffuse erosions simulating red lesions may be seen in early or healing vesiculobullous diseases such as pemphigus vulgaris, lupus erythematosus, lichen planus, and benign mucous membrane pemphigoid.

Exophytic Lesions

Torus Palatinus and Torus Mandibularis
Torus palatinus and torus mandibularis occur in up to 10% of people. They are excessive, lobulated growths of bone in the midline of the palate and on the lingual surface of the mandible respectively. They grow slowly and seldom cause problems unless the overlying thin mucosa is injured, exposing bone and causing pain. Removal is unnecessary except in preparation for wearing dentures.

Squamous Cell Carcinoma
Squamous cell carcinoma is the most frequent malignancy of the oral mucosa, accounting for 1 to 3% of all cancers. It occurs in older individuals and especially in those who use tobacco and alcohol. Up to 80% of intraoral carcinomas occur in the floor of the mouth and ventral surface of the tongue, although they can occur elsewhere. The clinical presentation is variable, but generally these lesions are hard, with central granular and ulcerated surfaces of red or red and white tissue. Because oral cancer mimics the clinical appearance of many ulcerative white and red lesions, positive differentiation from other lesions is made only by biopsy. Oral cancers spread to regional lymph nodes readily; therefore, examination of the neck as well as the mouth is necessary. Treatment is by surgery or radiation therapy and results in an overall 5-year survival rate of over 50%.

Traumatic Lesions
Soft tumors are generally less likely to be malignant than firm ones. The most common lesions are overzealous responses to injury. Traumatic fibromas are 5- to 15-mm, pink, mobile tumors that occur near the commissure. They enlarge when injured, as in biting. *Pyogenic granulomas* are granular-surfaced, soft red lesions that bleed easily upon manipulation. They may be found anywhere in the mouth but most commonly are seen on the gingiva. Pregnant females with poor oral hygiene frequently have these lesions. The lesions must be totally removed.
    An *abscess* from an infected tooth or periodontal disease may drain to the outside through a mass of the gingiva called a parulis (gum boil). These lesions are soft red masses with traces of pus on the surface. They ordinarily regress when the tooth or periodontal pocket is treated.

Salivary Gland Tumors

Pleomorphic adenoma, the most common benign tumor, occurs in major glands as a firm, well-circumscribed mass that is painless and mobile. Complete surgical removal is the treatment of choice. Significant numbers of malignant salivary gland tumors occur in the minor salivary glands, especially in the lateral portions of the hard palate, the floor of the mouth, and the lips. Ulcerations over masses in these areas, plus pain and/or paresthesia, strongly suggest malignancy.

Referral

When referrals are considered necessary, most should be to dermatologists, since they are familiar with all of the major dangerous diseases of the oral cavity. If cancer is suspected, the referral can be directly to an ear, nose, and throat specialist.

Hooley JR, Whitacre RJ. *Principles of Biopsy: A Self-Instruction Guide to Oral Surgery* (2nd ed.). Seattle: Stoma, 1980.
  Illustrates recommended biopsy principles and techniques for oral mucosa.
Roitt IM, Lehner T. *Immunology of Oral Diseases.* Oxford: Blackwell, 1980.
  A textbook incorporating current information on immunology with application to oral lesions and conditions.
Stanley HR. Management of patients with persistent recurrent aphthous stomatitis and Sutton's disease. *Oral Surg* 35:174–179, 1973.
  Clinically acceptable suggestions of treatment regimens for these conditions.
Graykowski EA, Kingman A. Double-blind trial of tetracycline in recurrent aphthous ulceration. *J Oral Pathol* 7:376–383, 1978.
  A publication stemming from a wide research effort to identify successful treatments for aphthous ulcers.
Decker J, Goldstein JC. Risk factors in head and neck cancer. *N Engl J Med* 306(19):1151–1155, 1982.
  Statistical analysis of numerous factors relating to oral cancer.
Weathers DR, Griffin JW. Intraoral ulcerations of recurrent herpes simplex and recurrent aphthae. *JAMA* 82:81–88, 1970.
  Outline of the clinical differences between herpetic and aphthous lesions.
Silverman S, Griffith M. Studies on oral lichen planus. *Oral Surg* 37:705–710, 1974.
  Study of 200 patients giving clinical characteristics and addressing the question of malignant transformation.
Lehner T. Steroids and oral disease. *Br J Dermatol* 94(Suppl 12):59–60, 1976.
  Explanations of the usefulness of steroids in specific oral lesions.
Cawson RA. Premalignant lesions in the mouth. *Br Med Bull* 31(2):164–168, 1975.
  Clinical, etiologic, and managerial information about lesions that have significant risk of becoming squamous cell carcinoma.
Buchner A, Calderon S, Ramon Y. Localized hyperplastic lesions of the gingiva: A clinicopathological study of 302 lesions. *J Periodontol* 48:101–104, 1977.
  A review of a biopsy service experience with tumor-like proliferations.

V. LOWER RESPIRATORY PROBLEMS

Asthma is a complex disorder with many precipitating causes and pathophysiologic abnormalities. It can appear at any age, from infancy to old age. The prevalence is about 3% at all ages. Older classifications were based on the age of onset (childhood versus adult) and apparent cause (extrinsic, provoked by inhaled allergens versus intrinsic, usually infection-related). These dichotomies are not useful because the majority of patients fall into a mixed category. Of the childhood asthmatics, over 50% "outgrow" the disease, 25% have mild, intermittent symptoms, and 25% have a chronic illness.

Symptoms
Patients characteristically complain of intermittent wheezing. Other symptoms suggesting asthma include chest tightness, cough, and breathlessness. The last two symptoms may be the sole presenting complaint in some patients with asthma, and some may have dyspnea without wheezing. Other patients with chronic cough but a normal physical examination and spirometry have been found to have bronchospasm on methacholine challenge and to respond to asthma therapy.

Asthmatic patients sometimes complain of nocturnal dyspnea, wheezing, or cough. Multiple mechanisms have been proposed, including diurnal variations in circulating catecholamines, autonomically mediated changes in bronchomotor tone, inadequate blood levels of short-acting therapeutic agents, and exposure to allergens in the bedding. Clinical studies have demonstrated wide swings in peak flow rates with lowest values at 4 to 6 AM; this correlates with the observation that asthmatic deaths occur most commonly in the early morning hours.

In adults, aggravation of asthma often follows a viral upper respiratory tract infection or exposure to air pollution. These conditions stimulate irritant receptors, fine nerve endings found beneath tight junction or epithelial cells, that are capable of producing bronchoconstriction by vagal reflexes. Antigen exposure can produce asthma in atopic individuals, so that seasonal variation and/or exacerbation following exposure to recognized allergens (e.g., cat danders, ragweed pollen) are usual. In some adults, aspirin ingestion provokes asthma, apparently by inhibiting the synthesis of prostaglandins that are bronchodilators. Other prostaglandin inhibitors such as indomethacin and ibuprofen, as well as tartrazine yellow, a dye present in foods and medications, can also cause this syndrome. Beta-blockers can provoke asthma even when given in small doses, such as eye drops.

Physical Findings
During mild attacks, characteristic findings include inspiratory and expiratory wheezes and prolongation of expiratory time. The latter is measured by timing a forced expiration performed as rapidly as possible following a full inspiration; the normal value is 3 seconds. During severe asthma attacks, a paradoxical pulse is a useful sign because it suggests significant obstruction and rapidly disappears or diminishes following successful therapy. On the other hand, wheezing is not a precise sign in assessing severity or response to therapy; it may persist for long periods or not be heard during severe attacks with very low flow rates. Because signs and symptoms are at times unreliable in asthma, objective measurements are frequently necessary.

Laboratory Evaluation

Pulmonary Function Studies
Pulmonary function studies, including spirometry and peak flow rates, are an indispensable part of the clinical evaluation of asthma. Simple office spirometry is used to establish the diagnosis of asthma, determine the severity of impairment, evaluate the response to therapy, assess the need for hospitalization, and determine disability status.

A diagnosis of asthma can be made by the presence of a decrease in expiratory flow rates that reverses or improves following the administration of bronchodilators. The obstructive pattern includes a decrease in the ratio of forced expiratory volume in 1 second to forced vital capacity (FEV_1/FVC; normal is 75% or more). A decrease in FEV_1 is the most useful parameter in assessing severity: 60 to 80% of predicted indicates mild obstruction, 50 to 60% indicates moderate obstruction, and less than 50% indicates severe obstruction. Patients with an FEV_1 of less than 50% following acute therapy may require hospitalization, despite symptomatic improvement. The patient's subjective impression of improvement may be deceptive; studies have shown that 15% of patients failed to detect the presence of marked airway obstruction (reduction of FEV_1 to 50%) induced by methacholine. Patients who rebound to the emergency room or office following initial therapy often have more severe obstruction than the physician estimated on clinical grounds. The obstruction in some patients involves mucosal edema, inflammation, and mucous secretions, which may require long-term therapy before pulmonary function returns to normal. Therefore, serial measurements are necessary, particularly when evaluating therapeutic response to agents like corticosteroids, where the response is delayed.

The peak expiratory flow rate (PEFR), widely used in the United Kingdom, is another inexpensive but accurate measurement of mechanical lung function. Criteria for assessing severity in normal-sized adults are as follows: 200 L per minute or greater reflects mild obstruction, which can be treated with outpatient therapy; 100 to 200 L per minute indicates moderate obstruction, which can be treated in a holding area; 60 to 100 L per minute indicates severe obstruction with a need to hospitalize. Serial PEFRs can be obtained readily in the physician's office to evaluate the response to therapy. In hospitalized patients, improvement in PEFR correlates well with improvement in arterial blood gases, and painful arterial punctures can be avoided when PEFR is greater than 100 L per minute. Daily measurements at home with a "mini-peak" flow meter may predict a need to adjust medications. In a select group of patients, daily measurement of PEFR is useful for behavior modification.

Absolute Eosinophil Counts

Absolute eosinophil counts can be useful in regulating corticosteroid therapy and monitoring asthma activity. Counts in normal subjects average $122/mm^3$, in patients with asthma they are usually greater than $350/mm^3$, and in asthmatics on steroids they are less than $85/mm^3$. When corticosteroids are being used, a dosage sufficient to lower the eosinophil count below $85/mm^3$ is desirable. Also, when corticosteroids are being tapered, an increase in the eosinophil count correlates with deterioration in pulmonary function and therefore reflects activity of asthma. The relative utility of serial eosinophil counts versus serial measurements of PEFR or FEV_1 is not known.

Sputum Evaluation

Sputum evaluation is useful during exacerbations. Purulence does not necessarily indicate infection because eosinophils can impart a yellow-green color to sputum. Gram's stains are often negative because most infections are viral. However, it is diagnostically useful to know if there are large numbers of eosinophils on Wright's or Hensel stain of sputum. So, too, is a simple wet mount of sputum that reveals eosinophils with granules and eosinophil breakdown products (such as Charcot-Leyden crystals and Curschmann's spirals), which may indicate that the appropriate treatment is corticosteroids and not antimicrobials.

Other Studies

The asthmatic patient's baseline purified protein derivative (PPD) status should be documented, particularly if corticosteroids may be used subsequently. Also, a routine chest radiograph is worthwhile on the initial visit as a baseline measure. Repeat x-rays are not necessary for most acute attacks unless fever is present, symptoms are prolonged, or the attack is severe.

Arterial Blood Gases

Arterial blood gases (ABG) are essential for accurately assessing a severe attack. The usual ABG patterns in asthma attacks are as follows:

Mild attack: PaO_2 slightly decreased, $PaCO_2$ markedly decreased, pH alkalotic
Moderate attack: PaO_2 moderately decreased, $PaCO_2$ slightly decreased, pH slightly alkalotic

Severe attack: PaO_2 less than 60 mm Hg (or < 90% saturation), $Paco_2$ greater than 45 mm Hg, pH acidotic

Serial measurements of ABG are necessary in status asthmaticus or if the PEFR or FEV_1 remains very low or fails to improve during treatment for an attack. In the ambulatory setting, serial PEFR or FEV_1 is usually more useful and less invasive than serial ABGs.

Differential Diagnosis
Usually the diagnosis of asthma is straightforward and is established by the presence of wheezing plus spirometry demonstrating a low FEV_1 that improves following bronchodilators. However, considerable overlap exists between asthma and irreversible chronic obstructive pulmonary disease (COPD). Many patients with COPD have a reversible asthmatic component to their impairment, while many asthmatics appear to have an irreversible component to the obstruction that may require steroids or prolonged therapy before improvement in FEV_1 is apparent. Clues to COPD are a history of cigarette smoking, longer duration of illness, and decreased single-breath diffusing capacity on pulmonary function testing. Other anatomic problems that produce wheezing include bronchogenic carcinoma, aneurysms, and fixed upper airway obstruction due to laryngeal or tracheal stenosis (particularly in patients with prior intubation or tracheostomy). These are ruled out by chest x-ray or bronchoscopy. Wheezing due to pulmonary edema ("cardiac asthma") must be considered, especially in older patients. Acute hyperventilation does not cause wheezing but some patients with a form of conversion reaction have a functional disorder of the vocal cords that mimics asthma.

Fischl, MA, Pitchenik A, Gardner LB. An index predicting relapse and need for hospitalization in patients with acute bronchial asthma. *N Engl J Med* 305: 783–789, 1981.
The authors developed a predictive index useful for the assessment of acute asthma so that physicians can identify patients needing hospitalization.
Irwin RS, Carrao WM, Pratter MR. Chronic persistent cough in the adult: The spectrum and frequency of causes and successful outcome of specific therapy. *Am Rev Respir Dis* 123:413–417, 1981.
The authors demonstrate that chronic cough may be the presenting sign of asthma and that the cause of cough can be approached logically.
Williams MH. Asthma and airway reactivity. *Semin Respir Med* 1:283–339, 1980.
This monogram presents an in-depth overview of asthma, including natural history pathogenesis, pathophysiology, clinical features, and treatment.
Mathison DA, Stevenson DD, Simm RA. Asthma and the home environment. *Ann Intern Med* 97:128–130, 1982.
Aeroirritants and allergens in the home aggravate asthma. Simple preventive measures can be taken to minimize exposure.
Baibelman W, et al. Sputum and blood eosinophils during corticosteroid treatment of acute exacerbations of asthma. *Am J Med* 75:929–936, 1983.
Numbers of blood and sputum eosinophils reflect the response of an acute exacerbation of asthma to corticosteroids.
Asthma at night (editorial). *Lancet* 1:220–222, 1983.
An overview of the nocturnal difficulties asthmatics encounter, with suggestions for treatment.

23. ASTHMA: TREATMENT
James F. Donohue

The goal of outpatient asthma therapy is to identify and avoid any specific inciting cause, if possible, and then to select the most effective and innocuous pharmacologic agents that control symptoms, maintain improvement in lung function, and prevent subsequent attacks.

Mild, intermittent asthma is usually treated with a β_2-adrenergic aerosol. Chronic or persistent asthma often requires the combined use of a β_2-aerosol with oral theophylline, an oral β_2-agent, or both. In more severe asthma, a short course of corticosteroids is added, followed by aerosol steroids and/or cromolyn.

Adrenergic Agents

Adrenergic agents are potent bronchodilators that prevent mediator release and improve mucociliary clearance. The β_2-adrenergic drugs are preferred because of a more selective effect on the bronchi and fewer side effects.

Beta$_2$-drugs are administered by oral, parenteral, and inhalational routes. The benefits of the aerosol route are prompt onset of action, smaller dose requirements, preferential deposition on airway receptors, less systemic absorption, and less undesirable side effects of tachycardia, tremor, and anxiety. Freon-propelled, metered-dose, pressurized inhalers are convenient for outpatients. Solutions are also available for use in hand nebulizers or in air-compressor–powered nebulizers. Intermittent positive pressure breathing (IPPB) has no role in the therapy of bronchospasm.

Disadvantages of aerosols are that they may be used improperly and may penetrate poorly to distal airways during an exacerbation. Concern that overuse of inhalant drugs leads to paradoxical bronchoconstriction, tolerance, and status asthmaticus has not been substantiated. Rather, it has been found that progressively waning responsiveness or seemingly excessive patient use is often associated with increasingly severe airway obstruction, requiring corticosteroids and hospital admission. The occasional patient who has a paradoxical bronchostriction response can usually be identified by pre- and postmedication spirometry.

Proper administration of aerosols is accomplished as follows: After exhaling completely, the patient takes a slow, deep breath to total lung capacity (to promote distribution of the drug), simultaneously activating the valve of the inhaler. Then, after holding his breath for 10 seconds, the patient exhales. Although maximal improvement in lung function is observed when the second and third puffs are taken sequentially at 10- to 20-minute intervals, this is impractical. Most patients take the second puff within a few minutes of the first. Patients must be thoroughly instructed in the proper use of aerosol devices through the use of demonstration placebo when the initial prescription is written. To reinforce proper technique, patients should demonstrate their technique with the metered inhaler during subsequent visits. As many as one-half of them experience difficulty. The elderly and children, in particular, fail to get the knack of activating the device at the right time. Recently developed tube spacers, aerochambers, and collapsible resevoir bags have been attached to the metered dose inhaler, improving delivery and reducing errors in technique.

When given by the oral route, β_2-agents have a long duration of action, are useful in preventing exercise-induced and nocturnal asthma, and theroretically are carried by the pulmonary circulation to receptors inaccessible to aerosols. However, up to 20% of patients experience side effects when therapy is initiated, commonly including muscle tremors, tachycardia, anxiety, palpitation, and dizziness. These side effects are substantially reduced when lower doses are used to initiate therapy and full doses are added later, after a period of stabilization. Tolerance to muscle tremors develops rapidly, while bronchodilator action persists. Although oral β_2-agents are the initial choice of some physicians, the more common practice in this country is to combine a β_2-aerosol with theophylline and add oral β_2-drugs if symptoms persist. See Table 23-1 for dosages and details of these drugs.

Theophylline

Theophylline is used by many physicians as the initial agent for asthma or added when aerosol adrenergic agents fail to control symptoms. Because xanthines and β_2-adrenergic agents increase cyclic adenosine monophosphate (AMP) in mast cells, but by different mechanisms, they are synergistic.

In addition to bronchodilation and inhibition of mediator release, the pharmacologic actions of theophylline include positive inotropic and chronotropic cardiac effects, increased coronary blood flow, stimulation of the central nervous system and respiratory center, and a mild diuretic effect. Tolerance has been reported for the diuretic effects, but not for bronchodilation or central nervous system stimulation. The goal of therapy with theophylline is to achieve optimal improvement in bronchial hyperactivity without undue toxicity.

Products
There are over 200 theophylline-containing products in various concentrations as solutions, elixirs, plain tablets, enteric coated tablets, sustained-released tablets and capsules, rectal suppositories and enemas, and combination preparations. There are important differences among them in absorption, bioavailability, and theophylline content. Oral solutions, elixirs, and uncoated tablets are completely and rapidly absorbed with peak concentrations at 2 hours after ingestion. Many, but not all, sustained-release tablets and capsules are completely absorbed, with peak concentrations occurring 1 to 3 hours following ingestion. In addition, each product's theophylline content varies greatly. Physicians should choose a particular product on the basis of flexibility of dosage and cost. Sustained-release preparations that are completely absorbed offer the advantage of longer dosing intervals, which should improve patient compliance, and less fluctuation of serum concentration in chronic therapy. While elixirs and solutions have excellent bioavailability, they may be unpalatable and contain up to 20% alcohol. Rectal suppositories are not recommended because of erratic and incomplete absorption, as well as proctitis, but theophylline rectal solutions can be used in patients who cannot take oral medicines because of vomiting (from causes other than theophylline toxicity) or when fasting before surgery.

In addition to interproduct variability, there is considerable interpatient variability in theophylline dosage requirements, chiefly as the result of varying rates of hepatic biotransformation. Children and young adult cigarette smokers metabolize theophylline much more rapidly than do adults and older people; the serum half-life in young children may be less than 4 hours and in older adults more than 10 hours. Theophylline elimination can be decreased by cirrhosis, congestive heart failure, viral upper respiratory tract infections, pneumonia, severe COPD, and, at times, obesity and/or malnutrition. Recent administration of influenza vaccine impairs theophylline clearance, as does concurrent use of drugs such as cimetidine, erythromycin, high doses of allopurinol, and propranolol. Physicians must lower the theophylline dosage in these circumstances until serum levels are available. Smoking, low-carbohydrate high-protein diet, and the use of phenobarbital and phenytoin may increase theophylline clearance and necessitate high dosages.

Combination Drugs
Combination drugs containing fixed dosages of theophylline, ephedrine, barbiturates, and expectorants, although convenient, are not recommended. Adjustments in theophylline dosage are more difficult when combinations are used. In addition, barbiturates alter the hepatic metabolism of theophylline, decrease the response to corticosteroids, and are associated with dangerous respiratory center depression in severe asthma. The theophylline/ephedrine combination offers no advantages because toxicity is additive and tolerance to ephedrine's bronchodilating effect develops rapidly.

Theophylline Serum Levels
Theophylline serum levels must be monitored both because the drug's half-life varies greatly and because a standard dose may not always produce the desired concentration (see Chap. 140). Serum concentrations ranging from 10 to 20 µg/ml coincide with therapeutic efficacy, although a few patients seem to do well at lower doses. Increasing serum levels are associated with improvement of forced expiratory volume in 1 second (FEV_1), but also with signs and symptoms of toxicity. Nausea and vomiting characteristically occur with levels above 20 µg/ml. Headaches and nervousness occur with levels above 25 µg/ml. Cardiac arrythmias may develop with levels above 30 µg/ml and convulsions at 40 µg/ml and above.

Initiating Therapy
Ambulatory patients should be started on low theophylline doses; many experience nausea and vomiting at first, presumably because of caffeine-like effects and local gastrointestinal toxicity. This problem subsides within the first or second day of treatment. Patients who are not acutely ill can be started at 200 mg twice a day and the dosage is gradually increased over weeks. In more symptomatic patients, the usual loading dosage, calculated to achieve a therapeutic serum level around the clock, is approximately 0.5 mg/kg per hour. This is accomplished by using either 3 mg/kg every 6 hours with a short-acting preparation or 4 mg/kg every 8 hours or 6 mg/kg every 12 hours with sustained-release formulations. Because theophylline is not distributed in

Table 23-1. Adrenergic Agents

Agent	Route	Dosage	Pharmacodynamics			Comments
			Onset	Peak	Duration	
Metaproterenol	Aerosol solution (5%)	1–3 puffs q4–6h 0.3 cc in 2.5-cc saline q6h	5 min	30–90 min	5 hr	Minimal side effects from aerosol administration
	Oral	10–20 mg tid	30 min	2.0–2.5 hr	5 hr	Less consistent bronchodilation from oral dose
Terbutaline	Oral	2.5–5.0 mg q8h	30 min	2–4 hr	4–6 hr	20–30% of patients will have tremors at the 5-mg dose; treatment usually initiated at 2.5 mg q8h; tremors usually subside in several days
	Subcutaneous	0.25 mg, repeated 1 time in 30 min				At this dose, has approximately same side effects as epinephrine and can be used interchangeably
Albuterol	Aerosol	2 puffs q6h				Highly beta selective, so less cardiac stimulation, slightly more potent, longer acting than others; also more expensive
	Oral	2–4 mg q8h				Not approved for use in pregnancy

Drug	Form	Dose	Onset	Peak	Duration	Comments
Isoproterenol	Aerosol	Several preparations with concentration 0.075 mg–0.125 mg/puff: 2 puffs q3h (4–6 times qd)	3 min	30 min	1–3 hr	Less expensive than beta-selective agents, short-acting, more side effects, higher reported abuse potential
	Solution (1:200) Solution (1:100)	5 inhalations qid 3 inhalations qid				
Isoetharine	Metered aerosol Solution	2 puffs q4–6h 0.5 ml diluted 1:3 with saline	5 min 5 min	60 min 60 min	1.5–3.0 hr 4 hr	Short-acting (onset 5 min, peak 60 min, duration 1.5–3.0 hr) Fewer side effects than isoproterenol
Epinephrine	Aerosols		1.5 min	90–120 min	2–3 hr	Widely used over the counter (Primatene); short-acting, alpha-beta, adrenergic; side effects are common, tolerance develops
	Subcutaneous	1:1000 solution 0.3 cc, repeated in 15–30 min	10–15 min	1 hr	4 hr	Has limited usefulness in patients with cardiac disease, hypertension, respiratory acidosis
Ephedrine			60 min	1.0–3.5 hr	3–5 hr	Works indirectly via secretion of norepinephrine; barbiturate required because of CNS stimulation, tachyphylaxis

body fat, dosages for obese patients should be calculated on the basis of ideal body weight.

A serum level should be obtained after equilibration has occurred, usually in 72 hours. The goal of therapy is a level of 10 to 20 μg/ml. If a loading dose is used initially, from 5 to 25% of patients will have levels above or below this range, and appropriate adjustments must be made. When short-acting preparations are used, it is sometimes necessary to draw blood for a peak serum level 2 hours after a dose and a trough level 1 hour prior to the next scheduled dose to insure levels that are both adequate and safe. With sustained-release preparations, blood is drawn 4 to 6 hours after a dose but can be measured any time because the peak-trough difference is less than 5 μg/ml. However, a follow-up level is necessary because the sustained-release drugs may insidiously accumulate during the first weeks of therapy. If the initial doses fail to control symptoms, the dosage can be cautiously adjusted upward, but levels should never exceed 20 μg/ml.

Corticosteroids

When daily therapy with theophylline and beta-adrenergic agents has not alleviated symptoms or prevented deterioration of pulmonary function in moderate to severe persistent asthma, corticosteroids are especially effective. They lessen obstruction through direct effects on bronchial smooth muscle, mucosa, and vasculature, as well as having powerful anti-inflammatory actions. The decision to initiate, maintain, or terminate corticosteroids is based on weighing the benefit of impressive symptomatic relief against the risk of side effects. To minimize risk, the principles of therapy include trials of short courses (7–14 days), single daily (morning) dosing, alternate-day therapy when feasible, employment of short-acting preparations, use of objective tests of pulmonary function to assess results, surveillance for complications, concomitant therapy with bronchodilators, and rapid taper using alternate-day and/or aerosol steroids. The usual starting dosage for ambulatory patients is 40 to 60 mg per day for 3 days, tapering over a period of 2 weeks. The withdrawal of steroids may be accompanied by exacerbation of asthma or, in chronic users, steroid withdrawal syndrome: fatigue, malaise, fever, arthralgias, depression, or adrenal insufficiency.

Inhaled Steroid Aerosols

Inhaled steroid aerosols are safe and effective with primarily topical actions in the airway and little effect on the adrenal glands except at higher dosages. Beclomethasone dipropionate is sometimes used in conjunction with oral and aerosol bronchodilators as the primary steroid in persistent asthma; more often, it is given to patients taking oral corticosteroids to reduce their oral dosage. When initiating aerosol steroids in steroid-dependent patients, oral dosages should be slowly reduced. Usually 1 to 2 weeks of overlapping therapy is needed, with longer periods of combined therapy depending on the duration and dosage requirements of the oral steroids. Beclomethasone is inhaled at a dosage of 2 puffs (50 μg) four times daily. Larger dosages of 800 μg (4 puffs qid) or higher can be used but are associated with a higher rate of oral candidiasis.

Inhaled steroids have been used with varying success in weaning patients off oral corticosteroids. The likelihood of eliminating oral steroids is inversely related to the prednisone requirement; there is a high probability of successful weaning if the daily dose is 10 mg or less. Inhaled steroids are of no benefit in acute asthma when oral or parenteral forms are needed. Since inhaled steroids are not systemically absorbed at conventional dosages, full replacement with systemic steroids is necessary at times of stress or surgery.

Principal side effects of inhaled steroids include oral candidiasis (easily treated with topical antifungal mouthwashes), hoarseness, mild dysphonia, and throat irritation. Although the local toxicity can be a nuisance, there is no evidence that invasive tracheobronchial *Candida* infection occurs. The most serious complication as oral steroids are replaced by the inhaled agents is adrenal insufficiency.

Other Therapies

Disodium Cromoglycate (Cromolyn)

Cromolyn prevents asthma in some patients when given before exposure to agents that provoke bronchoconstriction. It is inhaled in a dry powder form through a Spinhaler apparatus. It is thought to work by stabilizing mast cell membranes and preventing mediator release. Cromolyn is not a bronchodilator and should not be used during an acute attack because of its irritant properties. Inhaling an adrenergic aerosol before cromolyn may decrease the irritation.

Cromolyn is usually added to the preexisting regimen in moderate asthma in an attempt to gradually reduce the dosage of corticosteroids if they were being used. A 4-week trial of the drug, inhaled four times daily, is necessary to assess its effectiveness. Pretreatment with cromolyn is particularly useful in patients with exercise-induced asthma. Although this drug is relatively nontoxic, clinical improvement is observed in less than one-third of adult asthmatics; better results are achieved in adolescents.

Immunotherapy
Immunotherapy may benefit some allergic individuals who have not responded to bronchodilators and conventional therapy. It has been proved in well-controlled, double-blind studies to be effective in allergic rhinitis and asthma due to cat dander. However, since allergic mechanisms are estimated to account for only 25% of asthma attacks, immunotherapy will not control symptoms in the majority of patients.

General Measures
Adequate hydration (3–4 quarts daily) is necessary to replace excessive respiratory water loss and to promote expectoration of the thick, tenacious mucus. Adequate pulmonary toilet is needed; postural drainage following aerosol bronchodilators promotes expectoration of mucus, but percussion and vibration alone are not effective. Intermittent positive pressure breathing with saline or ultrasonic nebulization has not been proved beneficial and may in fact provoke irritation and bronchoconstriction. The home and work environment should be controlled: known allergens such as animal danders, dusts, and feathers are avoided, as are irritants like air pollution, cooking odors, cigarette smoke, and aerosol hair sprays. Air conditioning, with frequent changes of the air filter, decreases exposure to airborne pollens and pollution. A food diary may identify products known to provoke asthma (e.g., milk, eggs, nuts, wines, seafood) so that they can be eliminated from the diet.

Infection, particularly sinusitis, should be treated promptly. Antibiotics are not otherwise useful in asthma, because bacterial pathogens rarely produce attacks. Yearly influenza immunization is recommended. Upper respiratory problems (e.g., nasal polyps, nasal obstruction, deviated septum) may aggravate asthma and require aggressive medical-surgical management. Antihistamines, useful in treating allergic rhinitis, have not been effective for asthma and are contraindicated in acute disease because of their drying effect. Expectorants, mucolytics, and cough suppressants are not proved effective in most patients.

Physical fitness is important in controlling asthma; exercise, particularly swimming, is encouraged (after premedication with a bronchodilator and cromolyn). Although asthma is not purely a psychosomatic problem, emotions can modulate the disease. Suggestion can override powerful pharmacologic agents and produce paradoxical effects (e.g., isoproterenol can cause bronchoconstriction). A reassuring physician can employ suggestion in a positive, therapeutic way. The benefit of recently popular modalities offered to help cope with asthma (transcendental meditation, hypnosis, biofeedback) is not known, but relaxation with slow, deep breaths is encouraged. Clearly, patients should be well educated about the disease, methods of avoiding attacks, and strategies for treating exacerbations. The key to self-help is confidence in one's own ability to exert control; this is a reasonable goal in the care of asthmatics.

Asthma in the Elderly
At times asthma in the elderly is obscured by the presence of other long-standing problems or age-related disability. Other conditions that produce cough and wheezing in this age group (beta-blocking drugs, tuberculosis, bronchogenic carcinoma, chronic obstructive pulmonary disease) must be ruled out by history, PPD, chest radiogram, and spirometry. However, if reversible obstruction is detected, anti-asthma therapy may be indicated.

Therapy is more complicated in elderly patients because of potential toxicity with adrenergic drugs from age-related arrhythmias, cardiovascular impairment, and tremors. Theophylline is associated with a great deal of local gastrointestinal toxicity, including gastritis, reflux due to gastroesophageal incompetence, and central nervous system stimulation contributing to insomnia and anxiety. Steroids may be associated with acceleration of degenerative conditions (e.g., osteoporosis and cataract formation) and may uncover latent diabetes or contribute to vascular necrosis of the femoral head. Nonetheless, treatment can have a favorable risk-benefit ratio.

Simple dosage schedules are needed because of patients' possible memory lapses. Small doses of steroids are used on alternate days or by aerosol. Although aerosol therapy has less side effects, many elderly patients cannot use the freon-propelled devices properly.

Management of the Acute Asthma Attack

Patients with acute asthma are treated with nasal oxygen at a flow rate of 2 to 3 L per minute; with an adrenergic agent administered subcutaneously, either epinephrine, 0.3 ml (1 : 1000), or terbutaline, 0.25 mg (can be repeated once after 20-minutes); and with an adrenergic aerosol, either metaproterenol, 0.3 ml in 2.5 ml of saline, isoetharine, 0.5 ml in 2.5 of saline, or isoproterenol. Adding the adrenergic aerosol does not cause more toxicity than using epinephrine alone, produces a large improvement in FEV_1, and may lead to a more rapid discharge from the emergency department.

For patients who do not respond to this regimen, aminophylline is added. The aminophylline loading dose, based on ideal body weight, is 6 mg/kg given in 100 ml of 5% dextrose over 30 minutes. A full loading dose is not necessary and may actually be dangerous if the patient has taken a short-acting theophylline in the past 12 hours or a long-acting one within 18 hours. The maintenance dosage varies: 0.5 mg/kg per hour in healthy nonsmoking adults; 0.2 to 0.3 mg/kg per hour in older patients and those with congestive heart failure, cor pulmonale, or liver disease; and 0.8 mg/kg per hour in young adult smokers. If the last dose of oral theophylline was taken in the last 24 hours by a young patient who can tolerate somewhat higher blood levels, a loading dose of 2.9 mg/kg per hour of aminophylline can be used while waiting for theophylline levels.

After 2 hours of acute therapy, a disposition decision is made based on the initial response to therapy. Helpful clues for the need for hospitalization include continued dyspnea, accessory muscle use, wheezing, pulse rate over 120 per minute, respiratory rate over 30 per minute, pulsus paradoxicus above 18 mm Hg, and a peak expiratory flow rate below 120 L per minute, FEV_1 below 1.6 (pretreatment less than 0.6), PaO_2 below 60 mm Hg, or $PaCO_2$ above 45 mm Hg. Additional considerations favoring admission are (1) history of prior episodes of serious asthma, (2) repeat emergency room or clinic visits within the past 2 days, (3) symptoms for over 1 week, or (4) maximal dosages of outpatient medicines.

Rossing TH, Fanta CH, McFadden ER. A controlled trial of the use of single drug versus combined drug therapy in the treatment of acute episodes of asthma. *Am Rev Respir Dis* 123:190–199, 1981.
  The combination of epinephrine plus inhaled bronchodilators or aminophylline was more effective and no more toxic than ephinephrine alone when used in patients in the emergency room.

Lichtenstein LM. An evaluation of the role of immunotherapy in asthma. *Am Rev Respir Dis* 117:191–197, 1978.
  An editorial reviewing the data and controversy surrounding the use of immunotherapy in asthma. Since many asthma attacks are not of immunologic etiology, candidates for this therapy should be selected carefully.

Patterson JW, Woolcock AJ, Shenfield, GW. Bronchodilator drugs. *Am Rev Respir Dis* 120:1149–1188, 1979.
  In-depth review of beta-adrenergic agents and theophylline.

Williams MH. Beclomethasone dipropionate. *Ann Intern Med* 95:464–467, 1981.
  A review of the topically effective corticosteroid.

Bernstein IL, Johnson CL, Tse, CS. Therapy with cromolyn sodium. *Ann Intern Med* 89:228–233, 1978.
  A review of this inhaled agent, useful in preventing some symptoms of asthma.

Weinberger M, Hendeles L. Slow release theophylline rationale and basis for product selection. *N Engl J Med* 308:760–764, 1983.
  The dosage of theophylline in the ambulatory patient is best determined by slow clinical titration.

Hillen FC, Wilson FJ. Evaluation and management of acute asthma. *Med Clin North Am* 67:669–684, 1983.
An overview of the assessment and management of acute asthma.

24. CHRONIC OBSTRUCTIVE PULMONARY DISEASE: EVALUATION
James F. Donohue

Chronic obstructive pulmonary disease (COPD) is characterized by chronic limitation of air flow, usually manifested by a decrease in expiratory flow rates on spirometry. The general term includes three separate but closely related conditions: chronic bronchitis, emphysema, and bronchospasm (asthma). For the purposes of treatment and prognosis, an attempt should be made to differentiate the reversible components, that is, asthma and acute bronchitis, from the irreversible component, emphysema.

Emphysema is described in anatomic terms as permanent, abnormal enlargement of acini accompanied by destructive changes. Chronic bronchitis is a clinical concept defined by chronic excessive secretion of mucus leading to persistent cough productive of sputum on most days for 3 or more months per year over at least a 2-year period. Chronic mucus hypersecretion by itself, with chronic cough and frequent respiratory infection, does not necessarily result in significant airway obstruction; however, some of these patients develop chronic obstructive bronchitis, with rapid deterioration of pulmonary function and early death.

Three respiratory system responses determine the consequences and natural history of COPD: responsiveness of the respiratory center to elevation of arterial carbon dioxide tension, reactivity of the pulmonary vascular bed in response to alveolar hypoxia, and the response of the lung to harmful enzymes. Genetic susceptibility apparently plays a role in these responses. Although many inhaled irritants can produce COPD, tobacco smoke is the most prevalent. It is estimated that 10% of smokers are susceptible to its irritant effects and develop COPD.

Chronic obstructive pulmonary disease affects between 8 and 9 million people in the United States, of whom 1 million have limited activity and 500,000 receive Social Security disability (second only to coronary artery disease). Since 1968, COPD has been the fastest rising major cause of death in the United States. It currently affects more males than females, but the prevalence of COPD in women is rising rapidly, presumably because of increased smoking rates in women.

Clinical Course
The typical smoker who develops COPD is asymptomatic for the first 10 to 20 years of smoking. After 20 years, mild cough and dyspnea on exertion are characteristic, and abnormalities in the small airways can be detected on pulmonary function testing. Usually sometime after age 40, following 20 to 30 years of smoking, productive cough, dyspnea, and physical signs are apparent and spirometry demonstrates a decrease in forced expiratory volume in 1 second (FEV_1). The FEV_1 has been shown to fall gradually throughout life, at a rate of 20 to 30 ml per year in most nonsmokers and many nonsusceptible smokers, so that clinically significant air flow obstruction never develops in these people. However, the rate of decline in susceptible patients who smoke is approximately 60 ml per year. When people stop smoking, they will not recover most of the lost function, but the rate of decline in FEV_1 approaches that in nonsmokers.

Symptoms
Early in their disease, patients with primarily chronic bronchitis have a morning cough productive of clear sputum. During upper respiratory infections, the sputum turns a yellow or greenish color, and there is episodic dyspnea, wheezing, and coughing. As the disease progresses, constant dyspnea aggravated by exertion, incessant mucus production, and nocturnal wakenings due to choking and coughing are common. With far-advanced disease, structural changes result in chronic alveolar hypoxia, which in turn produces pulmonary hypertension and cor pulmonale. Patients at this

stage are described as "blue bloaters"; when severely affected, they have cyanosis, edema, cardiomegaly, recurrent respiratory failure, reactive airways, polycythemia (a compensation for chronic hypoxemia occurring at night), loss of carbon dioxide ventilatory response with alveolar hypoventilation, and carbon dioxide retention. These patients require frequent hospitalization and have a poor prognosis.

Patients with predominantly emphysema complain of mild dyspnea in the early stages, but have little cough. Later, these patients have severe dyspnea and are referred to as "pink puffers" because they maintain relatively normal arterial oxygen and carbon dioxide tensions until late in their course by maintaining high minute ventilation. Patients tend to be thin and barrel-chested and are neither cyanotic nor edematous until the terminal stage of disease. However, most patients fall into a "mixed" clinical category.

Signs

The measurement of forced expiratory time is a useful, simple maneuver for evaluating the degree of air flow limitation. After a full inspiration, the patient exhales with the mouth wide open until air flow ceases, as judged by listening at the mouth or by stethoscope over the trachea. The normal duration is 3 seconds; in COPD the time is prolonged because of increased resistance to air flow or decreased elastic recoil.

Evaluation of the chest configuration and musculature may indicate the degree of hyperinflation. The accessory muscles of respiration (scalenes, sternomastoids) contract in inspiration during periods of increasing ventilation and are palpably hardened when there is overinflation of the chest and decreased flow rates. These muscles are probably used because the diaphragm and intercostal muscles are unable to develop the pressures required for adequate ventilation because of a loss of mechanical efficiency. The presence of tracheal descent with inspiration, felt by resting the tip of the index finger on the thyroid cartilage, and inward costal margin movement (Hoover's sign) correlate with long-standing overinflation that causes the rib cage and diaphragm to change shape. The length of the trachea, measured in finger breadths above the sternal notch at the end of inspiration, varies from 3 to 4 in normal persons to 0 in patients with COPD. In patients with hyperinflation, the most prominent palpable and/or auscultatory cardiac contraction is often in the epigastrium, rather than the fourth left intercostal space. Excavation of the suprasternal space and supraclavicular fossa and recession of the intercostal spaces durin   inspiration are due to a phase lag between the generation of large negative pleural   ressures and the resultant change in lung volume because of high airway resistance. (auscultation, breath sounds are distant and augment poorly with deep breathing;   nd expiratory wheezes are heard on forced expiration.

Laboratory Evaluation

Office Spirometry
Office spirometry can detect clinically significant disease and is an excellent prognostic indicator. Also, two studies have shown that patients with spirometric abnormalities were motivated to stop smoking following testing, suggesting that it is useful as a behavior modification tool.

The earliest change in bronchitis and emphysema is a decrease in the maximum mid-expiratory flow rate, suggesting obstruction in the small airways or loss of elastic recoil. However, wide variability in this parameter limits its usefulness in the office. The hallmark of COPD is a ratio of FEV_1 to forced vital capacity (FVC) below 70%, which does not completely return to normal following therapy. The FEV_1, expressed as a percent of predicted, is the most useful parameter in assessing severity of ventilatory impairment: 60 to 80%, mild; 50 to 60%, moderate; and below 50%, severe obstruction.

The FEV_1 is used in Social Security disability determinations, for prognosis, and to document both the progress of the disease and response to therapy. Roughly 50% of patients with an FEV_1 of 1.0 L per second die within 5 years, and mean survival is less than 2 years in those with an FEV_1 of 0.5 L per second or less. Spirometry should be repeated 30 minutes after inhaling a bronchodilator; if there is a 15% or more increase in FEV_1, there is a bronchospastic component to the obstruction. Spirometry is repeated after 2 weeks of therapy to determine the effects of therapy and to document the irreversible component of obstruction.

At times dyspnea is not correlated with changes in FEV_1. In such cases, it is useful to refer patients to a pulmonary function laboratory for measurement of lung volumes and diffusing capacity in order to characterize the type of COPD (e.g., emphysema) and estimate the degree of functional derangement more precisely.

The chest radiograph is not particularly useful, relative to other tests, in diagnosing COPD; it is normal in the early stages. Increased lung markings in the lower lobes, the so-called dirty lungs, and peribronchial thickening are seen in chronic bronchitis. The findings in emphysema include hyperinflation (low, flat diaphragm; enlarged retrosternal space), hypovascularity, areas of hyperlucency and bullae formation, and a small cardiac silhouette.

Arterial Blood Gases
Arterial blood gases should be measured in patients with COPD to determine gas exchange and need for oxygen therapy (PaO_2), alveolar ventilation ($PaCO_2$), and overall acid-base state (pH). Baseline values are useful benchmarks for comparison during subsequent exacerbations. Blood gases during the early stages of COPD show only mild hypoxemia. Later in the course of COPD, low ventilation-perfusion ratios can cause severe arterial hypoxemia and respiratory acidosis. Secondary polycythemia often results from chronic hypoxemia, which appears to be more pronounced during sleep. An elevated $PaCO_2$ (above 44 mm Hg), if attributable to mechanical abnormalities, is usually seen with an FEV_1 of 0.8 L per second or less. If the FEV_1 is higher, another mechanism to account for hypoventilation should be sought, such as sedative use or sleep apnea. Arterial blood gases during exercise can be helpful in evaluating some patients because hypoxemia can contribute to dyspnea on exertion.

Serum Electrolytes
Serum electrolytes should be measured in patients with COPD and carbon dioxide retention and in those on corticosteroid and diuretic therapy, because of the likelihood of chloride and potassium deficiency leading to a superimposed metabolic alkalosis with hypokalemia.

Electrocardiogram
The electrocardiographic changes of COPD are nonspecific. With severe disease, the changes of right ventricular hypertrophy occur, and atrial arrhythmias are common during acute illness.

Serum α_1-Antitrypsin
Serum α_1-antitrypsin levels should be determined in those COPD patients with disease onset before the age of 45, with clinical emphysema, or with a family history of COPD. Serum α_1-antitrypsin deficiency accounts for 1 to 2% of patients with emphysema. This information is useful for the purposes of patient and family counseling, especially in light of the considerable combined risks with smoking. Approximately 5% of the population is heterozygous; the relationship of heterozygotes to risk of COPD has not been established. In α_1-antitrypsin deficiency, the chest radiograph shows lower lobe predominance of disease.

Stubbing DG, et al. Some physical signs in patients with chronic airflow obstruction. *Am Rev Respir Dis* 1225:549–552, 1982.
The authors demonstrate that certain physical signs in COPD should not be regarded as inferior to tests of pulmonary function, but rather physical examination and spirometry are complementary.

Taser I, Speizer FE. Role of infection in chronic bronchitis. *N Engl J Med* 292:563–571, 1975.
An excellent review of the controversy surrounding the relationship of respiratory infections to COPD.

Fletcher C, Peta R. The natural history of chronic airflow obstruction. *Br Med J* 1:1645–1648, 1977.
A prospective epidemiologic study of London working men showing the various patterns of rates of decline in FEV_1 over a lifetime and the effects of smoking and of smoking cessation.

Hugh-Jones P, Whimster W. The etiology and management of disability emphysema. *Am Rev Resp Dis* 117:343–371, 1978.

  An excellent overview of the pathologic features, etiology, pathophysiology, diagnosis, and medical management of emphysema.

Snider GI. Pathogenesis of emphysema and chronic bronchitis. *Med Clin North Am* 65:647–665, 1981.

  A comprehensive overview of the various causes of emphysema.

Matthay RA. Obstructive lung disease. *Med Clin North Am* 65:543–709, 1981.

  An up-to-date review of many aspects of COPD including pathogenesis, epidemiology, treatment, and rehabilitation.

Morris JF. Spirometry in the evaluation of pulmonary function. *West J Med* 125:110–118, 1976.

  A concise review of spirometry including indication, equipment, interpretation, and predictive normograms.

25. CHRONIC OBSTRUCTIVE PULMONARY DISEASE: TREATMENT
James F. Donohue

Health Maintenance Measures
The management of chronic obstructive pulmonary disease (COPD) involves measures to prevent exacerbations and deterioration as well as specific treatment of bronchial disease and cor pulmonale.

Avoidance of Irritants
Avoidance of irritants that will further damage the tracheobronchial tree or lead to an exacerbation of symptoms is a top priority. Cessation of cigarette smoking can definitively alter the course of the disease. In one study, patients who stopped smoking experienced a decrease in cough and sputum production plus improvement in lung function over 30 months of observation. Most important, the discontinuation of smoking slows the disease process, and the rate of decline in forced expiratory volume in 1 second (FEV_1) returns toward normal. Techniques and programs available to aid in smoking cessation are discussed in Chapter 13.

Patients with COPD are cautioned to avoid areas of high air pollution or, if they cannot, to curtail physical activities during air pollution alerts. Sulfur dioxide, nitrogen dioxide, and particulate matter can exacerbate symptoms. Likewise, occupational exposure to cereal grain dusts, fumes, vapors, and irritants (e.g., formaldehyde) can cause worsening of symptoms. Smoking should not be allowed in patients' homes, and they should avoid poorly ventilated places where others smoke.

Avoidance of Respiratory Infections
Avoidance of respiratory infections, most of which are viral, may be aided by refraining from contact with crowds during viral epidemics and "flu" season and by keeping away from people with colds. Patients should receive immunizations each fall with polyvalent influenza vaccine. Amantadine hydrochloride is useful if started within 48 hours of exposure to influenza A and can protect highly susceptible individuals during the 2-week latency period before the vaccine is effective (see Chap. 118). Polyvalent pneumococcal vaccine should be given once.

On the basis of currently available data, it seems that prophylactic antibiotic therapy (e.g., tetracycline, 250 mg twice daily) does not lessen symptoms, arrest functional deterioration, or decrease the number of days of hospitalization. An exception may be a highly selective group with multiple exacerbations every winter for many years. Respiratory therapy and oxygen equipment used in the home should be carefully cleaned to prevent bacterial colonization and subsequent infection with pathogens.

Avoidance of Potentially Harmful Drugs
Antihistamines tend to cause inspissated mucus and can even depress ventilation in the seriously ill. Likewise, sedatives, tranquilizers, and narcotics prescribed for pain

relief or cough suppression must be used with caution in patients with COPD and are contraindicated in those with carbon dioxide retention because they may cause ventilatory suppression. Aspirin can provoke bronchospasm in sensitive patients, especially those with nasal polyps. Beta-blockers given for concomitant angina, hypertension, or glaucoma can worsen symptoms in COPD, particularly in patients with a "reactive" component, that is, bronchodilator responsiveness. Although selective β_1-blockers have been given in low dosages to patients with angina and fixed irreversible obstruction to air flow, these agents are not selective at higher doses and are best avoided.

Psychosocial Stresses

Patients who are chronically short of breath experience a great deal of stress. Anxiety can in turn lead to an increase in oxygen consumption and an increase in the work of breathing and can thereby aggravate symptoms. In addition to medical therapy, training in relaxation methods and counseling about self-care can increase patients' feelings of autonomy in the control of dyspnea and are useful in coping with and controlling anxiety. Because rapid breathing can lead to air trapping, an increase in the work of breathing, and more dyspnea, the patient is instructed to take slow, deep breaths, the most efficient breathing pattern. Progressive exercise may decrease the unrealistic fear of activity and dyspnea. Education, support, and reassurance are essential components in the psychological management of patients with COPD. Well-informed family members and patient discussion groups are useful resources; frequent follow-up visits can consolidate gains.

Other Measures

Susceptible patients are advised to avoid food and beverages that provoke bronchorrhea and bronchospasm, such as dairy products, spicy foods, wine, and other alcohol-containing products.

Extremes of temperature can cause symptoms and should be avoided. High altitude can pose problems for hypoxemic patients. Other practical measures include aggressive treatment of upper respiratory problems that can aggravate symptoms, including rhinitis and postnasal drip.

Training Programs

Training programs recommended for the patient with COPD include general physical reconditioning and breathing exercises. Inactivity and deconditioning are accompanied by increased lactate production with high ventilatory drive and dyspnea on exertion. Patients with chronic bronchitis become increasingly disabled and frustrated by breathlessness on exertion as their disease progresses. Moderate exercise training by walking and graded stair climbing has been shown to be useful. In some patients, breathlessness is not dangerous, and sustained moderate dyspnea resulting from exercise improves overall endurance, strengthens the respiratory muscles, and increases exercise capability.

Slow abdominal diaphragmatic breathing with exhalation against pursed lips helps not only to relieve dyspnea subjectively but also to decrease respiratory rate and minute ventilation while increasing tidal volume, thereby improving arterial blood gases.

Alteration of Secretions

It is generally believed that thinning secretions and increasing the volume expectorated are desired goals, although this premise has not been validated by research on patients with COPD. Sputum liquefaction is attempted when mucus is thick, tenacious, or excessive. Unfortunately, there are no drugs to accomplish this safely and effectively. Most evidence suggests that commonly used expectorants, including glyceryl guaiacolate, terpin hydrate, and potassium iodide, have little or no effect on expectoration in most patients. Efforts to increase mucociliary transport by aerosol deposition of N-acetylcysteine and detergents have not been successful and sometimes result in bronchospasm. Likewise, there is no evidence that inhaling bland aerosols of water, saline, or steam by themselves improves pulmonary mucociliary clearance or promotes expectoration of viscous secretions. The most useful techniques are adequate hydration, bronchodilators that improve mucociliary clearance, chest physiotherapy, and postural drainage. There is a clinical impression that the development of viscid secretions can be prevented by ensuring a fluid intake of 2 to 3 L per day and maintaining home humidity above 50%.

Intermittent Positive Pressure Breathing
Long-term use of intermittent positive pressure breathing (IPPB) in patients with secretions causes no benefits other than those derived from the bronchodilators themselves. Adrenergic bronchodilators can be adequately delivered with an air compres-
sor–powered nebulizer and with less side effects (e.g., inspissated secretions, infections)
than with IPPB.

Physiotherapy and Cough
Changes in cough, sputum production, and sputum characteristics can signal the need
for additional therapy or evaluation. However, coughing itself is not necessarily bad in
COPD; in fact, cough serves as a major mechanism for removal of secretions from the
large airways. Smoking, infection, and reduction of flow rates due to poor mechanical
function interfere with effective cough and clearance. Properly performed chest physiotherapy can assist cough and clear retained tracheobronchial secretions. Therefore, encouragement of deep abdominal breathing, education in proper coughing techniques,
and instruction in postural drainage and chest percussion with clapping or vibration
are important. Although gravity does not affect mucus flow in normal subjects, postural drainage is extremely important when the mucus is thick, as in patients recovering from surgery or patients with cystic fibrosis, bronchiectasis, or chronic bronchitis.
Vigorous, repetitive, hard coughing causes airway collapse, is inefficient, and can cause
additional bronchospasm by vagal reflexes. Gentle cough against pursed lips is more
efficient.

   Therefore, the usual sequence of pulmonary toilet in patients with chronic bronchitis
and thick mucus is inhalation of bronchodilators, followed by postural drainage with
percussion if someone is available to do it. Immediately afterward the patient takes
three or four deep inhalations with pursed-lip exhalation, followed by three short, gentle coughs.

Specific Treatment

Bronchodilators
Selective β_2-adrenergic agents, including metaproterenol, terbutaline, isoetharine, and
albuterol, are discussed in Asthma: Treatment, but a few specific points relative to
their use in COPD deserve emphasis. Failure of expiratory flow rates to increase after
the inhalation of bronchodilators should not be interpreted as absolute evidence of non-
responsive airways. While the amount of bronchodilation may be smaller in COPD
compared to asthma, adrenergic aerosols also enhance clearance of retained secretions
and decrease air trapping, thereby relieving the sensation of dyspnea. Therefore, these
agents have a major role in therapy. Since patients with COPD are older and may
have concurrent heart disease, toxicity is more likely, and it may be necessary to give
these agents in smaller doses. More active patients usually prefer the hand-held, freon-
propelled adrenergic inhalers. However, many of the more severely impaired patients
are so weak that they have difficulty using the freon-propelled nebulizer and require
mechanical nebulizers (e.g., DeVilbuss) to deliver a solution of adrenergic agents. In
mechanical nebulization the time of delivery is increased, so that approximatey 10
times more drug is administered. The drug may be better distributed to the distal
airways. Most patients require treatments only on arising and before bedtime; others
need supplementary treatment at 4- to 6-hour intervals with either hand-held aerosols
or inhaled solutions. Metaproterenol is given in a standard dose of 0.3 ml diluted in 2
ml of saline, and the aerosol treatment is followed by postural drainage.

   The use of nebulized atropine (0.05 mg/kg) for COPD is presently under investigation. When added to adrenergic agents during exacerbations, additional bronchodilation results. Side effects with inhaled atropine are less than with parenteral forms, but
dry mouth, tachycardia, and urinary retention occur.

Theophylline
It is often difficult to document improvement in flow rates after theophylline administration, but subjective improvement is seen. Theophylline improves the strength of
diaphragmatic contractility in COPD and may improve ventilatory function. However,
toxicity is a problem, and serum level and clinical response must be closely monitored.
Lower maintenance doses are needed in cor pulmonale and congestive heart failure.

Oral adrenergic preparations (e.g., albuterol, terbutaline, metaproterenol) can be used in place of theophylline but more commonly are added if aerosol adrenergics and theophylline do not suffice.

Systemic Steroids

Systemic steroids clearly lessen airway obstruction in asthma, but their value for ambulatory patients with severe COPD remains uncertain. Impressive results are seen with acute exacerbations. In contrast, only a minority of stable patients with COPD benefit from long-term oral corticosteroids. However, since the results are occasionally quite dramatic, an attempt should be made to identify steroid responders. Responsive patients tend to have blood and sputum eosinophilia, response to inhaled bronchodilators, positive skin reactions to common antigens, and history suggesting allergy or asthma. However, these criteria are not very precise, and the only way to identify definitively patients who will respond to corticosteroids is by a therapeutic trial. Usually 32 mg per day of methylprednisone or 40 mg per day of prednisone is given for 2 weeks, and the response is assessed by spirometry. Approximately 15 to 30% of patients show a 15 to 20% improvement in FEV_1. In responders, oral steroids produce a more definitive improvement than inhaled steroids; efforts to convert patients to aerosol corticosteroids have not been as successful in COPD as in asthma.

Treatment of Infectious Complications

Patients with bronchitis appear to have a high frequency of respiratory infections. It is estimated that one-third of exacerbations are noninfectious, one-third are viral or mycoplasmal, and one-third are bacterial. The relationship between bacterial infection and exacerbation is confused by the fact that patients with chronic bronchitis are sometimes colonized with bacteria that are present in the sputum between exacerbations and are not eradicated by antibiotics. Also, viral infections predispose to bacterial infections, and bacterial infections are often accompanied by severe symptoms and many provoke respiratory failure. Studies of antibiotic use fail to resolve this dilemma; six placebo-controlled studies of the effects of antimicrobial agents during exacerbations show no benefit in four and a significant advantage in two. Most physicians treat exacerbations with antibiotics.

Microscopic examination of the sputum during an excerbation can guide the selection of treatment. A purulent appearance may reflect the presence of large numbers of eosinophils and indicates the need for steroids rather than antibiotics. The presence on Gram's stain of a predominant organism associated with numerous neutrophils can help to determine therapy. Large numbers of neutrophils without organisms suggest a virus, *Mycoplasma,* or *Legionella,* and erythromycin may be an appropriate choice of antibiotic. Sputum cultures are usually unnecessary unless the exacerbation occurred while the patient was already on antimicrobials or there is no response after 72 hours. The bacterial pathogens most commonly found in bronchitic sputum are *Hemophilus influenzae* and *Streptococcus pneumoniae.* Gram-negative organisms are more common in recently treated or hospitalized patients. Ampicillin, amoxicillin, tetracycline (2 gm daily), and trimethoprim/sulfamethoxazole are effective agents.

Supplemental Oxygen Therapy

Patients with documented hypoxemia benefit from long-term, low-flow oxygen therapy. Candidates for home oxygen therapy include those with a resting PaO_2 of 55 mm Hg or less, patients with a PaO_2 of 55 to 59 mm Hg with evidence of erythrocytosis or cor pulmonale, and those with documented hypoxemia during exercise or sleep. Hypoventilation and low ventilation-perfusion ratios, particularly during sleep, lead to alveolar hypoxia, which in turn causes increased pulmonary artery pressure, right heart dilatation, peripheral edema, and polycythemia. Oxygen reverses this vicious cycle. In one study, patients given low-flow oxygen for 15 hours daily had better survival rates than those given no oxygen. A recent multicenter study found that patients with hypoxemic COPD, particularly those with more severe derangements of lung and brain function, had a lower mortality rate if they were treated by continuous rather than nocturnal (12 hours) oxygen therapy.

Low-flow oxygen (1–2 L per minute) can be readily administered from a variety of sources, such as compressed oxygen gas cylinders, liquid oxygen reservoirs, or oxygen concentrators. Liquid oxygen "walkers" are particularly useful for ambulatory patients who have hypoxemia with exercise. The goal of therapy is a PaO_2 of at least 60 mm Hg or 90% saturation. Most COPD patients do not require this expensive ($300 per month) treatment.

Treatment of Cor Pulmonale

Digoxin

Digoxin is indicated for patients with COPD only if they have atrial tachyarrhythmias or concomitant left ventricular failure. Inotropic agents are not usually helpful in cor pulmonale. The majority of patients with COPD do not have evidence of left ventricular dysfunction at autopsy. Furthermore, digoxin has substantial toxicity in COPD because of an unexplained prolongation of half-life and increased sensitivity to the drug in the setting of hypokalemia, hypoxemia, and concomitant adrenergic therapy.

Diuretics

Hypoxia and acidosis cause pulmonary hypertension and right heart failure with sodium retention and expansion of the extracellular fluid volume. A triad of prerenal azotemia, hyponatremia, and low cardiac output develops. Therefore, patients benefit from loop diuretics. Side effects of diuretics used for cor pulmonale include reduced cardiac output and metabolic alkalosis with increased plasma bicarbonate from contraction of extracellular volume and loss of chloride. Small doses of furosemide, accompanied by potassium chloride supplements, are recommended, along with restriction of sodium and close monitoring of fluid intake.

Phlebotomy

Some patients with chronic bronchitis develop erythrocytosis to compensate for chronic hypoxemia. The consequences of polycythemia are determined by a tenuous balance between increased oxygen transport versus high viscosity and increased pulmonary artery pressure. Although phlebotomy is rarely indicated, a trial is sometimes necessary to determine its effect on heart failure. Only a moderate decrease in hematocrit is necessary; there is no reason to lower the hematocrit below 50%.

Mendella LA, et al. Steroid response in stable chronic obstructive lung disease. *Ann Intern Med* 96:17–21, 1982.
   A small percentage of stable COPD patients showed a significant improvement in FEV_1 following a 2-week trial of steroids.
Nocturnal Oxygen Therapy Trial Group. Continuous nocturnal oxygen therapy in hypoxemic chronic obstructive disease: A clinical trial. *Ann Intern Med* 93:391–398, 1980.
   Continuous oxygen therapy is associated with lower mortality than nocturnal oxygen therapy.
Dudley DL, et al. Psychological concomitants to rehabilitation in chronic obstructive lung disease. *Chest* 77:413–420, 544–550, 677–684, 1980.
   A three-part series exploring the psychosocial concomitants to COPD with emphasis on anxiety and depression and the role of the primary physician.
Hudson LD, Pierson DJ. Comprehensive respiratory care for patients with COPD. *Med Clin North Am* 67:629, 1981.
   Very readable, up-to-date review.
Green LH, Sith TW. The use of digitalis in patients with pulmonary disease. *Ann Intern Med* 87:459–465, 1977.
   Patients with lung disease are more susceptible to the toxic effects of digoxin.
Heinemann HO. Right-sided heart failure and the use of diuretics. *Am J Med* 67:367–370, 1978.
   This review assesses the effects of diuretic therapy in COPD.
Block AJ. Dangerous sleep: Oxygen therapy for nocturnal hypoxemia. *N Engl J Med* 306:166–167, 1982.
   The presence of nocturnal oxygen desaturation may determine which patients with COPD develop cor pulmonale.

26. ACUTE LOWER RESPIRATORY TRACT INFECTION
C. Glenn Pickard, Jr.

The spectrum of acute, infectious, lower respiratory tract disease in adults ranges from minor, self-limited tracheobronchitis to severe and sometimes fatal lobar pneumonia. The usual discussion of these diseases differentiates "bronchitis" from "pneumonia." This differentiation, based primarily on pathologic changes in the lung, does not correlate well with patterns of clinical management. In practice, the severity of the illness, specifically the height of the fever and the presence or absence of dyspnea and tachypnea, is a better determinant of management strategy. Less seriously ill patients can be managed in the ambulatory setting; more seriously ill patients usually require hospitalization.

Although the less seriously ill patients will usually have acute bronchitis, many have areas of "pneumonia," often inapparent on clinical examination, that can be detected only by chest x-ray. Radiographically these areas appear as segmental or subsegmental patchy infiltrates or peribronchial cuffing. Patients with acute bronchitis and less seriously ill patients with these x-ray findings are usually managed similarly. More seriously ill patients, many of whom have lobar pneumonia, require hospitalization for diagnostic procedures, administration of parenteral medications and fluids, and oxygen therapy.

Causes
The causes of acute adult lower respiratory disease are difficult to determine because of problems in obtaining accurate cultures. False-positive cultures occur because the normal upper respiratory passages are frequently colonized by *Streptococcus pneumoniae* and occasionally *Hemophilus influenzae,* the organisms thought to be the primary bacterial pathogens in lower respiratory tract disease. Because expectorated sputum is almost always contaminated with nasopharyngeal secretions, it is difficult to be certain that pathogens recovered in sputum represent true lower tract pathogens. False-negative results have been reported in patients with lobar pneumonia and pneumococcal bacteremia. In these patients, sputum cultures obtained at the same time as blood cultures fail to grow pneumococci approximately 45% of the time.

In studies performed on inpatients with pneumonia, direct lung puncture has been shown to produce the highest yield of single pathogens, and transtracheal aspiration has been found to be superior to culture of expectorated sputum. Studies of expectorated sputum in which the sputum was graded based on the number of neutrophils versus the number of buccal squamous epithelial cells present showed that "high-quality" sputum specimens (numerous neutrophils and few squamous cells) gave results comparable to transtracheal aspiration.

Studies using these approaches on ambulatory adults with acute lower respiratory infections have not been reported. Thus, one can only speculate about the probable causes, using the best data from inpatient and community surveillance studies obtained by conventional techniques in patients with a diagnosis of pneumonia. The great majority of cases are probably caused by viruses, and the next most frequent cause is probably mycoplasma. Bacteria, primarily *S. pneumoniae* and to a lesser extent *H. influenzae,* account for only a small minority of the cases.

Factors that decrease the mucociliary cleansing of the tracheobronchial tree may make patients more susceptible to lower respiratory tract infection. These include chilling, cigarette smoking, and consumption of alcohol. Preceding viral infection is also believed to make bacterial infection more likely, although this commonly held belief has been challenged.

Evaluation

General Assessment
Early in the course of pneumonia the physical examination and chest x-ray may be normal, and a general assessment of the severity of the illness may therefore be the only clue to serious disease. Ill-appearing patients with fever of 39°C or more, tachypnea, tachycardia, pallor or cyanosis, flaring of the alae nasi, or mental confusion should be hospitalized regardless of the findings on chest examination or chest x-ray.

History
Most patients present with an illness of less than 2 weeks' duration characterized by low-grade fever, sore throat, rhinorrhea, mild malaise, and initially a dry, nonproductive cough. Frequently, the visit to the physician is precipitated by a slight worsening of the symptoms, with the development of a productive cough and purulent sputum. This is commonly believed to be due to bacterial superinfection of a viral illness; however, evidence to support this belief is scanty.

Physical Examination
Inflammation of the nasal mucosa and pharynx is commonly present. In bronchitis, percussion of the chest is normal. Coarse rhonchi that clear or shift with cough are the hallmark of bronchitis. Often the presence of small areas of pneumonia cannot be detected by physical examination.

Chest X-Ray
Not all patients with acute bronchitis and/or small areas of pneumonia require a chest x-ray for safe and effective management. The decision to use antibiotics is probably best guided by the severity of illness and the presence or absence of purulent sputum rather than by the detection of otherwise inapparent small areas of pneumonia. Chest x-rays are indicated for patients who appear more ill or for whom the diagnosis is uncertain.

Laboratory
If the sputum is purulent, a Gram's stain may yield useful information, particularly if one has any reason to suspect an unusual or opportunistic pathogen.

It has been shown that "grading" of the quality of sputum can greatly increase the likelihood that one is analyzing lower respiratory tract exudate with little upper airway contamination. Once a good-quality specimen has been obtained and gram-stained, several key observations can be made. *S. pneumoniae* can be differentiated from other gram-positive organisms with a high degree of reliability, and *H. influenzae* and other gram-negative rods can be detected when they are the predominant organisms. The absence of significant pathogens on Gram's stain should make one suspect *Mycoplasma, Legionella,* or other nonbacterial pathogens.

Sputum cultures are seldom, if ever, indicated in patients with straightforward illness because cultures done in the routine manner may miss important pathogens, fail to indicate the dominant organism, and frequently reveal only "normal respiratory flora."

In patients with lower respiratory tract infection, white blood counts with or without differential and erythrocyte sedimentation rates have also been found to distinguish poorly between bacterial and viral infection. Although cold agglutinins are frequently present in the serum of patients with *Mycoplasma* infection, this test is seldom done in the ambulatory setting because attempts to distinguish mild to moderate *Mycoplasma* infection from other causes of bronchitis are usually relatively unimportant. Serologic studies, including those for *Legionella,* can only provide retrospective confirmation of infection and are therefore primarily useful in epidemiologic surveillance studies.

Treatment

Expectorants
Oral hydration and humidification are probably the most effective agents to thin the mucoid sputum and aid the patient in clearing bronchial secretions. There is no evidence that any of the orally administered agents, such as guaifenesin, are efficacious. Saturated solution of potassium iodide (SSKI) and other iodides may have a slight mucolytic action, but their use is limited by the frequent development of iodide hypersensitivity with skin rash.

Cough Suppressants
Use of cough suppressants is controversial. There are no good clinical studies to establish whether they do more good than harm. It is conventional wisdom that coughing aids in clearing secretions and should hasten resolution. Others argue that cough suppression may encourage persistent or more severe infection by diminishing the

Table 26-1. Antibiotic choice based on Gram's stain of sputum

Gram's stain	Antibiotic and dosage
No pathogen seen (presumably viral or *Mycoplasma*)	Erythromycin, 250–500 mg PO qid for 10–14 days *or* Tetracycline, 250–500 mg PO qid for 10–14 days
Gram-positive diplococci (presumed streptococcal pneumonia)	Penicillin V, 500 mg PO qid for 10–14 days *or* Ampicillin, 500 mg PO qid for 10–14 days *or* Erythromycin, 250–500 mg PO qid for 10–14 days
Gram-negative coccobacilli (presumed *H. influenzae*)	Ampicillin, 500 mg PO qid for 10–14 days *or* Erythromycin, 250–500 mg PO qid for 10–14 days

clearance of sputum. However, the suppression of a severe, dry, hacking, nonproductive cough can provide relief to a suffering patient, and there is little evidence of harm in these circumstances.

Dextromethorphan (DM) and codeine are effective cough suppressants when given in adequate dosages (see Chap. 16). Many clinicians favor codeine even though there is no sound evidence that it is superior. The agent in which the cough suppressant is delivered makes little difference because the primary effect is centrally mediated. Most patients, however, prefer a syrup to codeine tablets.

Antibiotics
The presence of purulent sputum is frequently used as a guide to the use of antibiotics. Years of clinical tradition support this approach; however, a clinical trial in which patients with acute bronchitis with cough and purulent sputum were randomly assigned to treatment with an antibiotic or placebo showed no difference in the outcome of the two groups. If there is clinical or radiographic evidence of pneumonia, even with minimal involvement, then most physicians advocate treatment with antibiotics. The choice of specific antibiotic is usually made on the basis of a Gram's stain of the sputum (Table 26-1).

Because common organisms can develop antibiotic resistance, physicians must keep abreast of developing patterns in their own community and modify initial treatment accordingly. Resistance of *S. pneumoniae* to penicillin and *H. influenzae* to ampicillin has been reported but is present in only a very small percentage of organisms.

Follow-Up
Clinical improvement should begin within 24 to 36 hours. If the patient becomes completely asymptomatic, no clinical or radiographic follow-up is necessary. Patients should be encouraged to contact their physician promptly if they do not improve significantly or if they worsen. Persistence of symptoms beyond 2 to 3 weeks should prompt further clinical evaluation. Symptoms persisting 6 weeks mandate a chest x-ray and other studies depending on the clinical situation.

Sullivan RJ Jr, et al. Adult pneumonia in a general hospital. *Arch Intern Med* 129:935, 1972.
An excellent study of patients hospitalized for pneumonia in a large urban teaching hospital. Of greater interest for this chapter would be the equal number of patients who were treated as outpatients during the time of study.

Macfarlane JT, et al. Hospital study of adult community-acquired pneumonia. *Lancet* 2:255–258, July 1982.

> *Another excellent study of hospitalized patients with pneumonia. S. pneumoniae accounted for 76% of cases. Legionnaires' disease was second most common (15%). Good bibliography.*

Foy HM, et al. *Mycoplasma pneumoniae* pneumonia in an urban area: Five years of surveillance. *JAMA* 214:1666–1672, 1970.

> *Classical surveillance study from Group Health Cooperative of Puget Sound. Good data on the incidence of pneumonia in the population, and specific data on* Mycoplasma *including clinical syndrome and response to treatment.*

Barrett-Connor E. The nonvalue of sputum culture in the diagnosis of pneumococcal pneumonia. *Am Rev Respir Dis* 103:345–348, 1971.

> *A good study on the problems of sputum culture in the diagnosis of the etiology of pneumonia. Includes the data on sputum culture–negative patients with pneumococcal bacteremia.*

Davidson M, Tempest B, Palmer DL. Bacterial diagnosis of acute pneumonia, comparison of sputum, transtracheal aspirates and lung aspirates. *JAMA* 235:158–163, 1976.

> *Demonstrates the relative value of each technique, and provides excellent references to the literature prior to this article.*

Geckler W, et al. Microscopic and bacteriological comparison of paired sputa and transtracheal aspirates. *J Clin Microbiol*, pp. 396–399, Oct. 1977.

> *Discusses the value of "grading" the quality of sputum based on number of buccal squamous cells versus the number of leukocytes in determining if specimens are indeed of lower tract origin.*

Rein, MF, et al. Accuracy of Grams' stain in indentifying pneumococci in sputum. *JAMA* 239:2671–2673, 1978.

> *Demonstrates reliability of identifying pneumococci on sputum smear. False-negative results (38% by this study) remain a problem.*

Stott NCH, West R. Randomized controlled trial of antibiotics in patients with cough and purulent sputum. *Br Med J* 2:556–559, 1976.

> *An excellent study of 212 adults with cough and purulent sputum randomly treated with doxycycline versus placebo. There were no clinically significant differences in outcome.*

27. SOLITARY PULMONARY NODULE

Raymond F. Bianchi

A solitary pulmonary nodule (SPN), also known as a coin lesion, is round to oval and less than 6 cm in diameter; a diameter greater than 6 cm signifies a pulmonary mass. Nodules are radiographically described as homogeneous, free of infiltrate, and separated from the mediastinum and pleura by lung parenchyma.

The SPN is usually discovered on a chest x-ray obtained in an asymptomatic patient. The dilemma for both radiologist and clinician lies in determining whether the lesion is benign or malignant.

Based on a review of over 1700 patients, 53.9% of SPNs will be granulomas, 28.3% primary malignancies (usually adenocarcinoma), 6.6% hamartomas, 3.5% metastasis (nearly always located in the outer third of the lung), and 2.0% bronchial adenomas. The proportion of benign disease is higher in the Midwest and Southwest, where histoplasmosis and coccidioidomycosis are endemic. Carcinoma is more likely in those with a long history of cigarette smoking. The risk of cancer increases with age: 25 to 50% in those over age 50, compared to less than 1% in those under age 35.

Diagnostic Tests

Chest X-Rays

A benign process is favored by the absence of pulmonary symptoms, distinct nodule margins, and the presence of satellite lesions. However, these findings cannot clinically eliminate a diagnosis of malignancy. The only two radiographic criteria for benign lesions are absence of nodule growth and presence of calcium within the nodule. If old chest x-rays confirm that the nodule size has been stable for at least 2 years, the lesion is considered benign. This is based on the observation that doubling time for pulmonary malignancies is between 1 and 16 months. Doubling time refers to the change in volume: a nodule doubles in size when its radius increases by a factor of 1.26 (volume = $\pi[r^3]$).

Calcium within a nodule is nearly diagnostic of a benign process. The calcium may be deposited in concentric rings (histoplasmosis), in a popcorn pattern (hamartoma), or in a dense central nidus. Small flecks of calcium may be seen in malignant nodules, the source being either scar or granulomatous material that has been engulfed by a spreading neoplasm. Detection of calcium within a nodule by conventional radiography may be difficult, particularly when it is distributed in a homogeneous pattern. Tomography assists in identifying this type of calcification.

CT Scanning

CT scanning is currently being evaluated for use in SPN. Although inferior to tomography for identifying calcification, scanning is excellent for measuring nodule density: the denser the nodule, the more likely it is benign. The density of benign nodules comes from tight cellular organization and the deposition of calcium. Preliminary results suggest that SPNs with a representation density greater than 164 Housfield units (4 standard deviations above the mean found for malignancies) are benign. Malignancy should be considered if the value is less than 164 Housfield units or if the nodule demonstrates an "edge effect," that is, the edge of the lesion has the greatest density. (Benign lesions tend to be most dense in the middle.) Faulty technique has resulted in artificially low density and hence diagnoses of benign lesions as malignant. However, there have been no reports of artificially high densities and therefore no cancers misdiagnosed as benign.

Cytologic Analysis

Cytologic analysis of sputum is simple and noninvasive but an insensitive means of discovering malignancy. Analysis of three or more sputum samples is positive for tumor cells in only 20 to 30% of malignant SPNs.

Flexible Fiberoptic Bronchoscopy

Flexible fiberoptic bronchoscopy is recommended if sputum cytologies are nondiagnostic. The combination of fluoroscopic-guided bronchoscopic brushings and biopsy is diagnostic in 28 to 64% of SPN cases. The larger the nodule, the greater the opportunity for tissue diagnosis. Proximal lesions tend to be easier to obtain specimens from, but peripheral nodules larger than 2 cm have an equally good yield. Primary malignancies are most likely to be identified by bronchoscopy, because benign nodules and solitary metastases do not usually originate in the bronchus.

Needle Biopsy

If bronchoscopy is unrevealing, or if the SPN is peripheral and less than 2 cm in diameter, percutaneous needle aspiration biopsy should be attempted. The accuracy of skinny-needle aspiration biopsy is similar to that of bronchoscopy for diagnosing primary lung cancers larger than 2 cm, and it is superior for dealing with smaller primary malignancies and metastases. The risk of pneumothorax is approximately 25%, with about one-half of the cases requiring chest tube drainage. Serious morbidity (hemorrhage, air embolism) occurs in less than 2% of biopsies. The spreading of tumor cells or inflammatory disease along the needle tract is rare and has been associated only with larger cutting needles or with neoplasms so advanced that the seeding has no effect on the course of disease.

Thoracotomy

Thoracotomy has low mortality and morbidity, plus the benefit of early resection of a carcinomatous nodule and the peace of mind that accompanies excision of benign lesions. When the nodule is neither calcified nor demonstrated to be of stable size, resection is often the first diagnostic maneuver in patients over age 35 who are felt to be good operative risks.

Diagnostic Strategy

When an SPN is first discovered, it is often not possible to be certain of the diagnosis, short of an invasive procedure. The following recommendations represent a reasonable compromise between unnecessary diagnostic testing and failure to discover important diseases.

First, previous chest x-rays should be compared for nodule growth. A nodule of stable size for at least 2 years can be considered benign. If old chest x-rays are not available, the nodule should be evaluated for calcification. Observation of the plain film or tomography is at present the best way to examine for calcium. The workup can stop if the calcium pattern indicates the nodule is benign. Measuring nodule density by means of CT scanning may be useful at this point, but the evidence to date is inadequate to be certain.

When malignancy cannot be excluded on the basis of prior films or calcium deposition, patients under age 35 can be followed with chest x-rays every 3 months for 2 years. If there is no growth, the evaluation stops. However, if the nodule is neither calcified nor demonstrated to be stable in size, thoracotomy is indicated, particularly in patients over age 35 with a smoking history. If, considering all the relevant clinical information, it seems that immediate surgery should be avoided, a nonsurgical diagnostic approach begins with sputum cytology. A positive cytology can make the diagnosis, but since this test is of low sensitivity, a negative sputum cytology requires further evaluation. Flexible fiberoptic bronchoscopy or skinny-needle biopsy-bronchoscopy should be used for a centrally located nodule and needle biopsy for peripheral nodules or lesions less than 2 cm in diameter. Cytologic or biopsy specimens positive for malignancy indicate the need for surgery. In these cases, mediastinoscopy is generally recommended before thoracotomy. Negative cytologic or biopsy specimens are reassuring, but the patient must still be followed with serial chest x-rays.

Lillington GA. The solitary pulmonary nodule—1974. Am Rev Respir Dis 110:699–707, 1974.
  Comprehensive review of the SPN, with outline of management protocol.
Sieleman SS, et al. CT of the solitary pulmonary nodule. AJR 135:1–13, 1980.
  Benign SPNs tend to be denser than malignancies; density can be ascertained by CT scanning. Guidelines are offered for following (presumed) benign nodules without invasive tissue diagnosis.
Radke JR, et al. Diagnostic accuracy in peripheral lung lesions: Factors predicting success with flexible fiberoptic bronchoscopy. Chest 76:176–179, 1979.
  Nodule size is a critical factor in diagnostic yield from flexible fiberoptic bronchoscopy. Bronchoscopic biopsy of peripheral lesions larger than 2 cm is advocated, whereas smaller lesions should be approached by fine-needle aspiration or thoracotomy.
Mark JBD, Marglin SI, Castellino RA. The role of bronchoscopy and needle aspiration in the diagnosis of peripheral lung masses. J Thorac Cardiovasc Surg 76:266, 1978.
  Fine-needle aspiration is preferred in the diagnosis of peripheral lung lesions; bronchoscopy is additive, and both procedures can be performed with the same anesthesia. The diagnostic yield was highest for primary pulmonary malignancy.
Sagel SS, et al. Percutaneous transthoracic aspiration needle biopsy. Ann Thorac Surg 26:399–404, 1978.
  Percutaneous needle aspirate biopsy is considered as effective as cutting needle biopsy for diagnosis of suspected malignancy. Although cell type differentiation is superior with the cutting needle, the risks are greater.
Kaga AR, Steckel RJ, Braun R. Asymptomatic peripheral lung nodule. AJR 135:417–420, 1980.
  Effectiveness and relative safety of percutaneous needle biopsy are discussed. Operator and cytologist skills are emphasized.
Ray JF, et al. The coin lesion story: Update 1976. Twenty years' experience with thoracotomy for 179 suspected malignant coin lesions. Chest 70;332–336, 1976.
  This article argues that SPNs suspected of malignancy, particularly if under 2 cm should be removed by early thoracotomy. Twelve malignancies were discovered in 179 patients. An 83% five-year survival was cited, while mortality and morbidity from the thoracotomy were low.

Whitcomb ME, et al. Indications for mediastinoscopy in bronchogenic carcinoma. *Am Rev Respir Dis* 113:189–195, 1976.
The indications for mediastinoscopy are based on tumor location and tissue type. All centrally located tumors require mediastinoscopy prior to resection, whereas histologic tumor type influences whether parenchymal or peripheral lesions need further evaluation prior to resection.

Nathan MH. Management of solitary pulmonary nodules. An organized approach based on growth rate and statistics. *JAMA* 227:1141–1144, 1974.
"Watchful waiting" is the underlying message, with emphasis on conservative evaluation, particularly serial x-rays and sputum cytologies. The basis for this approach is the opinion that 42% of malignant nodules have metastasized to the mediastinum when first discovered, and excision 6 to 12 months after discovery offers as good a prognosis as does excision in less than 6 months.

Wallace JM, Deutsch AL. Flexible fiberoptic bronchoscopy and percutaneous needle lung aspiration for evaluating the solitary pulmonary nodule. *Chest* 81;665–671, 1982.
The combination of flexible fiberoptic bronchoscopy and needle aspiration provided a diagnosis in 88% of patients who were found to have a malignant solitary pulmonary nodule. Neither procedure was diagnostic in patients with benign nodules.

28. OCCUPATIONAL LUNG DISEASES
Mario C. Battigelli

Occupational disorders are adverse health effects caused by exposure to an occupation, industry, or trade. The manifestations may be primarily physical or emotional; more often, both occur together. Some occupational disorders, such as rhinitis from solvents, are self-limited and trivial. Others, such as cancers and pneumoconioses, are progressive and even fatal. The wide spectrum of organs and tissues that may be involved depends, among other factors, on portal of entry and, most critically, on the dose and rate of the exposure. For instance, mercury vapors affect principally nervous tissue, producing tremor and irritability when the exposure is of low magnitude and prolonged, but fulminant pneumonia can result when the exposure is acute and massive (e.g., fires involving mercury).

Recognition
Only a few occupational disorders, other than accidents, present with clinical features indicating their specific nature. In most instances, occupationally related diseases are clinically indistinguishable from similar diseases not related to occupational exposure. For example, a case of lung cancer in a chemical worker exposed to bis-chloromethyl ether is clinically and pathologically indistinguishable from cancer of the lung in a nonexposed individual. Similarly, industrial bronchitis that occurs in a foundry worker after sustained dust exposure cannot be differentiated from bronchitis occurring in people who smoke cigarettes. There is often a long latent period, sometimes measured in decades, between the onset of exposure and first recognition. In general, the less acute a clinical problem is, the less characteristic will be the diagnostic features that suggest an occupational etiology.

It follows that the diagnostician cannot use pattern recognition in identifying cases of occupational diseases. Often the existence of a relationship between an occupational exposure and disease can only be recognized by carefully executed research; this information can then be used to assess the plausibility of occupational disease in individual patients.

Type and Frequency
Table 28-1, which is based on over 64,000 occurrences reported in California during 1977, indicates the most common categories of occupational disorders encountered in

Table 28-1. Relative frequencies of occupational disorders*

Disorder	%
Dermatologic conditions	39.0
Eye disorders	29.6
Chemical burns	8.9
Respiratory, including pneumoconiosis	5.1
Toxic, systemic	2.9
Infective and parasitic	0.9
Others (digestive, cardiovascular, etc.)	12.8

*43,888 occurrences reported in California, 1977.
Source: From The Division of Labor Statistics. *Occupational Disease in California, 1977*. San Francisco: California Department of Industrial Relations, Aug. 1981.

medical practice. Most reports were for skin and eye conditions while systemic intoxications were relatively uncommon. For example, disorders that result from inhalation of carbon monoxide or toxic gases amount to 2% of the total. The severity of disability (work time lost of any duration) ranged from 15% in cases of hearing loss to 76% in occupational infectious diseases. About 2.4% of the entire group of occupational diseases reported in that year (1977) required hospitalization.

Only a small proportion of occupational disease is reported. Therefore, the data in Table 28-1 greatly underestimate the frequency of these disorders. Also, the apparent relative frequencies of various manifestations are likely to be determined by the ease with which they are recognized and reported, rather than their true occurrence.

Cause and Effect
A vast array of agents can cause injury and illness in exposed people (Table 28-2). Official surveys indicate that over 63,000 chemicals are in use in industry today. Three factors determine whether exposure to an occupational agent results in disease: the dose, the specific biological reactivity of a given agent, and the exposed individual's susceptibility to injury. Any agent may cause an occupational disorder when experienced in adequate strength (i.e., dose). For inhalation, dose is commonly defined by two factors: concentration and duration. In practice, however, the duration of exposure is more easily documented than the concentration. The nature of the agent suspected of being the cause of injury helps in the analysis of an exposure-injury connection. For example, a simple irritant, such as graphite dust, may be responsible for aggravating symptoms in an asthmatic, but it would not be likely to explain a devastating fibrotic process of the lung. Individual susceptibility to an agent also determines whether disease will ensue. For instance, bronchial hyperreactivity that is present prior to exposure may explain a dramatic response to an agent that, at the same dose, may not affect individuals free of this hyperreactivity.

Diagnosis
The history must elicit information about specific occupational tasks, materials handled, and work environment experienced. This must include both recent and past history. Some agents result in injury directly, but others initiate a process that does not result in manifest disease until many years after the initial exposure. The nature of the contact with the material handled must be specified (e.g., direct or remote contact, amount processed, physical nature of the material [whether solid, liquid, gas], protective garments used). Evidence of risks endured at work may be supported by reports of fellow workers complaining of symptoms consistent with those presented by the patient.

Table 28-2. Agents of injury

Agent of injury	Examples of injury
Physical	
Electricity	Electrocution
Ionizing radiation	Cancer
Noise	Deafness, vocal cord nodules
Pressure	Barotrauma
Temperature extremes	Heat casualties, frostbite
Ultraviolet light	Cataracts, cancer
Vibration	Raynaud's phenomenon
Chemical	
Inhalation exposure agents	
Vapors, gases, fumes, mist	Inhalation casualties
Dust and fibers	Asthma, pneumoconiosis
Agents acting through the skin	Dermatosis
Ingested agents	Lead poisoning, paraquat
Biologic	
Infectious agents—bacteria, mycobacteria, rickettsia, virus	Sanitation work casualties
Parasites	Ankylostomiasis
Others: plant and animal products	Asthmatic syndrome
Stressors	
Effort and fatigue	Repeated motion trauma
Psychological agents of injury or stress	Burnout syndromes

Route and Physical Form of Exposure

Inhalation, skin absorption, and ingestion are, in order of importance, the ways in which exposures take place. The physical characteristics of an airborne contaminant must be known, as well as its chemical nature and its biological reactivity. Coarse particles, greater than 10 μ, usually have an effect limited to the surfaces of the upper respiratory system (e.g., wood dust affects paranasal sinuses). Water-soluble chemicals, once airborne, also tend to affect preferentially the upper respiratory surfaces (e.g., chromic acid mists cause nasal septal ulcer). Conversely, small particles and less soluble chemicals involve most characteristically the deepest portions of the respiratory system (e.g., oxides of nitrogen, fine-particle aerosols, oily mists cause brancheolitis, alveolitis, edema). For skin penetration, high solubility, neutrality, and an elevated lipid-water partition are the main factors of absorption. Furthermore, concentration, extent and duration of contact, as well as skin conditions, including anatomical site (palpebral, axillary, volar, and abdominal surfaces), are all important elements favoring the uptake of a substance through the skin.

Quantitative Assessment of Exposure

Report of mere exposure to a potentially harmful agent or condition cannot be considered sufficient evidence for injury. The dose of exposure is the most important information for establishing causation; a low dose is a less likely cause of injury and disease than a substantial dose. Once the quantitative estimate of exposure is obtained, the likelihood that it will cause disease can be assessed by using reference guides such as the *Threshold Limit Values* published by the American Conference of Governmental Industrial Hygienists. This assessment is greatly helped by measurements at the work environment, such as those provided by an industrial hygiene survey or by data on file concerning the specific work setting.

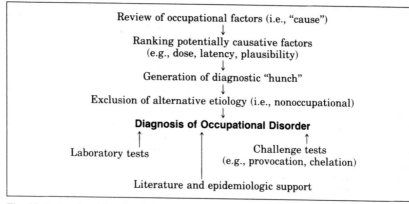

Fig. 28-1. An algorithm for diagnosing occupational diseases.

Special Diagnostic Tests
In order to verify and/or strengthen the evidence for a cause-and-effect relationship, specific diagnostic procedures can sometimes be employed. These include the patch test for dermatologic problems, inhalation of the suspected agent in respiratory asthmatic disorders, and the chelation test with certain heavy metals. The last allows an estimate of body burden by monitoring urinary elimination of certain substances (i.e., metals) during chelation treatment.

Diagnostic Algorithm
An orderly series of steps is followed in assessing the probability of an occupational cause for disease (Fig. 28-1). The sequence starts with the selection of a "pivot" feature which characterizes the clinical presentation. This is matched against the list of possible causes present at work. The list is derived from the inventory of the work environment/history and is arranged in order of probability of injury. More plausible or common factors of causation, such as those pertaining to nonoccupational categories (e.g., common infections, tobacco smoke effects), are considered and excluded. The most probable match of a pivot clinical manifestation with the pertinent exposure dose is explored. Laboratory verification by analysis of tissues and biological fluids (e.g., blood, urine) further supports the occupational cause of a disorder. Epidemiological information obtained from the literature or from work records, such as reports of additional occurrences of related problems, particularly when observed in the recent past at the same and/or similar locations, often helps in strengthening the diagnostic conclusions.

Treatment and Prevention
The basic corrective measure is avoidance. This is best accomplished, in the long run, by reduced exposure at its source. Methods include improved industrial hygiene (e.g., ventilation, enclosure) and monitoring exposure by either medical surveillance or environmental control (e.g., air sampling), or both. Personal protective devices are appropriate for high-intensity, brief exposures. However, they are often uncomfortable or inconvenient, so that compliance with them is likely to be low; therefore, they are not a long-term solution. Workers should be educated about work practices as soon as they are exposed to a particular risk, and this training should be reviewed periodically.

Legal Responsibility
Special statutes regulate the reporting and compensation of occupational disorders. In certain states, it is mandatory that compensable diseases be reported to the state agencies with pertinent jurisdiction.

The elements of compensation vary according to the different statutes, but all include the identification, by the reporting physician, of a state of disability (interference with fitness to work), a specific causality (occupational cause-and-effect relationship), and a quantitative assessment of the extent and type of impairment observed, whether partial or total, temporary or permanent.

Records or transactions related to a workman's compensation evaluation are usually considered free of the privileged information restriction. The information can be made available to the employer and/or the investigating agency without specific consent by the worker.

Division of Labor Statistics. *Occupational Disease in California, 1977.* San Francisco: California Department of Industrial Relations, Aug. 1981.

This report reflects the experience of the state of California, which provides the only tabulation of actually reported disorders of occupational nature. The frequencies cited are affected by the reporting compliance and should not be directly extrapolated to the experience of other states.

NIOSH-OSHA. *Pocket Guide to Chemical Hazards, USDHHS.* Washington, DC: Government Printing Office, 1980.

This truly pocket-sized guide, available on request from NIOSH, is a valuable quick reference giving basic elements of hazard for an array of chemicals, listed alphabetically.

Rom WN. *Environmental and Occupational Medicine.* Boston: Little, Brown, 1983.

This book assembles, with reasonably succinct descriptions, a range of disorders of occupational nature. Additional items of management and control of environmental hazards are presented by a wide variety of authors. It also includes examples of inhalation provocation tests and patch testing and offers a brief discussion of casualties of stress and related subjects.

Taking the occupational history. *Ann Intern Med* 99:641–651, 1983.

This 10-page synopsis was prepared with the specific aim of assisting the internist in obtaining an occupational history.

VI. CARDIOVASCULAR PROBLEMS

C. Stewart Rogers

There is no sharp distinction between "normal" and "abnormal" blood pressure (BP). The correlation between BP and the most prevalent cardiovascular disorders (atherosclerosis, heart failure, and stroke) begins well within the normal range and continues into the range we call "hypertensive." This chapter reviews what is known about the effects of treating various kinds of people with various patterns and levels of BP.

The Risk of Hypertension
Studies of the natural history of hypertension have established that

1. High blood pressure causes direct mechanical morbidity (e.g., hemorrhagic stroke, aortic dissection, congestive heart failure) and contributes to the progression of atherosclerosis, retinopathy, and renal failure in a more prolonged and indirect manner.
2. While both diastolic (DBP) and systolic (SBP) pressures are highly correlated with morbidity, systolic pressure is the stronger predictor of morbid outcomes.
3. Hypertension interacts with other risk factors—especially cigarette smoking, cholesterol levels, and diabetes— so that their risk together is greater than the sum of their risks individually. The magnitude of risk varies enormously with age, sex, and the presence of other risk factors (see Chap. 128).
4. All BP is labile; higher pressures are more labile than lower ones. There is no safety in lability and no evidence that a "basal pressure"—usually meaning the lowest pressure one can obtain—is a better predictor of risk than is a casual reading or an average of several measurements.
5. Women do not tolerate hypertension better than do men. Direct mechanical damage from hypertension is equally prevalent in men and women at any age. Symptomatic atherosclerosis in women is generally delayed beyond menopause, but thereafter the effects of hypertension are similar.
6. The elderly do not have a special tolerance for hypertension. Instead, the relation of morbidity to BP actually accelerates with advancing age. This is true for both diastolic and isolated systolic patterns of hypertension.
7. In the United States, black men and women have higher mean BPs than whites at every age and a higher prevalence of hypertension. Likewise, blacks have much higher rates of hypertensive complications, especially strokes, cardiac failure, and nephrosclerosis.

The Value of Treatment
It has long been accepted that malignant hypertension should be treated. Sound evidence on the value of treating lesser degrees of chronic hypertension became available in the late 1960s and after with the development of effective oral antihypertensive drugs. Trials of treatment have used DBP (usually disappearance of the fifth Korotkoff sound) as their criteria, so DBP is our point of comparison even though SBP is more closely related to morbid events.

Severe Hypertension
The first large, placebo-controlled trial was undertaken by the Veterans Administration and concluded in 1970. It was clear that for subjects entering the study with DBP greater than 105 mm Hg, active treatment effected a marked reduction in morbidity. For example, in the group with a DBP of 105 to 114 mm Hg, active treatment resulted in a 75% reduction in morbid cardiovascular events compared to placebo. Stroke, congestive heart failure, and accelerated hypertension were observed almost exclusively in the placebo group, while the study was inconclusive for myocardial infarction. Elderly patients profited from active therapy to the same extent as did younger ones. The drugs used (hydrochlorothiazide, reserpine, and hydralazine) were clearly effective in lowering BP even in patients with severe hypertension. The drugs were also well tolerated, with major side effects (including peptic ulcer and depression) being equally observed in placebo and treatment groups. Finally, even partial reduction of pressure conferred major benefit. Of the maximal benefit observed with full control of DBP,

about 75% was achieved in patients who were actively treated but whose DBP remained above 90 mm Hg.

The VA study was limited to compliant male veterans without other important disease, and its results can not necessarily be generalized to other kinds of patients.

Mild Diastolic Hypertension

It is well established that people with DBP greater than 105 mm Hg should be treated. Twenty million Americans (70% of all hypertensives) have DBP of 90 to 104 mm Hg. These people are clearly at risk, but can they benefit from treatment? Potential benefits of treatment must be weighed against several costs: the investment of money and time, potential adverse psychological effects accompanying the diagnosis ("labeling"), and the possible debilitating effects of antihypertensive drugs.

Three large, community-based trials of treating less severe elevations of DBP have been reported since 1979, and a fourth is in progress. These studies support the following general conclusions:

1. Hypertension can be controlled in most of the general population. A majority of patients requires two or more drugs, and considerable cost and drug morbidity are encountered, even in the mildly hypertensive group.
2. Most benefits of treatment within the total "mild" group accrue to patients with the higher DBPs (e.g., patients with a DBP of 100–110 mm Hg suffered more excess morbidity than those with a DBP of 90–100 mm Hg).
3. Patients with lesser degrees of hypertension (e.g., 90–100 mm Hg) are most likely to benefit from treatment if they are among those whose BP subsequently rises to higher levels. In one study, only a small fraction of those placed on *placebo* advanced during 4 years follow-up to a DBP greater than 100 mm Hg, and this small group accounted for all of the 30% excess morbidity as compared to the active treatment group.
4. Benefits from active treatment require continuous adherence to the protocol.

Factors other than BP must be weighed in the decision to treat hypertension. Other risk factors, including SBP, age, sex, cardiovascular status, and renal function, exert an amplifier effect on the danger of increased BPs, as do other atherosclerotic risk factors such as smoking, diabetes, and high cholesterol. It is reasonable to assume that reducing mildly elevated BP in persons with these other factors is especially useful. Likewise, the presence of existing atherosclerotic disease can be taken as evidence of individual susceptibility and grounds for aggressive management. Evidence that hypertension accelerates retinopathy in diabetics suggests that hypertension should be treated more vigorously in these patients. For most others with a DBP in the mildest range (85–100 mm Hg), a period of surveillance, diet, and education may be pursued for several months. Thereafter, only those with a DBP exceeding 100 mm Hg would be treated with drugs, and the rest would be followed indefinitely with that therapeutic threshold in mind.

Systolic Hypertension

Systolic hypertension usually coexists with diastolic hypertension but may be predominant or even isolated (e.g., 220/80 mm Hg). Isolated systolic hypertension is a major disease pattern in older patients, reaching a prevalence of 30% in the eighth decade. While balanced hypertension can usually be treated in the same way as diastolic hypertension, we presently have no firm basis for directing treatment of systolic hypertension, since no study has selected subjects for systolic hypertension or has targeted a goal SBP. Reasons for giving less attention to SBP are based on several conceptions of systolic hypertension in the elderly, which have led some to discount its importance. Systolic blood pressure is said to be highly labile. It has been said to reflect cardiac function rather than the arteriolar resistance that is so important to theories of chronic essential hypertension. More cogently, systolic hypertension is argued to be the result of established central atherosclerosis and so a marker of existing disease rather than a cause. The fatalist viewpoint that systolic hypertension cannot be effectively treated unless we can reverse the underlying vasculopathy is supported by the difficulties in controlling isolated systolic hypertension without compromising orthostatic adjustments or coronary perfusion.

These arguments may contain some truth but do not in themselves justify abandoning efforts at treatment. Everything we have learned about lowering BPs promises long-term benefits if we can avoid short-term costs. Although no data can be cited, it seems advisable to lower systolic pressure over 180 mm Hg, with an initial goal of 10% reduction and eventual normalization if tolerated.

The treatment of isolated systolic hypertension is especially difficult because it so often occurs in the elderly, whose treatment is complicated by varying degrees of atherosclerosis, other systemic disease, impaired cardiac and renal function, and concurrent drug therapy. In addition, treatment of the elderly is most likely to be complicated by postural hypotension because of reduced aortic compliance, a hemodynamic pattern of high peripheral resistance with low plasma volume, and a reduced baroreceptor sensitivity. Coronary occlusive disease renders patients especially sensitive to falls in diastolic perfusion pressure, while left ventricular failure obviates myocardial depressant drugs, such as reserpine and beta-blockers. Lastly, the contracted plasma volumes of the elderly predispose to prerenal azotemia with diuretic use.

Thus, although it is desirable in the long run to treat hypertension in elderly patients, there is greater potential for short-term harm, and regimens must be closely monitored. Specific treatment guidelines are described in Chapter 31.

Kannel WB. Some lessons in cardiovascular epidemiology from Framingham. *Am J Cardiol* 37:269–282, 1976.
An excellent history of this great project and succinct review of the major findings and their implications for practice of preventive medicine.

Freis ED, et al. Effects of treatment on morbidity in hypertension (the VA trial). Part I, *JAMA* 202:116–122, 1967; Part II, *JAMA* 213:1143–1152, 1970.
A classic in modern internal medicine, the basis of our motivation to treat hypertension. Should be read by all practitioners of adult medicine to dispel any doubts about need for therapy, for historic perspective, and as an elegant example of clinical investigation.

Hypertension Detection and Follow-up Program Cooperative Group. Five year findings of the hypertension detection and follow-up program, Parts I and II. *JAMA* 242:2562–2571, 1979.
A huge American field trial of two systems of primary care with special attention to mild hypertension. Clearly proves that a highly structured and totally sponsored clinic system reduces mortality (cardiovascular and noncardiovascular) compared to the mix of health care resources in our communities. It is unclear what it proves about mild hypertension.

Report by the Management Committee. The Australian therapeutic trial in mild hypertension. *Lancet* 1:1261–1267, 1980.
A placebo-controlled mild hypertension trial, which seems to demonstrate value of therapy. Should be read along with Dr. Ram's editorial (see below) for critical qualification.

Ram CVS. Should mild hypertension be treated? *Ann Intern Med* 99:403–405, 1983.
A concise review of the major trials of mild hypertension, including the Multiple Risk Factor Intervention Trial which has led to a re-evaluation of the costs and benefits of treating DBP 90–100.

Gifford RW Jr, et al. The dilemma of "mild" hypertension. *JAMA* 250:3171–3173, 1983.
This is a rebuttal of the conservative viewpoint on mild hypertension. The several major trials are reviewed yet again and the treatment of DBP 90–100 is strongly supported. This should be read with Dr. Ram's editorial for balance.

Kannel WB, Dawber TR, McGee DL. Perspectives on systolic hypertension. *Circulation* 61:1179–1182, 1980.
Review of the Framingham data, which has led authors to maintain a consistent focus on systolic hypertension as a major risk factor. Addresses the question of whether systolic hypertension is merely a marker of atherosclerosis.

Kirkendall WM, Hammond JJ. Hypertension in the elderly. *Arch Intern Med* 140:1155–1161, 1980.
Comprehensive review and bibliography of epidemiology and therapy of hypertension in older patients, including the issues of systolic hypertension. Contains an excellent review of the indirect evidence favoring treatment and a long bibliography.

Gifford RW Jr. Isolated systolic hypertension in the elderly. *JAMA* 247:781–785, 1982.
A brief subject review, incorporating relevant data from recent mild hypertension trials and setting the stage for the more definitive intervention trials currently underway that specifically target elderly patients and systolic hypertension. Includes a brief, practical section on therapy.

30. HYPERTENSION: INITIAL EVALUATION
Edward H. Wagner

When a patient is first found to have an elevated blood pressure (BP), the clinician confronts three questions in planning an evaluation: Does this patient have hypertension? If so, what information should be collected to determine if it is essential or secondary hypertension? If it is essential hypertension, what information should be collected to help plan management? The answers to these questions will determine the extent and content of the initial evaluation.

Confirming Elevated Blood Pressure
There are many reasons why a given individual may be found to have an elevated BP on a single determination, only one of which is sustained hypertension. Errors in measurement can result from the use of unstandardized aneroid manometers or from faulty procedures. Indirect BP can be falsely elevated, by as much as 10 to 30 mm Hg, if the patient's arm is obese and a large cuff is not used. In addition, arterial pressure varies in response to many stimuli; for example, pressures are generally higher during the day than at night, in a clinic than at home, outside the hospital than in, and during periods of stress compared to periods of tranquility. If BP is measured during a moment of relative elevation, an erroneous impression of the basal BP may be obtained. Depending on the extent of an initial elevation, as many as 40% of individuals with a single elevated BP will be found to be normotensive on repeat examination. This phenomenon, termed regression to the mean, results from the fact that individuals selected for re-examination because of an elevation on a single occasion include some who happened to have been caught at a moment when their BP was higher than usual.

Thus, to avoid the risk of committing a normotensive patient to a diagnosis that has rather grave implications, physicians must ensure that BP measurements are accurate and insist on multiple BP elevations before the diagnosis is confirmed. Current consensus recommendations seem prudent and appropriate: "After screening, the diagnosis of hypertension is confirmed when the average of multiple blood pressure measurements made on at least two subsequent visits is 90 mm Hg or higher" (The Joint National Committee on Detection, Evaluation, and Treatment of High Blood Pressure, 1980).

Detecting Secondary Hypertension
It has generally been taught that a substantial proportion of hypertension occurs secondary to known causes, many of which are reversible, and that the identification and correction of such causes avoid the necessity of lifelong treatment in some patients. Such causes include surgically correctable lesions, such as renal artery stenosis, pheochromocytoma, hyperaldosteronism, and coarctation, and the use of drugs like oral contraceptives, appetite suppressants, sympathomimetics, and large quantities of licorice. Of these, renovascular hypertension constitutes the great majority, while aldosterone-secreting tumors make up most of the rest.

Whether the search for secondary hypertension should be part of a routine evaluation depends on its frequency, the accuracy and cost of diagnostic procedures for detection, and the response of surgically correctable lesions to conventional medical treatment.

Frequency
Conventional teaching, based on a single important study of patients visiting a large referral center, has been that approximately 10% of adult hypertensive patients have

a secondary cause of their hypertension and perhaps half of those will have a surgically correctable cause. More recently, however, it has become apparent that in more unselected populations, such as in primary care practice or in the community, the prevalence of surgically correctable hypertension is about 0.7%, approximately one-tenth that reported from referral centers.

The lesser prevalence of secondary causes in unselected settings reduces the efficiency of diagnostic efforts in two ways. First, the yield of diagnostic evaluations will be negative more frequently and the costs of detecting a patient with surgically correctable disease will increase. Second, when individual patients are tested, the likelihood that a positive test represents disease (the "positive predictive value") declines as the prevalence of disease among those tested falls. For example, with a prevalence of renovascular hypertension of 1%, 94% of all positive intravenous pyelograms (IVPs) would be false positives.

Improving the Yield of Tests

How can the prevalence of secondary hypertension be increased among those tested? Physicians can reduce the number of hypertensives considered to be "at risk" of surgically correctable hypertension by confining the diagnostic workup to those with a higher likelihood (prevalence) of having a surgically correctable cause.

Certain findings from history, physical examination, and laboratory tests increase the likelihood of surgically correctable hypertension. Young age of onset, absence of a family history, and recent onset appear to be somewhat more common in patients with renal artery stenosis, for example. Unfortunately, they are also relatively common among patients with essential hypertension as well.

More specific clinical evidence in deciding which patients to study more thoroughly is indicated in Table 30-1. Reliance on the presence of these few clinical clues, mostly obtained by an appropriate history and physical examination, will reduce by a factor of 10 or more those patients who may require further evaluation.

Once the determination is made to proceed with further workup, the selection of subsequent tests is controversial. Chest x-ray, followed by aortography, is appropriate for coarctation. Although there is no consensus on other testing, the following have the broadest empiric support: rapid-sequence IVP for renal artery stenosis, plasma catecholamines or urinary metanephrines for pheochromocytoma, and serum potassium and serum aldosterone after sodium loading for aldosterone-producing adenoma.

Results of Treatment

How important is it to diagnose surgically treatable hypertension? Many patients with one of the four most prevalent surgically correctable causes of hypertension respond to conventional pharmacologic therapy. There are no clear guidelines at present for the

Table 30-1. Clinical clues to surgically correctable hypertension

Diagnosis	Clinical clues	Prevalence for hypertension specific diagnoses (%)	Prevalence in unselected hypertensives (%)
Renal artery stenosis	Abdominal bruit	70	10
	Grade III or IV retinopathy	25	10
Pheochromocytoma	Adrenergic attacks	80	Presumably low
	Orthostatic hypotension	60	Presumably low in untreated patients
Aldosterone-producing adenoma	Hypokalemia (<3.6 mEq/L)	80	10
Coarctation	Diminished distal BP levels	Reported to be common	Presumably rare

optimal management of functionally significant renal artery stenosis. Many experts take the view that only patients not responding to conventional medical therapy should be exposed to surgical intervention. The recent developments of angioplasty and captopril further complicate decision-making. Although a variety of factors differentiate low-risk from high-risk surgical candidates, there is no clear evidence that patients who respond to medical therapy achieve greater benefits from surgical intervention.

Similar uncertainty may pertain to the choice of therapy in hyperaldosteronism. For pheochromocytoma and coarctation, however, surgical therapy remains the treatment of choice despite some responsiveness to medical therapy, because of the occurrence of malignancy and catecholamine myocardial disease in the former and endocarditis, dissection, or intracranial hemorrhage in the latter.

In summary, except for pheochromocytoma or coarctation, there may not be compelling reasons to search for surgically correctable hypertension. For this reason, many feel that the strongest indication for a more aggressive diagnostic approach to search for surgically correctable disease would be accelerating or severe hypertension in the face of adequate medical therapy, taken as prescribed.

Planning Management

Information collected during evaluation may influence the selection of therapy. Relative contraindications to various drugs, such as a history of heart failure or asthma (beta-blockers), depression or peptic ulcer (reserpine), or angina (hydralazine), will prompt the selection of alternative agents. Similarly, elevated BP in a young woman who uses oral contraceptives should, in most instances, lead to the recommendation of another method of birth control.

Measures of plasma renin activity (PRA) have been advocated as useful to "tailor" antihypertensive therapy to the pathophysiologic state of the individual patient. Randomized trials that have examined the relative efficacy of beta-blockers versus diuretics in low-renin and high-renin patients have not confirmed that these subgroups of hypertensive patients respond differently to these two classes of agents. Thus, at present, the use of PRA as a routine baseline measure does not appear to be warranted.

Table 30-2. Recommended initial workup of the hypertensive patient

History
    Beliefs and attitudes about hypertension and its treatment
    Duration of elevated BP
    Previous treatment
    Use of drugs (oral contraceptives, appetite suppressants, sympathomimetics)
    Health behaviors
    Muscle weakness or polyuria
    Attacks of headaches, palpitations, sweats

Physical examination
    Sitting and standing
    BP determinations
    Height and weight
    Fundoscopic
    Neck veins
    Carotid auscultation
    Cardiac examination
    Abdominal examination, including auscultation
    Peripheral pulses, including radial/femoral lag
    Neurologic (if warranted)

Laboratory tests
    Urinalysis
    Serum potassium
    Serum creatinine (BUN)
    Serum cholesterol
    Blood glucose
    Serum uric acid
    Electrocardiogram

The Initial Workup

Table 30-2 lists procedures appropriate for the routine initial evaluation of the new hypertensive (following appropriate confirmation of the diagnosis) that provide information that might alter the diagnostic or therapeutic approach. These recommendations coincide closely to current consensus guidelines of the Joint National Committee on Detection, Evaluation, and Treatment of High Blood Pressure (1980). The recommended workup includes a relatively complete history and physical examination with special emphasis given to clues suggesting secondary causes. Of special note is the limited extent of the laboratory evaluation.

Perhaps the most critical aspect of the initial evaluation is the unhurried exchange of information about the disease and the establishment of a long-term relationship based on mutual understanding of priorities and concerns between patient and physician. Many patients harbor beliefs and fears about hypertension and antihypertensive therapy. These patterns of beliefs may well influence the hypertensive patient's response to the illness and the prescription of therapy. The systematic assessment of a patient's concerns about the disease, and mutual discussion in light of known facts, may be an essential early step in long-term management. The selection of laboratory tests may be trivial by comparison.

Hypertension Detection and Follow-up Program Cooperative Group. Patient participation in a hypertension control program. *JAMA* 239:1507, 1978.
This early paper from a major hypertension intervention randomized trial demonstrates the importance of multiple BP measurements after an initial elevation because of the large proportion of patients whose BP becomes normal on subsequent readings.

The Joint National Committee on Detection, Evaluation, and Treatment of High Blood Pressure. The 1980 report of the Joint National Committee on Detection, Evaluation, and Treatment of High Blood Pressure. *Arch Intern Med* 140:1280, 1980.
This paper outlines and discusses consensus guidelines for hypertension management; it is thoughtful and worth the attention of all primary care physicians.

Gifford RW. Evaluation of the hypertensive patient with emphasis on detecting curable causes. *Milbank Mem Fund Q* 47:170, 1969.
This now classic paper carefully describes the distribution of secondary hypertension in a referral setting.

Berglund G, Anderson O, Wilhelmsen L. Prevalence of primary and secondary hypertension: Studies in a random population sample. *Br Med J* 2:5543, 1976.

Rudnick KV, et al. Hypertension in a family practice. *Can Med Assoc J* 17:492, 1977.
These papers describe the prevalence of secondary hypertension in a community sample (Berglund et al.) and a community primary care practice (Rudnick et al.), demonstrating much lower rates than seen in referral practice.

Simon N, et al. Clinical characteristics of renovascular hypertension. *JAMA* 220:1209, 1972.
These reports from a large collaborative study of renovascular hypertension provide useful information regarding the diagnostic utility of various clinical features and radiologic procedures.

Grim CE, et al. Sensitivity and specificity of screening tests for renal vascular hypertension. *Ann Intern Med* 91:617, 1979.
This useful study compares the sensitivities and specificities of various tests used to diagnose renal artery stenosis.

Bravo EL, et al. Circulating and urinary catecholamines in pheochromocytoma. *N Engl J Med* 301:682, 1979.
This careful study assesses the utility of various measures of catecholamines and their metabolites in the diagnosis of pheochromocytoma.

Carey RM. Screening for surgically correctable hypertension caused by primary aldosteronism. *Arch Intern Med* 141:1594, 1981.
This report sheds some light on the confusing array of metabolic indicators used in the evaluation of suspected hyperaldosteronism.

Yamauchi H. Screening hypertensive patients for surgically reversible causes: Unsettled issues. *Heart Lung* 10:261, 1981.
This provocative review seriously questions the wisdom of aggressively evaluating patients for secondary hypertension.

Rudnick MR, Bastl CP, Narins RG. Diagnostic Approaches to Hypertension. In BM

Brenner and JHJ Stein (Eds.), *Hypertension*. New York: Churchill Livingstone, 1981. P. 270.

This comprehensive and balanced review of diagnostic questions in hypertension is worth reading both for its insights and the bibliography.

Woods JW, et al. Renin profiling in hypertension and its use in treatment with propranolol and chlorthalidone. *N Engl J Med* 294:1137, 1976.

Holland OB, Fairchild C. Renin classification for diuretic and beta-blocker treatment of black hypertensive patients. *J Chronic Dis* 35:179, 1982.

These two well-designed therapeutic trials show that tailoring therapy based on plasma renin levels offers no therapeutic advantage.

Kasl S. A social-psychologic perspective on successful community control of high blood pressure: A review. *J Behav Med* 1:347, 1978.

This thoughtful and comprehensive review of psychosocial issues in community hypertension control has many valuable insights for the primary care provider.

31. HYPERTENSION: TREATMENT

C. Stewart Rogers

Current treatment of hypertension involves choices among many possible interventions. Most physicians follow a "stepped care" strategy in which they begin with relatively simple, safe interventions and proceed to more powerful, complex, and potentially toxic ones. This approach is usually followed regardless of baseline severity of disease or its specific causes or biochemical markers.

Step One

General Considerations

Once the diagnosis of lasting hypertension has been made, patient education is essential. Issues to be stressed are as follows:

1. Hypertension is, with few exceptions, a lifelong condition that is usually asymptomatic.
2. There is excellent evidence that treatment reduces the risk of complications.
3. A tolerable therapeutic regimen can almost always be found because there are a great many options.
4. Patients play a critical role in maintaining their own health.

The message should be kept simple: follow the prescribed regimen, and stay in touch. Advice that is either less beneficial, less realistically achievable, or more discouraging (e.g., weight loss, cessation of smoking, and exercise) can be addressed during or after establishment of the basic regimen.

Diet

Salt restriction and weight reduction (in obese patients) both lower blood pressure (BP). Salt restriction is often downplayed because it is intrusive and is considered unnecessary with the potent oral diuretics available. However, growing awareness of drug costs and toxicity, interest in nutrition, and the desire of many patients to assert more responsibility for health maintenance has countered this trend. Many Americans habitually consume more than 200 mEq of sodium daily. General reduction of a few high-sodium items in the diet (e.g., packaged meats, canned soups, snack foods, pickles, tomato juice) will drop most diets below 200 mEq of sodium per day (see Chap. 141).

Diuretics

Diuretics are routinely suggested for step one because they are relatively cheap, are effective taken once a day, require little titration, and have very few contraindications or serious adverse effects. They are effective for hypertension of all degrees of severity and prevent the renin-mediated fluid retention provoked by most nondiuretic hypotensive agents.

The cheapest diuretic is hydrochlorothiazide (HCTZ). It maintains its full hypotensive effect consistently for over 24 hours and is thus effective in daily dosing even though its plasma half-life and duration of enhanced diuresis are short.

Several other thiazides, as well as chlorthalidone, metolazone, and loop diuretics (furosemide, ethacrynic acid), are widely used as step-one diuretics. These are much more expensive and share most of the metabolic side effects of HCTZ (hypokalemia, hyperuricemia, hyperglycemia). Of these drugs, only thiazides raise serum calcium, but the elevation is usually mild, transient, and clinically unimportant. The only reasons for choosing nonthiazide diuretics are drug allergy and the presence of renal failure (creatinine clearance below 30 ml per minute) or heart failure, in which loop agents are usually required for effective diuresis.

The metabolic side effects are not cause to avoid diuretics. Hyperuricemia may occasionally provoke gout, but this is easily recognized and treated. Asymptomatic hyperuricemia need not be treated. Diuretics can unmask diabetes but do not cause it or precipitate crises and complications. However, hypoglycemic therapy may require adjustment when diuretics are started or stopped.

Most patients with uncomplicated hypertension treated chronically with usual dosages of diuretics will manifest some fall in serum potassium, but less than 10% will develop clinically important potassium depletion. Most people remain asymptomatic and unharmed by serum potassium of 3.0 to 3.5 mEq/L unless they are taking digitalis. If potassium falls below this level, the possibility of hyperaldosteronism should be considered and a careful dietary history should be done to estimate sodium and potassium intake. A large salt intake requires large natriuresis, which obligates a larger loss of potassium. Lowering sodium intake may solve the problem and may even achieve further reduction of BP.

When supplemental potassium is given to patients taking diuretics, it must be as a chloride. Medicinal potassium chloride is packaged as various bitter liquids, fizzy tablets, and slow-release tablets. Prices of the various preparations do not differ much. Combination products containing HCTZ and a potassium-sparing diuretic may prevent hypokalemia and are comparable in price to the two drugs separately; these include Dyazide (contains triamterene), Aldactazide (contains spironolactone), and Moduretic (contains amiloride). It is dangerous to prescribe both potassium supplements and potassium-sparing diuretics together, and the potassium-sparing diuretics should not be used in renal failure. Any means of maintaining serum potassium adds $10 to $20 per month to the regimen as well as complexity and bother, which are reasons for dropping out of care. Therefore, this should be undertaken only in the minority of patients who require it.

Beta-Blockers

Beta-blockers produce sustained benefit in about half of patients when used alone and block the reflex fluid retention by suppressing renin release. They are therefore an alternative choice for a step-one drug. Disadvantages compared to diuretics alone are their much greater cost, the enormous dose-response range (which at times requires a long titration process), and a number of serious toxicities for susceptible persons. However, if the hypertension coexists with angina, essential tremor, migraine, or a recent myocardial infarction, a beta-blocker can treat the two conditions at once.

Step Two

Almost half of patients with essential hypertension require a second drug to achieve BP control. Most physicians add a sympathoplegic, for which the costs, bother, and side effects are major concerns. All the sympathoplegics must be used with a diuretic to block reflex fluid retention.

Reserpine

Reserpine was the sympathoplegic used in the landmark VA trials on which our therapy of moderate hypertension is based. It has several advantages: it is considerably cheaper than alternate sympathoplegics, it is given once a day, and it reaches nearly full effect at the starting dose of 0.125 mg per day, so that little or no titration is needed. Reserpine is not a particularly toxic drug. There is no acceptable evidence that reserpine actually causes or exacerbates peptic ulcer disease or breast cancer. In the VA trial, most adverse effects (including depression) occurred with similar frequency in both active drug and placebo groups. Reserpine may cause more nasal congestion than other drugs and shares with beta-blockers a negative inotropic effect. Depression has been reported with reserpine and several other antihypertensive medications. Likewise, sedation and impotence may occur with most sympathoplegics. There are no sound studies comparing the frequency of side effects of the several sympathoplegics.

Methyldopa and Clonidine

Methyldopa and clonidine both act in the central nervous system to modify sympathetic outflow. They cause sedation when they are first given, which usually improves after a few days. In rare instances, methyldopa causes toxic hepatitis, and a transaminase should be checked if suspicion of acquired liver disease arises. Clonidine and methyldopa have both been reported to induce a withdrawal syndrome after abrupt discontinuation, with hyperadrenergic discomforts and rapid reversion to pretreatment BP. This may be more common with clonidine, especially in doses greater than 0.8 mg per day.

Beta-Blockers

Beta-blockers reduce BP by reducing cardiac output, and secondary fluid retention is lessened by inhibition of renin release. They may be used alone in hypertension but are usually more effective when combined with a diuretic. There are five beta-blockers on the American market: atenolol and metoprolol are semispecific for β_1 receptors, propranolol and timolol reduce mortality after myocardial infarction, and atenolol and nadolol are approved for once daily dosing.

Beta-blockers have an enormous dose-response range, and, as with the sympathoplegics (except reserpine), several office visits may be required to ascertain the effective dosage. Because of their physiologic effects, beta-blockers should not be given to patients with some common chronic problems. Congestive heart failure, atrioventricular block, and bradycardia are all worsened by beta-blockers and may be unmasked by these drugs. A true bronchospastic disorder is a contraindication to any beta-blocker, although emphysema that does not involve bronchospasm may not be affected by a β_1 specific blocker. Patients with Raynaud's phenomenon and some with peripheral vascular disease should not use nonselective blockers, and vasospastic angina can theoretically be aggravated by leaving alpha-constrictor tone unopposed. The adrenergic response to insulin-induced hypoglycemia is masked, leaving the tightly controlled diabetic with no warning of impending neuroglycopenic coma.

Although beta-blockers reduce cardiac output, most patients can easily tolerate this; however, the elderly and patients with compromised left ventricular function may notice decreased exercise tolerance. These drugs do not cause sedation, but they tend to be enervating. Central nervous system effects, especially disturbed sleep and depression, develop insidiously and are probably unusual.

One reason for using beta-blockers in hypertension is the presence of a coexisting disease also treated with these drugs, such as angina, essential tremor, migraine, and certain arrhythmias, and for the prevention of death in recent survivors of acute myocardial infarction.

Prazosin

Prazosin is a sympathoplegic drug that blocks postsynaptic alpha-receptors. It has one unique precaution: syncope can occur with first use or with dosage increments. This can be prevented with small doses and small changes and by taking the first dose at bedtime to avoid orthostatic effects. Prazosin should be used with a diuretic and can be combined with another step-two drug. Because it results in balanced venodilation and afterload reduction, prazosin may have a special advantage for hypertensive patients with chronic congestive heart failure.

Hydralazine

Hydralazine is a direct vasodilator with no sympathoplegic action. When it is used alone, the drop in blood pressure is followed by sympathetic reflex tachycardia, which in susceptible persons may provoke angina. For this reason, hydralazine is usually added as a step-three drug after sympathetic blockade is established.

Many elderly patients with decreased left ventricular function develop symptoms of fatigue when cardiac output is further reduced by cardiodepressant drugs (especially reserpine and beta-blockers). In these patients, hydralazine is especially helpful because it raises cardiac output by reducing peripheral resistance. Many elderly patients also have blunted baroreceptor sensitivity and will not manifest a reflex tachycardia. Persons who may benefit from hydralazine can be identified by cautious trial.

One-fifth of persons taking over 200 mg of hydralazine daily will develop the minor manifestations of systemic lupus erythematosus: lupus rash, arthralgia, serositis, and a positive antinuclear antibody. These will remit when the drug is discontinued.

Step Three

Before adding a third drug, every effort should be made to ascertain dietary and medication compliance. A determination of 24-hour urine sodium and creatinine may be helpful at this point: more than 150 mEq of sodium, with creatinine indicating a complete collection, suggests that dietary changes would improve BP control. Clues to patient noncompliance include inability to describe the therapeutic regimen, complaints about cost or side effects, missed appointments, variable control at different visits, long intervals between refills, no side effects, no reduction in BP, and no fall in serum potassium. It is clearly futile to add a third drug when the first two are not being taken; worse, it is dangerous, because the patient may suddenly comply fully and become hypotensive.

The usual three-drug regimen comprises a diuretic, a sympathoplegic, and hydralazine. There is no good reason to vary from this scheme except for intolerance to the components. Other options include (1) intensifying volume depletion with high-dose loop diuretics, with or without another diuretic (thiazide, metolazone, or spironolactone); the limitation is decreased renal perfusion as signified by prerenal azotemia; (2) use of two concurrent sympathoplegics, usually a beta-blocker plus either methyldopa, clonidine, or prazosin; (3) substitution of guanethidine for the initial sympatholytic, titrating up to tolerance or benefit; (4) substitution of minoxidil for hydralazine; or (5) trial of captopril with or without a diuretic. These newer drugs are potent and potentially toxic, and the physician should either learn the details and precautions of their use or seek consultation.

Drug Dosage

Choice of drugs within the stepped-care scheme depends on physician preference, cost, specific contraindications, and sometimes the opportunity to treat a coexisting disorder with the same medication. Once daily dosing is believed to improve compliance. Recent studies suggest two or three times daily dosing for many hypotensive agents. However, besides the drugs established for once daily dosing (reserpine, guanethidine, chlorthalidone, atenolol, and nadolol), there are published studies showing once daily dosing to be effective with hydrochlorothiazide, methyldopa, propranolol, and metoprolol as well. Clonidine loses effect after 18 hours, and hydralazine and prazosin taken once daily have not been studied.

Combination drugs may also simplify the regimen. Hydrochlorothiazide is available in combination with reserpine, methyldopa, prazosin, propranolol, and hydralazine.

It is usually assumed that antihypertensive drug therapy is permanent. However, when medication is discontinued for a trial period, between 5 and 20% of patients go on to lasting normotension. Doubtless some of these patients were never truly hypertensive, and some may have lowered their blood pressure by losing weight or decreasing sodium intake. If any of these factors is present, a trial off medication is reasonable; if it fails, then treatment should be considered lifelong.

Orthostatic hypotension can occur with any of the drug regimens described and probably accounts for considerable morbidity among elderly patients. The best approaches to this problem are conservative dosing, asking frequently about dizziness, and checking supine and upright pressures. Intercurrent dehydrating illnesses and unusually hot weather are major risk factors, and the antihypertensive regimen should be relaxed at such times.

Nondrug Management

Behavioral approaches to hypertension control include biofeedback, meditation, psychotherapy, exercise, hospitalization, placebo tablets, and environmental adjustments.

Briefly, everything that has been tried works in at least some settings and in small, short-term, noncontrolled trials.

These approaches require a trained, committed therapist and a receptive patient. Only a minority of patients have the mental and social resources to implement these regimens. At present, drug therapy is far more cost-effective, but in settings with special resources and selected patients, behavioral management may serve well for primary or adjunctive management.

The Joint National Committee on Detection, Evaluation, and Treatment of High Blood Pressure. The 1980 report of the Joint National Committee on Detection, Evaluation, and Treatment of High Blood Pressure. *Arch Intern Med* 140:1280–1285, 1980.
Current official state-of-the-art of hypertension care. Especially good overview of drug therapy.

MacGregor GA, et al. Double-blind randomized crossover trial of moderate sodium restriction in essential hypertension. *Lancet* 13:351–355, February 1982.
Latest of many small, well-done demonstrations showing that reducing daily sodium by about one-half can achieve a 6 to 8 mm Hg fall in mean BP (enough to avoid or reduce drug use in mild hypertension).

Reisin E, et al. Effect of weight loss without salt restriction on the reduction of blood pressure in overweight hypertensive patients. *N Engl J Med* 298:1–6, 1978.
Successful treatment of obesity reduces BP even without salt restriction. Might allow some use of salty diet foods in selected cases.

Finnerty FA. Initial therapy of essential hypertension: Diuretic or beta blocker. *J Fam Pract* 11:199–205, 1980.
A toss-up. Either choice achieves goal for 50% of patients. Choice depends on cost and individual patient factors.

Lutterodt A, Nattel S, McLeod PJ. Duration of antihypertensive effect of a single daily dose of hydrochlorothiazide. *Clin Pharmacol Ther* 27:324–328, 1980.
No falloff in hypertension control during 24 hours after daily dose, despite short diuretic action.

Kassirer JP, Harrington, JT. Diuretics and potassium metabolism: A reassessment of the need, effectiveness and safety of potassium therapy. *Kidney Int* 11:505–514, 1977.
Classic review of subject. Defends thesis that routine use of potassium or potassium-sparing drugs is unnecessary and dangerous.

Finnerty FA, et al. Step 2 regimens in hypertension. *JAMA* 241:579–581, 1979.
Ramdomized, single-blind trial of 3 two-drug regimens: thiazide in all plus reserpine (0.125–0.25 mg), methyldopa (500–2000 mg), or propranolol (80–320 mg). Thiazide/reserpine was the superior regimen for efficacy and acceptability, as well as cost and convenience.

Veterans Administration Cooperative Study Group on Antihypertensive Agents. Propranolol in the treatment of essential hypertension. *JAMA* 237:2303–2310, 1977.
A large VA cooperative trial, demonstrating that propranolol in various combinations works in hypertension—almost as well as reserpine and with comparable toxicity. This is must reading for anyone who believes beta-blockers have replaced reserpine for routine step-two use.

Wright JM, McLeod PJ, McCullough RN. Antihypertensive efficacy of a single bedtime dose of methyldopa. *Clin Pharmacol Ther* 20(6):733–737, 1976.
Total daily dose can be given at once at bedtime with 24-hour effect and less sedation.

Veterans Administration Cooperative Study Group on Antihypertensive Agents. Comparison of prazosin with hydralazine in patients receiving hydrochlorothiazide. *Circulation* 64:772–779, 1981.
Six-month trial of prazosin or hydralazine used with a diuretic but without a sympathoplegic. The regimens were moderately and equally effective, and hydralazine produced fewer side effects. Hydralazine did not produce reflex tachycardia in this trial.

Gifford RW, Tarazi RC. Resistant hypertension: Diagnosis and management. *Ann Intern Med* 88:661–665, 1978.
A classic analysis of the causes of treatment failure, including patient and physician factors in pharmacologic and nutritional management. Especially thorough presentation of drug resistance and interactions.

Shapiro AP, et al. Behavioral methods in the treatment of hypertension. *Ann Intern Med* 86:626–636, 1977.

Review article of experience with behavioral approaches to hypertension—many mildly effective techniques with limited present application, some with future promise.

32. ANGINA PECTORIS
Andreas T. Wielgosz

The term *angina pectoris* refers to chest pain resulting from coronary ischemia. The certainty with which coronary disease is considered the cause of chest pain depends on the character of the pain. "Typical" or "definite" angina conforms to a convincing, classic description: onset with exertion or emotion, location substernal or precordial, with radiation to the arms and neck, and subsiding over several minutes with rest and faster after nitroglycerin. Less classic symptoms are referred to as "probable" or "atypical" angina. Variant angina occurs at rest, often nocturnally, and is associated with ST segment elevation during pain. It is caused by coronary spasm, with or without atherosclerosis.

Unstable angina, also described as "crescendo" or "preinfarction" angina, refers to an increase, over a few weeks' time, in the frequency and/or severity of pain; generally the pain is present at rest. Electrocardiographic changes are reversible, and cardiac enzymes are not elevated. This pattern of angina is associated with an increased risk for myocardial infarction (12% over the several weeks following onset).

Angina pectoris is the initial manifestation of coronary heart disease in 32% of men and 56% of women. It occurs at a rate of 1% per year in middle-aged men and women. About 9% of elderly adults have angina pectoris.

Nearly all ischemic pain is caused by coronary atherosclerosis, coronary spasm, or both; the relative frequencies appear to be 78%, 2%, and 20%, respectively. Rarely, vasculitis causes coronary ischemia. Angina can be unmasked or aggravated by conditions that increase cardiac work, such as aortic stenosis, severe hypertension, or anemia. The risk factors for angina pectoris are those for atherosclerosis in general (see Chap. 128).

Prognosis
Patients who begin to have angina pectoris may die suddenly or may live for decades experiencing remissions and recrudescences in their symptoms. In one longitudinal study, spontaneous remission of angina pectoris of at least 2 years' duration occurred in 32% of men and 44% of women. After the onset of angina, the incidence of acute myocardial infarction is 5% per year, and the risk of sudden death is increased fourfold over that of the general population. The overall annual mortality rate is about 4% per year.

The prognosis for an individual patient with angina pectoris depends on several factors. Persistence of symptoms is associated with a worse prognosis than short-term angina pectoris, presumably because of advanced atherosclerotic disease. The extent of underlying coronary artery disease—that is, the number of coronary arteries involved and the functional state of the left ventricle—also alters the prognosis. In one study, the 5-year cardiac mortality for patients with one-, two-, and three-vessel disease and left main coronary artery disease treated medically was 4%, 14%, 30%, and 61%, respectively. Involvement of the left main coronary artery is present in 5 to 10% of patients with chronic angina and associated with a worse prognosis, particularly when there is also depression of left ventricular function. Other factors associated with a worse prognosis are related to either coronary atherosclerosis, left ventricular function, or both; these include systemic hypertension, diabetes mellitus, congestive heart failure, and cardiac enlargement.

Diagnosis

Differential Diagnosis
Causes of chest pain other than angina pectoris include anxiety, other cardiovascular disorders such as premature beats and pericarditis, and gastrointestinal problems in-

cluding reflux esophagitis, hiatus hernia, and esophageal spasm. Esophageal pain can resemble ischemic pain, presumably because the structures are innervated by the same visceral nerves as the heart. Other causes include pulmonary embolism or neuromuscular problems such as neurovascular compression at the thoracic outlet, costochondral inflammation (Tietze's syndrome), or the early phase of herpes zoster.

Objectives

In the initial evaluation of patients with chest pain, the first task is to determine the cause. If coronary disease is found, it is then useful to know the anatomic distribution of the disease, because certain groups of patients (those with left main coronary artery stenosis or three-vessel disease) have unusually high mortality that can be reduced by coronary bypass surgery. Unfortunately, noninvasive diagnostic tests are crude ways of determining whether these high-risk conditions are present.

History

Factors favoring coronary pain include typical angina, male sex, advanced age, and other manifestations of atherosclerosis (e.g., cerebral or peripheral vascular disease). However, the symptoms of angina pectoris are so widely known, and the prospect of coronary disease is so feared, that patients may exaggerate angina-like symptoms, and physicians may be prompted to pursue such symptoms unnecessarily.

Physical Examination

A normal cardiovascular examination does not preclude angina pectoris and when abnormalities are found they are not specific for angina. Auscultation during an episode of pain may disclose a new gallop sound, regurgitant murmur of papillary muscle dysfunction, rales, wheezing, or extrasystoles. Attacks of angina are usually associated with a rise in blood pressure; a hypotensive response suggests extensive coronary disease. The examination should include a search for other evidence of atherosclerosis in carotid and peripheral vessels.

Electrocardiogram

A resting electrocardiogram (ECG) is usually obtained; although it is normal in 50 to 70% of patients with ischemic heart disease, it is informative if abnormal. If possible, the ideal time to record the ECG is during an actual episode of pain, when ST segment depression is usually present. Ambulatory electrocardiography, using a 24-hour Holter monitor, is a more sensitive way of detecting ischemic changes, as well as associated supraventricular tachycardias, bundle branch block, and atrioventricular block. Transient elevation of the ST segment during pain implicates coronary artery spasm.

Treadmill Exercise Test

The treadmill exercise test is especially useful in people who are believed to have an intermediate probability of coronary disease prior to the test (e.g., 10–80%). If the probability of coronary disease is already high, a positive test provides little additional information, and a negative test is likely to be falsely negative. When the chance of coronary disease is low, positive tests are infrequent, and negative tests simply strengthen the original impression.

A positive test, indicative of ischemia, is characterized by a horizontal or downsloping ST segment depression of at least 1 mm for a duration of 80 msec. Depression of the ST segment by more than 2 mm magnitude at a heart rate below 120 beats per minute, continuing beyond 5 minutes after cessation of exercise, is generally indicative of severe triple-vessel disease or left main coronary artery stenosis. Resting ECG abnormalities, especially if drug induced (e.g., digitalis), may preclude interpretation of the stress test.

The exercise test provides useful information other than the presence or absence of ischemia. If the patient develops the usual pain, there is an opportunity to describe it. Exercise tolerance can be observed and measured objectively. Blood pressure usually rises with exercise and during angina; a fall in blood pressure is a bad prognostic sign. Arrhythmias, either at rest or during exercise, are also associated with a worse prognosis, although perhaps not independently of other findings.

Radionuclide Studies
Exercise thallium imaging can provide further evidence of ischemia when the interpretation of ECGs is impaired by left ventricular hypertrophy, left bundle branch block, nonspecific ST–T wave abnormalities, and the Wolff-Parkinson-White syndrome. A recent multicenter study found that rest or exercise thallium imaging was abnormal in 92% of patients with coronary artery disease; the ECG studies alone detected only 73%. Gated blood pool scanning is best used for an evaluation of the extent of disease, particularly as it affects left ventricular function. Regional wall motion abnormalities along with a subnormal ejection fraction response are predictive of advanced coronary disease, with high sensitivity and specificity.

Echocardiography
The two-dimensional echocardiogram is particularly useful in assessing areas of abnormal left ventricular motion and left ventricular size. It is also often possible to visualize the ostium of the left main coronary artery.

Coronary Arteriography
Coronary arteriography demonstrates the location and extent of coronary disease; it is useful if surgery is contemplated. Arteriography should be done for patients in whom significant multivessel coronary disease is indicated by noninvasive tests and for patients whose pain is not controlled by medication; however, criteria for undertaking the procedure are more liberal in some centers. The relative contribution to myocardial ischemia of occlusive disease and coronary vasospasm can also be assessed using provocative testing with ergonovine maleate. Mortality for the procedure is about 0.07%.

Treatment
The management of angina pectoris has as its primary goal palliation—allowing the patient to return to his or her normal daily activities. Another goal is to prevent the consequences of the underlying disease process, that is, myocardial tissue necrosis and ultimately death.

The standard therapeutic modalities are nitrates, beta-blockers, and more recently, calcium blocking agents. Surgery is reserved for those who do not respond to medication and for a subgroup of patients whose subsequent mortality can be reduced (see Coronary Artery Bypass Surgery below).

Unstable angina, characterized by a recent increase in frequency or intensity of pain, can often be managed with an increase in appropriate medications without hospital admission. On the other hand, if there is prolonged and severe pain, patients are usually hospitalized for ECG monitoring. The benefits of urgent surgery have not been demonstrated, and even the correct medical approach is controversial.

Changing Life-Style
Common sense dictates that patients with angina pectoris get adequate rest and avoid excesses in food, drink, and exertion. Patients should particularly avoid those activities that in their experience induce pain. It is also important that patients be educated about their condition, thus allowing them to be active participants in their own therapy.

Sublingual Nitrates
Sublingual nitrates are taken during attacks; the initial dose is ordinarily 0.3 mg. Longer acting nitrates can be used to prevent attacks and are available in 2% ointment, sustained-release oral tablets and capsules, and transdermal patches as well as intravenous forms. Choice of preparation is a matter of personal perference. Sublingual nitroglycerin appears in the blood within 30 seconds, reaches a peak at 2 minutes, and is barely detectable by 20 minutes. The hemodynamic effects of nitroglycerin ointment are maximal between 60 and 90 minutes after its application and persist for at least 4 to 6 hours. Transdermal patches provide a plasma concentration of nitroglycerin equivalent to that of ointment but require less frequent application. Patients should be reassured that nitroglycerin is not habit-forming and that headaches are common side effects, which usually disappear as tolerance develops.

Beta-Blockers
Propranolol should be initiated along with nitrate therapy. A starting dosage of 20 to 40 mg four times daily can be doubled or tripled if necessary. Alternatively, one may choose a longer-acting beta-blocker or one that is cardioselective. One convenient way of assessing the adequacy of beta-blockade is to see that the pulse is at the lowest tolerated rate, usually around 50 beats per minute. Contraindications to beta-blockers are discussed in Chapter 31.

Diuretics
Diuretics may raise the angina threshold when congestive heart failure contributes to the angina through an increase in heart size.

Calcium Blocking Agents
Calcium blocking agents, such as verapamil (80–120 mg tid–qid) and nifedipine (10 mg tid), are as effective as beta-blockers in the treatment of effort angina. Calcium blocking and beta-blocking drugs can be used together, and their effect on angina is additive. However, their side effects—decreased cardiac contractility, atrioventricular conduction disturbance, and sinus bradycardia (verapamil)—are also additive. These drugs are also the preferred treatment for classic variant angina. Because fixed stenosis may contribute to the angina along with vasospasm, nitrates are given with calcium blocking agents. Beta-blockers are also given, although use of them alone is contraindicated in classic variant angina.

Coronary Artery Bypass Surgery
Coronary artery bypass surgery is used in the management of angina pectoris for two purposes. First, it relieves pain in the great majority of patients. Surgery is not undertaken for this purpose until medical therapy has had a fair trial. From 29 to 75% of patients have a recurrence in symptoms within 5 years following surgery, related to perioperative myocardial infarction, postpericardiotomy syndrome, and abnormalities at the stenotic site. Second, surgery reduces subsequent mortality in some patients. This benefit has been demonstrated thus far only for patients with significant (> 50%) stenosis of the left main coronary artery or of all three vessels. For such patients, surgery reduces mortality by about 20% over the first few years following surgery.

Percutaneous Transluminal Coronary Angioplasty
The benefits of percutaneous transluminal coronary angioplasty (PTCA) are currently being evaluated in an international collaborative study. Only about 15% of patients have lesions that can be managed in this way. Patients with unstable angina and primarily one-vessel disease (LAD) are the best candidates for PTCA. Thus far, good results have been obtained with dilation of graft as well as native vessels in approximately 60% of selected patients; in 30% the obstruction cannot be traversed, and in 10% dilation cannot be achieved due to rigidity of the plaque.

Intracoronary Streptokinase
Early intracoronary streptokinase offers promising results in the preinfarction state, although the ideal time to initiate therapy from onset of symptoms is as yet unclear.

Christie LG, Conti CR. Systematic approach to evaluation of angina-like chest pain: Pathophysiology in clinical testing with emphasis on objective documentation of myocardial ischemia. *Am Heart J* 102:897, 1981.
  The subject is well treated by this overview. A broad differential diagnostic list is considered.
Kannel WB, Sorlic PD. Remission of angina pectoris: The Framingham Study. *Am J Cardiol* 42:119, 1978.
  Patients with remission of their angina pectoris have a better prognosis than patients with persistent angina pectoris.
Harris PJ, et al. Outcome in medically treated coronary artery disease. Ischemic events: non-fatal infarction and death. *Circulation* 62:718, 1980.
  A description of the incidence of events in 1214 patients over a period of 7 years following angiography. Progressive chest pain, number of diseased vessels, left main ste-

nosis, and left ventricular function were found to be the most important prognostic indicators of death and nonfatal infarctions.

Ritchie JL, et al. Myocardial imaging with thallium-201: A multicentre study in patients with angina pectoris or acute myocardial infarction. *Am J Cardiol* 42:345, 1978.
This is a widely quoted study, from five centers, of the sensitivity of nuclear imaging compared with rest and exercise ECG findings and angiographic assessment. Rest/exercise thallium and electrocardiography detected disease in 91% of patients.

Read L. Tests for coronary artery disease: How cost-effective? *J Cardiovasc Med* 7:471, 1982.
A good introduction to the yield of various diagnostic tests. The predictive value of tests, pre- and post-test probabilities of disease, and dollar costs are some of the issues considered.

Brown BG. Coronary vasopasm. *Arch Intern Med* 141:716, 1981.
A good overview, which also looks at the interaction between coronary atherosclerosis and vascular smooth muscle contraction in different coronary ischemic syndromes.

Bertrand ME, et al. Frequency of provoked coronary arterial spasm in 1089 consecutive patients undergoing coronary arteriography. *Circulation* 65:1299, 1982.
Describes the incidence of spasm in patients with typical and atypical angina, with recent myocardial infarction and valvular disease or congestive cardiomyopathy.

Russel RO Jr, et al. Unstable angina pectoris: National cooperative study group to compare medical and surgical therapy: IV. Results in patients with left anterior descending coronary artery disease. *Am J Cardiol* 48:517–524, 1981.
A prospective, randomized comparison of intensive medical therapy with urgent coronary bypass surgery for patients with unstable angina showed no significant difference in early or late mortality and incidence of myocardial infarction.

Rahimtoola SH. Coronary bypass surgery for chronic angina—1981. *Circulation* 2:224, 1982.
This is a state-of-the-art treatise on the subject. There is an extensive reference list of the major studies to date.

Kent KM, et al. Percutaneous transluminal coronary angioplasty: Report from the registry of the National Heart, Lung and Blood Institute. *Am J Cardiol* 48:2011, 1982.
A report from 34 centers on 631 patients who underwent PTCA.

33. CONGESTIVE HEART FAILURE
Laurence O. Watkins

Congestive heart failure (CHF) is a clinical syndrome, the essential feature of which is the failure of the heart to deliver an adequate supply of oxygenated blood to meet the metabolic needs of the tissue, both at rest and during exercise.

Causes
Congestive heart failure occurs at a rate of about 5 cases per 1000 a year after age 50, somewhat more frequently in men than women. Most patients (75%) have a history of hypertension, often in association with coronary artery disease (29%). Other risk factors for CHF are elevated serum cholesterol, cigarette smoking, and obesity. Fewer cases are caused by rheumatic heart disease and even fewer by the cardiomyopathies (dilated and restrictive) or constrictive pericarditis.

Pathophysiology
The hemodynamic characteristics of CHF are decreased cardiac output and elevated ventricular filling pressure (end-diastolic pressure). Low cardiac output is the basis for patients' complaints of weakness, lethargy, and easy fatigability. If left ventricular end-diastolic pressure cannot be maintained at normal levels, the pulmonary capillary wedge pressure rises, which can result in interstitial and alveolar edema and decreased

pulmonary compliance. These are the basis for exertional dyspnea, orthopnea, and paroxysmal nocturnal dyspnea (PND). If the filling pressure of the right ventricle is high, the resulting elevation of central venous pressure is associated with hepatic congestion, pedal edema, and in severe cases, ascites and anasarca. The congestive symptoms result from responses in both the venous and arterial circulations to compensate for chronic reduction of cardiac output. Decreased renal perfusion stimulates the renin-angiotensin-aldosterone system, which results in augmented sodium and fluid retention. This mechanism serves to maintain cardiac output by increasing ventricular preload. In the early stages of CHF, increases in systemic vascular resistance (afterload) serve to maintain an adequate tissue perfusion pressure in the face of decreased cardiac output. Later, further arteriolar constriction acts to preserve regional flow to the heart and brain even at the expense of reduced flow to other organs, such as the kidneys, and at the cost of increased cardiac work.

Diagnosis

Congestive heart failure is frequently misdiagnosed. On the one hand, CHF may cause only subtle complaints so that the diagnosis is not considered. On the other hand, symptoms and signs of CHF are also caused by other common diseases (e.g., obstructive lung disease, obesity, and venous insufficiency) so that a diagnosis of CHF may be made in error.

Criteria

One large study of heart disease, the Framingham Study, used major and minor criteria for CHF that reflect current clinical judgment. Major criteria were paroxysmal nocturnal dyspnea or orthopnea, neck vein distention, rales, cardiomegaly, acute pulmonary edema, S_3 gallop, increased venous pressure ($>$ 16 cm H_2O), circulation time $\geq$ 25 seconds, and hepatojugular reflux. Minor criteria were ankle edema, night cough, dyspnea on exertion, hepatomegaly, pleural effusion, vital capacity decreased by one-third from maximum, and tachycardia (rate $\geq$ 120/min). Weight loss $\geq$ 4.5 kg in 5 days in response to treatment was considered either a major or minor criterion. The diagnosis of CHF required the presence of 2 major or 1 major and 2 minor criteria.

In a study of clinical criteria for chronic CHF in patients with coronary artery disease referred for catheterization, CHF was associated with two clinical findings: cardiomegaly (cardiothoracic ratio greater than 0.48 on chest x-ray) and the presence of a third heart sound (S_3). This criterion for the cardiothoracic ratio is derived from a study of predominantly white patients, and may not apply for blacks of West African descent because they have relatively smaller thoracic diameter. Dyspnea on exertion was a sensitive indicator of CHF, and the specificity of this symptom was higher if either orthopnea or PND was present. Pulmonary rales, peripheral edema, tachycardia (heart rate greater than 100 per minute at rest), and neck vein distention were present only infrequently, since many patients with these signs were already being treated for CHF. However, if present, these findings were highly specific for CHF. Similarly, radiographic findings of pulmonary venous cephalization, interstitial edema, and Kerley's B lines were infrequent; they were absent if heart size was normal. Cardiomegaly, an S_3, or other clinical findings of CHF correctly identified 53% of patients with LVEDP greater than 15 mm Hg and 73% of patients with LVEDP greater than 12 mm Hg.

Strategy

To establish the diagnosis of CHF, the clinician should inquire about dyspnea, decreased exercise tolerance, and peripheral congestion, either current or past. Unfortunately, patient complaints may not reflect accurately the degree of cardiac dysfunction. There is generally poor agreement between the New York Heart Association clinical classification of patients on the basis of exertional symptoms and objective assessment of exercise performance. Because pulmonary disease often underlies exertional dyspnea, a history of cigarette smoking, chronic sputum production, wheezing, or asthma should be sought. Attempts should also be made to determine the cause of cardiac dysfunction, by seeking a history of hypertension, exertional chest pain, palpitations, rheumatic fever, or murmur. Physical examination should be directed particularly toward determining whether there is congestion in the peripheral or pulmonary circulation, cardiomegaly, and abnormal heart sounds (S_3, S_4) or murmurs. The presence of the last would suggest valvular disease, either congenital or acquired.

Investigation
If CHF is suspected, a chest x-ray should be obtained, both to obtain an accurate estimate of cardiac size and to determine whether there is pulmonary vascular congestion
or evidence of intrinsic pulmonary disease. An electrocardiogram may suggest the
presence of heart disease. Occasionally, if the cause of CHF remains unclear, echocardiography may be warranted. In some patients, the presence of chest pain or murmurs
may suggest that a surgically correctable lesion is present. In these cases, referral for
further, invasive evaluation should be considered.

Prognosis
The prognosis of patients with CHF is poor. In the Framingham Study, of the 142
patients who developed CHF, 62% of the men and 42% of the women died within 5
years, despite treatment with diuretics and digitalis. In a study of CHF associated with
coronary artery disease, 40% of those with either cardiomegaly or an S_3 died within 36
months, regardless of whether medical or surgical therapy was applied.

Treatment
Many different modalities are available for the treatment of CHF. The imbalance between cardiac output and peripheral tissue demands can be corrected by maneuvers
directed either to decreasing tissue demand or to altering the factors that affect cardiac
output, namely preload, afterload, and myocardial contractility. The choice of therapy
should be guided by the underlying cardiac abnormality and the ensuing pathophysiologic adaptations. For example, patients with pulmonary and visceral congestion and
peripheral edema require different therapy from patients whose major problem is low
cardiac output. If CHF is new or recently worse, precipitating causes should be sought
and treated first. While the underlying cause of CHF may be myocardial contractile
failure, worsening may be due to uncontrolled hypertension, arrhythmias, side effects
of antiarrhythmic or other drugs, excessive salt intake, poor medication compliance, or
metabolic factors such as hypoxemia, hypercapnea, acidosis, hypokalemia, or hypocalcemia.

Activity
The ambulatory patient who experiences symptoms on mild or marked exertion should
be advised to avoid isometric exercise. In more severely compromised patients, periodic
bed rest will allow increased renal (instead of muscular) perfusion and consequent diuresis, with relief of congestive symptoms.

Salt Restriction
For patients whose symptoms result from peripheral or pulmonary congestion, ventricular preload should be reduced. Restriction of dietary salt to 2 gm per day opposes the
tendency to renal salt and water conservation and reduces intravascular volume and
ventricular filling pressures.

Diuretics
A diuretic should be added if symptoms do not resolve with salt restriction alone. A
daily dose of a thiazide diuretic such as hydrochlorothiazide (50–100 mg) promotes
sodium and water excretion if renal function is normal. If CHF is moderate or severe,
or if the serum creatinine exceeds 2.5 mg/dl, a more potent, loop diuretic such as
furosemide (usually 40–240 mg per day, maximal dose 300 mg bid) may be necessary.
Bumetanide (usually 1–6 mg per day) and ethacrynic acid are as potent as furosemide;
there is little to choose among them, except that furosemide and bumetanide should be
avoided in patients who are allergic to sulfonamides. In some patients, 20 to 40 mg of
furosemide will enhance the maximal diuresis obtained with thiazides, and addition of
furosemide, rather than substitution, may be effective. The natriuretic effect, and
hence the dosage, of the loop diuretics depends on renal plasma flow, which varies
markedly among CHF patients. Their duration of action is 6 to 8 hours in normal
individuals but is usually prolonged in CHF. In some patients, a single daily dose
reduces congestive symptoms, although in others twice or thrice daily administration
is necessary. Metolazone (5–10 mg qd) is effective in patients with marked renal insufficiency. The addition of metolazone often produces brisk diuresis in patients refractory to maximal recommended doses of furosemide.

It is doubtful whether total body potassium depletion, other than that attributable to increased age or decreased muscle mass, is a characteristic of CHF patients treated with diuretics. Hypokalemia (serum potassium 3.5 mEq/L or less) is rarely observed in CHF patients treated with 50 to 100 mg per day of hydrochlorothiazide or 40 to 80 mg per day of furosemide. It may occur more commonly when higher doses of potent diuretics are used, but accurate estimates of incidence are not available. It is prudent to measure serum potassium before and 2 months after institution of diuretic therapy and to give supplemenatary potassium only if hypokalemia develops. Treatment of hypokalemia is especially important if digitalis glycosides are being used, because hypokalemia makes digitalis-associated arrhythmias more likely. Addition of the potassium-sparing diuretic amiloride (5–10 mg per day) is more effective than potassium chloride supplements of 40 to 80 mEq per day. Triamterene (100 mg qd–100 mg qid) and spironolactone (25–100 mg qid) also spare potassium.

Preload Reduction

Long-acting nitrates diminish congestive symptoms by reducing preload. They decrease venous return by inducing pooling in venous capacitance vessels; they are unlikely to be effective in patients whose severe peripheral edema restricts venous distention. Isosorbide dinitrate (5–10 mg sublingually or 20–40 mg po every 4–6 hours) reduces preload, causes mild arteriolar relaxation, and usually reduces systemic blood pressure. Dosage should be titrated so that the systolic blood pressure difference between the supine and the upright position is less than 20 mm Hg.

In patients whose major symptoms reflect a low output state, the aim of therapy is to increase the cardiac output. This may be achieved by either increasing myocardial contractility or decreasing afterload.

Digoxin

Myocardial contractility can be improved by a number of oral inotropic agents. Digoxin is the most commonly used. It is particularly useful if atrial fibrillation is present and should be used to decrease the ventricular response to 60 to 90 per minute. The utility of chronic oral digoxin therapy for CHF has been questioned, particularly for patients in sinus rhythm with normal cardiac size. However, in a recent randomized, double-blind, crossover trial, 14 of 25 CHF patients (56%) with normal sinus rhythm obtained benefit from digoxin. These patients had more severe CHF, greater left ventricle size, and an S_3. Persistence of an S_3 after maximal diuretic therapy was an excellent predictor of response to digoxin (sensitivity 100%, specificity 90%). In patients whose renal function is normal, the usual maintenance dose is 0.25 mg per day, and a loading dose is not necessary. If renal function is impaired (e.g., serum creatinine > 1.5 mg/dl), digoxin should be reduced to 0.125 mg per day or 0.25 mg every other day.

Afterload Reduction

Hydralazine, a direct arterial vasodilator, and prazosin, an alpha-adrenergic antagonist, are commonly used for decreasing afterload in patients with severe low-output failure. The daily dosage required to attain optimal effects on cardiac output varies markedly (100–800 mg of hydralazine, 4–30 mg of prazosin). It is difficult to establish an optimal regimen with these drugs in ambulatory patients without serial assessment of exercise performance. However, use of these drugs is more frequently guided by clinical judgment; the systolic blood pressure should be maintained at 90 to 100 mm Hg, and alleviation of symptoms or improved exercise tolerance should be used as clinical end points. These agents are particularly useful if hypertension or valvular regurgitation accompanies cardiac dysfunction. They should be used with caution in patients with coronary artery disease because of the theoretic concern that vasodilatation in normal areas of the coronary bed may lead to diminished flow in post-stenotic areas.

Hydralazine has the advantage that it improves renal perfusion and enhances the effect of furosemide. A test dose of 25 mg may be given, and if blood pressure does not fall, the drug can be continued at this dosage every 6 hours. Increments of 25 mg every 6 hours can be employed until maximum improvement in symptoms occurs. At dosages greater than 200 mg per day, chronic hydralazine therapy may cause a lupus-like syndrome. Since oral nitrates have predominantly venodilator effects, they can be used concurrently with hydralazine to treat congestive symptoms and often decrease the requirement for large doses of hydralazine.

Prazosin combines both arterial and venous dilating effects and is not used in combination with other vasodilators. A test dose of 1 mg should be used, and if orthostatic hypotension does not develop, the dosage may be increased to a maximum of 5 to 10 mg every 6 hours. Attenuation of the hemodynamic effects of prazosin has been observed in studies of resting patients after chronic use, but the beneficial effects on exercise tolerance usually persist. If exercise tolerance worsens, a small increase in dosage or a 2-week interruption of therapy appears to result in renewed benefit.

Other Drugs
There is only limited experience with minoxidil (20 mg every 12 hours), captopril (25–100 mg tid), and nifedipine (10–20 mg tid) as vasodilators for treating CHF. Nifedipine may become the preferred therapy if CHF is the result of coronary artery disease because of the theoretical potential for adverse effects on coronary blood flow resulting from both prazosin and hydralazine.

Choosing Therapy
An appropriate therapeutic regimen for individual patients should reflect such factors as patient convenience, ease of monitoring, and risks of chronic therapy. The effectiveness of therapy can be assessed periodically by determining whether symptoms of congestion, poor exercise tolerance, or fatigue has diminished. Blood pressure and weight should be measured at each visit and therapy adjusted if these change inappropriately. Evidence of drug side effects or toxicity should be sought and alternative drugs substituted if these are troublesome.

McKee P, et al. The natural history of congestive heart failure: The Framingham Study. *N Engl J Med* 285:1441, 1971.
  Standard diagnostic criteria: data on incidence, causes, and prognosis.
Harlan WR, et al. Chronic congestive heart failure in coronary artery disease: Clinical criteria. *Ann Intern Med* 86:133, 1977.
  Relates clinical diagnostic criteria to left ventricular function.
Zelis R, Flaim SF. The circulations in congestive heart failure. *Mod Concepts Cardiovasc Dis* 51(2):79, 1982.
  Summarizes physiologic adaptations; describes ideal vasodilator.
Morgan DB, Burkinshaw L, Davidson C. Potassium depletion in heart failure and its relation to long-term treatment with diuretics: A review of the literature. *Postgrad Med J* 54:72, 1978.
  Reviews methodologic problems and finds no evidence of total body potassium depletion.
Lawson DH, et al. Potassium supplements in patients receiving long-term diuretics for edema. *Q J Med* 45:469, 1976.
  No significant fall in plasma potassium occurred when supplements were withdrawn. If diet and gastrointestinal tract are normal, routine potassium supplementation is unnecessary.
Gifford RW. A guide to the practical use of diuretics. *JAMA* 235:1890, 1976.
  A concise guide to agents, clinical applications, and side effects.
Nomura A, et al. Effect of furosemide in congestive heart failure. *Clin Pharmacol Ther* 30:177, 1981.
  Natriuresis and diuresis enhanced by hydralazine.
Lee DC, et al. Heart failure in outpatients: A randomized trial of digoxin versus placebo. *N Engl J Med* 306:699, 1982.
  Suggests that long-term digoxin therapy is clinically beneficial in some patients with heart failure unaccompanied by atrial fibrillation.
Franciosa JA. Effectiveness of long-term vasodilator administration in the treatment of chronic left ventricular failure. *Prog Cardiovasc Dis* 24:319, 1982.
  A review.
Parmley WW, Rouleau JL, Chatterjee K. Vasodilators in heart failure secondary to coronary artery disease. *Am Heart J* 103:625, 1982.
  Hydralazine and prazosin may have adverse effects on the myocardial oxygen supply.
Franciosa JA, et al. Survival in men with severe chronic left ventricular failure due to either coronary heart disease or idiopathic dilated cardiomyopathy. *Am J Cardiol* 1983; 53:831.

High mortality despite "modern" management: Prognosis worse in patients with CAD, and those with worse symptoms and hemodynamic abnormalities.

34. REHABILITATION AFTER MYOCARDIAL INFARCTION
Thomas Kottke, Mark A. Hlatky, Michael C. Hindman, Robert M. Califf

The aim of rehabilitation after myocardial infarction (MI) is to return patients to full productive lives. This is a major challenge, for many patients do not return to work after a myocardial infarction, and often many more are needlessly restricted in less dramatic ways.

A cardiac rehabilitation program must address five problems: (1) return to physical activity, (2) concerns about sexual activity, (3) psychological adjustment, (4) return to work, and (5) prevention of reinfarction and death. A prerequisite for effective rehabilitation is control of the physiologic problems of angina pectoris, arrhythmias, hypertension, and congestive heart failure.

Return to Physical Activity
Since prolonged bed rest for the MI patient was abandoned in the early 1950s, mobilization has come earlier and earlier in the course of recovery. Current practice is to begin ambulation in the coronary care unit and progressively increase activity under direct supervision until discharge from the hospital. Activity recommendations after myocardial infarction should be tailored to the individual patient.

To assure both patient and physician that home activities immediately after discharge can be tolerated, hospitalized patients can be readily asessed by monitoring symptoms, heart rate, blood pressure, and electrocardiogram (ECG) during walking or climbing stairs. Low-level formal exercise testing is often performed prior to discharge to provide more detailed information for counseling and post-discharge exercise prescription. The patient should be carefully monitored during exercise testing for the first signs of ischemia, insufficient cardiac output, or arrhythmia. A heart rate at least 10 beats per minute lower than this threshold should be set as the safe maximum for activity, since it has been shown that most complications occur in patients who have marked ischemic responses and who have exceeded the threshold heart rate.

After discharge, patients should progressively resume their former levels of activity. Formal cardiac rehabilitation programs can speed conditioning and assist psychological adjustment and risk factor modification, particularly in high-risk patients. Unsupervised progressive conditioning is suitable for selected patients, such as those with normal blood pressure response to exercise, no signs or symptoms of myocardial ischemia at heart rates below 120, no evidence of congestive heart failure, and no complex ventricular arrhythmias.

Unsupervised activity is best guided by teaching the patient to take his pulse and not exceed the determined safe maximum for exercise heart rate. Initially, short periods of walking two or three times daily with rest periods in between are usually well tolerated. If no symptoms occur, both higher levels and longer durations of activity should gradually be attempted.

A maximum (symptom-limited) exercise test performed 6 to 12 weeks after discharge can give both the physician and the patient an objective assessment of physical work capacity and can identify those patients who should be considered for invasive evaluation. Exercise testing is also useful for reassuring the patient about physical activity. However, if arrhythmia is suspected, the 24-hour rhythm monitor is more sensitive than the exercise test.

Many patients who have had an MI have been sedentary and are poorly conditioned. For them, programs aimed at increasing exercise capacity may be useful. Attaining a training effect allows the same level of external work to be achieved at a lower heart rate and blood pressure, reducing the demands on the heart. Thus, activities that would otherwise precipitate angina can be performed comfortably. A conditioning program usually consists of dynamic exercise with large muscle groups (e.g., walking, jogging, swimming) at adequate heart rates (e.g., 60–80% of the maximum safe heart rate) for sufficient duration (15–60 minutes) and frequency (at least three times a week) to achieve and sustain a training effect.

Sexual Activity

The return to sexual activity is a primary concern of a large proportion of cardiac patients of all ages. In one Veterans Administration study, 49% of MI patients reported concerns about sexual activity, usually fear of chest pain, impotence, or death during intercourse. To forestall sexual dysfunction resulting from such fears and to indicate that sexual activity is an appropriate topic for discussion, the physician should make a point of inquiring whether the patient expects changed sexual activities as a result of heart disease.

The estimated peak heart rate during sexual activity is about 120 per minute and is sustained for only about a minute. Thus, as a guideline, the cardiac stress of intercourse can usually be tolerated if a rise in heart rate to 120 per minute causes no symptoms. For the patient with continued anxiety about sexual activity, Holter monitoring during intercourse may be a method of demonstrating that the activity is safe.

Symptoms can also be averted by lessening the metabolic demands of sexual intercourse, for example, by pausing intermittently, changing position, and emphasizing foreplay. Sexual activity in the morning or after a nap may be less likely to cause cardiac symptoms than after a long day or a heavy meal. Angina medications should be accessible; if angina is expected during sexual activity, nitroglycerin should be taken before starting.

Psychological Adjustment

An acute MI is usually a crisis for the patient and family. Thoughtful explanation of the nature of the illness and the expected course can help to dispel many unwarranted fears and concerns. Well-designed pamphlets are available through the state affiliates of the American Heart Association; these may be useful during a period when patients have many questions and anxieties about their illness.

Early and progressive ambulation helps combat the anxiety, depression, and low self-esteem common after an MI. Exercise testing and training may also help allay fears about activities by establishing safe limits, thus avoiding both inappropriate restrictions and dangerous excesses. Formal cardiac conditioning programs may be particularly helpful for anxious patients, who find reassurance from the structured approach and support from interaction with other post-MI patients. Additional counseling and therapy may be necessary for the occasional patient with prolonged or excessive depression or anxiety after an MI.

Return to Work

Returning the patient to gainful employment is a major goal of post-MI rehabilitation. Whether this goal is achieved is often affected by socioeconomic factors such as the patient's age, type of employment, job satisfaction, ability to control the work schedule and pace, and financial necessity for continued employment. The patient's symptoms and functional capacity certainly must dictate the feasibility of resuming work. Clearly, the physical demands of the occupation must not exceed the limits imposed by symptoms. Exercise testing may aid decision-making by providing objective evidence concerning functional capacity. Physician advice may prove decisive in borderline cases. Workers in sedentary occupations may return as soon as 6 weeks after uncomplicated MI and convalescence, while laborers may have to delay returning to work for several months. Because their stamina may be low, patients should work part-time for the first few weeks, if possible.

The patient can be prepared psychologically for returning to the job by the physician's emphasizing, early in the course of rehabilitative treatment, that most MI patients go back to work. Physicians should also be prepared to speak with employers who may be reluctant to rehire the patient. If the patient needs to be retrained, contacting the state's vocational rehabilitation program while the patient is still in the hospital will speed this process.

Prevention of Reinfarction and Death

Patients suffering an acute MI are at higher risk of death over the first year, and particularly over the first few months, following the event. Prevention of recurrent infarction and cardiac death should be an integral component of cardiac rehabilitation. However, programs to prevent reinfarction and sudden death may have to treat up to a hundred patients to prevent death in one. The efficiency of these efforts would be increased if it were possible to identify high-risk patients. A variety of tests are being investigated as a means of identifying patients who are at high risk and of choosing the appropriate intervention to reduce that risk.

Vigorous efforts to control the cardiac risk factors should be intensified after an MI. Several risk factors are harmful in patients with coronary disease, apart from any role in promoting atherosclerosis. Elevated blood pressure increases cardiac work and aggravates ischemia. Smoking has adverse hemodynamic and metabolic effects that may precipitate myocardial ischemia. Obesity increases the strain of any activity on both muscles and heart. Excessive psychological stress adds further burdens to a diseased heart.

Beta-Blocking Agents

Beta-blocking agents have been shown to reduce subsequent coronary events after MI by three methodologically sound, randomized clinical trials. A beta-blocker is therefore recommended for all patients without specific contraindications. There is evidence that the improved prognosis depends on treatment being started early; most experts recommend starting patients on beta-blockers before hospital discharge. However, the optimal agent, dosage, and length of treatment after MI remain uncertain.

Smoking

There is strong and consistent evidence from observational studies that smoking is an important risk factor for subsequent coronary events after MI and that stopping smoking reduces risk. Patients should be advised to stop smoking while in the coronary care unit, when they may be particularly susceptible to such advice. This advice should be repeated on follow-up visits; failure to ask the patient about smoking may imply that it is no longer an important issue. Special smoking cessation programs may be effective (see Chap. 131).

Exercise Training

Exercise training has also been shown to reduce the mortality after MI in several trials, but because of the small numbers of patients enrolled in these studies, the differences have not been statistically significant. Thus, recommendations regarding exercise after MI should be guided more by the expected effect on symptoms than by any potential effect on mortality. It is uncertain whether beta-blockers prevent exercise from inducing a training effect. However, it is clear that maximum exercise capacity can be increased, even on beta-blockers. Therefore, post-MI patients should be continued on beta-blockers during exercise rehabilitation.

Social Reinforcement of Risk Modification

Patients are faced daily with social and visual cues to return to their previous lifestyles. Rehabilitation efforts must therefore emphasize skills, social supports, and the availability of choices to maintain behavioral changes. Dietary adherence will probably be improved by having the whole family adopt a low-sodium, low–saturated fat cuisine by learning skills in food buying and preparation and in choosing satisfactory foods while dining out. Smoking cessation will be facilitated if other household members also stop smoking and all smoking paraphernalia is discarded. The spouse should participate in the patient's walking or exercise program. In addition to making adherence easier for the cardiac patient, this strategy allows the physician to introduce other family members to healthy habits.

Wenger NK, Hellerstein HK (Eds.). *Rehabilitation of the Coronary Patient* (2nd ed.). New York: Wiley, 1984.
   Contains much useful material, including details for rehabilitation program delivery and planning and facilitation of return to work.

Pollock ML, Ward A, Foster C. Exercise Prescription for Rehabilitation of the Cardiac Patient. In ML Pollock and DH Schmidt (Eds.), *Heart Disease and Rehabilitation.* Boston: Houghton Mifflin, 1979. Pp. 413–445.

A detailed description of the post-discharge exercise conditioning regimen used by a major center, with a survey of methods used by 31 other programs.

Williams RS, et al. Guidelines for unsupervised exercise in patients with ischemic heart disease. *J Cardiac Rehab* 1:213–219, 1981.

Discusses the rationale and selection criteria for supervised and unsupervised exercise conditioning after MI.

Miller DH, Borer JS. Exercise testing, early myocardial infarction. Risks and benefits. *Am. J. Med.* 72:427, 1982.

A critical review of the role of exercise tests after myocardial infarction.

McLane M, Kròp H, Mehta J. Psychosexual adjustment and counseling after myocardial infarction. *Ann Intern Med* 92:514–519, 1980.

The most recent review emphasizing resumption of sexual activity after MI.

Davidson DM, Taylor CG, DeBusk RF. Factors influencing return to work after myocardial infarction or coronary bypass surgery. *Cardiac Rehab* 10:1–4, 1979.

A concise review of studies relating to resumption of employment after an MI.

May GS, et al. Secondary prevention after myocardial infarction: A review of long-term trials. *Prog Cardiovasc Dis* 24:331–352, 1982.

A complete and concise review of long-term trials that have tried to influence post-MI mortality through lipid-lowering agents, antiarrhythmic drugs, anticoagulants, platelet-active dugs, beta-blockers, and physical exercise.

Committee on Exercise. *Exercise Testing and Training of Individuals with Heart Disease or at High Risk for Its Development. A Handbook for Physicians.* Dallas: American Heart Association, 1975.

Authoritative guidelines for exercise testing and training.

35. PAROXYSMAL SUPRAVENTRICULAR TACHYCARDIA

Ross J. Simpson, Jr.

Paroxysmal supraventricular tachycardia (PSVT) is a rapid (140–220 beats per minute), regular, narrow-QRS tachycardia that usually occurs without obvious precipitating cause. The interval between attacks varies widely.

Paroxysmal supraventricular tachycardia is a common rhythm disturbance that is present on approximately 0.6% of electrocardiograms (ECGs). Most PSVT is caused by reentry within the atrioventricular (AV) node itself (50% of patients) or by AV reciprocation involving either a manifest AV connection (the Wolff-Parkinson-White [WPW] syndrome, 30% of patients) or concealed AV connection (10% of patients). The remaining 10% of patients have PSVT because of reentry within the atrium or sinus node or have an ectopic atrial tachycardia.

The electrophysiologic basis for PSVT is ultimately either or acquired dual-conducting pathways between the atrium and ventricle. In AV nodal reentry, division of the AV node into two separate pathways by congenital or degenerative changes results in potential reentry circuits for PSVT. The tachycardia is generally initiated by a premature atrial beat that blocks in one pathway and conducts slowly down the alternate pathway. By the time the slowly conducting impulse reaches the distal connection of the pathway, sufficient time has elapsed to allow retrograde conduction back up the previously blocked pathway. The atrium is then depolarized, and conduction down the antegrade pathway occurs again.

Diagnosis

The clinical manifestations of PSVT depend on the presence or absence of structural heart disease and the rate of the tachycardia.

Symptoms

The most common clinical symptom is the sudden onset of palpitations, light-headedness, weakness, or shortness of breath. If preexisting heart disease is present, congestive heart failure or angina pectoris may occur as a consequence of the rapid heart rate. Most patients without structural heart disease tolerate rapid PSVT without incapacitating symptoms.

Clinical Signs

At heart rates of over 180, systolic blood pressure falls, and diastolic filling pressures rise, even in patients with normal hearts. The pulse is regular and rapid, and mechanical pulsus alternans may occur if there is heart failure or a very rapid heart rate. Polyuria begins after 4 to 6 hours but is not seen in patients with mitral stenosis or chronic left ventricular failure. If the arrhythmia persists for several days, salt and water retention occurs, even in patients with normal hearts.

Documentation of PSVT

The occurrence of paroxysmal, rapid, regular palpitations cannot be used to diagnose PSVT because paroxysms of atrial fibrillation and ventricular tachycardia can produce identical symptoms. An electrocardiogram of the tachycardia is essential for diagnosis.

In most instances, the ECG of PSVT is characteristic. The QRS is typically narrow (less than .10 sec in duration) and monotonously regular (except at the beginning and end of the tachycardia, when variation in the rate is expected), and there should be no evidence of AV dissociation. Often, the P wave is not visible because it occurs synchronously with the QRS. Less frequently, a retrograde P wave (negative P wave in leads II, III, aV_F) is visible following or preceding the QRS. Atypically, the QRS may be widened during PSVT due to a rate-dependent bundle branch block. Patients with accessory AV connections have faster rates during PSVT and a greater tendency toward wide-QRS tachycardia than patients with AV nodal reentrant tachycardia.

Patients with infrequent episodes may require other procedures to diagnose the cause of their symptoms. A Holter monitor rarely documents PSVT because of the unpredictable frequency of attacks, and a treadmill exercise test only rarely induces PSVT. An ECG telephone transmitter has become the standard technique to document infrequently occurring, nonsustained arrhythmias. Patients suspected of PSVT are given this device, which they can carry in a purse or briefcase; during an attack, they connect the leads, dial a central number, and use the device to transmit an ECG. If this fails, cardiac pacing techniques are successful in inducing the arrhythmia in almost all patients prone to PSVT.

Differential Diagnosis

Differential diagnosis of a rapid, regular, narrow-QRS tachycardia includes sinus tachycardia, atrial flutter with 2:1 block, rapid atrial fibrillation, and paroxysmal atrial tachycardia with block. Normal sinus P waves (upright P waves in leads I, II, III) before the QRS suggest sinus tachycardia; an irregular ventricular response suggests atrial fibrillation. Atrial flutter with 2:1 block may resemble PSVT if the flutter is atypical and the two P waves for each QRS cannot be readily separated from the ST segment and T waves. Paroxysmal atrial tachycardia with block is seen in digitalis intoxication and resembles atrial flutter except that the atrial rate is slower, the degree of AV block may be greater than 2:1, and escape or accelerated junctional beats may be present. When the QRS is widened, ventricular tachycardia is a likely diagnosis and is confirmed by AV dissociation or fusion or capture beats on long rhythm strips of lead II or V_1 (see Chap. 36).

If the rhythm is not obvious from the ECG, positioning an esophageal electrode or a catheter in the right heart may be required for definitive diagnosis. An additional advantage of these invasive procedures is that the tachycardia can be broken by pacing through the electrode.

Treatment

Most episodes of PSVT will terminate spontaneously. However, because episodes may last for days and cause major hemodynamic changes, termination of the tachycardia is recommended even in asymptomatic patients. The following maneuvers, listed in order of preference, are commonly used to interrupt PSVT.

"Vagal" Maneuvers

Because sympathetic tone can maintain the tachycardia and counteract the parasympathetic effect of vagal maneuvers, the patient should be placed in the reclining position. Carotid sinus massage is performed by providing even, firm pressure on one carotid body at the carotid artery below the angle of the jaw. This maneuver should not be done in patients with bruits in either carotid. The Valsalva maneuver is performed by asking the patient to take a deep breath and bear down as if to have a bowel movement. The physician places a hand on the abdomen to provide opposing pressure. The diving reflex is performed by having the patient turn on his side and, while holding his breath, immerse his face in ice water. A physician should be present during this maneuver.

Verapamil

Verapamil, 0.10 to 0.15 mg/kg, is administered as a rapid (15–60 seconds) intravenous bolus and may be repeated in 30 minutes if the arrhythmia is not broken. Verapamil is reported to be effective in over 90% of patients who have not responded to vagal maneuvers. Verapamil should not be given to patients with heart failure, acute myocardial infarction, or hypotension. It may accelerate the ventricular response of atrial fibrillation in WPW and should be avoided in these patients.

Other Drugs

Intravenous edrophonium (10 mg), propanolol (0.15 mg/kg), or digoxin will also terminate PSVT. Digitalis has been implicated as a cause of death in patients with WPW syndrome and should not be given to these patients. Vasopressor agents should not be used because of the possibility of precipitating pulmonary edema or other cardiovascular complications.

Electrical Pacing

Electrical pacing, involving catheterization of the right atrium, is safe and effective but is rarely needed because of the usual success of pharmacologic therapy. Electrical direct current (DC) conversion synchronized to the QRS complex is recommended if the patient appears hemodynamically unstable, is having angina, is hypotensive, or has evidence of impaired cardiac output. Usually only 25 to 50 watt-sec are required to convert PSVT.

Prevention

The natural history of PSVT is not known. Except in patients with structural heart disease or WPW syndrome, it does not appear to shorten life. However, in patients with chronic heart disease, PSVT may precipitate angina, congestive heart failure, or syncope. Patients with WPW and a history of rapid PSVT, atrial fibrillation, or short antegrade refractory periods of the accessory pathway may in rare instances die suddenly.

It is difficult to predict how the frequency of PSVT will change with age. Infants and young children may "grow out" of their arrhythmia, while adults tend to have the propensity to PSVT for decades or for life.

Drug Therapy

Drug therapy is usually helpful in preventing recurrent episodes of tachycardia. However, patients with infrequent PSVT (e.g., less than one occurrence per year) or PSVT that causes only mild symptoms may not require long-term treatment. Chronic therapy is also not recommended following the first episode of PSVT in such patients.

Before beginning long-term therapy, the patient's history, physical examination, chest film, and ECG should be reviewed to assess ventricular function, to determine if ventricular preexcitation (WPW syndrome) from a manifest AV connection is present (shortened PR interval, widened QRS, and ST and T abnormalities), and to evaluate underlying structural heart disease. Hypokalemia, congestive heart failure, unexplained heart murmurs, or other medical conditions should be investigated and treated.

Possible goals of long-term therapy in the treatment of PSVT are to decrease or eliminate recurrent episodes and to modify the severity or ease of termination of episodes. All of the drugs outlined below may abolish frequent episodes of PSVT. However, because the frequency of occurrence of PSVT varies over time and a particular drug may increase, decrease, or have no effect on the frequency of episodes, prolonged observation and blood levels of drug are necessary to establish efficacy.

Drugs that prolong conduction and refractoriness in the antegrade direction of the AV node (e.g., digoxin, beta-blockers, verapamil) are particularly useful in the treatment of PSVT, because if they do not prevent PSVT, they slow the rate of the tachycardia and aid in terminating PSVT. They also have a low frequency of side effects. These drugs are generally the standard of therapy of AV nodal reentrant PSVT. Digoxin, and probably verapamil, should not be used in WPW.

Digoxin, because of its long half-life and infrequent side effects, is often the initial therapy in patients who do not have WPW syndrome. If digoxin in therapeutic plasma concentrations does not offer protection from PSVT or is contraindicated, either a beta-sympathetic blocking drug or verapamil should be used. If beta-blockers are used, the dosage is adjusted to achieve beta-blockade. If verapamil is used, the dosage is generally 120 mg three times a day. Most patients require a combination of drugs to prevent recurrences. The combination of digoxin and a beta-sympathetic blocking drug is particularly effective for patients with AV nodal reentry.

If drugs that slow the AV node are not successful in preventing attacks of tachycardia, a quinidine-like drug (e.g., quinidine, procainamide, or disopyramide) should be given. These act by slowing conduction and prolonging refractoriness in the accessory or retrograde pathway in the AV node. They may reduce the frequency of attacks but often do not change the rate of the tachycardia if it occurs. If atrial flutter or ectopic atrial tachycardia is suspected, these drugs should be administered in combination with a drug that prolongs the refractory period of the AV node, because alone they have the potential to increase the ventricular response rate.

Diagnostic Cardiac Pacing Studies
Diagnostic cardiac pacing studies should be performed in patients who have PSVT despite drug therapy, who have unexplained syncope, or who have had an episode of atrial fibrillation in the setting of WPW syndrome. Rare patients in whom drugs cannot modify the tachycardia are recommended for surgery, endocardial catheter ablation of an AV connection or implantation of an antitachycardia pacemaker.

Wu D, et al. Clinical electrocardiographic and electrophysiologic observations in patients with paroxysmal supraventricular tachycardia. *Am J Cardiol* 41:1045–1051, 1978.
Reviews the electrophysiology and ECG characteristics of PSVT.
Wood P. Polyuria in paroxysmal tachycardia and paroxysmal atrial flutter and fibrillation. *Br Heart J* 25:273–282, 1963.
Classic description of hemodynamic consequences of PSVT.
Pritchett ELC, et al. Supraventricular tachycardia dependent upon accessory pathways in the absence of ventricular pre-excitation. *Am J Med* 64:214–220, 1978.
Mechanism of PSVT. Describes concealed accessory AV connections causing PSVT.
Denes P, et al. Dual atrioventricular nodal pathways: A common electrophysiological response. *Br Heart J* 37:1069–1076, 1975.
Reviews clinical and electrophysiologic characteristics of PSVT caused by dual AV nodal pathways.
Gallanger JJ, et al. The preexcitation syndromes. *Prog Cardiovasc Dis* 20(4):285–327, 1978.
Reviews Wolff-Parkinson-White syndrome.
Waxman MB, et al. Vagal techniques for termination of paroxysmal supraventricular tachycardia. *Am J Cardiol* 46:655–664, 1980.
Reviews effectiveness of vagal maneuvers in terminating PSVT.
Sung RJ, Elser B, McAllister RG. Intravenous verapamil for termination of re-entrant supraventricular tachycardias: Intracardiac studies correlated with plasma verapamil concentrations. *Ann Intern Med* 93:682–689, 1980.
Effect of plasma levels of verapamil on PSVT.
Swiryn S, et al. Effects of oral disopyramide phosphate on induction of paroxysmal supraventricular tachycardia. *Circulation* 64(1):169–175, 1981.
Use of disopyramide in PSVT.
Gettes LS, Foster JR, Simpson RJ. Clinical Use of Antiarrhythmic Drugs. In B Hoffman and M. Rosen (Eds.), *Cardiac Therapy*. The Hague: Marlinus Myhoff, 1983.
Review of pharmacology of antiarrhythmic drugs.
Hammill SC, Pritchett EC. Simplified esophageal electrocardiography using bipolar recording leads. *Ann Intern Med* 95:14–18, 1981.
Describes a useful method to detect P wave activity during tachycardia.

36. PREMATURE VENTRICULAR CONTRACTIONS
Ross J. Simpson, Jr.

Premature ventricular contractions (PVCs) can cause unpleasant symptoms and are associated with increased risk of sudden cardiac death in some patients. Physicians often administer potent antiarrhythmic drugs in an attempt to suppress these arrhythmias, although there is no compelling evidence that such treatment prevents death.

Prevalence
Premature ventricular contractions are found in apparently healthy individuals as well as in patients with severe structural heart disease. In patients without apparent heart disease, PVCs are present in 30 to 50% during a 24-hour period and are found in approximately 0.8% of routine electrocardiograms (ECGs). They are more common in older people. Complex forms are not rare: in a study of 50 normal medical students, 25 had at least one PVC in 24 hours, and of these, 6 had multiform PVCs, 3 had R-on-T PVCs, 1 had a couplet, and 1 had a five-beat run of ventricular tachycardia at a rate of 136 beats per minute. The frequency and complexity of PVCs are not necessarily related to each other.

Premature ventricular contractions are found more frequently in the presence of structural heart disease. During the early phase of acute myocardial infarction (MI), virtually 100% of patients have PVCs, approximately 10% of patients have R-on-T PVCs, and 15% of patients have ventricular tachycardia. The prevalence of PVCs decreases rapidly after the MI but increases again following discharge from the hospital. Patients with chronic angina pectoris or previous MI have a high prevalence of PVCs, and 5 to 10% of patients have asymptomatic, short-duration ventricular tachycardia during a 24-hour period. Premature ventricular contractions also occur frequently in other types of heart disease, including hypertensive and valvular heart disease, idiopathic hypertrophic subaortic stenosis (IHSS), sarcoidosis, and mitral valve prolapse.

Relationship to Sudden Cardiac Death
Not all patients with PVCs are at increased risk for sudden death. Factors that increase risk include the presence of heart disease, the frequency and complexity of the PVCs, concurrent drug use, and the presence of other diseases. If none of these is present (i.e., the patient is otherwise clinically healthy), the occurrence of simple PVCs is not known to increase the risk of death.

In contrast, patients with ischemic heart disease and PVCs may be at increased risk of sudden death, particularly if ventricular contractility is decreased. For example, the combination of complex PVCs and congestive heart failure (CHF) is associated with a sixfold increase in risk of sudden cardiac death and most deaths in the first 6 months following an MI occur in patients with a low ejection fraction (less than 0.4) and complex PVCs.

Certain complex forms are related to greater risk of subsequent mortality. Multiform PVCs and R-on-T PVCs appear to pose the greatest risk. Frequent PVCs, bigeminal patterns, and repetitive beats, although they mark an excess risk, are not independently associated with early mortality following an MI. Prolongation of the QT interval also predisposes to ventricular fibrillation.

Drug-Induced PVCs
Drugs, particularly digitalis, can cause PVCs and ventricular fibrillation. Others include quinidine, procainamide, disopyramide, the phenothiazines, and tricyclic antidepressants. Patients with heart disease as manifested by CHF, digitalis use, hypokalemia, and prolonged QT intervals are at greatest risk. Factors that predispose to drug-induced ventricular arrhythmias include the type and amount of drug, the extent of the underlying cardiac disease, and the individual myocardial sensitivity to the drug. However, because many of these drugs are used to treat PVCs, and because physicians expect patients with ventricular arrhythmias to die suddenly, an excess mortality caused by these drugs may go unnoticed.

Diagnosis

Symptoms and Signs
Patients with frequent or complex PVCs may be asymptomatic or may complain of palpitations, light-headedness, syncope, or atypical chest pains.

Symptoms of ventricular tachycardia are related to the rate and the underlying mechanical reserve of the heart. Ventricular tachycardia may be a stable rhythm for some patients for days or even weeks. Some patients may be relatively asymptomatic and feel only palpitations, light-headedness, or other symptoms similar to those occurring with paroxysmal supraventricular tachycardia. Others, with more rapid ventricular rates or more depressed cardiac contractility, may have syncope, profound hypotension, diaphoresis, and impaired tissue perfusion. The pulse is regular and rapid, and physical findings of atrioventricular (AV) dissociation, including venous cannon A waves and variation in the intensity of the first heart sound, may be present.

Electrocardiogram
A PVC is premature, wide, and often bizarre in appearance. The ST segment and T wave are abnormal and often in the opposite direction from the QRS. There is usually no P wave preceding the QRS, and the pause following a PVC is often fully compensatory. Occasionally, a PVC captures the atrium, resets the sinus node, and causes a less than compensatory pause. Interpolated PVCs (when the PVC is squeezed in between two normally occurring sinus beats) occur at slow rates when early-cycle PVCs do not reset the sinus rate or interfere with AV conduction of the subsequent normal beat. The coupling interval between PVCs and sinus beats may be "fixed"; for short periods there is less than a 0.06-second variation in the coupling interval of the QRS of the sinus beat to the PVC.

Ventricular tachycardia is defined as three or more consecutive PVCs. The rate varies from 100 to over 200 beats per minute, and the rhythm may be regular (like paroxysmal supraventricular tachycardia [PSVT]) or slightly irregular. Consecutive PVCs at a rate of less than 100 per minute are usually referred to as accelerated idioventricular rhythm. Sustained ventricular tachycardia may be difficult to distinguish from PSVT with bundle branch block or conduction aberration; however, AV dissociation and ventricular capture and fusion beats identify ventricular tachycardia. Occasionally, AV dissociation may be absent or incomplete because of intermittent atrial capture by the ventricles. Other, less reliable electrocardiographic features of ventricular tachycardia include a QRS duration of greater than 0.14 seconds, extreme left axis deviation, or certain abnormal QRS configurations (e.g., a mono- or biphasic right bundle branch block–shaped QRS complex in V_1).

Other Studies
Most PVCs can be diagnosed from the standard ECG. Lewis leads or esophageal leads may aid diagnosis by detection of AV dissociation. If necessary, intracardiac electrodes can be inserted for definitive diagnosis.

Treatment
Deciding whether to treat PVCs is difficult since not all patients with PVCs are at risk of sudden death and treatment is often disruptive or dangerous. Moreover, the frequency of PVCs varies so greatly that very large reductions in observed PVCs in an individual patient must be observed before it is reasonable to conclude that treatment, rather than spontaneous variation, is responsible for the change. Finally, a reduction in frequency or complexity of PVCs is often used as a marker of successful treatment, although this reduction in PVCs is not known to be associated with reduction in the incidence of sudden cardiac death.

In general, treatment is considered if the patient is symptomatic, has ventricular tachycardia, is within 6 months of an MI, or has heart failure, angina, mitral prolapse, IHSS, sarcoidosis, valvular heart disease, poor left ventricular function, or other types of structural heart disease.

Because of the possibility that antiarrhythmic drugs may worsen the arrhythmia, many cardiologists admit patients to the hospital prior to beginning therapy. Hypokalemia, CHF, and coronary ischemia are treated. Cardiac drugs are often discontinued and the patient is monitored to estimate PVC frequency and complexity. Often 48 hours of monitoring are necessary to document frequency adequately. The following are often determined: the effect of exercise on the arrhythmia and an estimation of cardiac contractility (by echocardiogram, nuclear angiography, or cardiac catheterization). An antiarrhythmic drug is then administered, and the efficacy of the drug is evaluated by continuing ECG monitoring and treadmill exercise testing. An electrophysiologic cardiac pacing study is considered for patients with sustained ventricular tachycardia or those resuscitated from sudden cardiac death since the arrhythmia can be reproduced and treated by this method in a high percentage of patients.

Drug Therapy

It is best to think of the antiarrhythmic drugs according to their effect or specific characteristics on the cardiac action potential. One scheme divides the drugs into those that act like the prototype drugs: quinidine, lidocaine, verapamil, or propranolol. Because there is considerable individual variability in drug responsiveness, absorption, and half-life, therapy with these drugs should be guided by serum drug levels.

Quinidine-like Drugs

Quinidine-like drugs (quinidine, procainamide, and disopyramide) are the most commonly used antiarrhythmic drugs in the treatment of chronic PVCs. They slow the upstroke of the action potential and decrease cellular excitability by depressing the rapid sodium-dependent channel. Quinidine-like drugs decrease conduction velocity in both normal and abnormal fibers. The most serious side effect of these drugs is the potentiation of life-threatening ventricular arrhythmias. This complication is most likely to occur if the QT interval is excessively prolonged.

Quinidine is available as the sulfate salt. The usual dosage is 200 to 400 mg every 6 to 8 hours. Longer-acting preparations are available as a gluconate salt or as a time-release tablet. Quinidine has negligible depressant effects on left ventricular function, but other side effects include diarrhea, tinnitus, thrombocytopenia, and hypotension. As many as 25% of patients given quinidine may have to discontinue it because of side effects.

Procainamide is available as an immediate-release preparation administered 200 to 750 mg every 3 to 4 hours or as a slow-release preparation administered every 6 to 8 hours. Nausea is not infrequent with procainamide. Antinuclear antibodies are positive in a high percentage of patients, but a lupus-like syndrome occurs in only a small number of these patients. As with quinidine, the depressant effect on left ventricular contractility is small.

Disopyramide is administered as 100 to 120 mg every 6 to 8 hours. Side effects include urinary retention, dry mouth, hypotension, exacerbation of CHF, and depression of left ventricular contractility.

Lidocaine-like Drugs

Lidocaine-like drugs are unlike the quinidine-like drugs in that they selectively depress the rapid sodium current in partially depressed fibers. This difference in effect on the action potential may partially explain the relatively low reported incidence of lidocaine-potentiated arrhythmias. Orally administered lidocaine-like drugs will be available for clinical use in the next few years.

Calcium Blocking Drugs

Calcium blocking drugs like verapamil may be effective in treating certain types of ventricular arrhythmias, particularly in preventing the ventricular tachycardia associated with coronary artery spasm or in treating exercise-potentiated ventricular arrhythmias.

Beta-Sympathetic Blocking Drugs

Beta-sympathetic blocking drugs are effective in controlling catecholamine-potentiated ventricular arrhythmias, including those induced by anesthetic agents, thyrotoxicosis, and digitalis excess and those associated with cardiac ischemia. Beta-sympathetic drugs are particularly useful in treating patients with exercise-induced ventricular tachycardia.

Propranolol is administered in a dosage of 20 to 80 mg every 6 to 8 hours. Side effects include fatigue, lethargy, impotence, exacerbation of CHF, potentiation of bradyar-rhythmias in patients with preexisting sinoatrial disease, and bronchospasm in pa-tients prone to asthma. Because these drugs significantly depress left ventricular func-tion, the combination of propranolol and disopyramide should be avoided. The water-soluble beta-blocking drugs, including atenolol and nadolol, need less dose titration and less frequent dosing intervals.

Moss AJ. Clinical significance of ventricular arrhythmias in patients with and without coronary artery disease. *Prog Cardiovasc Dis* 23:33–52, 1980.
Excellent review of the prevalence and significance of PVCs in clinical practice.

Brodsky M, et al. Arrhythmias documented by 24 hour continuous electrocardiographic monitoring in 50 male medical students without apparent heart disease. *Am J Car-diol* 39:390–395, 1977.
Frequency and complexity of PVCs in a normal population.

Hiss RG, Lamb LE. Electrocardiographic findings in 122,043 individuals. *Circulation* 25:947–961, 1962.
Electrocardiographic abnormalities in normal subjects.

Kostis JB, et al. Premature ventricular complexes in the absence of identifiable heart disease. *Circulation* 63:1351–1356, 1981.
Twenty-four–hour Holter monitor study of apparently normal subjects.

Winkle RA, et al. Arrhythmias in patients with mitral valve prolapse. *Circulation* 52:73–81, 1975.
Prevalence of PVCs and other arrhythmias in mitral prolapse.

Schulze RA Jr, et al. Ventricular arrhythmias in the late hospital phase of acute myo-cardial infarction: Relation to left ventricular function detected by gated cardiac blood pool scanning. *Circulation* 52:1006–1011, 1975.
Relationship of PVCs to cardiac contractility.

Schulze RA, Strauss HW, Pitt B. Sudden death in the year following myocardial in-farction: Relation to ventricular premature contractions in the late hospital phase and left ventricular ejection fraction. *Am J Med* 62:192–199, 1977.
Relationship of PVCs and cardiac contractility to mortality.

Gettes LS, Foster JR, Simpson RJ. Clinical Use of Antiarrhythmic Drugs. In B Hoff-man and M Rosen (Eds.), *Cardiac Therapy*. The Hague: Marinus Nijhoff, 1983.
Clinical pharmacology of the antiarrhythmic drugs.

37. PACEMAKERS
Andreas T. Wielgosz

Although management of patients with implanted cardiac pacemakers is often super-vised by a cardiologist, other clinicians must be able to recognize complications as they occur. Over 250,000 patients in the United States have artificial pacemakers. The de-vices are produced by 27 companies worldwide, many featuring several models. In spite of increasing technologic complexities, there remain three basic characteristics for each pacemaker: sensing, power, and capture. Sensing is the receiving and processing of electrical signals generated by the heart. Power is the ability of the pacemaker to provide stimulation as required. Capture describes the appropriate stimulation of the heart by the pacemaker. All pacemakers have a built-in replacement indicator, and most units implanted today are also programmable.

Complications

Local Complications
Infections around the implanted pacemaker are now very uncommon because of im-proved techniques. Most occur within 3 months of surgery and may present with con-

stitutional symptoms as well as local inflammation. Tenderness and shifting or erosion at the pacemaker site can also occur without infection.

Not uncommonly patients with pacemakers have muscular distress. The most common syndrome is diaphragmatic stimulation, usually from phrenic nerve activation (because of its proximity to the apex of the heart). Less often, the pectoralis muscle is stimulated. If muscular stimulation occurs around the pacing wires or near the pacemaker of a bioplar system, it usually indicates an electrical leak.

Pacemaker Failure

About 10% of all failures (i.e., any deviation from intended function) are reported within the first week of implantation. After 1 week, only 10% of failures are accompanied by the return of symptoms; most are asymptomatic when they are first detected. In one study of 340 pacemaker failures occurring in 1,705 patients over 4 years, 50% of the failures were due to lead-related problems (mainly dislodgement), 41% were battery failures, and 5% were electronic component failures. Dysrhythmias unrelated to the pacemaker occurred in 4% of failures.

Poor sensing may be due to reception of an inadequate cardiac signal, either because the lead is malpositioned or because there is an increase in threshold at the electrode-myocardial interface. Failure to sense may be accompanied by failure to capture. Usually the lead is implanted through the cephalic, subclavian, or jugular vein into the right ventricular endocardium. New lead systems allow active (screw mechanisms) or passive (barb) fixation. A dislodged or fractured lead may be detected by x-ray. When no radiologic abnormalities are seen, analysis of the stimulus artifact is a sensitive way of detecting wire fracture or failure secondary to insulation disruption.

Oversensing is a response of the pacemaker to undesired stimuli. The pacemaker may inappropriately sense normal cardiac electrical events, such as T waves, electromagnetic interference from a microwave oven, or small potentials from contraction of pectoralis muscle underlying the pulse generator. Myo-potential inhibition of demand pacemakers can be caused by electrical stimuli generated by skeletal muscle. This phenomenon has been reported in 11 to 85% of patients with unipolar lead systems and favors the use of bipolar lead systems.

Failure to capture may be due to lead interruption, exit block, subthreshold generator output, and battery exhaustion.

Power failures can be due to either disturbances in the electronic circuitry, which tend to be a random event, or battery depletion, which is usually a function of time. Beyond 5 years, battery depletion is the leading cause for pacemaker failure. A decline in rate below the fixed setting of the implanted unit is the usual indicator of power source depletion. A small or moderate decline in rate (less than 10% of set rate) usually requires no intervention. However, if the decline continues, the battery needs replacement. Fluctuation in the rate usually indicates instability of the electronic circuit and should be monitored closely. Rate variations can also occur with fever, particularly in lithium-powered units. In most systems, battery depletion is indicated by alterations in pulse width and rate.

Patient Monitoring

Every patient should be educated about the pacemaker while still in the hospital. Most centers provide an instruction book. Important information, such as the model type and serial number of the implanted pacemaker unit, should either be kept in the book or typed on a special card. This will help identify the specific characteristics of the system that will be needed in case of complications or manufacturer recall.

After the first visit, 2 weeks postimplantation, two additional visits at 3-month intervals are customary, followed by annual checks. After the fifth year, patients with lithium-powered units should be seen every 3 months. The life expectancy of mercury cells is shorter, but these units are no longer implanted. Newly introduced, programmable, dual-chamber pacemakers (which can stimulate both atria and ventricles) may require more frequent checks while more experience with them accumulates. Multiprogrammable pacemakers permit noninvasive analysis of problems; this is best done by a specialist.

Besides inquiring about general health, the physician should specifically ask about signs and symptoms of heart failure, syncope, respiratory insufficiency, coronary insufficiency, skin reactions, and accompanying pain, hematomas, and thrombosis. It is important to be attentive to the psychological adjustment after implantation and to provide reassurance. Following a thorough physical examination, the patient should have an electrocardiogram (ECG) taken both with and without the application of a magnet to assess rate, sensory, power, and capture functions of the system. The magnet turns a demand pacemaker into a fixed-rhythm pacemaker.

Many specialized clinics have the facilities for monitoring pacemaker systems by transmitting an audible tone by telephone. Usually the entire ECG, both with and without the magnetic mode, is relayed over the telephone. From this, pulse width and rate can be measured. Newer, more sophisticated systems provide additional electronic analysis. Primarily, telephone monitoring is used to confirm the presence of pacemaker stimulation and subsequent capture and to assess the power reserve from the magnetic mode rate.

Vera A, Klein C, Mason DT. Recent advances in programmable pacemakers. *Am J Med* 66:473, 1979.
  The indications, mechanisms, and significance of these units are discussed.
Furman S. Cardiac pacing and pacemakers: VIII. The pacemaker follow up clinic. *Am Heart J* 94:795, 1977.
  A leading authority on the subject reviews the experience of several pacemaker clinics and provides guidelines for follow-up of patients with implanted pacemakers.
Mantini EL, et al. A recommended protocol for pacemaker follow up; analysis of 1705 implanted pacemakers. *Ann Thorac Surg* 24:62, 1977.
  Based on a 4-year follow-up of 1705 patients with implanted pacemakers, a clinical protocol is offered for monitoring such patients.
Furman S. Newer modes of cardiac pacing: I. Desciption of pacing modes. *Mod Concepts Cardiovasc Dis* 52:1, 1983.
  The major stimulation modes of dual chamber pacemakers are described, and the new five-position ICHD code is explained.
Furham S. Newer modes of cardiac pacing: II. Intraoperative evaluation and selection of pacemakers for bradyarrhythmias. *Mod Concepts Cardiovasc Dis* 52:7, 1983.
  The author discusses the selection of the appropriate dual chamber pacing system in order to restore normal physiologic, atrioventricular function.
Josephson ME. Key references—pacemakers. *Circulation* 63:230, 1981.
  Although not annotated, this is the most comprehensive bibliographic list readily available on the subject. References are listed under 13 major headings.
Parsonnet, V, Bernstein, AD. Cardiac pacing in the 1980s: Treatment and techniques in transition. *J Am Coll Cardiol* 1:339–54, 1983.
  An excellent, objective discussion of the current use of pacemakers. This well-referenced article also provides a good evaluation of dual-chamber pacemakers, which show promise of being the predominant pacemaker of the immediate future.

38. HEART MURMURS
Park W. Willis IV

Careful auscultation in quiet surroundings frequently reveals cardiac murmurs in healthy individuals and patients without diagnosed heart disease. The distinction between an innocent and pathologic murmur can usually be made by a history and thorough cardiovascular examination. The amplitude, location, and timing of a murmur are important; however, diagnosis also depends on examination of carotid, jugular venous, and precordial pulses and heart sounds.

Systolic Murmurs
Under optimal conditions, systolic murmurs are audible with a stethoscope in 50 to 70% of normal children and adolescents. In early adulthood systolic murmurs are less

frequently detected, but the prevalence of systolic murmurs gradually increases, to reach approximately 50% over age 50.

Midsystolic (ejection) murmurs begin after the first heart sound (S_1), terminate before the related semilunar valve closure, and have a crescendo-decrescendo contour. These murmurs are caused by turbulence of flow as blood is ejected from the ventricle, across the aortic or pulmonic valve into a great vessel. The amplitude of a midsystolic ejection murmur varies with stroke volume; it may be diminished with premature beats and increases after long diastolic filling periods following a premature beat or during atrial fibrillation.

Pansystolic (regurgitant) murmurs are caused by turbulent flow from a high- to a low-pressure chamber. These murmurs begin with S_1 and continue through the related semilunar valve closure sound. Unlike ejection murmurs, pansystolic regurgitant murmurs do not change significantly in amplitude with changes in diastolic filling period length.

Late systolic murmurs begin in mid or late systole and continue up to and sometimes through S_2.

Early systolic murmurs begin with S_1 and end in mid or late systole before S_2. These murmurs are caused by the same lesions responsible for pansystolic murmurs. However, because of conditions in the chamber accepting the regurgitant volume, the pressure rises to equal that in the donor chamber in late systole, decreasing retrograde flow and causing the murmur to diminish before S_2.

Innocent Murmurs

An innocent murmur occurs in the absence of any abnormality of cardiac structure or function. Murmurs associated with an abnormally large cardiac output and those caused by a selective increase in flow through a valve, such as midsystolic ejection murmurs associated with aortic regurgitation or atrial septal defect, are not considered innocent.

Innocent systolic murmurs are midsystolic and usually grade $^{1-2}/_6$ in amplitude. They may be louder in thin children and young adults when the stethoscope on the chest wall is close to the source of the murmur and when the cardiac output is increased by anemia, anxiety, fever, or pregnancy. Innocent murmurs are usually best heard at the left sternal edge in the second and third intercostal spaces and tend to decrease, or disappear, with upright position. A common form of innocent systolic murmur (Still's murmur) is twanging, vibratory, or grunting in quality and loudest at the lower sternal border and midprecordium. This murmur is usually found in children. In the majority of cases, it disappears during puberty but may persist into adulthood.

The cardiorespiratory murmur is an unusual type of innocent systolic murmur. It is loudest during inspiration and markedly reduced, or absent, during expiration and with breath-holding. The murmur is high frequency and is heard best at the left sternal edge or apex. It is probably caused by the heart compressing and decompressing a portion of lung or bronchus so that the murmur is actually a breath sound.

If a systolic murmur is innocent, the carotid, jugular venous, and left ventricular apex pulses are normal; S_1 is of normal amplitude; S_2 shows physiologic splitting; and there are no abnormal extra sounds, or diastolic murmurs.

Midsystolic Murmurs in Middle and Old Age

Midsystolic murmurs in middle and old age are common and are similar to the innocent murmurs of younger individuals. They are maximal at the left sternal edge or aortic area but are often heard best at the apex. The murmurs frequently reach grade $^{2-3}/_6$ amplitude. Because they are usually associated with some minor underlying cardiac abnormality, they are not truly innocent. Age-related thickening of the base of the aortic valve cusps (aortic sclerosis), hypertension, and dilation of the aortic root are frequent causes. In the absence of other disease the carotid pulse is normal. When there is associated left ventricular hypertrophy, the cause of a midsystolic murmur may be calcific aortic stenosis.

Pathologic Midsystolic Murmurs

These are caused by aortic or pulmonic stenosis or atrial septal defect and may be confused with innocent murmurs in children and young adults.

Semilunar valve stenosis of mild degree is almost always associated with an ejection sound. These are discrete, high-frequency sounds that follow S_1 by about 0.04 to 0.06

second. Aortic ejection sounds are widely transmitted over the precordium and are usually loudest at the apex, while pulmonic ejection sounds are localized to the left sternal edge and show respiratory variation, increasing in amplitude with expiration and decreasing or disappearing with inspiration. When the degree of semilunar valve stenosis is mild, the murmurs are maximal in midsystole, similar to an innocent murmur. With increasing obstruction to blood flow, they become longer and reach maximal amplitude later in systole. Important valvular stenosis causes hypertrophy of the related ventricle, which can be detected as a sustained apical impulse or parasternal lift. S_2 is normal in mild aortic stenosis. The pulmonic component (P_2) is delayed and often diminished in amplitude in valvular pulmonic stenosis.

In adults with moderate to severe aortic valvular stenosis, there may be no ejection sound, and the S_2 may diminish because cusp excursion is limited by calcification. Although the midsystolic murmur of valvular aortic stenosis is typically heard best at the aortic area, in elderly patients it is frequently loudest at the apex. When S_2 is diminished and not well transmitted to the apex, it may be difficult to decide whether the murmur is mid- or pansystolic. When premature beats are present, a murmur louder after long diastolic filling periods is an important clue to outflow tract obstruction. The carotid pulse is abnormal in most patients with significant left ventricular outflow obstruction.

Hemodynamically significant atrial septal defects are associated with large right ventricular stroke volumes and a midsystolic pulmonic ejection murmur that is identical in character to an innocent murmur. However, other clues to the correct diagnosis are often present. A prominent right ventricular impulse at the left sternal edge is usually palpable. S_1 is often widely split because of increased blood flow over the tricuspid valve and delayed tricuspid closure, and S_2 is usually widely split with little respiratory variation. In children and young adults with significant left-to-right shunts, a mid-diastolic rumble is usually audible at the lower left sternal edge.

The systolic murmur in IHSS is midsystolic and usually loudest at the left sternal edge, rather than at the aortic area. The murmur is often associated with a sustained left ventricular apex impulse and an S_4. Response of the murmur to physiologic maneuvers provides specific information. The strain phase of Valsalva's maneuver, standing from a squatting position, and inhalation of amyl nitrite all increase the midsystolic murmur of IHSS by causing an abrupt fall in systemic venous return, which leads to a decrease in left ventricular cavity size and augmentation of the subaortic left ventricular outflow tract gradient. The innocent midsystolic murmur decreases in amplitude with these maneuvers. Differentiation of IHSS from valvular aortic stenosis can be made by careful examination or graphic recording of the carotid pulse. In IHSS, the carotid upstroke is brisk and usually bisferious in contour. In most cases of valvular aortic stenosis the rate of rise of the carotid pulse is slow, with a palpable systolic vibration (carotid shudder).

Other causes of midsystolic murmurs include supravalvular aortic stenosis and fibromuscular subaortic stenosis. In these variants there is no ejection sound. With infundibular pulmonic stenosis, the midsystolic murmur is maximal lower along the left sternal border and there is no ejection sound. With valvular as well as infundibular pulmonic stenosis, the pulmonic component of S_2 is delayed and soft if the outflow gradient is significant.

Pansystolic Murmurs

These are always pathologic and are usually caused by mitral regurgitation, tricuspid regurgitation, or ventricular septal defect.

A pansystolic murmur maximal at the apex is evidence for mitral regurgitation. The pansystolic murmur of ventricular septal defects is usually loudest at the lower left sternal edge. Tricuspid regurgitation is most commonly a late complication of left-sided heart disease that has resulted in pulmonary hypertension. The murmur of tricuspid regurgitation is usually loudest at the lower left sternal edge, but when the right ventricle is dilated the murmur may be maximal in the fifth intercostal space in the midclavicular line. Audibility only during inspiration, inspiratory increase in intensity of the murmur, an abnormal systolic wave in the jugular venous pulse, and hepatic pulsation are helpful aids in recognizing tricuspid regurgitation.

Late Systolic Murmurs
The late systolic murmur of mild mitral regurgitation, resulting from mitral valve prolapse, usually maximal at the apex, may be audible only when the patient is sitting or standing. The murmur is often associated with solitary or multiple mid- or late systolic clicks.

Early Systolic Murmurs
Early systolic murmurs are uncommon. Trivial mitral and tricuspid regurgitation are two causes. In acute severe mitral regurgitation, the murmur may terminate before S_2, simulating a midsystolic ejection murmur. Echophonocardiographic studies can distinguish the murmurs when the clinical diagnosis is uncertain.

Diastolic Murmurs
Diastolic murmurs almost always indicate organic heart disease. Early diastolic decrescendo murmurs from aortic or pulmonic regurgitation begin with the appropriate semilunar valve closure sound and are usually loudest at the left sternal edge. Mid- and late diastolic murmurs are most often caused by mitral stenosis. However, they may also be caused by high volume antegrade flow over regurgitant atrioventricular valves, by premature closure of the mitral valve in severe aortic regurgitation (Austin Flint murmur), and by intracardiac shunts, especially atrial or ventricular septal defects.

Continuous Murmurs
Continuous murmurs begin in systole and persist through S_2 into diastole. The most common is the innocent venous hum, which is present in most children and many young adults. The murmur is usually loudest over the medial aspect of the right supraclavicular fossa with the patient sitting and the chin pulled upward and to the left. Deep inspiration may increase the amplitude of a venous hum, and the murmur can be abolished by firm pressure over the ipsilateral internal jugular vein.

Pathologic continuous murmurs can result from an aortopulmonary connection. The most common of these is patent ductus arteriosus, in which the murmur is loudest at the upper left sternal edge or under the left clavicle. Other causes of continuous murmurs are congenital, traumatic, or surgically constructed arteriovenous fistulae. Coarctation of the aorta and peripheral pulmonary stenosis cause systolic murmurs, but can result in continuous murmurs, loudest in systole, when there is very severe constriction.

Evaluation
When a soft, midsystolic murmur is heard in an asymptomatic child or young adult and the remainder of the cardiovascular examination is normal, there is a strong likelihood that the murmur is innocent. If the murmur disappears with standing or the strain phase of Valsalva's maneuver, the diagnosis of an innocent systolic ejection murmur is firm, and further studies are not necessary. Innocent murmurs are frequently louder with increased cardiac output caused by transient conditions such as exercise, anxiety, fever, anemia, pregnancy, or thyrotoxicosis. Therefore, repeated examination may be helpful.

When the history, physical findings, response to physiologic maneuvers, or an unusually loud murmur suggests an organic lesion, the 12-lead electrocardiogram (ECG) and chest x-ray are useful in assessing cardiac dimensions and hypertrophy. Echophonocardiography and pulse recordings are very useful when physical findings are equivocal. The greatest value of echocardiography is in the assessment of cardiac disease diagnosed by history, physical examination, chest x-ray, and ECG. Echocardiography is useful in confirming the location and severity of clinically detected valvular lesions. This information is often valuable as part of the initial evaluation and in the follow-up of patients with heart disease.

Leatham A. Auscultation of the heart. *Lancet* 2:703, 757, 1958. (This is a two-part article in separate issues.)
A classic discussion on auscultation and classification of heart murmurs.
Craige E. Echophonocardiography and Other Non-invasive Techniques to Elucidate

Heart Murmurs. In E Braunwald (Ed.), *Heart Disease* (2nd ed.). Philadelphia: Saunders, 1984. P. 68.

A comprehensive discussion of the diagnostic techniques of echophonocardiography and pulse recordings.

McLaren MJ, et al. Innocent murmurs and third heart sounds in Black schoolchildren. *Br Heart J* 43:67, 1980.

Of 12,050 children aged 2 to 18 years, 96% had physiologic S_3, 72% had innocent systolic murmurs, and 0.27% had innocent mid-diastolic murmurs.

Hancock EW. The ejection sound in aortic stenosis. *Am J Med* 40:569, 1966.

Aortic ejection sounds were uniformly present in patients with noncalcific aortic valve stenosis but absent in those with subvalvular or supravalvular stenosis.

Perloff JK. Clinical recognition of aortic stenosis: The physical signs and differential diagnosis of various forms of obstruction to the left ventricular outflow. *Prog Cardiovasc Dis* 10:323, 1968.

An extensive review of the subject.

Leatham A, Weitzman, D. Auscultatory and phonocardiographic signs of pulmonary stenosis. *Br Heart J* 19:303, 1957.

Study of 70 patients with valvular and infundibular stenosis.

Rees A, Farru O, Rodriguez R. Phonocardiographic, radiologic, and hemodynamic correlation in atrial septal defect. *Br Heart J* 34:781, 1972.

Auscultatory findings in 51 patients with atrial septal defect proved by cardiac catheterization.

Bruns, DL, VanDerHauwaert, LG. The aortic systolic murmur developing with increasing age. *Br Heart J* 20:370, 1958.

Systolic murmurs were present in 50% of 300 patients over 50 years of age.

Barlow J, Kincaid-Smith P. The auscultatory findings in hypertension. *Br Heart J* 22:505, 1960.

Of 100 patients with hypertension, 71% were found to have systolic ejection murmurs.

Tavel ME. Innocent Murmurs. In DF Leon and JA Shaver (Eds.), *Physiologic Principles of Heart Sounds and Murmurs*. New York: American Heart Association, 1975. Pp. 102–106.

An excellent discussion.

Dohan MC, Criscitiello MG. Physiological and pharmacological manipulations of heart sounds and murmurs. *Mod Concepts Cardiovasc Dis* 36:121, 1970.

A good review.

Sutton GC, Craige E. Clinical signs of severe acute mitral regurgitation. *Am J Cardiol* 20:141, 1967.

A case report and discussion of the pathophysiology underlying the clinical manifestations of acute severe mitral regurgitation.

Grimmer SFM, Tindall H, Hill JD. Diagnostic contribution of echocardiography. *Lancet* 1:440, 1982.

Only 5% of echocardiographic examinations revealed a diagnosis when there was no clinical cardiac diagnosis prior to the study.

Newburger JW, et al. Noninvasive tests in the initial evaluation of heart murmurs in children. *N Engl J Med* 308:61, 1983.

Routine ECG, chest x-rays, and M-mode echocardiography rarely improved upon the diagnosis made by qualified pediatric cardiologists on the basis of history and physical examination.

Rothman A, Goldberger AL. Aids to cardiac ascultation. *Ann Intern Med* 99:346, 1983.

A recent, critical literature review with emphasis on the sensitivity and specificity of physiologic and pharmacologic maneuvers commonly used to aid in cardiac auscultation.

39. MITRAL VALVE PROLAPSE

Sheldon M. Retchin and Robert A. Waugh

Mitral valve prolapse (MVP) is a common condition resulting from an abnormal systolic protrusion of the mitral valve leaflets into the left atrium. In most cases, the prolapse is probably due to fibromyxomatous degeneration of the leaflets, which less often may affect other valves. Usually MVP is discovered during a routine checkup or when evaluating symptoms referable to the chest.

Clinical Manifestations

A variety of symptoms—chest pain, dyspnea, fatigue, dizziness, syncope, palpitations, and anxiety—have been attributed to MVP; many think that together they constitute a syndrome. Although a majority of people with MVP eventually experience one or more of the above symptoms, it is not certain whether these complaints are found more often in people with MVP than in other patients.

Chest pain is often the most troublesome and frequent symptom attributed to MVP. The pain has been described as a poorly localized, dull ache, which is nonexertional, nonradiating, and unrelieved by rest or nitroglycerin. A variety of pathophysiologic explanations for the chest pain have been proposed, but none has been established. While dyspnea and fatigue are also frequent complaints, they rarely indicate the development of congestive heart failure. Mitral valve prolapse has also been associated with both ventricular and supraventricular arrhythmias and infrequently with dysautonomia. These conditions should be considered in patients with dizziness or syncope.

Prevalence

The prevalence of MVP largely depends on the diagnostic test used for detection. Studies using either M-mode or two-dimensional echocardiography have consistently found MVP to be present in about 6% of people. With cardiac auscultation, the prevalence of MVP ranges from 1 to 21%, depending on who is performing the examination. These estimates of prevalence are based on anatomic and physiologic criteria for MVP, which do not necessarily predict clinically important sequelae such as arrhythmias or endocarditis. Most published studies of MVP describe a 2:1 female predominance, but this may be an artifact, resulting from the greater frequency with which females visit physicians and the bias from early studies, which included only female volunteers.

Diagnosis

During the physical examination particular attention should be paid to findings suggested by the history. The patient's general appearance may suggest one of a variety of abnormalities of connective tissue disorders associated with MVP, the most common of which is Marfan's syndrome.

The spectrum of auscultatory findings in MVP is quite broad, ranging from one or more mid- to late systolic clicks, to a mid- to late systolic murmur with or without a click, to a holosystolic murmur with or without late systolic accentuation. Approximately one-third of patients have click(s) alone, one-third have click(s) and murmur, and one-third have a murmur alone.

The click is a high-pitched sound, which may be single or multiple and can be distinguished from ejection clicks by respiration (pulmonic diminishes with inspiration) and location (aortic louder along the outflow tract and base). The vast majority of mid- to late systolic nonejection clicks are due to MVP.

The murmur of MVP may begin with the first heart sound and be holosystolic (with or without late systolic accentuation) or may begin in mid- to late systole. Although the majority of murmurs with a late systolic crescendo are due to MVP, the absence of an associated click should prompt consideration of papillary muscle dysfunction or rheumatic heart disease.

Occasionally a provocative maneuver is necessary to bring out the typical auscultatory findings. Since MVP may be thought of as a condition in which the mitral valve is "too large" for the left ventricle, any maneuver that decreases the size of the ventricle will exaggerate the prolapse. Standing the patient up, a continued Valsalva strain, and amyl nitrite inhalation will all tend to move click and murmur closer toward S_1, making them easier to hear.

Echocardiography

Both M-mode and two-dimensional echocardiography are safe, accurate, and reliable ways of confirming MVP and are commonly used for that purpose. However, because most MVP is harmless, these tests are primarily useful for detecting a complication of MVP (e.g., ruptured chordae tendinae, endocarditis with vegetations) or ruling out other treatable conditions (e.g., idiopathic hypertrophic subacute stenosis) when they are suspected. Because of the frequency of MVP, the excellent prognosis in most cases, and the expense of the echocardiograms, these tests should not be used simply for confirmation. Similarly, neither angiography nor nuclear imaging has a place in the routine evaluation of MVP, except to rule in other disease (e.g., ischemic heart disease) or complications (e.g., severe mitral regurgitation).

Prognosis

While it is generally agreed that MVP can lead to endocarditis, arrhythmias or sudden death, congestive heart failure, and cerebrovascular accidents, the rates at which these happen are clearly low. It is likely that many published studies of prognosis included patients who were at unusually high risk for complications for reasons other than MVP (e.g., drug addiction, immunocompromised states) and probably overestimate the risk for unselected people.

Management

Most people with MVP are not at significantly increased risk of complications. However, clinicians frequently must decide what, if anything, should be done when the syndrome is found.

Asymptomatic Patients

A substantial proportion of patients with MVP are diagnosed on routine physical examination or while being seen for unrelated problems. For the great majority of these patients, the prognosis is excellent, and no further diagnostic tests or treatments are necessary. These patients should not suffer unnecessarily from the impression that they have an abnormal heart. The benign nature of MVP should be strongly emphasized in order to avoid needless anxiety.

Endocarditis

The American Heart Association currently recommends antibiotic prophylaxis to prevent bacterial endocarditis in patients with MVP who have mitral regurgitation. Usually this is decided by cardiac auscultation because there is no other noninvasive, inexpensive method for determining the hemodynamic significance of MR. Decisions about individual patients should be based on characteristics of the murmur.

Arrhythmias and Sudden Death

Numerous supraventricular and ventricular arrhythmias have been described in patients with MVP. However, a policy of extensively evaluating all MVP patients with dizziness or palpitations is clearly difficult to justify. Symptoms often fail to match arrhythmias seen on Holter monitoring, and spontaneous variation of rhythm disturbances makes response to antiarrhythmic drugs difficult to assess.

Although MVP has been associated with an increased risk of sudden death, the risk must be very small. In most autopsy series of sudden death, MVP is rarely cited. In general, the decision to evaluate or treat syncope should be made without regard to the presence of MVP, and MVP should not serve as a cue for treatment with antiarrhythmic agents.

Cerebrovascular Events

Several case series have linked MVP with cerebral ischemic events, particularly in young adults. However, the rarity of cerebrovascular events in this age group makes any risk from MVP extremely small. In addition, the proposed hypercoagulable state said to account for the association between cerebrovascular events and MVP is not substantiated by reports of associations with either thrombophlebitis or other extracerebral embolic events. Therefore, based on current data, the use of prophylactic anticoagulant drugs in patients with MVP is not warranted.

Barlow TB, et al. The significance of late systolic murmurs. *Am Heart J* 66:443–452, 1963.
Regarded as the original article demonstrating a structural cardiac defect in patients with auscultatory findings of click or late systolic murmur.

Procacci PM, et al. Prevalence of clinical mitral-valve prolapse in 1169 young women. *N Engl J Med* 294:1086–1088, 1976.
In 1169 women examined during a 2-week period for the presence of MVP, 74 (6.3%) had physical findings consistent with MVP and 60 (5.1%) also had positive echocardiograms.

Markiewicz W, et al. Mitral valve prolapse in one hundred presumably healthy young females. *Circulation* 53:464–473, 1975.
Twenty-one per cent were found to have systolic prolapse by echocardiography. Most clinical findings were remarkably similar in those with and without echocardiographic evidence of MVP.

Walsh PN, et al. Platelets, thromboembolism and mitral valve prolapse. *Circulation* 63:552–559, 1981.
Twenty-nine patients with MVP, including 17 who had a history of thromboembolic events or visual complaints. Platelet coagulant hyperactivity was highly associated with a history of thromboembolism.

Mills P, et al. Long-term prognosis of mitral-valve prolapse. *N Engl J Med* 297:13–18, 1977.
A retrospective follow-up of 53 patients detected 1 to 22 years previously as having a midsystolic click and/or late systolic murmur by phonocardiogram. Three developed bacterial endocarditis, 5 had progressive mitral valve regurgitation (2 required mitral valve replacement), and 1 had recurrent ventricular fibrillation. There were 2 deaths. The presence of a late murmur was considered a significant predictor of complications.

Perloff JK. Evolving concepts of mitral valve prolapse. *N Engl J Med* 307:369–370, 1982.
Perloff emphasizes the need to distinguish between "pathologic" and "normal" MVP. He refers to the pathologic variety as being strongly associated with connective-tissue disorders and the others as normal variants.

Clemens JD, et al. A controlled evaluation of the risk of bacterial endocarditis in persons with mitral-valve prolapse. *N Engl J Med* 307:776–781, 1982.
Using a case-control design, patients with MVP were estimated to have more than eight times the risk of endocarditis than the normal population.

Retchin, SM, et al. Endocarditis and mitral valve prolapse: What is the risk? *Int. J. Card.* 5:654, 1984.
Emphasizes that the risk of endocarditis with MVP is exceedingly small.

40. PROSTHETIC VALVES
Andreas T. Wielgosz

Prosthetic valve types today are either ball, tilting disk, or tissue valves. Numerous variations of these designs represent attempts to improve performance and minimize the risk of complications.

Survival in patients with prosthetic valves has improved markedly in recent years, in part due to improved design and in large part due to careful medical and surgical management.

Complications

Thromboembolism
Thromboembolism is the major complication of prosthetic valves. The introduction of cloth-covered prostheses and the use of tissue valves have substantially decreased the

frequency of systemic embolization. The risk is greater with artificial mitral valves (3–5% per patient per year) than with artificial aortic valves (1–3% per patient per year). Patients with an enlarged left atrium and inadequate anticoagulation are especially at risk for embolic events.

Thrombotic material can either rest on the valve, causing dysfunction, or embolize into the systemic circulation. The former may be accompanied by muffling or loss of prosthetic valve opening sounds or by new murmurs of regurgitation; knowledge of the character of the heart sounds in the early postoperative period may be crucial to detecting the buildup of thrombotic material.

Phonocardiography and echocardiography are used to evaluate prosthesis dysfunction. However, technical difficulties often limit the interpretation of these tests, especially for the aortic valve. Interpretation is more accurate when baseline records taken immediately after implantation are available. When other findings strongly suggest valve dysfunction from a thrombus, cardiac catheterization may demonstrate the exact cause; otherwise, the yield is low.

All patients with mechanical valves should be anticoagulated with warfarin indefinitely. Patients with tissue valves generally receive no anticoagulation unless they have an enlarged left atrium, atrial fibrillation, or a previous history of emboli. Taking aspirin or dipyridamole in addition to warfarin has not been shown to reduce the risk of embolization, except in patients with older Starr-Edwards prostheses. Patients with mechanical prostheses, especially older models, who have an embolic episode despite adequate anticoagulation therapy should be considered for reoperation and insertion of a tissue valve.

Endocarditis

The incidence of infective endocarditis with prosthetic valves has declined over the years to an overall rate of less than 4% per year. Early infection (i.e., within 2 months of insertion) usually occurs by contamination at the time of surgery. Staphylococcus is the usual organism; fungal or gram-negative organisms are less common. Mortality remains high (65–85%).

Late endocarditis, occurring at least 60 days after insertion, is most often a streptococcal infection. Mortality is 35 to 45%. Management is the same as for endocarditis affecting natural valves.

Because the symptoms of endocarditis are often nonspecific, suspicion is the key to early diagnosis. Any fever lasting more than 48 hours with a murmur (especially if new) should stimulate efforts to rule out endocarditis. Up to six samples of blood are sufficient to indicate bacteremia; the majority of positive cultures are obtained with the first two samples. In 10% of patients with endocarditis, cultures show no bacterial growth. When culture reports are negative, the decision to use antibiotics is difficult and should be made on clinical grounds.

Hemolysis

Hemolysis is uncommon with modern mechanical valves. When present, it may indicate a structural defect. Other factors contributing to hemolysis include perivalvular regurgitation and high transvalvular pressure gradient (i.e., disproportionate valve size). Iron deficiency anemia, even when secondary to hemolysis, may aggravate the hemolytic process. When hemolysis is mild, iron and folic acid supplements may suffice. In severe hemolysis, it may be necessary to replace the valve.

Mechanical Breakdown

Mechanical breakdown can occur, particularly with older valve models. The incidence of breakdown in new prostheses is less than 1% per year. The durability of tissue valves has not been established, a factor to be considered in younger patients. Other problems include ball variance found with Silastic rubber poppets, a cocked disk, fracture of balls or struts, and valve dehiscence (i.e., disruption of the suture line around the prosthesis). The resulting changes in clinical status may range from subtle (e.g., fatigue) to dramatic (e.g., acute congestive failure). Telltale findings are variations in intensity or loss of opening sounds, as thrombus accumulates on newly exposed surfaces, and murmurs of regurgitation due to incomplete closure of the valve or separation of the valve from the adjacent tissue.

Patient Monitoring

Follow-up
Follow-up of a patient with a prosthetic valve involves close monitoring not only of the valve itself, but also of the patient's overall cardiac function. Congestive heart failure, dysrhythmias, and coronary insufficiency must be treated as necessary. Patients with prosthetic valves undergoing general surgery require careful anticoagulation and bacterial endocarditis prophylaxis (see Chap. 41). During the first 3 months of pregnancy, subcutaneous heparin is recommended to avoid the teratogenic effects of warfarin; in the last 2 months, heparin is recommended to reduce the danger of bleeding. It can be stopped at the time of delivery. Bacterial endocarditis prophylaxis is recommended during the delivery.

Referral
Most large centers involved in the implantation of prosthetic valves have follow-up clinics to which patients should be referred when serious complications are suspected. Careful assessment of function and structural integrity of the valve may require diagnostic studies available only at such centers.

Kloster FE. Diagnosis and management of complications of prosthetic heart valves. *Am J Cardiol* 35:872, 1975.
  This article deals with the major short- and long-term complications seen in patients with prosthetic heart valves and makes recommendations for management.
Bonchek, LI. Indications for surgery of the mitral valve. *Am J Cardiol* 46:155, 1980.
  Indications for valvular surgery are often based on the experience gained at specific centers. This article reviews the practice at the Milwaukee Regional Medical Center.
Smith ND, Raizada V, Abrams J. Auscultation of the normal functioning prosthetic valve. *Ann Intern Med* 95:594, 1981.
  Reviews the auscultatory findings of the major types of prosthetic devices.
Rahimtoola SH. Valvular heart disease: A perspective. *J Am Coll Cardiol* 1:199, 1983.
  An excellent, well-referenced review of valve replacement. Several associated issues are discussed, e.g., concomitant bypass surgery.
Brandenburg RO, et al. Infective endocarditis—a 25 year overview of diagnosis and therapy. *J Am Coll Cardiol* 1:280–291, 1983.
  The authors review the epidemiologic changes seen in the last 25 years. Complications and indications for surgery are well presented. The use of echocardiography is well presented and well referenced.
Silverman NA, Levitsky S. Current choices for prosthetic valve replacement. *Mod Concepts Cardiovasc Dis* 52:35, 1983.
  A succinct review of the major types of prosthetic valves, relating advantages and shortcomings to published reports as well as personal experience.

41. ENDOCARDITIS PROPHYLAXIS
Park W. Willis IV

Infective endocarditis is an uncommon serious complication of cardiac disease that results from microorganisms proliferating on damaged or abnormal endothelium. Despite major advances in antibiotic therapy and cardiovascular surgery, the morbidity and mortality remain significant. Therefore, it is accepted practice to administer antibiotics to susceptible patients whenever they are subjected to a procedure that may cause bacteremia.

"At Risk" Patients
The incidence of infective endocarditis in the general population has been estimated to be 1.1 to 3.6 per 100,000 per year. Although only 50% of patients have known heart disease, many patients at risk of infective endocarditis can be identified.

Abnormal heart valves due to congenital or rheumatic disease are most commonly affected. The endothelium in the area of the jet lesion of a ventricular septal defect or patent ductus arteriosus may also be involved. It is recommended that patients receive prophylactic antibiotic therapy if they have ventricular septal defect, tetralogy of Fallot, bicuspid aortic valve, aortic stenosis or regurgitation, pulmonic stenosis, complex congenital heart disease, patent ductus arteriosus, idiopathic hypertrophic subaortic stenosis, mitral valve prolapse *with* mitral regurgitation, or rheumatic valvular disease. Patients with uncomplicated atrial septal defect do not require prophylaxis. Patients with prosthetic heart valves are at especially high risk and parenteral antibiotic therapy is generally recommended for them.

Table 41-1. Antibiotic regimens for prophylaxis of infective endocarditis after procedures involving the upper respiratory tract

Regimen A—for patients at risk, except those with prosthetic valves
1. Parenteral-oral combined
   Adults: Aqueous crystalline penicillin G (1,000,000 units IM) *mixed with* procaine penicillin G (600,000 units IM). Give 30 minutes to 1 hour prior to procedure, and then give penicillin V (formerly called phenoxymethyl penicillin) 500 mg orally every 6 hours for eight doses.
   Children: Aqueous crystalline penicillin G (30,000 units/kg IM) *mixed with* procaine penicillin G (600,000 units IM). Timing of doses for children is the same as for adults. For children less than 60 pounds, the dosage of penicillin V is 250 mg orally every 6 hours for eight doses.
2. Oral
   Adults: Penicillin V, 2 gm orally 30 minutes to 1 hour prior to the procedure and then 500 mg orally every 6 hours for eight doses.
   Children: Penicillin V, 2 gm orally 30 minutes to 1 hour prior to procedure and then 500 mg orally every 6 hours for eight doses. For children less than 60 pounds, use 1 gm orally 30 minutes to 1 hour prior to the procedure and then 250 mg orally every 6 hours for eight doses.
For Patients Allergic to Penicillin
   Use either vancomycin (see Regimen B)

   or

   Adults: Erythromycin, 1.0 gm orally 1½ to 2 hours prior to the procedure and then 500 mg orally every 6 hours for eight doses.
   Children: Erythromycin 20 mg/kg orally 1½ to 2 hours prior to the procedure and then 10 mg/kg every 6 hours for eight doses.
Regimen B—for patients with prosthetic heart valves
   Adults: Aqueous crystalline penicillin G (1,000,000 units IM) *mixed with* procaine penicillin G (600,000 units IM) *plus* streptomycin (1 gm IM). Give 30 minutes to 1 hour prior to the procedure, and then give penicillin V 500 mg orally every 6 hours for eight doses.
   Children: Aqueous crystalline penicillin G (30,000 units/kg IM) mixed with procaine penicillin G (600,000 units IM) *plus* streptomycin (20 mg/kg IM). Timing of doses for children is the same as for adults. For children less than 60 pounds, the recommended dosage of penicillin V is 250 mg orally every 6 hours for eight doses.
For Patients Allergic to Penicillin
   Adults: Vancomycin (1 gm IV over 30 minutes to 1 hour). Start initial vancomycin infusion ½ to 1 hour prior to the procedure; then erythromycin 500 mg orally every 6 hours for eight doses.
   Children: Vancomycin (20 mg/kg IV over 30 minutes to 1 hour). Timing of doses for children is the same as for adults. Erythromycin dosage is 10 mg/kg every 6 hours for eight doses.

Source: From E.L. Kaplan et al. Prevention of bacterial endocarditis. *Circulation* 56:139A, 1977.

"At Risk" Procedures

Respiratory Tract
Dental procedures are the most commonly recognized cause of transient bacteremia. Dental extraction is associated with a 60 to 90% incidence of bacteremia; periodontal surgery, fillings, and cleaning of teeth cause bacteremia less frequently. Prophylactic antibiotic therapy is recommended for all patients at risk having dental procedures that are likely to cause gingival bleeding. Other procedures, instrumentation, and operations involving disruption of the respiratory mucosa such as tonsillectomy, adenoidectomy, or bronchoscopy may cause bacteremia, and here antibiotic prophylaxis is also recommended.

Genitourinary Tract
Urethral or prostatic manipulation including cystoscopy, urethral dilation, prostatectomy, and transurethral biopsy of the prostate often causes bacteremia. For example, at the time of transurethral prostatectomy about 10% of patients with sterile urine have positive blood cultures; with infected urine the incidence of transient bacteremia is about 60%. Urethral catheterization can cause bacteremia whether the urine is infected or not. Because endocarditis has been reported to follow these procedures, antibiotic prophylaxis is recommended for susceptible patients.

Gastrointestinal Tract
Gastrointestinal (GI) tract and gallbladder instrumentation and surgery have been documented to cause bacteremia and endocarditis; therefore, antibiotic prophylaxis is generally recommended. However, certain other GI procedures have been associated with bacteremia but rarely, if ever, infective endocarditis. These include upper GI endoscopy without biopsy, percutaneous liver biopsy, proctoscopy, sigmoidoscopy, and barium enema. For these procedures, antibiotic prophylaxis is recommended only for patients with prosthetic heart valves.

Uterus
Uncomplicated vaginal delivery and minor gynecologic procedures, such as cervical dilation and curettage of the uterus and insertion or removal of intrauterine contraceptive devices, can cause bacteremia but rarely result in infective endocarditis. Except for patients with prosthetic heart valves, antibiotic prophylaxis is not recommended for patients undergoing these procedures.

Table 41-2. Antibiotic regimens for prophylaxis of infective endocarditis after procedures involving the gastrointestinal or genitourinary tract

---

Adults: Aqueous crystalline penicillin G (2,000,000 units IM or IV) *or* ampicillin (1 gm IM or IV) *plus* gentamicin (1.5 mg/kg [not to exceed 80 mg] IM or IV) *or* streptomycin (1 gm IM). Give initial doses 30 minutes to 1 hour prior to procedure. If gentamicin is used, then give a similar dose of gentamicin and penicillin (or ampicillin) every 8 hours for two additional doses. If streptomycin is used, then give a similar dose of streptomycin and penicillin (or ampicillin) every 12 hours for two additional doses.
Children: Aqueous crystalline penicillin G (30,000 units/kg IM or IV) *or* ampicillin (50 mg/kg IM or IV) *plus* gentamicin (2 mg/kg IM or IV) *or* streptomycin (20 mg/kg IM). Timing of doses for children is the same as for adults.
For Patients Allergic to Penicillin
Adults: Vancomycin (1 gm IV given over 30 minutes to 1 hour) *plus* streptomycin (1 gm IM). A single dose of these antibiotics begun 30 minutes to 1 hour prior to the procedure is probably sufficient, but the same dose may be repeated in 12 hours.
Children: Vancomycin (20 mg/kg IV given over 30 minutes to 1 hour) *plus* streptomycin (20 mg/kg IM). Timing of doses for children is the same as for adults.

Source: From E.L. Kaplan et al. Prevention of bacterial endocarditis. *Circulation* 56:139A, 1977.

Recommendations

Infective endocarditis is rare. Even though the population at risk is large and bacteremia occurs frequently during dental and medical procedures, the chance that organisms will localize on a damaged valve during a single bacteremic episode is very small. Therefore, controlled trials of the efficacy of antimicrobial prophylaxis are virtually impossible. Recommendations are based on what is known about the mechanisms of endocarditis, the bacteria involved, and the efficacy of antibiotics in animal models of infective endocarditis. The antibiotic regimens outlined below have been recommended by the American Heart Association Committee on Prevention of Rheumatic Fever and Bacterial Endocarditis.

These are general recommendations. Patients with significantly compromised renal function may require modified doses of antibiotics. In unusual circumstances, during prolonged procedures or in the case of delayed healing, it may be necessary to provide additional doses of antibiotics. Doses for children should not exceed recommendations for adults for a single dose or for a 24-hour period; for children, the total dose of vancomycin should not exceed 44 mg/kg/24 hours.

Dental and Surgical Procedures of the Upper Respiratory Tract

For dental and surgical procedures of the upper respiratory tract, the regimens described in Table 41-1 are recommended. Oral regimen A has been deemed sufficient for all patients at risk except for those with prosthetic heart valves, who should be given parenteral regimen B regardless of the procedure involved.

Some patients receiving long-term oral penicillin for secondary prevention of rheumatic fever have been found to have penicillin-resistant alpha-hemolytic streptococci in their oral cavities. It has been suggested that the doses described in Regimen A are high enough to be effective against these organisms. However, oral erythromycin or regimen B may be prescribed if there is concern about potential infection with penicillin-resistant alpha-hemolytic streptococci.

Gastrointestinal and Genitourinary Tract Procedures

For gastrointestinal and genitourinary tract surgery and instrumentation, the parenteral regimens described in Table 41-2 are recommended.

Weinstein L, Schlesinger JJ. Pathoanatomic, pathophysiologic and clinical correlations in endocarditis. *N Engl J Med* 291:832 and 1122, 1974.
  An excellent review article in two parts.
Everett ED, Hirschmann JV. Transient bacteremia and endocarditis prophylaxis: A review. *Medicine* 56:61, 1977.
  A complete review of procedures causing bacteremia.
Kaplan EL, et al. Prevention of bacterial endocarditis. *Circulation* 56:139A, 1977.
  The most recent report and recommendations of the American Heart Association Committee on Prevention of Rheumatic Fever and Bacterial Endocarditis.
Prevention of bacterial endocarditis. *Med Lett Drugs Ther* 26:3–4, 1984; 26:18, 1984.
  Recommends only 2 doses of antibiotics.

42. PULMONARY EMBOLISM

Bernard Lo

Pulmonary embolism (PE) poses a dilemma for clinicians. It is relatively common, potentially dangerous, and difficult to diagnose with certainty. The "gold standard" for diagnosis, pulmonary angiography, is sensitive and specific. However, since it is also invasive and expensive, it cannot be used in every patient suspected of having PE. On the other hand, alternative tests that are safe and less expensive lead to both false-positive and false-negative diagnoses.

The challenge for the physician is to plan the most efficient workup that yields the required diagnostic certainty. Clinical findings and laboratory tests are used in sequence, proceeding to more specific risky and costly ones. Negative results on several sensitive tests exclude the diagnosis of PE; positive results must be confirmed with additional, more specific tests.

PE is suspected far more often than it is diagnosed; in one series, only 6% of patients suspected of having PE had the diagnosis confirmed on extensive testing. When the clinical likelihood of PE is low, as it often is in outpatients, the strategy is to rule out the diagnosis by obtaining normal results on several sensitive tests or clinical findings.

Risk Factors

PE is considered more likely to occur in the presence of recent surgery, immobilization (e.g., from a stroke or myocardial infarction), previous thromboembolism, cancer, pregnancy, estrogen therapy, obesity, advanced age, and varicose veins. Because of the diagnostic difficulties already cited, precise estimates of the incidence of PE in various clinical situations are not available.

Clinical Evaluation

PE has a range of clinical presentations. At one extreme, a large PE in patients with prior cardiac or pulmonary disease may present with death, shock, or right heart failure. Physicians' beliefs about PE may be biased because many series and discussions emphasize these severe cases. At the other extreme, PE may be asymptomatic and diagnosed only by laboratory abnormalities. Most cases occur at the milder end of the spectrum, where symptoms and signs are usually not specific.

The most common symptoms of PE, found in a prospective, well-designed multicenter study (Bell et al, 1976), were chest pain (88%) and dyspnea (84%), while apprehension (59%), cough (53%), and hemoptysis (30%) were less common. On physical examination, tachypnea (respirations > 16/minute) occurred in 92% of patients with PE; hence, its absence helps exclude the diagnosis. Tachycardia, rales, increased second pulmonic heart sound, fever, and clinical signs of deep venous thrombosis were less frequent (32–53%). Surprisingly, only 45% of patients with PE had a pulse greater than 100 beats per minute; hence, the absence of tachycardia does not exclude PE.

Laboratory Studies

Routine blood tests, including white blood cell count, serum glutamic-oxaloacetic transaminase (SGOT), bilirubin, and lactic dehydrogenase (LDH) are usually not helpful in excluding or establishing the diagnosis. Although the *chest x-ray* is said to be frequently normal, recent studies have shown nonspecific (and often subtle) findings of effusion, atelectasis, infiltration, and elevated hemidiaphragm in 88% of cases. The *electrocardiogram* is abnormal in 87% of cases, but the usual findings of tachycardia and ST segment changes are not specific. Acute cor pulmonale, which is said to be diagnostic of PE, occurs in only 26% of cases.

An *arterial blood gas* shows a PO_2 of less than 80 mm Hg in 88% of cases, but hypoxemia is common as well among patients suspected of having PE. Thus, a normal PO_2 helps rule out PE, but a low PO_2 is not specific.

It has been suggested that PE might be diagnosed by measuring fibrin degradation products, platelet release factors, or plasma DNA. The accuracy of these tests, however, has not been rigorously demonstrated.

Most information from history, physical examination, and simple laboratory tests is neither sensitive nor specific and therefore must be interpreted with caution. If the clinical suspicion is low, normal results on sensitive tests (e.g., absence of tachypnea and normal PO_2) can rule out PE. However, abnormal findings are common in illnesses that predispose to or mimic PE. In such patients abnormal findings require further evaluation with more specific tests.

The next diagnostic step is a *perfusion lung scan.* Normal results on perfusion scan rule out PE: abnormalities, however, are not specific and must be evaluated further.

A *ventilation-perfusion* (V/Q) lung scan has been generally considered the next diagnostic test to perform. In this scan, ventilation images are obtained and compared with perfusion images. Patient cooperation is necessary.

A recent, well-designed prospective study (Hull et al, 1983) challenges the usefulness of V/Q scans. All patients with abnormal perfusion scans were scheduled for ventilation scanning and angiography; 63% of these patients were able to have both tests performed adequately. V/Q scans were helpful in patients with segmental or larger perfusion defects that were not matched by ventilation defects. Of such patients, 86% had angiograms that were positive for PE. Thus, this finding on a V/Q scan usually does not require confirmation by angiography.

Other findings on V/Q scan, however, were not diagnostic. It was formerly believed that patients with perfusion defects matched by ventilation defects had a low probability of PE. However, in this study, such patients had a probability of 19%. Moreover, some patients with matching perfusion and ventilation defects and negative angiograms had venograms that were positive for proximal deep venous thrombosis. Thus, in patients with matched defects, the overall incidence of thromboembolic disease requiring anticoagulation was 33%.

This study has changed our thinking about V/Q scans. If a V/Q scan would not be decisive, it is best to omit it and proceed directly to angiography. For example, a ventilation scan would not be helpful if perfusion defects are subsequential. In addition, patients with perfusion defects corresponding to to infiltrates on x-ray have a 17 to 40% probability of PE.

As was mentioned previously, pulmonary *angiography* is considered the "gold standard" for definitive diagnosis of PE. Intraluminal filling defects are diagnostic of the disease and a negative angiogram usually rules it out, since an angiogram shows clots as small as 5 mm. Falsely negative angiograms due to resolution of the embolus are rare if the test is performed within 48 hours of the onset of symptoms. The interobserver reliability of angiogram readings is very good, with diagreement in fewer than 6% of cases.

, Angiograms involve some risk to the patient. The mortality associated with angiography is less than 0.5%, with intractable shock in patients with elevated right heart pressures accounting for many deaths. Significant morbidity, such as cardiac arrest, symptomatic arrhythmias, right ventricular perforation, and anaphylaxis, occur in 1.6 to 2.3% of cases. These data were gathered at centers performing more than 80 procedures a year; the complication rate at less experienced centers is probably higher.

As an alternative to angiography, some have suggested that the need for anticoagulation can be inferred from the presence of deep venous thrombosis in the legs, demonstrated on venography or impedance plethysmography. Indeed venograms may show proximal thrombosis in 33% of patients with negative angiograms. Although such patients do not have PE, they still require anticoagulation. Venograms are safer, cheaper, and more readily available than angiograms. However, the venogram is negative in 30% of patients in whom PE is demonstrated by angiography. Hence, a negative venogram in a patient with suspected PE must be followed by angiography.

Risks, Benefits, and Uncertainty

Since the diagnosis of PE involves probabilities rather than absolute certainty, the physician and patient need to weigh risks, benefits, and uncertainty. The greater the perceived risk, the more certainty in diagnosis will be required.

The risk of missing the diagnosis of PE is the morbidity and mortality of untreated PE. Untreated PE tends to recur: in the multicenter study, no solitary PE was detected. Recurrent PE may have grave consequences: in the only controlled study comparing heparin to placebo, patients given placebo had a mortality rate of 25%.

On the other hand, the risk of overdiagnosing PE is the unnecessary cost, morbidity, and mortality of treatment. In four well-designed recent series, the risk of major bleeding from heparin was between 3 and 17%. Similarly, in three series major bleeding from warfarin occurred in 6 to 17% of patents. The risks of overdiagnosis are even greater in three situations: (1) The patient is at high risk for bleeding from anticoagulation because of advanced age, recent surgery, trauma or bleeding, or hemostatic defects. (2) Thrombolytic therapy, which increases the risk of major bleeding, is considered. (3) Interruption of the inferior vena cava is planned. In these situations, the physician or patient may desire more diagnostic certainty than even a high-probability V/Q scan affords, and angiography may be appropriate.

The diagnostic approach to PE should be individualized. Different physicians and patients will place different values on risks and uncertainty. Moreover, in a particular hospital, some tests may not be available, or the local results may not match those reported in the literature.

Bell WR, Simon TL, DeMets DL. The clinical features of submassive and massive pulmonary emboli. *Am J Med* 62:355–360, 1976.
Review of clinical presentation of PE.

Caster C, Gent M. The epidemiology of venous thrombosis. In RW Coleman, et al. *Hemostasis and Thrombosis*. Philadelphia: Lippincott, 1982. Pp. 805–819.

Robin ED. Overdiagnosis and overtreatment of pulmonary embolism: The emperor may have no clothes. *Ann Intern Med* 87:755–781, 1977.
Critique of lung scans in diagnosis of PE.

Hull RD, et al. Pulmonary angiography, ventilation lung scanning and venography for clinically suspected pulmonary embolism with abnormal perfusion lung scan. *Ann Intern Med* 98:891–899, 1983.
Well-designed prospective study in which all patients with abnormal perfusion scans were scheduled for ventilation scans and angiography. Thus, selection bias was reduced. The findings of this study contradict previously held beliefs about the usefulness of ventilation scans.

Biello DR, et al. Interpretation of indeterminate lung scintigrams. *Radiology* 133:189–194, 1970.
Study of lung scans in patients with x-ray infiltrates. If the perfusion defect was substantially smaller than the x-ray infiltrate, only 1 of 14 patients had PE on angiography, whereas 16 of 18 patients with unmatched perfusion defects substantially larger than the x-ray infiltrates had PE. However, the reliability of "larger" and "smaller" was not studied.

Griner PF, et al. Selection and interpretation of diagnostic tests and procedures. *Ann Intern Med* 94(4, Part 2):453–600, 1981.
Discusses sensitivity, specificity, and predictive value of tests, with application to the diagnosis of PE. Emphasizes how normal results on a sensitive test can rule out PE in a patient in whom the prior probability (clinical suspicion) is low.

Barritt DW, Jordan SC. Anticoagulant drugs in the treatment of pulmonary embolism. *Lancet* 1:1309–1312, 1960.
The only prospective, randomized study of anticoagulation in PE. Heparin reduced mortality from 25 to 6%. Despite methodologic flaws (diagnosis was established only on clinical grounds, the study was not blinded), it has led to the clinical practice that all patients with PE must be treated with anticoagulants.

Sherry S, et al. Thrombolytic therapy in thrombosis: A National Institute of Health consensus development conference. *Ann Intern Med* 93:141–144, 1980.
Review of thrombolytic therapy. However, the authors' claim that with adequate precautions risk of bleeding is no greater than with anticoagulation alone is not substantiated in published studies.

VII. PERIPHERAL VASCULAR PROBLEMS

It is customary to separate discussion of chronic venous disorders into insufficiency and primary varicose veins, although chronic venous diseases of the legs overlap extensively in pathogenesis and clinical features. Acquaintance with functional anatomy is basic to understanding both conditions.

Leg veins include (1) three pairs of deep calf veins merging at the knee to form the popliteal vein, (2) a network of superficial veins whose axial trunks are the long and short saphenous veins, and (3) several perforators that penetrate the fascia to connect deep and superficial systems. Each of these veins has endothelial valves at frequent intervals, oriented to prevent retrograde flow in the longitudinal trunks and centrifugal flow in the perforators. Chronic venous disorders result primarily from valvular incompetence in one or more of these systems.

Chronic Venous Insufficiency

Chronic venous insufficiency (CVI), or "postphlebitic syndrome," results, in most cases, from prior episodes of deep venous thrombosis (DVT). The deep veins provide most of the limb drainage, overcoming gravity by means of the pumping action of calf muscles. Blood is forced from contracting muscles into the deep veins and directed upward by the valves. Blood from cutaneous tissues collects in the saphenous system and drains into the deep veins through the valved perforators. Competent valves in deep and superficial trunk veins protect against gravitational pressures, and competent perforator valves protect the skin from the high pressures of the deep muscle pump.

Acute DVT often heals with recanalization of the thrombosed lumen, leaving permanent destruction of the valves. If the deep system is left open to gravity, the pressure in upright adults may reach 120 cm H_2O at the ankle. When perforator valves are destroyed, both gravity and pulsatile waves from misdirected muscle pump action are transmitted to the cutaneous tissues. The "venous hypertension" leads to chronic skin changes, chiefly due to edema, which impairs nutrition and normal healing.

Presentation

Clinically significant CVI affects 5 to 10% of older people, and of these about one-fifth will develop venous leg ulcers. About one-third of patients do not report prior DVT, but no other etiology is strongly supported, and many of these cases probably derive from inapparent episodes of DVT, such as in trauma (e.g., surgery, casted fractures).

Chronic venous insufficiency primarily affects the skin of the lower legs. There is usually dependent edema, a splotchy brown discoloration of the epidermis from hemosiderin deposits, and an eczema, which may be dry, scaly, and intensely pruritic, or denuded, wet, and inflamed. Secondary varicosities, usually not so striking as in primary varicose veins, may result from distention of the superficial veins.

The major clinical problems are leg pain on prolonged standing and venous ulcers. The pain is described as a "bursting" sensation and can be relieved by elevation or compression stockings. Ulcerations are most common above the medial malleolus and develop rapidly in the setting of chronic indurated edema. Ninety percent of low leg ulcers are caused by venous hypertension and the balance by arterial insufficiency and several rare diseases. Venous ulcers are usually painless, but if pain is present elevation affords relief, whereas this position exacerbates the pain of arterial ulcers.

Diagnosis

The diagnosis of CVI is based on the history and physical examination. It is unusual to need confirmation for routine management. Studies of the deep veins are indicated only if there is a question about the cause of edema, pain, or ulceration or if varicose veins are prominent and surgery is contemplated.

Noninvasive techniques are available to demonstrate occlusion or valvular incompetence. Doppler studies are simple, harmless, portable, and easy to repeat. Plethysmographic studies measure changes in leg volume, representing effects of arterial inflow and venous drainage. The rate of volume loss with muscle contraction measures effectiveness of the calf muscle pump, while the refilling rate is a sensitive indicator of deep and perforator incompetence.

Special studies may be needed to diagnose acute DVT against a background of CVI. The "gold standard" has been venography, which is widely available but expensive and uncomfortable. It allows direct visualization of venous occlusion, but discrimination of old, organized occlusions versus fresh thrombosis may be impossible, in which case combination venography (excellent sensitivity) and ^{131}I fibrinogen scanning (specific for active clotting) are used.

Therapy

The therapy of CVI is primarily nonoperative. Apart from in a few experimental reports, venous incompetence is not surgically correctable. The patient must therefore adopt a lifelong program aimed at control of edema. Management includes regular light exercise and defecation, as well as avoidance of constricting garments and obesity. Conscientious use of periodic elevation is particularly helpful. The legs should be above chest level at night and perhaps for an hour during the day. Pillows are usually not satisfactory, since the ankle should be higher than the knee, the knee higher than the hip, and the hip higher than the heart. Cinder blocks under the bed work well.

The mainstay of long-term management is use of compression stockings. Most authors advise 30 to 40 mm Hg; higher pressure hose are difficult to pull on and may compromise arterial flow. This pressure range cannot be achieved with department store "support-hose"; medical products are necessary, but newer weaving techniques allow use of standard sizes without individual fitting. Since the skin manifestations of CVI are usually confined to the lower legs, most authors advise knee-length stockings.

It is essential that the arterial circulation be assessed in every case and corrected if necessary. Ischemia retards healing and contraindicates any form of high-compression bandaging.

Eczema of the scaly, pruritic type may benefit from a bland ointment or a topical corticosteroid if severe. The raw, weeping form of dermatitis is treated with moist dressings, using a 0.25% solution of aluminum subacetate, boric acid, or saline. Definite cellulitis should be treated with systemic antibiotics.

Treatment of ulceration must control edema long enough to allow healing. Constant elevation for several weeks is effective, but impractical for most people. The method of choice is therefore Unna's paste boot, a bandage applied like an Ace wrap, which hardens to form a light cast. It should be applied to a leg drained by overnight elevation, directly over the skin (and ulcer) without ointments or other dressings. Begin at the base of the toes (angle to stay clear of the fifth toe) and wrap to the knee, covering with an elastic bandage to protect clothing. Normal activity is encouraged throughout the several weeks of healing. The boot is changed every 7 to 10 days. Small ulcers will heal completely, while larger ones (> 4 cm) may require grafting.

Varicose Veins

The superficial veins are thin-walled structures with little tissue support against distention. Varicosities result from incompetence of the proximal valves that interrupt gravitational pressure and/or perforator valves that shield against the calf muscle pump. As a result, distending pressures are allowed into the superficial veins. Varicose veins may be caused by genetic dysplasia, hormone effects, trauma, or phlebitis.

About 5% of adult Americans will develop varicose veins. They are twice as prevalent in women, who constitute a much greater proportion of those seeking treatment.

Clinical Presentation and Diagnosis

Simple varicosities range from clusters of cutaneous vessels to extensive tortuous and dilated masses.

If the deep veins and perforators are normal, varicose veins are usually asymptomatic, except for the cosmetic deformity. There may be mild symptoms of venous hypertension, with pain on prolonged standing, mild edema, and rarely an ulcer. These latter findings require studies of deep veins as outlined above: plethysmography should distinguish the contributions of deep and superficial systems.

When surgery is contemplated, the state of the deep venous system should be evaluated. In the rare instance that the deep veins are occluded, the saphenous may be the principal drainage, and removal would invite disaster. Most commonly, the deep veins are patent, but their valves are incompetent. Recurrences of varicose veins are likely in this setting. If only perforators are incompetent, these can be ligated at the time of vein stripping, with good likelihood of success. Procedures available for performing these evaluations include plethysmography of various types and Doppler techniques. Despite the value of these tests in predicting the outcome, in practice they frequently are not performed prior to surgery.

Therapy

Although most authors specify that varicose veins should be treated only for symptoms, it can be assumed that most complaints will be cosmetic. The role of the primary care physician is to counsel and refer, making sure that appropriate assessment of the deep system is performed. Two forms of definitive treatment are available: sclerotherapy and surgery. The literature contains widely discrepant opinions concerning these choices. In many American locales, only surgical management is available, while sclerotherapy is very popular in Europe.

The goal of sclerosing therapy is to create a fibrous adhesion at the junctions of incompetent perforators with the superficial varicosities. Small amounts (0.5 ml) of sodium tetradecyl sulfate are injected through a 25-gauge needle into a vein that has been emptied by elevation. Several veins can be treated at one setting, and the leg is tightly wrapped for 6 weeks to maintain apposition of the venous walls. Adverse effects are few and depend on the accuracy of injection and maintenance of tight bandaging long enough to assure fibrous adhesion rather than thrombosis.

Advantages are lesser cost and lesser risk, and the veins can be retreated if necessary. Success depends on skill and on the patient's cooperation with the compression. Sclerotherapy alone is an adequate approach for total incompetence of the proximal saphenous valves.

Surgery may be radical or an adjunct to sclerotherapy. In the latter instances, patients with demonstrable saphenofemoral incompetence (about half of patients) may require a simple ligation of the saphenofemoral junction, after which the incompetent calf perforators are sclerosed. Pure surgical approaches include some combination of (1) saphenofemoral ligation, (2) stripping of long and short saphenous veins, (3) flush ligation of incompetent perforators, and (4) excision of major varicose tributaries of the saphenous system. Surgery can be performed with ambulation and discharge the same day. The necessity of prolonged high compression is much less than with sclerotherapy, but the cost and risk are greater, and the saphenous veins are lost to future coronary bypass.

Two major trials have compared these techniques: both show excellent and comparable results at 1 year, while at 3 years, recurrences are much greater with sclerotherapy. The choice usually depends on the preference and expertise of each surgical community.

Hobb JT. *The Treatment of Venous Disorders.* Philadelphia: Lippincott, 1977.
  A current classic from a British surgeon with a balanced view of operative management and sclerotherapy. Primarily a compendium of international essays on management techniques with considerable redundancy, overlapping terminology, and discrepant conclusions. Chapter 19 by Haeger on leg ulcers is superb, especially the section on therapy.
Lofgren KA. Varicose veins. *Postgrad Med* 65:131–139, 1979.
  Generally speaking, this is the voice of America with minimal mention of sclerotherapy and major advocacy of operative management. Good discussion of symptoms and complications, although the distinction between superficial varicose veins and deep venous insufficiency is often hazy.
Ludbrook J, Jamieson GG. Disorders of Systemic Veins. In DC Sabiston, Jr (Ed.), *Textbook of Surgery.* Philadelphia Saunders, 1981. Pp. 1808–1827.
  A standard textbook chapter with excellent diagrams and the clearest distinction of primary varices and post-thrombotic syndrome in print. Plainly states the limited role of complex diagnostic techniques, and provides comparative statements about injection and operative management. Bibliography includes annotation for special entries.
Nabatoff RA. Ambulatory management of lower extremity venous disease in the aged. *Mt Sinai J Med* 47:218–223, 1980.
  Excellent brief discussion of therapy of skin problems, including choice of dressings,

techniques of application, and modifications for special problems in older patients (e.g., coexisting arterial disease). Practical aspects of injection therapy briefly reviewed, and indications for surgery presented.

Abramowitz HB, et al. The use of photoplethysmography in the assessment of venous insufficiency: A comparison to venous pressure measurements. *Surgery* 86:434–441, 1979.

A well-presented example of the many ingenious diagnostic studies available to distinguish primary varicose veins from deep venous insufficiency. What is not made clear in this or similar articles is whether these clever tests are superior to clinical assessment with or without venography in providing therapeutically useful information.

Jakobsen RH. The value of different forms of treatment for varicose veins. *Br J Surg* 66:182–184, 1979.

Report of a controlled trial of 512 patients assigned to three treatment groups for varicose veins and outcomes assessed at 3 months and 3 years. Assignment was not random, and the type of varicose vein disease is not defined. Radical surgery produced better long-term results than injection sclerotherapy or combination therapy.

Hobbs JT. The management of varicose veins. *Surg Annu* 12:169–186, 1980.

Detailed methodology of sclerotherapy and operative management from a British surgeon who uses both approaches. Reports outcome of a comparative trial with breakdown as to type of disease, and relates results to other studies including that of Jakobsen (above). Concludes with treatment recommendations based on clinical pattern of disease.

Arnesen H, Høiseth A, Ly B. Streptokinase or heparin in the treatment of deep vein thrombosis. *Acta Med Scand* 211:65–68, 1982.

Six year follow-up of a randomized, prospective study of streptokinase or heparin as initial treatment for DVT. Clinical abnormalities were significantly more common in the heparin-treated legs, extending the existing knowledge that streptokinase gives much better short-term venographic results.

44. ARTERIAL DISEASE OF THE EXTREMITIES
John S. Kizer

Peripheral vascular disease is a common illness. As many as 17% of the adult population aged 55 to 64 years old are afflicted by ischemic limb disease, and about one-third of these are disabled by their illness. Risk factors for the development of peripheral vascular disease include diabetes and cigarette smoking. Other risk factors for cardiovascular disease in general, such as hypercholesterolemia, hypertension, and male sex, appear to be less strongly correlated with the development of peripheral vascular disease. The presence of peripheral vascular disease, on the other hand, is strongly correlated with the presence of arteriosclerotic lesions throughout the cardiovascular system.

Natural History
The prognosis for patients with limb ischemia is reasonably favorable. The majority improve on conservative management in 6 to 12 months. About 10% of patients presenting with peripheral vascular disease require amputation within 5 years; in diabetics, the rate of amputation is nearly five times higher, and for diabetic single amputees, the risk of amputation of the remaining limb is also five times higher (50% at 5 years).

Survival is reduced in the presence of peripheral vascular disease. A few patients die as a result of gangrene and sepsis. Overall cardiovascular mortality of patients with claudication is twice that of a comparable population without claudication.

Clinical Syndromes

Acute Vascular Insufficiency
The course of ischemic peripheral vascular disease may be complicated at any time by acute symptoms related to either an in situ thrombosis or the lodgement of an embolus, leading to limb-threatening ischemia and gangrene.

Acute limb-threatening ischemia presents as the sudden onset of severe pain in the involved leg with associated weakness and numbness. The pain may be described as a deep, continuous ache and is often excruciating. Any attempt to walk or stand aggravates the pain, and the symptoms are not relieved by rest. On clinical examination, the involved limb is cool or cold, the pulses are markedly diminished or absent in the involved portion of the limb, and the limb may be either pale or cyanotic. Often these symptoms and signs are superimposed on those of chronic ischemic arterial disease, described below.

Chronic Vascular Insufficiency

Symptoms of chronic ischemic vasculopathy of the extremities include pain, intermittent claudication, loss of hair, poor healing, loss of sensation, weakness, and muscular atrophy. The level of limb involvement depends on the exact anatomic location of the critical arterial lesions. For example, pain in the feet and calves implies disease of the femoral-popliteal system, whereas pain, weakness of the hip, and impotence suggest distal aortic disease. End-stage chronic vascular disease leads to the syndrome of resting pain or pregangrenous ischemia, which is characterized by a continuous ache, incapacitating pain on exertion, and pain or rubor when the leg is dependent. Further progression of the disease leads to persistent pain at rest, muscular atrophy, and eventually gangrene.

Evaluation

In evaluation of the patient with either acute or chronic arterial insufficiency of the extremities, diseases simulating peripheral vascular disease, such as Raynaud's disease or systemic vasculitis, and disease that may exacerbate limb ischemia, such as polycythemia, hyperviscosity syndromes, anemia, and recurrent embolization from proximal sites in the vascular tree, must be excluded or treated. Administration of beta-blockers to patients with previously stable chronic peripheral vascular disease can increase symptoms of ischemia. Furthermore, before impotence is attributed to peripheral vascular disease, antihypertensive medication as a cause for the impotence must be excluded.

The diagnosis of peripheral vascular disease and evaluation of its course are based on clinical observation. If the clinical findings are confusing, ultrasound is useful to confirm the presence of obstruction to arterial flow and to localize areas of maximal obstruction. Standard Doppler techniques and spectral analysis of Doppler scans correlate well with direct arterial measures of blood flow. Ultrasound cannot be relied on to quantitate small degrees of improvement or decline. Arteriography should be reserved for patients in whom surgery or angioplasty is contemplated.

Management of Acute Arterial Insufficiency

The acute onset of limb-threatening ischemia demands immediate intervention. There is no evidence that the administration of anticoagulants, vasodilators, or experimental therapies such as prostacyclin infusion are of value in treating this condition. Depending on the nature of the anatomic obstruction as determined by arteriography, the patient may be best suited for either bypass grafting of the occluded segments, catheter embolectomy, percutaneous transluminal angioplasty, or arterial streptokinase infusion. Acute catheter embolectomy or bypass grafting may save as many as 90% of the affected extremities. However, surgical mortality as high as 15% has been reported, due to the risk imposed by the concomitant presence of coronary and cerebral vascular disease. Following successful embolectomy, many institutions recommend the chronic administration of an oral anticoagulant, although firm data supporting the efficacy of such a regimen in preventing recurrence do not exist. Under certain circumstances, when sepsis and serious underlying illness are present, emergency amputation is necessary.

Management of Chronic Arterial Insufficiency

The treatment of peripheral vascular disease is palliative; medical therapy is preferred over surgery in the absence of incapacitating or limb-threatening ischemia. Of primary importance are attention to local skin care, avoidance of trauma, and prompt attention to localized infections. Ulcers must be treated promptly with vigorous sharp debridement and wet-to-dry dressings. In smokers, the progression of vascular disease and the rate of future amputation can be reduced by abstention from cigarette smoking. Although tighter control of diabetes mellitus by generally available methods may not halt the progression of peripheral vascular insufficiency, tighter glycemic control improves nerve conduction and may retard the development of peripheral neuropathy. If sensation in the distal extremities is preserved, the risk of trauma and local infection is lessened. Control of hypertension is recommended to reduce overall cardiovascular mortality; it is not clear whether control of hypertension halts the progression of peripheral vascular disease. Finally, although there is no clear relationship of diet and hyperlipidemia to the overall prognosis of peripheral vascular disease, dietary control and weight reduction may also reduce overall cardiovascular mortality.

Anticoagulant and Antiplatelet Drugs
Platelet microaggregates and the coagulation cascade have been implicated in the genesis of atherosclerotic lesions. However, there is no persuasive evidence, from available clinical trials, that either platelet antiaggregants or oral anticoagulants significantly alter the natural history of peripheral vascular disease. An exception is patients with recurrent arterial emboli, the majority of which originate from the left side of the heart; for these patients the administration of oral anticoagulants appears necessary to prevent recurrent distal embolization. In addition, the patient with recurrent in situ thromboses may benefit from oral anticoagulant therapy, although there is little firm information to support this approach.

Peripheral Vasodilators and Prostacyclin
Numerous clinical trials also provide little support for the use of vasodilators such as papaverine, isoxsuprine, cyclandelate, or nylidrin for the relief of symptoms from peripheral vascular insufficiency. Unlike the skin, muscles lack sympathetic vasoconstrictors; although pharmacologic or surgical sympathectomy may increase flow to the skin, it has little effect on blood flow to the deeper muscle bundles. Furthermore, it is likely that the arteries supplying exercising and ischemic muscles are already dilated to the fullest extent.

Beta-blockers can aggravate limb ischemia. Arteries supplying muscles possess β_2-adrenoreceptors mediating vasodilation, which can be blocked by propranolol or by high doses of relatively "selective" β_1-antagonists such as metoprolol, resulting in an augmentation of limb ischemia.

The role for the administration of prostacyclin or prostacyclin congeners in the treatment of advanced arteriosclerotic peripheral vascular disease has not yet been established.

Bypass Grafting and Embolectomy
In the event of limb-threatening or incapacitating limb ischemia, surgical intervention must be considered. Depending on the symptoms and the nature of the anatomic distribution of the arterial obstructions as determined by arteriography, the patient may be offered either bypass grafting of the occluded segments or embolectomy.

Surgery is not undertaken if palliation can be achieved in other ways. Mortality as high as 15% has been reported due to the risk imposed by the concomitant presence of coronary and cerebrovascular disease. Complications are also common. Following surgery, attention to the modification of risk factors is again important. Cessation of cigarette smoking may improve the patency rate following bypass grafting.

Transluminal angioplasty may offer a reasonable alternative to surgical bypass grafting in patients unfit for surgery or with an isolated stenosis or obstruction of the femoral or iliac arteries that is less than 8 m in length and that contains no calcium. Depending on the angiographer, primary success rates as high as 84% and 3-year patency rates of 70% (even in the presence of total obstructions) may be obtained in the femoral arteries; and primary success rates as high as 92% and 3-year patency rates of 83% may be obtained in the iliac arteries. The precise role of transluminal angioplasty in the management of vascular disease is as yet undefined. It is not clear what proportion of patients meet the exacting criteria for transluminal dilation. Also, there have not been clinical trials comparing surgery to angioplasty for the palliation of peripheral vascular disease. Finally, there are no controlled trials that indicate that postoperative or postangioplasty platelet antiaggregant or anticoagulant therapy is a useful adjuvant.

At present there is little role for vascular surgery in the treatment of impotence resulting from peripheral vascular disease. In fact, impotence may result from surgical attempts to correct obstructive or aneurysmal disease of the aortoiliac junctions. For a few patients, transluminal angioplasty of the internal iliac arteries may prove useful in the treatment of impotence.

Amputation

When all else fails, surgical amputation is necessary to remove parts of extremities destined to become gangrenous. Amputation below the knee is preferred when possible because rehabilitation is more often successful than for patients with amputations above the knee.

Thromboangiitis Obliterans

When peripheral vascular disease is found in a patient under age 40, particularly when involving both lower and upper extremities, thromboangiitis obliterans (Buerger's disease) is suspected. The disease is rare, is associated with heavy cigarette smoking, and occurs in men more often than women. It is characterized by focal, inflammatory lesions of small- and medium-sized arteries and veins. Management of the peripheral vascular disease for these patients is essentially the same as that outlined above. Lesions of thromboangiitis obliterans may regress on discontinuation of smoking and recur when cigarette smoking is resumed.

Richards RL, Bray TB. Long-term anti-coagulant therapy in atherosclerotic peripheral vascular disease. *Vasc Dis* 4:27–35, 1967.
  One of few controlled trials of oral anticoagulants in the prevention of progression of vascular disease. No treatment effect was observed.
Hegyeli RS (Ed.). *Atherosclerotic Reviews,* Vol. 7. New York: Raven, 1980.
  Excellent source for epidemiologic data concerning the prevalence and incidence of various types of atherosclerotic vascular disease.
Clyne CAC. Non-surgical management of peripheral vascular disease: A review. *Br Med J* 281:794–797, 1978.
  Succinct review of current accepted medical palliation of peripheral vascular disease.
Kammel WB, Shurtteff D. The Framingham Study: Cigarettes and the development of intermittent claudication. *Geriatrics* 28:61–68, 1973.
  Correlation of cigarette smoking with risk of peripheral vascular disease is greater than the correlation with risk of coronary or cerebrovascular disease.
Thompson JE, Garrett WV. Peripheral arterial surgery. *N Engl J Med* 302:491–503, 1980.
  Overview of the field of surgical palliation of arterial vascular disease.

45. THROMBOPHLEBITIS
Richard A. Davidson

Thrombophlebitis is the obstruction to venous flow by clotting. Stasis of blood flow in the bedridden patient, release of tissue thromboplastin by surgery or trauma, and injury of the vessel wall all contribute to the formation of thrombi.

The frequency of thrombophlebitis in the general population, or in office practice, is unknown. Studies of the prevalence of deep venous thrombophlebitis (DVT) in hospitalized patients suggest that 18% of patients with myocardial infarction, 18% of gynecologic patients, 28% of urologic patients, 30% of general surgery patients, and 50% of orthopedic patients develop clinically significant thrombophlebitis. Risk factors in addition to immobilization and surgery include malignancy (Trousseau's syndrome), estrogen use, congestive heart failure, disseminated intravascular coagulopathy, localized infection, and polycythemia vera. Nearly all clinically important thrombophlebitis occurs in the lower half of the body, specifically the lower extremities.

Diagnosis

Signs and Symptoms
When DVT is suspected, it is almost always because of signs of inflammation in the lower extremity: pain, swelling, warmth, and redness. A low-grade fever is sometimes present. Other purportedly more specific signs include a palpable cord in the course of the saphenous vein and Homans' sign (calf pain on dorsiflexion of the foot, attributed to stretching the inflamed vein). However, depending on these findings for a definitive diagnosis is often misleading because many episodes of DVT cause few if any symptoms and because the "classic" symptoms and signs can result from other conditions. One study collected 11 articles comparing venograms with the clinical diagnosis and found a mean false-positive rate of the clinical diagnosis of 51%. Even when multiple symptoms are grouped together, such as swelling, erythema, palpable cord, and Homans' sign, authors have found accuracy to be less than 60%.

Conditions that can be confused with DVT include superficial thrombophlebitis, usually presenting as a palpable, tender red cord; lymphangitis, with erythematous lymphatic channels; cellulitis, causing more diffuse erythema of the skin, often with a margin; ruptured Baker's cyst, which is most frequently associated with arthritis but may occur spontaneously; ruptured plantaris tendon, which is of sudden onset; and postphlebitic syndrome. Less common conditions are unilateral edema secondary to congestive heart failure or malignancy and myositis.

Clots confined to below the knee are thought not to be associated with clinically important emboli, although they may propagate proximally, where they are a risk.

Venography
Venography is the standard of accuracy for the diagnosis of DVT. A recent study found false-negative reports to be infrequent. Of 160 patients with clinically suggested DVT and negative venograms followed for 3 months, no patients died or developed pulmonary embolism, although 2 (1.3%) developed documented DVT within 5 days of venography. While the more recent introduction of dilute contrast material has decreased the complication rate, venography still causes phlebitis in 1 to 4% of patients. Also, the test is invasive and expensive and exposes the patient to risks of radiation and anaphylaxis. For these reasons, accurate noninvasive tests for DVT have been sought.

Doppler Ultrasound
Doppler ultrasound is performed by listening for blood flow through individual veins; it is, therefore, extremely dependent on the proficiency of the technician. This may account for the wide variation in reported accuracy of diagnosis using the Doppler. It is estimated that 75% of errors documented in the literature occur in misdiagnosis of calf vein thrombi.

In one review of 13 studies (1200 procedures), overall accuracy was 88% (range 49–95%). However, studies of the accuracy of Doppler have several flaws that are characteristic of the literature for other noninvasive methods. Results are based on those patients who happened to get both venograms and Doppler studies, thus excluding many possible false-negatives and falsely elevating the sensitivity; also most of these studies were done without blinding the technicians or radiologists to prior results. Because of these problems, it is difficult to describe the accuracy of noninvasive tests for DVT.

Impedance Plethysmography
Impedance plethysmography (IP), another widely used test for DVT, measures the electrical impedance within the column of blood filling leg veins, which changes as blood flows through the leg. Most studies have shown that IP is inaccurate below the knee (sensitivity 16–60%) and that a positive IP study above the knee is highly likely to be accurate (sensitivity 93–100%).

[125]I Fibrinogen Uptake Scanning
[125]I Fibrinogen uptake scanning (FUS) has been shown to be much more accurate below the knee than above. The test has the major disadvantage of requiring up to 3 days before results can be obtained, although some researchers are using modified 1-

day tests. In one study, the combination of IP (accurate above the knee) with FUS (accurate below the knee) was extremely accurate. Therefore, in some settings it may be reasonable to substitute these two for venography in the workup of DVT.

Other Tests
Other forms of testing that have been evaluated but have not been proved useful include fibrin degradation products, saline dilution tests, thermography, and urinary D-thromboglobulin levels.

Choice of Tests
For the clinician in practice, choice of tests for DVT depends on the accuracy of locally available tests. In many settings, where the accuracy of the noninvasive tests is unknown and where dilute contrast media are used, it may be preferable to do routine venograms in patients with a clinical suggestion of DVT. If the clinician has access to a vascular laboratory with accurate noninvasive testing facilities, other strategies may be developed, such as routine venograms in patients with negative IP or routine venograms in patients with positive Doppler examinations.

Treatment
The complications of iliofemoral DVT, other than acute symptoms, include pulmonary thromboembolism (see Chap. 42) and chronic venous insufficiency, or "postphlebitic leg" (see Chap. 43). The rate at which these occur is uncertain. It seems that most episodes of overt DVT are followed by some degree of chronic venous insufficiency, but most occurrences of venous insufficiency are not related to a preceding, recognized attack of DVT. Untreated iliofemoral DVT may be associated with 6 to 14% mortality from pulmonary embolism. Treatment is known to decrease the incidence of pulmonary embolism and is intended to decrease the rate of postphlebitic leg syndrome and recurrence as well.

General Measures
Bed rest to prevent embolization, elevation of the involved extremity to prevent propagation, and heat to reduce inflammation are usually recommended. Some maintain that the leg should be immobilized at first to prevent the clot from "shaking loose," while others believe movement, at least after the first few days, decreases stasis and thereby retards propagation. None of these recommendations has been studied by means of clinical trials to see if it does more good than harm.

Anticoagulation
Anticoagulation for DVT reduces the incidence of subsequent death from pulmonary embolism dramatically—in one study, from 6 to 14% to less than 1%. Standard therapy for DVT is usually 10 days of continuous intravenous haparin infusion followed by from 6 weeks to 6 months of anticoagulation with warfarin or subcutaneous heparin. The rationale for using intravenous heparin is to prevent propagation of the clot and for long-term anticoagulation to prevent recurrence. Both of these actions have been demonstrated in the literature.

Recommendations concerning the level and length of time of anticoagulation are based on our knowledge of coagulation and on clinical studies, which are mostly uncontrolled. Prothrombin time (PT) is used as a proxy measure of safe and effective anticoagulation with warfarin. It is ordinarily recommended that the prothrombin time be maintained at 1½ to 2 times control values; pulmonary embolus rarely occurs in patients who are in this range. A recent controlled trial has suggested that prothrombin times prolonged as little as 15 seconds (control 12 seconds) may be as effective in preventing emboli, and safer in avoiding bleeding, than more aggressive anticoagulation. It has been shown that most recurrences of DVT occur within 12 weeks of the onset of treatment, suggesting that therapy beyond these guidelines may not be indicated unless there is a prior recurrence.

Anticoagulant therapy leads to a 6 to 9% incidence of bleeding complications, of which half are serious enough to require hospitalization. The risk increases with age. Most authors agree, that a bleeding site from the gastrointestinal tract or pelvic organs, especially in patients in the therapeutic range of anticoagulation, requires an extensive workup for underlying causes. Generally, at least 50% of such patients will be found to have a previously unsuspected cause for the bleeding, such as malignancies or ulcers.

Anticoagulant therapy of isolated calf vein thrombi is controversial. It has recently been recognized that isolated calf DVT may not be associated with morbidity if the patient can be followed and evaluated for proximal extension. In one study, 11 patients with isolated calf DVT, symptomatic for over 1 week and documented by venography, were followed but not treated; none had extension or pulmonary emboli.

A major problem in outpatient anticoagulation is drug interaction with oral anticoagulants. Commonly used drugs that may interact with oral anticoagulants are listed in Table 45-1.

Thrombolytic Therapy
Unlike anticoagulant therapy, thrombolytic therapy is directed at lysis of existing clots. In DVT, the only documented advantage in using thrombolytic therapy is preservation of venous valvular function, the loss of which is believed to be a prognostic indicator of the postphlebitic syndrome and possibly of recurrent DVT. However, a follow-up of patients with DVT treated with streptokinase suggests that this effect must be small, because most patients have venous dysfunction several months after the attack. Streptokinase is most frequently used early in the hospitalization and followed by routine anticoagulation. Thrombolytic therapy is usually recommended in large-vein proximal DVT.

Superficial Venous Thrombophlebitis
Most authors agree that superficial venous thrombophlebitis (SVT) is not associated with an increased risk of pulmonary embolus or postphlebitic syndrome. Frequently the diagnosis is made easily because of signs of inflammation along the course of a palpable venous cord. Therapy consists of decreasing activity, warm moist soaks, and anti-inflammatory agents. Phenylbutazone in tapering dosage for 5 to 7 days is often recommended, but there is no sound evidence that this or other anti-inflammatory agents are helpful. Superficial venous thrombophlebitis or DVT occurring in multiple

Table 45-1. Commonly used drugs that may interact with oral anticoagulants

Drugs that may potentiate anticoagulation	Drugs that may inhibit anticoagulation
Acetaminophen	Barbiturates
Allopurinol	Cholestyramine
Chloral hydrate	Diphenylhydantoin
Chloramphenicol	Ethchlorvynol
Clofibrate	Griseofulvin
Dextrothyroxine	Oral contraceptives
Disulfiram	Parenteral alimentation preparations
Griseofulvin	
Nalidixic acid	
Neomycin	
Nortriptyline	
Phenylbutazone	
Quinidine	
Quinine	
Rifampin	
Salicylates	
Sulfonamides	
Sulfinpyrazone	

sites or recurring should raise the consideration of Trousseau's syndrome or malignancy-associated disseminated intravascular coagulopathy.

Prevention

Some clinical situations, particularly during bed rest for surgery, trauma, or leg edema, are associated with a high risk of DVT. In hip replacement surgery, venous thromboembolic disease is the leading cause of death. Elevation of the legs has been demonstrated not to be effective. Graded-pressure stockings were shown in two small but controlled studies to result in a significant reduction in DVT in patients undergoing general surgery and hip replacement. Data on early ambulation is incomplete, but one study has demonstrated a slight protective effect when early ambulation, pressure stockings, and physical therapy were combined in postoperative patients.

There is excellent evidence that the routine use of low-dose subcutaneous heparin (5000 units bid) in many groups of surgical inpatients prevents the complications of postoperative DVT and pulmonary embolus. Additionally, one study noted decreased thromboembolic complications in a group of myocardial infarction patients treated in this manner. Heparin-associated thrombocytopenia may occur with even low doses of heparin; routine, biweekly platelet counts are recommended for all patients on heparin therapy.

Because of bleeding complications from heparin and warfarin in patients undergoing hip surgery, a number of observers have studied aspirin prophylaxis in this subgroup. The results are mixed; aspirin in other settings has largely been found to be ineffective for prophylaxis.

Pogson GW, Conn RD. Bedside diagnosis of deep venous thrombosis: A myth exposed. *Mo Med* 76:203–206, 1979.
The overwhelming inaccuracy of the clinical examination is pointed out. In 11 studies, there were 51% false positives (range, 16–77%).
Coon WW, Willis PW III, Symons MJ. Assessment of anticoagulant treatment of venous thromboembolism. *Ann Surg* 170:559–567, 1969.
Confirmatory evidence of the efficacy of therapy. Suggests most recurrences happen within 12 weeks and that the best therapeutic level is below 30% (approximately two times control).
Coon WW, Willis PW III. Hemorrhagic complications of anticoagulant therapy. *Arch Intern Med* 133:386–392, 1974.
Bleeding occurred in 6.8% of 3,862 courses of anticoagulant therapy. There were 4 deaths. Over half who bled had recognizable lesions, many of which were previously unknown. Thus, patients who bleed should be investigated.
Davis FD, et al. Management of anticoagulation in outpatients. *Arch Intern Med* 137:197, 1977.
The authors set up a service to handle anticoagulation. Their therapeutic range was 1½ to 3 times control values. They noted an 8% overall complication rate and 4% major hemorrhagic morbidity.
Sumner DS, Lambeth A. Reliability of Doppler ultrasound in the diagnosis of acute venous thrombosis both above and below the knee. *Am J Surg* 138:205–210, 1979.
This generally favorable article suggests Dopplers may be used to diagnose and treat DVT. This is unusual, since the authors note other series with sensitivities and specificities as low as 39 and 59% respectively. Obviously strategies should be based on local accuracy.
Young AE, et al. Impedance plethysmography: Its limitations as a substitute for phlebography. *Cardiovasc Intervent Radiol* 1:223–239, 1978.
Using a scattergram technique, the authors failed to find a line of discrimination that could differentiate normal from phlebitic legs. False-negative results were found in 44%. They note other studies that demonstrate a high false-negative rate, especially those in which the readers were blinded. Their conclusion is that positive results are useful, negative results are not.
Hull R, et al. Replacement of venography in suspected venous thrombosis by impedance plethysmography and I^{125} leg scanning. *Ann Intern Med* 94:12–15, 1981.
A state-of-the-art prospective blinded trial that tested IP and FUS as diagnostic tests, demonstrating their safety as such in competent hands. Further, suggests that calf vein thrombi may not need therapy if the patients are carefully followed.

Sasahara AA, Sharma GV, Parisi AF. New developments in the detection and prevention of venous thromboembolism. *Am J Cardiol* 43:1214–1224, 1979.

An excellent overall review, suggesting on the basis of five studies that IP is accurate. The second half of the article contains a collection of prior work concerning low-dose heparin prophylaxis in surgical and myocardial infarction patients.

Hull R, et al. Cost effectiveness of clinical diagnosis, venography, and non-invasive testing in patients with symptomatic deep vein thrombosis. *N Engl J Med* 304:1561–1567, 1981.

Another study from the Hamilton group, which concludes that IP and FUS in combination are more cost-effective—but not by much—than outpatient venograms; in fact, in Canada, venograms would be more cost-effective.

Watz R, Savidge GF. Rapid thrombolysis and preservation of valvular venous function in high deep venous thrombosis. *Acta Med Scand* 205:293–298, 1979.

Ninety-two percent of patients treated with lytic therapy had normal functioning valves, compared to 13% treated with heparin.

Koch-Weser J, Sellers EM. Drug interactions with coumarin anticoagulants (two parts). *N Engl J Med* 285:487–498 and 547–557, 1971.

Comprehensive review of drug interactions.

Sack G, Levin J, Bell W. Trousseau's syndrome and other manifestations of chronic disseminated coagulopathy in patients with neoplasms: Clinical, pathophysiologic and therapeutic features. *Medicine* 56:1–30, 1977.

Encyclopedic review of the literature, plus a case series.

Sharma GV, et al. Thrombolytic therapy. *N Engl J Med* 306:1268–1276, 1982.

Excellent review of the development of, indicators for, and complications of thrombolytic agents, including usage in pulmonary embolus, acute myocardial infarction, arterial emboli, and venous thrombosis.

Hull R, Hirsh J. Long-term anticoagulant therapy in patients with venous thrombosis. *Arch Intern Med* 143:2061–2063, 1983.

A summary of the best, recent studies concerning (1) the choice of heparin versus warfarin, and (2) intensity of anticoagulation.

VIII. GASTROINTESTINAL PROBLEMS

Dysphagia is the subjective awareness that something has gone wrong with the active mechanical transport of food from pharynx to stomach. This symptom indicates esophageal disease and *demands* immediate and complete evaluation. Patients may describe dysphagia in a variety of ways, saying that food "sticks" or "slows down" or "doesn't go down right," or they may say that they choke when they swallow.

Dysphagia may be suggested in the patient who complains of the constant sensation of a lump in the throat that may disappear with swallowing. This condition, globus hystericus, occurs frequently in young to middle-aged patients, often women, in whom anxiety, depression, or obsessive features are also present. By means of a careful history, globus hystericus can be distinguished from true dysphagia, and an extensive evaluation may be avoided.

"Preesophageal dysphagia" occurs in patients with a variety of neuromuscular disorders. These patients have a problem initiating the act of swallowing or transferring food from the mouth to the esophagus.

In esophageal dysphagia, the sensation of food sticking is usually localized by the patient somewhere between the suprasternal notch and the xiphoid process. However, localization is not precise. The dysphagia that occurs with lesions at the lower end of the esophagus may be referred to the area of the suprasternal notch. On the other hand, it is very unusual for a lesion high in the esophagus to cause symptoms in the region of the xiphoid.

Causes

Two types of esophageal disease can cause dysphagia. One type produces dysphagia by obliteration or narrowing of the esophageal lumen; lesions such as esophageal carcinoma or peptic stricture are examples. Extrinsic lesions, such as mediastinal lymphoma, also can compress the esophageal lumen and lead to dysphagia. The other major category includes those diseases that cause motor failure of the esophagus, including achalasia and diffuse esophageal spasm. Scleroderma involving the esophagus initially presents as a motor abnormality, but peptic strictures may supervene.

Evaluation

History
Patients with lumen-obliterating lesions, whether intrinsic or extrinsic, characteristically have a progressive type of dysphagia. They first notice difficulty with solid foods, which progresses to difficulty with soft foods, and finally, liquids. In contrast, patients with primary motor disorders may have dysphagia with liquids as well as solids from the onset. Additionally, dysphagia of motor origin tends to be intermittent, whereas dysphagia secondary to mechanical obstruction tends to be constant and relentlessly progressive. The temperature of the ingested material has no effect on the dysphagia in obstructing lesions, but cold or iced liquids may aggravate the problem in patients with motor disorders, particularly diffuse esophageal spasm. Also, patients with mechanical narrowing of the esophagus who have an impacted bolus frequently have to regurgitate to obtain relief, whereas patients with motor disorders may pass the impacted material by "washing it down with liquids."

Physical Examination
The history is very important in patients with esophageal disease, and it should suggest the correct diagnosis. In contrast, the physical examination is usually normal and contributes little to the diagnosis. If abnormalities are present, they are, unfortunately, almost always manifestations of late disease, such as the systemic features of scleroderma, a palpable axillary or supraclavicular node, or recurrent laryngeal nerve involvement in inoperable or metastatic carcinoma of the esophagus.

X-ray and Other Studies

The complaint of dysphagia demands immediate investigation, which should not be considered complete without a careful upper gastrointestinal series, upper endoscopy with careful attention to the proximal stomach, and esophageal manometric studies. The upper gastrointestinal series is usually done first because it either makes the diagnosis or serves to focus the attention of the endoscopist to any abnormal or suspicious area. If the x-ray study is negative, endoscopy is indicated because small mucosal lesions or Schatzki's rings may not have been visible. Esophageal manometric studies may be necessary to verify and amplify x-ray findings, to complete the investigation in patients with negative x-rays and negative endoscopic examination, and to detect motor disorders that may have been missed by the other examinations.

Specific Clinical Conditions

Achalasia

Achalasia has been variously termed *cardiospasm, aperistalsis,* and *megaesophagus.* The cause of this disease in the United States and Europe is unknown. In South America, Chagas' disease causes the same radiographic and manometric features found in achalasia. In achalasia there is a decreased number of ganglion cells in Auerbach's plexus, in the body of the esophagus, and in the area of the lower esophageal sphincter. There are also reports of degeneration of the myelin sheath and breaks in the axon membrane of the vagus nerve, as well as decreased numbers of ganglion cells in the dorsal motor nucleus of the vagus nerve. These changes are reflected in the two characteristic features of the disease that lead to dysphagia: the absence of peristaltic activity and an increase in lower esophageal sphincter pressure with absent or incomplete relaxation. The fact that patients with achalasia respond in an abnormal fashion to the injection of mecholyl, a cholinergic drug, may be a reflection of these alterations in the nervous system and represents an example of Cannon's law of denervation.

Achalasia typically begins in middle age, although it has been diagnosed in early infancy and in the elderly. In addition to dysphagia, which is of the classic motor type, symptoms include regurgitation, and occasionally, chest pain and weight loss. There also may be symptoms indicative of aspiration, such as repeated bouts of pneumonitis. The physical examination is usually not helpful.

The chest x-ray suggests the diagnosis of achalasia if the fluid-filled esophagus is seen as a double density with an air-fluid level behind the heart. Other findings include the absence of a gastric air bubble, probably related to the abnormal lower esophageal sphincter, and an esophagus that is not completely empty. Barium examination shows a widely dilated esophagus tapering to a beak, delayed emptying of barium into the stomach, and absence of primary peristaltic waves.

Esophageal manometry demonstrates increased intraesophageal pressure (probably reflecting the retained secretions), complete aperistalsis with low amplitude waves, and a hypertensive lower esophageal sphincter with absent or incomplete relaxation. The mecholyl test is not useful in making the diagnosis of achalasia.

Endoscopy is mandatory to exclude secondary achalasia resulting from a variety of other lesions, such as carcinoma of the fundus of the stomach, which can invade the distal esophagus and produce a clinical picture similar to achalasia in all respects. Also, patients with achalasia have an increased incidence of esophageal carcinoma.

Nitrates and calcium channel blockers have been used to decrease symptoms in patients with achalasia. However, effective treatment depends mainly on disruption of the high pressure zone at the distal end of the esophagus, either by the use of a pneumatic dilator or, in certain instances, by thoracotomy and a Heller myotomy.

Diffuse Esophageal Spasm

The cause of diffuse esophageal spasm is unknown. It may occur in almost anyone, although it is more prevalent in middle-aged people and in women. In addition to dysphagia, symptoms include pain, which is prominent and distressing. The pain is often similar in location to angina pectoris, can be alleviated by nitroglycerin or long-acting nitrites, and at times is related to emotional stress. Because the pain is angina-like, patients are frequently evaluated for coronary artery disease. Regurgitation, weight loss, and symptoms suggesting aspiration are unusual. As in other motor disorders, dysphagia is observed with liquids as well as solids and may be aggravated by the ingestion of cold liquids. The fact that the pain can occur with swallowing (odynophagia) or can be spontaneous may be confusing, but the association of dysphagia with chest pain directs attention to the esophagus.

The radiologic appearance of the esophagus is quite characteristic; there are multiple areas of segmental spasm termed *pseudodiverticulosis of the esophagus* or *corkscrew esophagus*. Esophageal manometric results are also characteristic, demonstrating repetitive contractions in response to deglutition, as well as increased amplitude and duration of contractions. Many of the contractions are nonperistaltic; with repeated swallowing, however, some normal peristaltic contractions are seen. There also may be spontaneous activity noted in the body of the esophagus. The lower esophageal sphincter may or may not have increased pressure, but relaxation is usually complete. These patients may have a positive mecholyl test, and, occasionally, a patient with diffuse esophageal spasm eventually develops achalasia. There are many patients whose clinical presentation does not fit either the classic description of achalasia or diffuse esophageal spasm; their condition is best described as *nonspecific motor disorder of the esophagus* with appropriate modifiers.

Reflux Esophagitis with Peptic Stricture

Many factors contribute to the production of reflux esophagitis, including the competency of the antireflux mechanism (which consists mainly of the lower esophageal sphincter coupled with mechanical factors), the potency and volume of the refluxed material, esophageal emptying or dwell time, and tissue resistance. The lower esophageal sphincter is thought to be the most important barrier in preventing reflux of noxious material including acid, bile, and proteolytic enzymes into the esophagus. The function of the lower esophageal sphincter is governed by myogenic, neurohumoral, and mechanical factors. Hiatal hernia is *not* synonymous with reflux. Hiatal hernia may or may not be seen in association with reflux esophagitis, and reflux esophagitis may occur in the absence of a hiatal hernia. However, many patients with severe reflux esophagitis have an associated hiatal hernia.

The main symptom of reflux esophagitis is "heartburn" (pyrosis), a retrosternal burning pain that may begin in the epigastrium and end in the pharynx. It is usually promptly relieved by an antacid. When reflux proceeds to damage and scar formation, a stricture may form, leading to dysphagia. Barrett's esophagus (columnar-lined lower esophagus) is an acquired lesion related to gastroesophageal reflux. It is associated with esophageal ulcers and midesophageal strictures and is a precursor of adenocarcinoma of the esophagus in some instances. It demands continued surveillance.

It is not necessary to do an extensive evaluation of every patient with heartburn unless there is associated dysphagia, odynophagia, severe heartburn, or other worrisome features. Methods of evaluating the patient with reflux symptoms include upper gastrointestinal x-rays, esophageal manometry to document an incompetent lower esophageal sphincter, pH and potential difference recordings, Bernstein or acid perfusion test, esophagoscopy, and biopsy. Whether or not these are indicated is determined by the severity and chronicity of the complaints.

The medical treatment of reflux esophagitis is based on physical and mechanical maneuvers that prevent esophageal reflux, such as elevating the head of the bed 6 to 8 inches and not eating late in the evening. Agents known to decrease lower esophageal sphincter pressure—fats, chocolate, and drugs such as the estrogen-progesterone combinations and anticholinergics—should be avoided. Neutralization of acid with antacids remains the cornerstone of therapy. Other medications that may be helpful are alginic acid (Gaviscon), which provides an antacid foam barrier to reflux, and cimetidine (Tagamet), 300 mg orally four times a day, or ranitidine (Zantac) 150 mg twice a day. Drugs that increase lower esophageal sphincter pressure, such as bethanechol, 10 to 25 mg orally four times a day, or metoclopramide (Reglan), 10–20 mg orally one-half hour before meals and at bedtime, may be useful adjuncts. Metoclopramide may also improve gastric emptying. Surgical therapy of reflux is aimed at augmenting the lower esophageal sphincter, usually with some form of fundoplication. Indications for surgery include hemorrhage, severe reflux unresponsive to intensive medical therapy, stricture formation, and recurrent pulmonary aspiration. Patients in whom surgery is planned should have preoperative manometry, both for a baseline and to exclude a coexisting motor disorder of the esophagus.

Lower Esophageal Rings
Lower esophageal rings at the squamocolumnar junction, or Schatzki's rings, also may cause dysphagia. When the transverse diameter of the ring is less than 12 mm, patients usually experience dysphagia. Characteristically, the dysphagia is at first intermittent, giving rise to periodic bolus impaction. These patients have long symptom-free intervals, which over the years may become shortened, until eventually symptoms are continuous. The x-ray appearance is characteristic, but the radiologist should be alerted as these rings may be missed unless the esophagus is overly distended with barium or a bolus. Dilatation with mercury-filled bougies is curative.

Carcinoma
Dysphagia is the most common presenting complaint of patients with carcinoma of the esophagus. Classically, there is progressive dysphagia, initially for solids, with inexorable progression through semisolids and liquids. These symptoms are accompanied by weight loss. Odynophagia on occasion may be an initial symptom of esophageal cancer. Factors that predispose to esophageal cancer include smoking, alcohol, past history of lye stricture, achalasia, tylosis palmaris et plantaris, and Plummer-Vinson web. Columnar-lined lower esophagus (Barrett's esophagus) is associated with an increased incidence of adenocarcinoma of the esophagus, in contrast to the usual squamous cell carcinoma of the esophagus. The diagnosis of esophageal cancer is suggested by the characteristic x-ray appearance and confirmed by endoscopy and biopsy. If metastases have not occurred, treatment consists of preoperative irradiation followed by surgery. Unfortunately, the overall 5-year survival is 3 to 10%; it is higher in those patients resected for cure who have negative nodes.

Other Lesions
There is a long list of miscellaneous lesions that can lead to dysphagia. A partial list includes leiomyoma; mediastinal masses; radiation fibrosis; monilial infection of the esophagus; Plummer-Vinson web or upper esophageal webs, which may or may not be related to iron deficiency anemia; and thoracic aortic aneurysms.

Thorn GW, et al. (Eds.). *Harrison's Principles of Internal Medicine* (8th ed.). New York: McGraw-Hill, 1976. Pp. 203–205, 1487–1492.
A classic medical presentation of gastrointestinal diseases.
Sleisenger MH, Fordtran JS. *Gastrointestinal Disease* (2nd ed.). Philadelphia: Saunders, 1978. Pp. 196–199, 495–610.
A comprehensive subspeciality text dealing with the esophagus in all of its aspects.
Richter JE, Castell DO. Gastroesophageal reflux: Pathogenesis, diagnosis, and therapy. *Ann Intern Med* 97:93–103, 1982.
Discusses the role of the lower esophageal sphincter in preventing reflux. The value of the various tests to evaluate reflux is dealt with in an effective manner. The therapy is explained succinctly.
Bozymski EM, Herlihy KJ, Orlando RC. Barrett's esophagus. *Ann Intern Med* 97:104–107, 1982.
Barrett's esophagus, an acquired lesion secondary to chronic reflux, is probably more common than we appreciate. Radiographic features include high esophageal strictures and deep esophageal ulcers. The association of Barrett's esophagus with adenocarcinoma of the esophagus is discussed.
Sandler RS, Bozymski EM, Orlando RC. Failure of clinical criteria to distinguish between primary achalasia and achalasia secondary to tumor. *Dig Dis Sci* 27:209–213, 1982.
Three clinical criteria, onset at older age, significant weight loss, and short duration of symptoms, are reported to distinguish patients with achalasia secondary to tumor from patients with primary achalasia. Even though they are highly sensitive, they are not specific and their predictive value for distinguishing secondary achalasia from primary achalasia is exceedingly low.
Castell DO, et al. Dysphagia. *Gastroenterology* 76:1015–1024, 1979.
A good general discussion of the topic of dysphagia centered about a case presentation.
Petrokkubi RJ, Jeffreis GH. Cimetidine versus antacid in scleroderma with reflux esophagitis: A randomized double-blind controlled study. *Gastroenterology* 77:691–695, 1979.

Cimetidine was found to be more effective than antacid in controlling heartburn, and it also caused greater endoscopic improvement. Neither cimetidine nor antacid produced any improvement in esophageal strictures.

Vantrappen G, et al. Achalasia, diffuse esophageal spasm, and related motility disorders. *Gastroenterology* 76:450–457, 1979.

The authors have extensive experience with esophageal motor disorders and present a compilation of their data.

Cohen S. Motor disorders of the esophagus. *N Engl J Med* 301:184–190, 1979.

An excellent short review of the salient features of motor disorders of the esophagus.

47. ESOPHAGITIS
Sidney L. Levinson

Esophagitis is an inflammatory process involving the mucosa of the esophagus, usually resulting from retrograde flow of gastric contents above the gastroesophageal junction. The cardinal symptom of esophageal reflux is heartburn, which may be associated with esophageal inflammation ranging from macroscopic mucosal ulcerations to lack of a demonstrable esophageal lesion.

Esophagitis affects people of all ages, with no sex predominance. Reflux of gastric or duodenal contents into the esophagus occurs regularly in up to 10% of healthy people, and occasionally in up to 35%.

The pathogenesis of reflux esophagitis remains controversial. Many studies emphasize incompetence of the lower esophageal sphincter, both intermittently and persistently, in allowing acid-pepsin mixtures to bathe the squamous epithelial lining of the esophagus. Some authors suggest that impairment of normal esophageal peristalsis with resulting poor clearance of acid explains the development of esophagitis in patients in whom the frequency of reflux is not abnormal. Decreased gastric emptying with a resultant increase in postprandial gastric volume may also contribute to esophagitis. Less controversial is the involvement of hiatal hernia, an anatomic abnormality that by itself does not imply reflux. Although not all patients with hiatal hernia have esophageal reflux, most patients with severe esophagitis have coexistent hiatal hernia.

Clinical Presentation
Most patients with esophagitis consult a physician because of heartburn, a complaint of burning discomfort behind the lower sternum or in the midepigastrium, which frequently radiates upward. Heartburn typically increases soon after meals, particularly if the meals include spicy, fatty, or acidic foods. It is frequently aggravated by bending or stooping, particularly in association with lifting or straining. Patients also may complain of regurgitation of sour or bitter fluid, or of partially digested food, and they may even find fluid on their pillow on awakening in the morning. Heartburn occurs with greater frequency during recumbency, and patients with severe esophagitis are likely to awaken with nocturnal pain.

Odynophagia (pain on swallowing) may occur with the passage of large boluses of hot or cold liquids through an area of inflammation. Dysphagia (difficulty in swallowing) can occur with or without structural changes within the esophagus, as a result of either spasm associated within the area of inflammation or actual impedance of passage of a bolus by a stricture. Reflux esophagitis also must be considered in patients who present with chest pain not clearly of cardiac or musculoskeletal origin.

Certain factors may help to identify patients at risk for the development of esophagitis. Patients with previous acid-peptic symptoms or a family history of acid-peptic disease may be more likely to develop esophagitis, although acid secretory studies in patients with esophagitis do not differ significantly from results in healthy people. Obesity, pregnancy, and occupational bending or straining increase intra-abdominal pressure and predispose to reflux. Habitual use of acid stimulants or mucosal irritants such as caffeine, alcohol, and aspirin commonly contributes to the development of heartburn. Agents that decrease lower esophageal sphincter contraction and therefore increase reflux, such as tobacco, fatty foods, chocolate, and peppermint, also may cause heartburn. Although citrus juices or spicy foods incite symptoms by a direct irritant effect, they do not typically induce esophageal inflammation. Finally, patients with scleroderma frequently develop esophagitis.

Diagnosis

History
The presence of heartburn is diagnostic of esophageal reflux and raises the suspicion of esophagitis. The diagnostic reliability of historical findings is increased if the pain is postprandial, postexercise, and nocturnal, all of which are typical of pain from esophagitis. Smokers often note increasing symptoms soon after smoking, and patients frequently note more frequent symptoms when under stress.

The history should also be used to assess the likelihood of complications. Radiation of pain to the back, which is atypical, suggests spasms or posterior ulceration, whereas dysphagia suggests stricture. Heartburn that has been present for a long time and then decreases may herald the development of stricture or, occasionally, concomitant achalasia.

Physical Examination
Examination of patients with esophagitis is usually normal. Epigastric palpation may elicit tenderness or reflux symptoms. Occult bleeding or, infrequently, melena or hematemesis may indicate hemorrhage from ulcerations or erosions. Weight loss and cachexia are observed in some patients with benign strictures or in association with adenocarcinoma developing within Barrett's esophagus, a premalignant metaplastic mucosal change that can develop with long-standing reflux.

Laboratory Studies
Reflux esophagitis is confirmed by documenting reflux, histologic inflammatory changes, or both, depending on the extent of symptoms. Mild heartburn that resolves when acid stimulants are avoided and antacid therapy is begun requires no additional evaluation. Additional studies are warranted when reflux is suspected, but the history is not characteristic of reflux esophagitis; if initial measures do not completely resolve the patient's symptoms; or if dysphagia, weight loss, or occult bleeding is noted.

Upper gastrointestinal (UGI) x-rays are usually the first study obtained, in part because they are widely available and relatively inexpensive. Although relatively insensitive in detecting reflux (40%) and mild degrees of inflammation (22%), the UGI can be considered diagnostic when evidence for reflux is seen in concert with typical symptoms. Although normal x-ray findings do not rule out reflux esophagitis, they can exclude other conditions, such as peptic ulcer disease, malignancy, and complications of reflux, such as stricture or ulceration.

Endoscopy is a more accurate means of testing for the diagnosis of esophagitis than UGI x-rays, although interpretation of milder grades of inflammation is difficult. Mucosal biopsy increases the accuracy of this technique, but involves greater expense and risk. Investigation with endoscopy is warranted in patients with stricture or ulceration, with the search particularly geared toward evidence of malignancy or Barrett's esophagus. Endoscopy should be the first study performed when heartburn is seen in association with dysphagia or heme-positive stool.

The Bernstein acid infusion test is abnormal in up to 90% of patients with esophagitis and is the most sensitive nonhistologic study. It is readily performed in the office. A nasogastric tube is passed a distance of 30 cm, and with the patient sitting upright, solutions of normal saline and 0.1 NHCL are infused in a manner that allows changes to be made without the patient's knowledge. The test is considered positive if the patient's symptoms are reproduced twice during acid perfusion and relieved during saline perfusion. To avoid false-positive interpretations, discomfort produced by acid perfusion that does not mimic the patient's symptoms should not be considered a positive result. Because the Bernstein test allows the physician and patient to compare symptoms produced by acid perfusion with those experienced spontaneously, it is most useful in patients with multiple or atypical complaints. However, it does not actually measure acid reflux, nor does it confirm the presence of mucosal inflammation, which, if necessary, can be verified with endoscopy.

In difficult instances, or when surgery is considered, other studies are usually obtained after referral to a gastroenterologist. Esophageal manometrics can delineate abnormalities of peristalsis in achalasia, esophageal spasm, or scleroderma. Lower esophageal sphincter pressure measurements of less than 8 suggest reflux, although considerable overlap occurs between symptomatic and asymptomatic patients. The pH probe accurately reflects both spontaneous and provoked reflux, particularly after instillation of acid. Potential difference studies of the esophagus, which can be obtained with manometrics, demonstrate changes in epithelial function as a result of microscopic esophagitis, even when other modalities disclose no evidence for esophagitis. Gastroesophageal scintiscanning shows promise as a noninvasive technique for detecting reflux, but additional studies are needed to evaluate its efficacy.

Treatment
The typical course of esophagitis is one of intermittent exacerbations, many of which can be managed with a combination of nonmedical therapeutic modalities.

General Measures
Substances that stimulate acid production or that have been shown to be associated with symptoms should be avoided (see above). Measures that may decrease the occurrence of reflux during the day include weight loss (in the obese) and the avoidance of large meals, recumbency after eating, frequent bending, and tight-fitting garments. Elevation of the head of the bed 6 to 8 inches on concrete blocks decreases nocturnal reflux, and avoidance of late-night snacks decreases the availability of acid for reflux at bedtime. Drugs that may exacerbate reflux by decreasing lower esophageal sphincter pressure include anticholinergics, theophylline, alpha- and beta-adrenergic agents, diazepam, meperidine, nicotine, and the calcium channel blocking agents. The addition of either antacids or alginic acid (Gaviscon) to the measures described above effectively treats 75 percent of patients.

Drugs
For the 25% of patients who do not respond to the regimen described above, the addition of medication aimed at the pathogenetic mechanisms can increase healing of esophagitis. Several drugs have been used for this purpose.

Bethanechol, 25 mg four times a day, has been reported to increase lower esophageal sphincter pressure and improve esophageal acid clearing, but has achieved mixed success in symptomatic improvement. Whether it promotes healing of macroscopic disease is not well established.

Metoclopramide also has been shown to increase lower esophageal sphincter pressure, as well as to improve abnormal gastric emptying. Symptomatic relief and decreased antacid use have been demonstrated with a regimen of 10 mg four times a day. In a well-controlled double-blind cross-over study, patients receiving metoclopramide had a 57% improvement in symptoms, compared with a 33% improvement in the control group. In another study, however, one-third of patients reported neurologic or psychotropic symptoms with this dosage.

Cimetidine, which decreases gastric acid production, has also been shown to relieve symptoms of gastroesophageal reflux and, inconsistently, to improve healing of gross esophagitis. The usual dosage is 300 mg four times a day for 6 to 8 weeks.

It is reasonable to add cimetidine and either bethanechol or metoclopramide to the treatment of patients with esophagitis who fail to improve on nonmedical or antacid therapy. With maximal medical therapy, up to 90% of patients can be treated effectively.

The clinical course may be more complicated for patients who have demonstrated erosive esophagitis. Persistent heartburn may require ongoing antacid use. Complications of long-standing severe reflux esophagitis include strictures with weight loss and risk of food impaction, recurrent aspiration with resulting bronchopulmonary infections, and even oxygen-diffusion abnormalities. Gastrointestinal bleeding from esophagitis is usually occult.

Surgery
Prospective studies have demonstrated that modern surgical procedures improve heartburn in virtually all patients despite reflux demonstrable through pH probe. Postoperative complications, including pneumonia, infection, and atelectasis, are more com-

mon with the procedures that use a thoracic approach. Recurrence of severe esophagitis caused by operative failure is as low as 4% after 2½ years, but breakdown after more than 10 years may be more frequent. The choice of procedure depends on the skill and experience of the surgeon.

Dodds WJ, et al. Pathogenesis of reflux esophagitis. *Gastroenterology* 81:376–394, 1981.
A thorough review of the contributory mechanisms of esophageal reflux and esophagitis.

Richter JE, Castell DO. Gastroesophageal reflux: Pathogenesis, diagnosis, and therapy. *Ann Intern Med* 97:93–103, 1982.
A recent review, with practical advice about management.

Chernow B, Castell DO. Diet and heartburn. *JAMA* 241(21):2307–2308, 1979.
A discussion of foods that affect lower esophageal sphincter pressure and increase heartburn.

Behar J, Biancani P, Sheahan DG. Evaluation of esophageal tests in the diagnosis of reflux esophagitis. *Gastroenterology* 71:9–15, 1976.
The Bernstein test was more helpful than secretory studies or manometry in diagnosing esophagitis.

Castell DO. Medical therapy of reflux esophagitis. *Ann Intern Med* 93:926–927, 1980.
Most patients responded to a stepwise implementation of medical therapy.

Saco LS, et al. Double-blind controlled trial of bethanechol and antacid vs. placebo and antacid in the treatment of erosive esophagitis. *Gastroenterology* 82:1369–1373, 1982.
Bethanechol did not improve healing of gross peptic esophagitis.

McCallum RW, et al. A controlled trial of metoclopramide in symptomatic gastroesophageal reflux. *N Engl J Med* 296(7):354–357, 1977.
Metoclopramide improved patients' symptoms, although lower esophageal sphincter pressure did not correlate with symptomatic improvement.

DeMeester TR, Johnson LF, Kent AM. Evaluation of current operations for the prevention of gastroesophageal reflux. *Ann Surg* 180:511–525, 1974.
The Nissen procedure inhibited reflux adequately, with fewer operative complications than in the Belsey procedure.

Orlando RC, et al. Esophageal potential difference measurements in esophageal disease. *Gastroenterology* 83:1026–1032, 1982.
Potential difference studies accurately identified areas of esophageal disease.

Greenberger NJ. Peptic Esophagitis. In *Gastrointestinal Disorders*. Chicago: Year Book, 1980. Pp. 21–27.
A concise review of pathophysiologic mechanisms and evaluation measures in esophagitis.

48. FUNCTIONAL DYSPEPSIA
Douglas A. Drossman

Dyspepsia is a common symptom that defies precise definition or classification. We customarily use the term to refer to "indigestion," which is an abdominal fullness or pain that can be dull, gnawing, or burning in quality, or "gaseousness," which includes belching, abdominal distention, and audible borborygmus. The discomfort is usually localized in the upper abdomen or anterior chest, and eating may aggravate or relieve the discomfort. Associated symptoms may include anorexia, nausea, change in bowel habits, or dysphoric states such as anxiety and depression.

Dyspepsia can be experienced by patients with a variety of pathologic disorders, such as esophagitis, cholecystitis, or peptic ulcer. In this chapter, the term *functional dyspepsia* is used to denote symptoms in patients without structural abnormalities (i.e., with negative x-ray or endoscopic studies).

The true frequency of functional dyspepsia is difficult to establish because no precise clinical criteria are established and no demonstrable structural change or physiologic aberrations exist. It is believed to occur in at least 10% of the population, but its prevalence in clinical settings varies with the type of medical practice and the willingness of the physician to use symptomatic diagnostic categories. Although the incidence in a general medical outpatient population in Great Britain was reported to be as high as 26%, this diagnosis is rarely made in gastroenterology referral practices.

The correlation between the symptoms of functional dyspepsia and specific pathophysiologic abnormalities is generally poor. Endoscopic, radiologic, and surgical evaluation of patients with chronic dyspepsia identifies structural abnormalities in 13 to 86%. This wide variation is in part explained by the lack of precise symptom definition. Furthermore, dyspeptic symptoms and disease findings are not necessarily causally related. For example, gastric biopsies show inflammatory changes in 40 to 75% of patients with x-ray–negative dyspepsia, but the same proportion of asymptomatic subjects has similar pathology. Most patients and physicians believe that increased amounts of intestinal gas produce the pain and sensations of bloating and distention. However, the quantity and distribution of intestinal gas in these patients have been found to be no different from those of asymptomatic comparison groups.

Diagnosis
Dyspepsia, like pain, is accepted as present in any patient who complains of it. The physician's task is to decide whether additional diagnostic evaluation is needed to exclude specific disorders before instituting symptomatic treatment.

History and Physical Examination
The illness should be fully characterized, with attention to the diagnostic medical possibilities and the psychosocial factors influencing the experiencing and reporting of symptoms. Is the discomfort related to meals, change in bowel function, or exertion? Is it relieved by antacids or by rest? Is there dysphagia or shortness of breath? What was the setting of symptom onset? Was there associated anxiety or sadness?

Although perhaps the majority of patients presenting with dyspepsia in the primary care setting may be found to have no other pathologic diagnosis, the physician should consider in the differential diagnosis those disorders requiring specific treatment. These conditions include peptic ulcer disease (symptom is relieved by meals), cholecystitis, pancreatitis (symptom is often worse after meals), cardiac ischemia (symptom is worse during exertion), gastroesophageal reflux (symptom is worse when patient is straining or lying supine), diffuse esophageal spasm (associated with episodic dysphagia), irritable bowel syndrome (associated with changes in bowel function), and parasitic disorder such as that caused by *Giardia lamblia*. Psychological disorders to consider include anxiety (with or without aerophagia), conversion disorder, depression with somatization, and hypochondriasis.

Additional Studies
The need for diagnostic tests is determined by the findings on the history and physical examination. It is reasonable to include a complete blood count and to test the stool for occult blood. If these are negative, additional diagnostic study is usually not needed. However, evidence for occult bleeding suggests diagnoses such as esophagitis, gastritis, peptic ulcer, neoplasia, or infectious-inflammatory bowel disease, and requires additional diagnostic evaluation. An upper gastrointestinal series may be done if the patient has dysphagia, weight loss, vomiting, or a change in the pattern of symptoms with eating. These x-rays may disclose structural abnormalities (strictures, ulcers, tumor), but cannot identify esophagitis or superficial gastroduodenal erosions. Upper endoscopy, a more sensitive method for detecting mucosal abnormalities, has been recommended for evaluation of patients with continued unexplained symptoms. However, this examination does not prove cost-effective when there is no evidence for gastrointestinal blood loss and the upper GI series is normal. Esophageal manometry is indicated only if dysphagia, regurgitation, or evidence for aspiration suggests a motor disorder of the esophagus.

Electrocardiography, possibly with exercise testing, should be considered if the symptoms are related to exertion or are associated with dyspnea. Oral cholecystography is of uncertain diagnostic value in the patient with dyspepsia and no other clinical findings. Among patients referred for an oral cholecystogram, dyspepsia was equally frequent whether or not gallstones were present. Thus, if a patient complaining only of dyspepsia is found to have gallstones (within a functioning gallbladder), surgery may not clearly be indicated. However, if the patient has symptoms also suggestive of cholecystitis, choledocholithiasis, or cholangitis (intermittent postprandial pain localized to the right upper quadrant, vomiting after meals, fever, jaundice, or abnormal liver chemistries), more thorough evaluation of the biliary system is needed, and surgical intervention is recommended if disease is found. Sigmoidoscopy and possibly examination of the stool for ova and parasites should be done if the patient reports any associated change in bowel function. Finally, more thorough diagnostic evaluation such as barium enema may be needed in selected patient groups, such as patients over 45 years presenting with new symptoms.

Treatment
If the initial history and physical examination do not indicate the need for additional tests, or if the studies ordered are nondiagnostic, the physician may give reassurance, treat the patient symptomatically, and observe over time for any changes or new clinical findings. No one medication is of proven value in relieving symptoms of dyspepsia, but each physician develops a set of treatments that seems effective in many instances. Treatment should be relatively inexpensive, safe, and tailored to the amelioration of symptoms.

Dietary Changes
Patients should avoid foodstuffs known to affect acid secretions and intestinal motility adversely. These include tobacco, caffeine, and gas-producing substances such as beans and cabbage. A low-fat diet can be recommended for patients who report increased symptoms with fatty foods. These symptoms may occur because of the associated delay in gastric emptying caused by the endogenous release of cholecystokinin. The patient with lactase deficiency should avoid milk products.

Medications
Antacids can be tried for brief periods of time in an antiulcer schedule (i.e., 15–45 cc at 1 and 3 hours pc and hs). Simethicone, either in combination with an antacid or as chewable tablets, can be suggested to relieve symptoms of "gas." Although this surface-acting agent disperses gas bubbles, its efficacy in relieving patient symptoms is unproved. Most of these patients are believed to have a motility disorder rather than an increased accumulation of gas. There is also a subgroup of patients who are habitual air swallowers. They are observed to swallow air and belch when experiencing stress. For these patients treatment may involve reassurance and, on occasion, a short course of benzodiazepine agents (Valium, Librium). Metoclopramide, 10 mg one-half hour before meals and at bedtime, is reported to be of some value in patients with "functional" digestive disorders. Its effectiveness may be related to its ability to clear acid rapidly from the esophagus and stomach, or to its centrally mediated antiemetic effect. Side effects include drowsiness, dizziness, dystonia, and, on occasion, galactorrhea caused by stimulation of endogenous prolactin secretion. Other medications often used but of uncertain clinical benefit include cimetidine, cholestyramine, and anticholinergic agents.

Thompson WG. Functional Dyspepsia. In *The Irritable Gut: Functional Disorders of the Alimentary Canal.* Baltimore: University Park Press, 1979. Pp. 153–172.
  This well-written and enjoyable book reviews gastrointestinal disorders not associated with structural abnormalities.
Drossman DA. The Physician and the Patient: Review of the Psychosocial GI Literature with an Integrated Approach to the Patient. In MA Sleisenger and JF Fordtran (Eds.), *Gastrointestinal Disease: Pathophysiology, Diagnosis, Management* (3rd ed.). Philadelphia: Saunders, 1983. Pp. 3–20.
  This chapter reviews the GI disorders from a biopsychosocial perspective. Included are practical suggestions for the diagnosis and care of patients with "functional" complaints.
Joske RA, Finckh ES, Wood IJ. Gastric biopsy. *Q J Med* 24:269–294, 1955.
  Gastritis was found on biopsy in a high proportion of healthy, asymptomatic subjects.
Lasser RB, Bond JH, Levitt MD. The role of intestinal gas in functional abdominal pain. *N Engl J Med* 293:524–526, 1975.
  This important study reports no differences in the quantity or composition of intestinal gas between patients complaining of gaseousness and asymptomatic persons.

Schulze-Delrieu K. Metoclopramide. *Gastroenterology* 77:768–779, 1979.
  A comprehensive review of a relatively new drug that has become popular in the treatment of patients with motility disorders and "functional" complaints.

49. PEPTIC ULCER DISEASE OF THE DUODENUM
Eugene M. Bozymski

Duodenal ulcer disease has undergone some marked changes over the past decade. The increased understanding of the pathogenesis of duodenal ulcer and of the importance of hydrochloric acid production by the parietal cell, and the availability of medication to neutralize or inhibit acid production effectively, have led to changes in the clinical pattern of duodenal ulcer. The number of patients hospitalized for duodenal ulcer disease has declined considerably, as has the mortality. In spite of these decreases, the true incidence of duodenal ulcer disease may be stable, and the apparent changes may be a reflection of more effective therapy and changing diagnostic practices. One factor that points to some degree of stability in the duodenal ulcer disease population is the unchanging incidence of perforation.

Pathogenesis
Duodenal ulcers may be looked on as resulting from an imbalance of aggressive factors, such as acid and pepsin, and defensive factors.

Aggressive Factors
Of a variety of causal factors, hydrochloric acid is the most important. Duodenal ulcers virtually never occur in the absence of gastric acid. In general, patients with duodenal ulcers have a larger parietal cell mass and higher acid output than do unaffected people. Also, duodenal ulcers heal when gastric acid output is neutralized or reduced. Pepsin also plays a role; patients with elevated pepsinogen I levels have a greater risk for duodenal ulcer disease than do those with normal levels. A predisposition to duodenal ulcer in apparently normal siblings can be identified by finding elevated serum pepsinogen I level. Since many patients with ulcers secrete normal amounts of acid and have normal pepsinogen levels, other factors must be important in causing ulcers.

Defensive Factors
Factors that are protective and play a role in cytoprotection include bicarbonate production and disposal, local prostaglandins, cell repair and regeneration, mucus production, and mucosal blood flow, among others.
  There are many studies showing that the stomach and duodenum participate in the organism's adaptation to stress. Severe emotional tension and exacerbation of "usual" life stresses have been correlated with the onset of symptoms, and stress has been shown to cause ulcers in animals. However, no single "ulcer personality" has been defined.

Clinical Presentation
Pain is the most frequent complaint in patients with duodenal ulcer. It is described as sharp, gnawing, or burning, or as a hunger pain, and it usually is well localized in the high epigastrium, although it may occur anywhere in the epigastric area. Frequently the patient is able to point with one finger to the area of greatest discomfort. The pain may radiate to the back, particularly when the ulcer is posterior or penetrating. It often occurs when the stomach is empty, or awakens the patient from sleep an hour or so after midnight. The pain is usually improved by ingesting food or antacids; in some patients, however, eating makes the pain worse. Ulcer pain is characteristically intermittent, with periodic exacerbations and remissions over the years. Recurrences have been noted by some to be more common in the spring and fall but others find no seasonal variation.
  Vomiting can occur in the absence of outlet obstruction. This appears to be more common in patients with channel ulcers and may be related to alterations in antral motility.

Other symptoms occur with complications of duodenal ulcer which include obstruction, gastrointestinal bleeding, and perforation. At times, otherwise asymptomatic patients with duodenal ulcer present with symptoms of anemia secondary to chronic bleeding.

Evaluation
The history should include a search for evidence of the multiple endocrine adenoma syndrome (e.g., kidney stones or diarrhea) and any medication, particularly the antiinflammatory agents, that are known to cause mucosal irritation. Medical history is not sufficiently specific to distinguish patients with duodenal ulcers from those with gastric ulcer.

Physical Examination
The examination is usually entirely normal with uncomplicated duodenal ulcer. Sometimes there is an area of well-localized tenderness in the epigastrium. In the presence of complications, examination may disclose a tense, board-like abdomen and peritoneal signs suggesting a perforation, or a succussion splash suggesting gastric outlet obstruction.

There is no consensus regarding the need to investigate all patients with symptoms of duodenal ulcer completely with upper gastrointestinal x-rays or endoscopy. In people under 35 years of age who have symptoms consistent with *uncomplicated* duodenal ulcer, it is reasonable to proceed with antacid therapy; if the patient does well, x-ray studies need not be obtained. If the patient is older, or if there are recurrent, prolonged, or atypical symptoms, an investigation should be done. Many patients with "classic" ulcer symptoms are not found to have an ulcer when studied radiographically or endoscopically.

Laboratory Studies
Studies done should include a stool test for occult blood and hematocrit determination. A serum calcium determination is obtained if hyperparathyroidism or a multiple endocrine tumor is suspected.

Serum gastrin levels need be obtained only in patients with hyperparathyroidism, a family history of endocrine tumors, diarrhea, or evidence of increased secretion seen on upper gastrointestinal series. Gastrin levels also should be obtained to exclude an underlying gastrinoma in patients who have recurrent problems with peptic ulcer disease and in those who are to undergo surgery for peptic ulcer. In patients with ordinary duodenal ulcer disease, the fasting serum gastrin is normal. If the values are in the equivocal range, a secretin stimulation test will identify patients with gastrinoma.

X-rays
An upper gastrointestinal series with good air-contrast films is used to detect ulcers and identify other lesions that might masquerade as ulcers. If the duodenal bulb is markedly deformed because of previous ulcer disease, it is impossible for the radiologist to be certain if a crater is currently present, and one must rely on symptoms to judge activity.

Upper Gastrointestinal Endoscopy
There is no doubt that endoscopy provides a very accurate means of detecting the presence or absence of duodenal ulcers. However, the procedure is not necessary when the diagnosis is otherwise clear, nor is it necessary to monitor duodenal ulcer healing by either x-ray or endoscopy; symptomatic response is adequate. Endoscopy is useful and necessary to evaluate patients with serious complaints and negative x-rays, patients with bleeding, or those who are being considered for peptic ulcer surgery. Endoscopy is preferable to x-ray studies in the special instance of a pregnant woman with sufficient complaints to warrant investigation.

Gastric Secretory Testing
Although there is an increase in the average gastric acid output in patients with duodenal ulcer disease compared to controls, routine measurement of gastric acid output is not necessary. The average normal basal acid output (BAO) is 2 mEq per hour in normal people and twice that in the patient with duodenal ulcer. However, the discrim-

inatory power is poor because of overlap in the two groups. Acid output is normally greater in men than women and decreases with age. Gastric secretory testing is useful when Zollinger-Ellison syndrome or systemic mastocytosis is suspected, serum gastrin levels are elevated, or a recurrent ulcer follows ulcer surgery. Occasionally, patients with short-bowel syndrome or renal transplants have hypersecretion of gastric acid.

Gastric secretory studies are also helpful in establishing the achlorhydria associated with pernicious anemia and as a baseline in the patient with duodenal ulcer who is scheduled for surgery. Should recurrent ulcer occur after surgery, one can repeat the study and make inferences about the effectiveness of the surgery. If a vagotomy was part of the surgical procedure, and basal acid output is still greater than 1 mEq per hour, or the maximum acid output has not been reduced by more than 40% of the preoperative value, the vagotomy was not successful. The insulin (Hollander) test to check for vagal integrity is usually not necessary; if done, it requires *very careful* monitoring for hypoglycemic complications.

Complications

Hemorrhage, the most common complication of duodenal ulcer, occurs in 10 to 20% of patients. The blood loss may vary from massive gastrointestinal hemorrhage to chronic, occult bleeding leading to iron deficiency anemia. Occasionally, bleeding may be the first manifestation of duodenal ulcer. Once a patient has bled from a duodenal ulcer, the chance of rebleeding is 30 to 50%.

The role of agents such as aspirin, alcohol, corticosteroids, nonsteroidal anti-inflammatory drugs, and potassium supplements in initiating bleeding from duodenal ulcer is uncertain.

In patients with melena, it is important to aspirate the stomach. If blood is present, the bleeding site is above the ligament of Treitz. However, the absence of blood in the gastric aspirate does not exclude bleeding from a duodenal ulcer, because blood may be swept distally by peristalsis or may not have refluxed into the stomach. A past history of duodenal ulcer disease is no guarantee that the ulcer is the source of a present episode of gastrointestinal bleeding.

Endoscopy is the best way to identify the source of bleeding. Because most patients with upper gastrointestinal hemorrhage stop bleeding spontaneously, it is unclear whether upper endoscopy improves management of patients with bleeding. Many gastroenterologists believe that the care of the bleeding patient is improved when an accurate diagnosis has been made. Examples include bleeding from esophageal varices or the presence of a "visible vessel," which may be associated with continued bleeding, and may be found at endoscopy. This is invaluable information in the management of the patient and in planning surgery.

Bleeding may adversely affect the coronary or cerebral circulation, particularly in older patients. Prompt resuscitation, maintaining the hematocrit above 30%, is imperative to prevent transient ischemic attacks, stroke, angina, and infarction. Although it is clear that hemorrhage can be stopped by laser therapy, electrocoagulation, or embolization of various agents to the appropriate artery using angiography, their final role remains to be determined.

Penetration occurs when duodenal ulcers erode through the serosa, and free perforation is prevented by the inflammatory reaction and adjacent tissues such as the liver or pancreas. It is heralded by increasing pain, which may be intractable and radiates into the back. If penetration is into the pancreas, pancreatitis may ensue. Rarely, the penetration is into a hollow viscus, resulting in a fistula.

Perforation is a catastrophic event, accompanied by acute severe abdominal pain, rapid development of peritonitis, and rarely, bleeding. Increasing symptoms may be present for several days or weeks before the perforation. Free peritoneal air is best demonstrated on an upright abdominal or lateral decubitus film. Surgery remains the treatment of choice. If there are no contraindications, vagotomy and pyloroplasty can be done, to reduce subsequent acid secretion, in addition to closure of the perforation. If for some reason, such as recent myocardial infarction, surgery is contraindicated, medical treatment consisting of nasogastric suction, cimetidine, fluid and electrolyte replacement, and antibiotics has been successful.

Gastric outlet obstruction is less common than hemorrhage or perforation. With the "typical" presentation, a patient with long-standing ulcer symptoms develops constant pain and then vomiting. The vomiting may be severe and lead to weight loss, dehydration, and hypokalemic (and ultimately, hypochloremic) alkalosis. A succussion splash is often present. Upper gastrointestinal x-rays document the outlet obstruction; the cause can be confirmed by endoscopy.

The obstruction may be caused by edema and inflammation or by scar. The former may respond to medical therapy, whereas the latter requires surgery. Treatment includes hospital admission for nasogastric decompression, antacids, H_2 blockers, and avoidance of drugs that decrease gastric motility (e.g., anticholinergics).

Intractability has no strict definition. The ulcer is called "refractory" if a patient is on a good medical program while in the hospital and symptoms continue or recur shortly after discharge, or if relapses become longer and more severe and remissions, shorter. Symptoms that recur repeatedly under all but the most rigorous medical programs can also be termed refractory. One should always search for contributing causes such as gastrinoma, anti-inflammatory medications, alcohol, and psychiatric problems.

Medical Therapy
The goals of therapy are healing the ulcer, decreasing symptoms, and preventing complications and recurrences.

Diet
Many patients find that their symptoms are aggravated by certain foods. However, dietary therapy has not been shown to be effective in peptic ulcer disease, and there are no controlled studies to support any specific dietary regimen. Restriction of the use of caffeine-containing beverages and foods (e.g., coffee, tea, colas, and chocolate) and alcoholic beverages is prudent. Smoking should be avoided because it decreases pancreatic bicarbonate and is also associated with an increased rate of peptic ulcer and decreased healing. Aspirin and nonsteroidal anti-inflammatory drugs should be avoided, and theophylline-containing compounds monitored because of their effect on phosphodiesterase.

Antacids
Antacids remain the time-proven preference for patients with uncomplicated duodenal ulcer. A high-dose antacid regimen has been shown in a randomized controlled trial to heal substantially more ulcers than placebo. Important features in the choice of an antacid include neutralizing capacity, magnesium content (magnesium causes loose stool), aluminum content (aluminum is constipating), sodium content, taste, and cost. Calcium-containing antacids produce an acid-rebound and may lead to the milk-alkali syndrome; therefore, they should be avoided. Liquid antacids are preferable to tablets because they have greater neutralizing capacity. The usual dose is 20 cc of "concentrated" antacid or 30 cc of regular antacid approximately six times a day. Antacids are most effective when taken 1 and 3 hours after meals. Milk should not be advised; it contains a large amount of calcium and is not a satisfactory antacid. Antacids should not be given with other oral medications because they may bind them.

Histamine (H_2) Receptor Blockers
Cimetidine and ranitidine, H_2 receptor antagonists, are potent inhibitors of gastric acid secretion regardless of the stimulant used to increase secretion. They have been used extensively for duodenal ulcer. Cimetidine in doses of 300 mg four times a day with meals and at bedtime, and ranitidine 150 mg twice a day, have been shown in many controlled trials to enhance healing. They also have been shown to prevent recurrent duodenal ulcer when given in a single bedtime dose; this regimen can be continued for many months. The recurrence of ulcer after stopping H_2 blockers is not a rebound, but only a reflection of the natural history of peptic ulcer, which is expressed after gastric acid secretion returns to its usual rate.

High-dose antacid programs and H_2 blockers are equally effective in healing duodenal ulcer. One alternative for treating duodenal ulcer is to give antacids during the day and an H_2 receptor blocker at bedtime. The usual length of treatment for duodenal ulcer is approximately 6 to 8 weeks. If the ulcer disease has been severe or there have been complications, longer treatment may be necessary.

Overall, cimetidine is very well tolerated and has been used continuously for many years in patients with Zollinger-Ellison syndrome. However, several side effects have been described. Cimetidine has been associated with reversible confusion. This may occur with elevated blood levels, particularly in the elderly and those with underlying renal or hepatic dysfunction. Anti-androgenic effects, including gynecomastia, decreased sperm counts, and hyperprolactinemia, have been reported. Occasionally, neutropenia and elevation of serum SGOT and creatinine occur. Cimetidine affects hepatic microsomal enzymes (P-450), causing a variety of drug-drug interactions. One example is the reduction of the hepatic metabolism of warfarin, leading to increased blood levels and anticoagulant effects.

Ranitidine, a more potent, longer acting H_2 antagonist, given twice a day, does not seem to have as much effect on the hepatic microsomal P-450 system or androgen receptors. In hypersecretory states requiring high dose therapy, ranitidine is preferred because of fewer side effects with high doses, but side effects may occur.

Coating Agents

Some bismuth-containing compounds (e.g., Pepto-Bismol) and sucralfate coat the mucosa of the stomach and duodenum. Sucralfate (Carafate), a sulfated disaccharide, binds to the proteinaceous debris in the ulcer crater and blocks penetration of acid and pepsin and also binds bile acids. Sucralfate has been shown by controlled trials to be comparable to H_2 blockers in healing duodenal ulcers. Because sucralfate acts within the lumen and there is little absorption, it is apparently very safe and has few side effects. Constipation is noted occasionally, perhaps because sucralfate is an aluminum salt.

Anticholinergics

Anticholinergics inhibit gastric acid secretion and decrease the contractile force of smooth muscle. They have been found to prolong the effectiveness of antacids. It is apparently not necessary to push maximum dosage to achieve a beneficial effect. They can be given with antacids or histamine H_2 receptor antagonists to patients whose ulcer disease is difficult to control. Side effects include blurred vision, dry mouth, impotence, and difficulty in urinating. They are contraindicated in gastric outlet obstruction, reflux esophagitis, glaucoma, prostatic hypertrophy, and severe inflammatory bowel disease. They have been largely replaced by other agents.

Decreasing the Psychovisceral Component

Physicians should develop a strong working relationship with ulcer patients and allow sufficient time for discussing their problems. As in any chronic illness, the patient's ability to control stress is very important, and the physician can offer a great deal of support. Some patients benefit from mild antianxiety agents or antidepressants if indicated.

Surgery

When surgery is necessary, there are several options. Often the choice of operation depends on the past experience of the surgeon or the technical aspects of the situation. In general, operations can be divided into those that involve a partial gastrectomy with or without a vagotomy and those whose major emphasis is on interrupting branches of the vagus nerve. Presently most gastrectomies are coupled with vagotomy. These operations are associated with fewer recurrent ulcers, but more postgastrectomy complications. On the other hand, vagotomy with a drainage procedure is associated with a higher recurrence rate, but less postoperative morbidity. If partial gastrectomy with vagotomy is done, many surgeons and all gastroenterologists prefer a gastroduodenostomy (Billroth I) to a gastrojejunostomy (Billroth II), because the former is associated with fewer complications and alters gastrointestinal physiology to a lesser degree.

Selective proximal vagotomy (parietal cell vagotomy) without drainage is another surgical option for duodenal ulcer. It has several advantages. The hepatic, celiac, and antral fibers are preserved; the stomach is not entered, which reduces mortality and morbidity; and late complications (dumping, diarrhea, and bilious vomiting) are also less common. However, the rate of ulcer recurrence remains to be determined.

Grossman MI, et al. A new look at peptic ulcer. *Ann Intern Med* 84:57–67, 1976.
  A good discussion of the role of acid in duodenal ulcer disease. It also presents a discussion of superselective vagotomy as a means of denervating only the acid secreting portion of the stomach.
Grossman MI, et al. Peptic ulcer: New therapies, new diseases. *Ann Intern Med* 95:609–627, 1981.
  An excellent review that makes the point that peptic ulcer represents a heterogeneous

group of disorders in which multiple genetic and environmental causes play a role. Basic physiology and treatment are reviewed and the role of endoscopy is discussed.

Hollander D, Hollander PA. The role of diet in peptic ulcer disease. *Practical Gastroenterol* 5:60–64, 1981.

A very practical review of dietary factors in peptic ulcer disease.

Winship DH. Cimetidine in the treatment of duodenal ulcer: Review and commentary. *Gastroenterology* 74:402–406, 1978.

Reviews a number of studies that demonstrate the efficacy of cimetidine compared to placebo or antacid.

Korman MG, et al. Influence of Smoking on the Healing Rate of Duodenal Ulcer in Response to Cimetidine or High-dose Antacid. In DE Rogers, et al. (Eds.), *The Year Book of Medicine, 1982.* Chicago: Year Book, 1982. Pp. 381–384.

Carefully done studies indicate that there is an adverse effect of smoking on the healing rate of duodenal ulcer when treated by either cimetidine or Mylanta.

Vantrappen G, et al. Effect of 15(R)-15-methyl prostaglandin E_2 (arbaprostil) on the healing of duodenal ulcer: A double-blind multicenter study. *Gastroenterology* 83:357–363, 1982.

The study shows increased ulcer healing with prostaglandin E_2 to approximately the same degree as reported in most extensive studies with cimetidine.

Brogden RN, et al. Ranitidine: A review of its pharmacology and therapeutic use in peptic ulcer disease and other allied diseases. *Drugs* 24:267–303, 1982.

Ranitidine is a more potent H_2 receptor antagonist than cimetidine and does not appear to have the antiandrogenic effects of cimetidine, nor does it seem to impair the microsomal P-450 mixed function oxidase system and is comparable in efficacy to cimetidine in treating duodenal ulcer disease.

Marks IN, et al. Comparison of sucralfate with cimetidine in the short-term treatment of chronic peptic ulcers. *S Afr Med J* 57:567–573, 1980.

Sucralfate acts primarily as a coating agent binding to the proteinaceous debris in the ulcer base, and is shown to be comparable to cimetidine in producing healing of duodenal ulcers.

Sleisenger MH, Fordtran JS (Eds.). *Gastrointestinal Disease* (2nd ed.). Philadelphia: Saunders, 1978.

A comprehensive review of the pathophysiology, clinical manifestations and complications, and modalities of therapy of duodenal ulcers.

Peterson WL, et al. Healing of duodenal ulcer with an antacid regimen. *N. Engl J Med* 297:341–345, 1977.

In a randomized controlled trial, a large-dose antacid regimen was more effective than placebo in healing the ulcer.

Richardson CT. Sucralfate (editorial). *Ann Intern Med* 97:269–271, 1983.

A review of current evidence regarding sucralfate.

Collen MJ et al. Comparison of ranitidine and cimetidine in the treatment of gastric hypersecretion. *Ann Intern Med* 100:52–58, 1984.

Ranitidine-inhibited acid secretion in patients with hypersecretory states is safe at high doses, does not cause the antiandrogen effects frequently seen with high doses of cimetidine, and is more potent than cimetidine. Patients who were relatively resistant to cimetidine have proportional resistance to ranitidine.

50. IRRITABLE BOWEL SYNDROME
Douglas A. Drossman

The irritable bowel syndrome (IBS) is a physiologic disorder of unknown anatomic cause. The clinical course of patients with this disorder has not been well studied. Most adult patients report a long history of bowel-related difficulties going back to childhood.

The patients' complaints reflect the pattern of their bowel motility disorder: diarrhea (frequent, loose, or watery stools, usually of normal volumes), constipation (infrequent, hard stools) or, at different times, both. Abdominal pain is usually present, and is most often described as cramp-like and located in the mid to lower abdomen. Other nonspecific complaints include fatigue, nausea, and upper abdominal discomfort. Symptoms may be chronic and continuous or intermittent with flare-ups at times of stress, during travel, with medications, during menstrual cycles, or with dietary indiscretion—or with no apparent precipitants. There are no known complications of the disorder itself, although some patients become dependent on laxatives or analgesics.

Patients with IBS are commonly seen in primary care practices and account for 40 to 70% of referrals to gastroenterologists. Three times as many patients are hospitalized for IBS as for inflammatory bowel disease; medical costs and time lost from work because of IBS are considerable.

The prevalence of people with bowel dysfunction compatible with the IBS in the general population is about 15%. The disorder is most often seen in young adults, with a female to male ratio of 2:1. However, in countries in which men seek health care more readily than women, the ratio is reversed. These data suggest that sociocultural factors help determine which persons with the irritable bowel syndrome seek health care. The role of psychosocial factors in the causation of this disorder is still not clarified. Psychological stress affects bowel function in all people, and it is unclear whether people with the IBS are more susceptible. Physicians can often identify antecedent psychological and environmental events at the time of symptom onset and exacerbation. Psychometric tests of patients with the IBS show them to be more neurotic than healthy subjects, but less so than psychiatric patients. Psychiatric interviews disclose a high prevalence of depression, hysterical personality traits, hypochondriasis, and anxiety, but no particular personality pattern is characteristic. Whether these observations are unique to the disorder itself or reflect a subgroup of persons with the IBS who seek health care remains to be established.

Diagnostic Evaluation

Because no pathologic marker for the IBS exists, diagnosis depends on identifying historical data typical for the disorder. It recently has been shown that a cluster of several symptoms is reported significantly more often by patients with the IBS than by those with other gastrointestinal disorders. These include abdominal distention, loose or frequent stools with the onset of pain, relief of pain with defecation, mucus in the stool, and the experience of incomplete evacuation after defecation. Furthermore, the greater the number of these items present, the more likely is the clinical diagnosis to be correct. Identification of these symptoms by clinicians therefore places the diagnosis on a firmer basis.

A major effort of the diagnostic evaluation is to exclude conditions that may mimic IBS. Lactase deficiency is manifested as cramp-like abdominal pain and loose, frequent stool following the ingestion of milk. If this disorder is suspected, the diagnosis can be confirmed by a lactose tolerance test, but it is also reasonable to gauge clinical response to restriction of milk-containing foods. Other conditions to be considered include intestinal neoplasia, infectious or inflammatory disease, and malabsorption.

The physical examination helps mainly to exclude other medical disorders. However, localized tenderness elicited over the sigmoid colon or reproduction of the patient's pain during sigmoidoscopic examination suggests that the symptoms are bowel-related, and is consistent with IBS. An abdominal mass, rebound tenderness, and organomegaly are not typically found in the IBS.

It is difficult to know "how far to go" in the workup. The medical evaluation depends on the results of the complete history and physical examination, and must be individualized. A younger patient with a brief course of symptoms probably requires a minimum of diagnostic studies. Conversely, findings not characteristic of the IBS should prompt a more thorough workup. Such findings include the recent onset of symptoms in an older patient, reporting of blood or grease in the stool, fever, considerable weight loss, nocturnal awakening with pain, pain unrelated to changes in bowel function, or evidence suggesting metabolic disturbances. Stools should always be examined for blood; often for parasites, polymorphonuclear leukocytes, and pathogenic bacteria; and occasionally, for fat. Sigmoidoscopy (and in a patient over 40 years of age, barium enema) is usually indicated. Other studies often clinically indicated include CBC, sedimentation rate, serum amylase, liver chemistries, and urinalysis.

Recent electrophysiologic studies of the rectosigmoid colon in patients with the IBS suggest an increased prevalence of 3-cycle-per-minute basal electrical activity (BER) compared to the electrical pattern of healthy people. The clinical importance of this observation is uncertain, and electrophysiologic evaluation is therefore not yet recommended for diagnosis.

Treatment

Once the diagnosis is established, or it is at least determined that no additional studies are indicated, treatment should be directed toward amelioration of the symptoms, identification and modification of factors that aggravate the disorder, and encouragement of patient adaptation to what can be a chronic or relapsing condition.

General Approach

Because patients with this disorder may have chronic or recurring symptoms, an essential feature of treatment is the establishment of an ongoing physician-patient relationship. Frequent brief visits initially and during exacerbations are recommended, with the goals of reducing the patient's discomfort and providing psychosocial support. As with any chronic disorder, removal of symptoms is not always the goal of treatment. During periods of quiescence, the physician should set up one or two brief visits per year. This reinforces the physician's long-term commitment and, because of the patient's knowledge that there is a doctor familiar with the problem, minimizes the tendency of some patients to make late-night calls or "emergency" visits.

During visits, attempts should be made to modify identified environmental stress factors or the patient's attitude toward these factors. It is usually helpful to explain that the IBS is a very real disorder in which the intestine is overly sensitive to a variety of stimuli, such as food (type or quantity), hormonal changes (e.g., menses), or stress. Patients may benefit from a discussion of the relation between altered bowel physiology (e.g., segmental spasm of the colon) and clinical symptoms (pain, constipation). Patients are also reassured to learn that the condition is not associated with malignancy or shortened life expectancy and does not require surgery. In addition, the fact that the IBS may have an important psychological component in the absence of specific physical findings should not undermine the legitimacy of the patient's very real complaints. Any implication that the problem is all "emotional" is taken as a rejection by the patient.

Diet

The use of increased fiber in the form of bran (½ oz/day) or commercially prepared psyllium seed products (e.g., Metamucil, Effersyllium, 2 tsp bid) is strongly recommended because of their empiric effectiveness, low price, and virtual absence of side effects. Fiber has been shown to shorten the intestinal transit time, which is of benefit for patients with constipation, and may decrease symptoms in patients with the IBS. The presumed mechanism is one of increasing stool bulk, which minimizes the effects of the nonpropulsive segmental contractions of the colon. Patients should be informed that they may experience transient symptoms of gaseous discomfort during the first few days. (See Chap. 142 for additional information on high-fiber diets.) Food substances known to stimulate bowel action (e.g., caffeinated beverages) or produce increased intestinal gas (e.g., beans, cabbage) should be avoided. Patients with lactase deficiency who develop abdominal cramps and diarrhea when ingesting lactose should be told to avoid milk-containing products.

Drugs

Anticholinergic medication, such as dicyclomine (Bentyl), glycopyrrolate (Robinul), or propantheline bromide (Pro-Banthine), may reduce colonic segmental spasm and is recommended for symptomatic treatment of patients with predominant pain and constipation. It should be given ½ to 1 hour before meals and at bedtime. No particular agent has been shown to be superior. Dosage is based on the manufacturer's recommendations, the limiting factor being the development of side effects such as dry mouth and blurry vision. Sedative tranquilizers, particularly of the benzodiazepine family, have gained much popularity. These drugs have no effect on colonic motility but can be individualized to the emotional needs of the patient. Many physicians employ an antianxiety-anticholinergic combination drug with empiric success (Librax, Combid). Antidepressants may be of some help in patients whose symptoms are manifestations of depression.

Physical Measures

The use of baths, hot water bottles, exercise, relaxation techniques, and periods of rest can be of benefit when individualized to the patient's needs.

Drossman DA, Powell DW, Sessions JT Jr. The irritable bowel syndrome. *Gastroenterology* 73:811–822, 1977.
  A complete review of the epidemiologic, physiologic, and psychosocial aspects of the disorder. Practical suggestions for diagnosis and patient care are offered.
Drossman DA, et al. Patterns of bowel function in subjects not seeking health care. *Gastroenterology* 83:529–534, 1982.
  A report of the prevalence and characteristics of a nonpatient population with bowel dysfunction.
Snape WJ, Carlson GM, Cohen S. Colonic myoelectric activity in the irritable bowel syndrome. *Gastroenterology* 70:326–330, 1976.
  This study shows that patients with the IBS have a pattern of colonic smooth muscle electrical activity that is different from that of a healthy comparison group.
Manning AP, et al. Towards positive diagnosis of the irritable bowel. *Br Med J* 2:653–654, 1978.
  A more confident diagnosis of IBS can be made when specific items are obtained from the history.
Burkitt DP, Walker ARP, Painter AS. Effect of dietary fiber on stools and transit times, and its role in causation of disease. *Lancet* 2:1408–1411, 1972.
  A classic paper that reports the role of fiber in colonic function.
Manning AP, Heaton KW, Harvey RF. Wheat fiber and the irritable bowel syndrome: A controlled trial. *Lancet* 2:417–418, 1977.
  A high-fiber diet decreases symptoms in patients with IBS.

51. DIVERTICULAR DISEASE OF THE COLON
Douglas A. Drossman

Although almost unheard of 100 years ago, diverticular disease of the colon has now become a common, sometimes life-threatening, disorder of the elderly. Diverticulosis and diverticulitis are discussed separately because of differences in pathogenesis, presentation, and treatment.

Diverticulosis

The anatomic abnormality in diverticulosis is a pseudodiverticulum, produced by herniation of mucosa and submucosa through the serosa of the colonic wall. In the rare true diverticulum of the cecum, there is an abnormal outpouching of all wall layers. The prevalence of diverticulosis increases with age; it is found in 30% of people over age 60. However, it is estimated that only 20% of the population with diverticulosis develop symptoms. Typical symptoms include abdominal pain and tenderness and bowel irregularity, which are believed to develop from nonpropulsive colonic contractions that produce abnormally high intraluminal pressures. Patients with symptoms of diverticulosis often have thickening of the circular smooth-muscle layer of the sigmoid colon (myochosis), which is seen radiologically as narrowing and irregular distortion of the sigmoid lumen. This appearance is at times difficult to distinguish from carcinoma or inflammatory bowel disease.

Three to five percent of patients with diverticular disease may at some time develop diverticular bleeding. The bleeding is characteristically brisk and painless, and is usually right-sided in origin. Blood loss can at times be massive and require emergency surgery, but it is more often self-limited. The chance of recurrence is only approximately 20%.

The pathogenesis of diverticulosis is not yet fully established, although epidemiologic data and the results of animal studies suggest a strong association with dietary deficiency of fiber. Autopsy studies show a progressive increase in the disorder, beginning with the milling of wheat flour in the 1880s and the associated decreased consumption of crude cereal grains. Presently, the prevalence of diverticulosis is higher in Western industrialized nations, in which fiber consumption is much less than in the Third World countries. Diverticulosis has been produced in laboratory animals fed a diet deficient in fiber content. Additional studies in humans are needed to determine if eating a high-fiber diet can prevent the development of diverticulosis or its complications.

Diagnosis

In many instances, the diagnosis of diverticulosis is made incidentally during barium x-ray examination done for other reasons. However, symptomatic diverticulosis should be suspected in the older patient presenting with lower abdominal pain, localized tenderness, and episodes of constipation or diarrhea. Fever, leukocytosis, and/or peritoneal signs are more likely to indicate diverticulitis or other intra-abdominal infections or inflammatory conditions.

Evaluation of the older patient with recent onset of symptoms compatible with diverticulosis should include stool examination for occult blood, complete blood count, sigmoidoscopy, and barium enema. These are done to exclude polyps, carcinoma, inflammatory or ischemic bowel disease, or other serious medical disorders. Depending on the clinical presentation, other studies might include serum amylase, liver chemistries, and examination of the stool for inflammatory cells, bacteria, or parasitic pathogens. Recent weight loss or the presence of occult blood in the stool of a patient with x-ray-proven diverticulosis may require additional evaluation with colonoscopy to exclude carcinoma.

Diverticular bleeding should be suspected in the older patient who presents with the spontaneous passage of bright red or maroon-colored stools. The differential diagnosis includes angiodysplasia (arteriovenous malformations), polyps/carcinoma, hemorrhoids, or, in the presence of pain, ischemic colitis. The diagnostic evaluation of painless rectal bleeding in the older patient depends on the rapidity of the bleeding. With massive hemorrhage, resuscitative measures and arteriographic evaluation in preparation for possible emergency subtotal or segmental colonic resection are indicated. Barium enema should not be done because the opacified colon would obscure arteriographic localization of the bleeding source. In the more stable patient with moderate bleeding, arteriography, ^{99}Tc-labeled sulfur colloid, or red-cell scintiscan can help localize the site of bleeding. Colonoscopy is becoming more popular with episodic low-grade bleeding because of its greater diagnostic accuracy for mucosal lesions. The patient who has a single diverticular bleed that stops usually does not require surgery, and the approach can be more conservative; barium enema or colonoscopy should be done to exclude other disorders. If the examination is negative, no additional evaluation is needed unless another bleeding episode develops.

Treatment

A high-fiber diet has been recommended for patients with asymptomatic diverticulosis because of indirect evidence linking fiber deficiency to the disease. Bran has been shown to decrease intestinal transit time and to lessen pain in patients with diverticular disease. (See Chap. 142 for additional information on high-fiber diets.) The diet is inexpensive, may be effective in preventing progression of the disease, and has few immediate side effects. Some patients initially experience gaseous distention and nausea for several days. Patients with symptomatic disease, particularly those with pain and constipation, should take 15 to 30 gm of unprocessed bran per day, the dietary equivalent (2 oz bran cereal, 10 mg whole meal bread), or 2 to 4 teaspoons of a powdered psyllium seed preparation as a dietary supplement.

Anticholinergic drugs, such as dicyclomine (Bentyl), glycopyrrolate (Robinul), or propantheline bromide (Pro-Banthine), may be of additional benefit for treatment of pain, but are not recommended on a long-term basis. Mild analgesics can be used; narcotic agents are contraindicated, however, because of the chronic nature of the disorder. Furthermore, morphine and its congeners increase high-pressure nonpropulsive contractions in the colon, thus possibly increasing symptoms. Some surgeons advocate sigmoid colon resection or myotomy in patients with long-standing painful diverticular disease. However, this is not generally recommended because there are no data from controlled trials that support a good clinical response.

Diverticulitis

Diverticulitis occurs in 10 to 25% of patients with known diverticulosis. It develops from a micro- or macroperforation of a diverticulum and subsequent spillage of fecal contents outside the bowel wall. The resulting inflammatory process is usually confined to the pericolic space, where it is walled off by fat, mesentery, or adjacent organs. Diverticulitis most often occurs in the sigmoid colon, possibly because of the large number of diverticula and the presence of more formed stool to produce obstruction at the diverticular neck. The severity of the clinical symptoms and signs depends on the extent of the extradiverticular inflammation. Characteristically, patients complain of acute or subacute left-lower-quadrant pain, fever, and possibly, nausea, vomiting, and constipation. In some instances, the inflammation produces symptoms of partial or complete colonic obstruction, or, if the ureter is involved, may simulate a urinary tract infection. Older patients or those taking steroid preparation may present with minimal symptoms. Diverticulitis does not cause gross GI bleeding. However, on occasion the stool may be positive for occult blood.

Diagnosis

On physical examination, there is localized left-lower-quadrant discomfort and, possibly, a palpable mass or localized peritoneal signs with rebound tenderness. Rectal examination may reveal tenderness on the left or even a mass effect caused by a pelvic abscess. Laboratory studies invariably show leukocytosis and, if the ureter or bladder is secondarily involved, microscopic hematuria and pyuria. Electrolyte disturbances may occur, depending on the presence of vomiting or sepsis. Flat and upright x-rays of the abdomen must be done to evaluate for a perforated viscus or intestinal obstruction. Sigmoidoscopy should be performed to exclude a distal mass or inflammatory process. The stool is usually Hemoccult-negative. Barium enema is contraindicated in the acutely ill patient, particularly if free perforation is expected. In the patient with milder symptoms, barium enema can help demonstrate the site of the disease process, identify any complications such as abscess or fistula formation, and exclude other disorders such as carcinoma, Crohn's disease, or ischemic colitis. Care should be taken to instill the barium slowly, under low pressure. Some radiologists prefer to use a water-soluble contrast medium (Gastrografin), which gives less radiographic resolution but avoids the risk of barium spilling into the peritoneum. If the patient has an abnormal urinary sediment, an intravenous pyelogram (IVP) should be done to identify possible fistulization to the ureter or bladder.

Treatment

The management of acute diverticulitis is directed toward bowel rest and treatment of the infection. Acutely ill patients require hospitalization and should be placed at bed rest with nasogastric suction and IV fluid replacement. Parenteral antibiotics should be adequate to cover the normal enteric flora (*Escherichia coli,* enterococci, anaerobic bacteroids). Clindamycin and an aminoglycoside, or one of the newer broad-spectrum cephalosporins, can be used and adjusted pending the results of blood culture studies. The patient should be observed carefully with frequent abdominal examination, appropriate roentgenograms, and blood studies, so that developing complications are detected early. With clinical improvement, antibiotics should be continued for a total of 10 to 14 days. When the patient is clinically well, barium enema or colonoscopy is needed to confirm the diagnosis and exclude other disorders requiring additional treatment.

Many clinicians treat "mild" diverticulitis without hospitalization. In general these patients have little or no fever, do not appear toxic, and have minimal findings on physical examination (e.g., good bowel sounds and little or no rebound tenderness). They are placed at bed rest on a low-residue or liquid diet and given oral antibiotics, such as ampicillin or tetracycline. This approach is often successful; however, the similarity of this clinical presentation to that of noninflammatory painful diverticular disease and the lack of adequate controlled studies of patients treated for mild diverticulitis make it difficult to be certain if treatment is responsible for the improvement. It is important for the clinician to follow the patient closely for progression of symptoms or the development of complications.

Surgical consultation is required for all patients who are hospitalized. Emergency surgery is recommended if a serious complication develops, such as generalized peritonitis, an enlarging abdominal mass suggesting abscess, or fistulization to the bladder or other vital organs. Thirty percent of patients with diverticulitis develop a recurrent attack, usually within the first few years. Elective surgery should be considered in this group, because recurrences are associated with increased morbidity and mortality.

Almy TP, Howell DA. Diverticular disease of the colon. *N Engl J Med* 302:324–331, 1980.
  A complete and authoritative review.
Tedesco FJ, et al. Colonoscopic evaluation of rectal bleeding: A study of 304 patients. *Ann Intern Med* 89:907–909, 1978.
  In patients with lower GI bleeding, the presence of diverticula on barium edema is not sufficient for diagnosis. These authors report that colonoscopy revealed other important abnormalities in half the patients.
Levinson SL, et al. A current approach to rectal bleeding. *J Clin Gstroenterol* 3(1):9–16, 1981.
  This paper offers an algorithmic approach to the evaluation of patients with lower intestinal bleeding.
Burkitt DP, Walker ARP, Painter NS. Effect of dietary fiber on stools and transit times, and its role in causation of disease. *Lancet* 2:1408–1411, 1972.
  A classic paper that associates changes in dietary fiber with bowel function.
Brodribb AJM. Treatment of symptomatic diverticular disease with a high-fiber diet. *Lancet* 1:664–666, 1977.
  Pain symptoms improved in patients treated with high-fiber diets.

52. INFLAMMATORY BOWEL DISEASE

R. Balfour Sartor

Ulcerative colitis and Crohn's disease (regional enteritis, ileitis, or granulomatous colitis) are chronic inflammatory bowel diseases (IBD) of unknown cause. The incidence of Crohn's disease in industralized countries has increased in the past 30 years from 1 to 6 per 100,000 a year, whereas the incidence of ulcerative colitis has remained relatively stable at 6 to 8 per 100,000 a year. Because these disorders often present in young adults, persist, and are not cured by medical therapy, their prevalence is high: 30 to 117 per 100,000 population for ulcerative colitis and 34 to 106 per 100,000 for Crohn's disease.

Evaluation

History
The symptoms of inflammatory bowel disease often have an insidious onset and tend to wax and wane spontaneously. As a result, they frequently are ignored by the patient and misdiagnosed by the clinician until complications develop. In Crohn's disease, the mean length of time from the onset of symptoms to correct diagnosis is 3 to 5 years. The chronicity of symptoms helps to distinguish IBD from common bacterial and viral infections. Diarrhea persisting for more than 10 days or accompanied by considerable weight loss or bleeding should be fully investigated.

Bloody mucoid diarrhea, tenesmus, and malaise are characteristic of ulcerative colitis. Lower abdominal cramping pain and fever suggest extensive involvement. Patients with ulcerative proctitis may be constipated because of spasm of the distal colon but invariably have blood and mucus coating the stools. The most common symptoms of Crohn's disease are abdominal pain, diarrhea, and weight loss, followed by fever and perianal disease. Gross rectal bleeding can help differentiate these disorders. In the absence of perianal disease, bleeding is uncommon in Crohn's disease but almost invariable with ulcerative colitis.

Between 15 and 35% of patients with IBD have a family history of either Crohn's disease or ulcerative colitis.

Physical Examination

The examination is frequently nonspecific. An abdominal mass in the right lower quadrant is common in Crohn's disease and represents inflammation, possibly with abscess or adherent loops of bowel. Partial small-bowel obstruction is suspected when distention and/or palpable bowel loops are present along with abnormal bowel sounds. Perianal disease, such as fistulas, abscesses, and fissures refractory to therapy, occur in approximately one-third of patients with Crohn's disease; when found in young people, they mandate an extensive search for underlying bowel disease. Perianal disease is unusual in ulcerative colitis.

Clubbing, pallor, weight loss, extraintestinal disease, and fever help differentiate chronic inflammatory bowel disease from functional disorders such as irritable bowel syndrome. Extraintestinal manifestations, such as arthritis, dermatitis, liver disease, eye lesions, and aphthous stomatitis, occur in approximately 25% of patients with IBD. Others conditions that are less common but strongly suggest IBD, especially in the presence of diarrhea, are sclerosing cholangitis, pericholangitis, ankylosing spondylitis, nodular episcleritis, erythema nodosum, and pyoderma gangrenosum.

Proctosigmoidoscopy is the single best method for diagnosing ulcerative colitis; the disease involves the mucosa of the colon only and always involves the rectum. On the other hand, Crohn's disease is a transmural process most frequently affecting the ileocecal area and is seen in the rectum in only 16% of patients. In active ulcerative colitis, the mucosa appears diffusely granular, friable, and erythematous. In advanced disease, pseudopolyps up to 4 cm in length and confluent ulcerations may be present. Crohn's disease is characterized by nodularity, normal mucosa adjacent to areas that are obviously involved, and longitudinal ulcers 0.5 to 2 cm in length. Sigmoidoscopy should be performed without an enema so that trauma does not interfere with interpretation. Rectal biopsies are indicated only when visible disease is present and only if the diagnosis is in question, because the histologic appearance is nonspecific in ulcerative colitis and abnormal in only 10% of biopsies taken from patients with Crohn's disease when sigmoidoscopy is normal.

Laboratory Tests

Tests that are helpful in excluding other causes of diarrhea include a complete blood count with differential, sedimentation rate, amoeba serodiagnosis, and examination of fresh stool for ova and parasites, leukocytes, and enteric pathogens. Abnormalities of the CBC and sedimentation rate or the presence of fecal leukocytes excludes functional disorders, including irritable bowel syndrome. The chronicity of symptoms in most instances of IBD rules out infection with *Salmonella, Shigella,* and enteric viruses. However, *Yersinia* can cause a clinical syndrome of several weeks' duration that is indistinguishable from Crohn's ileocolitis, and *Campylobacter* can mimic ulcerative colitis. These organisms can be identified from stool cultures using special techniques. They should be sought when symptoms have been present for 3 months or less. Invasive amebiasis is detected by multiple fresh stool examinations and serodiagnosis. Enteric tuberculosis is now rare in developed countries, but it can produce a syndrome inseparable from Crohn's disease by clinical or radiographic criteria. Therefore, a chest x-ray and TB skin test are mandatory before use of steroids. When antibiotics have been used before the onset of bowel symptoms, antibiotic-associated colitis may be present. In the absence of pseudomembranes on sigmoidoscopy, a stool assay for *Clostridium difficile* toxin can help detect this condition.

Complications of IBD can be found before they are clinically suspected, through the CBC, and determinations of electrolytes, albumin, and alkaline phosphatase. Anemia is a frequent finding of IBD. The most common causes are iron deficiency in ulcerative colitis and anemia of chronic disease in Crohn's disease. Hypokalemia, metabolic alkalosis or acidosis, and hyponatremia are frequently present with protracted diarrhea. Serum albumin and total lymphocyte levels are sensitive indicators of malnutrition and protein-losing enteropathy. The alkaline phosphatase determination is the most sensitive test in screening for sclerosing cholangitis and pericholangitis.

X-rays

The diagnosis of IBD is confirmed by barium contrast radiography. When Crohn's disease is suspected, the entire gastrointestinal tract should be evaluated with both an upper GI series with small bowel follow-through and an air-contrast barium enema. In

Crohn's disease, the small intestine alone is involved in 30 to 40% of instances, the ileocolic area in 40 to 55%, and the colon only in approximately 20%. Duodenal abnormalities are shown on upper GI x-rays in up to 20% of patients.

Ulcerative colitis is diagnosed by sigmoidoscopy, but a barium enema helps establish the extent of disease, excludes Crohn's disease by visualizing the terminal ileum, and screens for coexistent carcinoma. An air-contrast barium enema is best for evaluating mucosal detail in IBD but does not allow reflux into the terminal ileum as readily as a full column study.

During active disease, mild laxatives and gentle enemas or oral electrolyte solutions (Go-Lytely) are given for bowel preparation prior to barium enema examination or colonoscopy. The usual cathartics are contraindicated, because they can cause hypovolemia, electrolyte abnormalities, and toxic dilatation. Barium enemas should not be done during acute exacerbations unless the results are expected to be immediately helpful because of the danger of precipitating toxic dilatation of the colon (toxic megacolon).

Fiberoptic endoscopy is rarely necessary in IBD. Colonscopy with biopsy may be useful in differentiating Crohn's disease from ileocecal lymphoma, constricting adenocarcinoma, and ischemic strictures, and in evaluating postoperative patients who have diarrhea for evidence of recurrent disease. Duodenoscopy may be helpful in distinguishing peptic ulcer disease from Crohn's duodenitis, although findings and biopsies are frequently nonspecific. The primary usefulness of colonoscopy in ulcerative colitis is in screening long-term patients for adenocarcinoma and dysplasia rather than in diagnosis.

Clinical Course

Patients generally experience spontaneous relapses and remissions of unpredictable duration. Although symptom-free intervals sometimes last for many years, periodic exacerbation is almost invariable. Morality rates are two to three times normal in both types of IBD. The majority of deaths occur postoperatively within a few years of diagnosis. Later in the course of the disease, death is from carcinoma of the digestive organs. In ulcerative colitis, the clinical course varies with the extent of disease. Pancolitis has a higher mortality rate and risk of colectomy than proctosigmoiditis. Only 10% of patients with disease initially confined to the rectum develop more extensive involvement. Approximately 60 to 90% of patients with Crohn's disease eventually require surgical intervention, compared with 10 to 30% of patients with ulcerative colitis. In a 20-year study of 174 patients with Crohn's disease, patients averaged 2.5 abdominal operations, and their mortality rate was 1.5 times normal; however, almost all surviving patients were leading a normal life. Patients who develop IBD disease in childhood or adolescence may have a more aggressive form of disease, require more surgery, and have higher mortality and morbidity rates than those whose disease is diagnosed later in life.

Therapy

Because Crohn's disease is a chronic illness with no medical or surgical cure and with frequent and diverse complications, most patients require close interaction with a primary care physician, gastroenterologist, and surgeon. This collaborative team provides the clinical judgment and experience to manage the complicated patient most effectively. There is no medical cure for IBD, but medications can improve symptoms in the majority of patients.

Crohn's Disease

Both prednisone and sulfasalazine (Azulfidine) are effective in decreasing symptoms of active Crohn's disease; their effect on the long-term progression of disease is unknown, however. Neither prednisone nor sulfasalazine prevents recurrences.

Sulfasalazine is most effective when the colon is involved but is often used initially for disease at any site. Approximately 50% of patients with active Crohn's disease experience symptomatic remission after 8 weeks of therapy. Fifteen to twenty percent of patients experience some toxicity on therapeutic dosages, but only 6% develop severe complications, such as overt hemolysis, leukopenia, or drug fever. Nausea and dyspepsia occur in 10% of patients; they can be minimized by giving the drug after meals and by initiating therapy at 500 mg once a day and then increasing the dosage by 500 mg a day until the full therapeutic dosage of 3 to 4 gm per day is reached. Patients who experience a rash frequently tolerate desensitization. After a drug-free period of 2 weeks, 1 mg per day sulfasalazine suspension is begun, and the dosage doubled daily as tolerated until reaching therapeutic amounts.

Corticosteroids are most effective for patients with small intestinal involvement. The response to corticosteroids is more rapid than the response to sulfasalazine, but serious side effects are more frequent. Patients with active disease who need immediate therapeutic intervention (e.g., those with small bowel obstruction) or those who do not respond to or cannot tolerate sulfasalazine should be started on 40 to 60 mg prednisone daily. Approximately 75% of patients enter a remission after 8 weeks of prednisone therapy. Once symptoms respond to therapy, the dosage is tapered as tolerated, with the goal of completing weaning the patient from steroids. However, a considerable number of patients require 5 to 15 mg of prednisone chronically because of flare-ups of disease when the drug is stopped. In approximately 30% of patients, it is necessary to decrease the dosage because of side effects.

Azathioprine and 6-mercaptopurine are reserved for patients whose disease is refractory to conventional therapy. A recent report of 6-mercaptopurine as primary therapy was encouraging; however, prolonged treatment (up to 6 months) was necessary before results were seen. Long-term metronidazole (Flagyl) has recently been shown to be effective in over 50% of people with perianal Crohn's disease and as effective as sulfasalazine in Crohn's colitis and ileocolitis. This drug in the dosage of 250 mg 3 to 4 times per day may be useful in patients who cannot tolerate or respond poorly to sulfasalazine or prednisone.

Nutritional repletion is an essential part of patient management of IBD. Weight loss occurs in 85% of Crohn's patients as a result of decreased food intake, malabsorption, and protein-electrolyte loss through the ulcerated mucosa. Correction of malnutrition prevents growth retardation in children and decreases the rate of complications following surgery.

Patients should be encouraged to eat a well-balanced diet; they should avoid dairy products if they are among the approximately 10% of IBD patients with lactose intolerance. A low-residue diet is useful only for patients with partial small-bowel obstruction or with very active disease. Multivitamins are indicated for patients with decreased food intake and weight loss. Zinc supplementation may be necessary for some patients with voluminous diarrhea or enterocutaneous fistulas. Vitamin B_{12} injections are required in patients with deficiencies caused by resection or extensive inflammation of the terminal ileum. Folic acid supplementation may be warranted in patients undergoing chronic sulfasalazine therapy, because the drug induces folate malabsorption.

Up to 90% of patients with Crohn's disease eventually require surgery. There is a 60 to 85% recurrence rate postoperatively. Because of this high recurrence rate, surgery is reserved for complications of the disease, such as small-bowel obstruction, fistulas, bleeding refractory to conservative measures, and intra-abdominal abscesses, or for patients who do not respond to maximal medical therapy.

Ulcerative Colitis

In general, patients with ulcerative colitis respond to medication more rapidly and the local complication rate is lower than in patients with Crohn's disease. Sulfasalazine (1 gm qid), the drug of first choice, also has been shown to decrease the rate of relapse and should be continued prophylactically at 2 to 3 gm per day during periods of remission.

If therapeutic dosages of sulfasalazine are not effective within 2 to 3 weeks, or if severe colitis is present, corticosteroids should be used. Hydrocortisone enemas are effective in two-thirds of patients with distal colitis and minimize the systemic side effects of steroids. If necessary, oral prednisone (30–60 mg per day) can be used to induce a remission, but this drug should be tapered and stopped when the disease becomes quiescent because corticosteroids do not prevent recurrences.

Because proctocolectomy cures ulcerative colitis, surgery has a role in patients who respond poorly to medical therapy. Because of the high risk of cancer in patients with long-standing ulcerative colitis, those with extensive disease of over 10 years' duration should be strongly considered for surgery, as should those who require chronic steroid therapy. Recent attempts to achieve bowel continence after total proctocolectomy, using the Kock pouch and ileoanal anastomosis, have been moderately successful; the methods, however, are technically difficult, and conventional ileostomy remains standard in most communities.

Complications

Patients with IBD, particularly those with ulcerative colitis, have an increased risk of carcinoma of the intestine. Approximately 2% of all patients with chronic ulcerative colitis develop adenocarcinoma of the colon. The risk is related to duration and extent of disease but not to activity of inflammation. Patients with involvement of the entire colon develop an increased risk of cancer after 10 years of symptoms; the risk is 4.5% at 15 years after onset of symptoms, 13% at 20 years, and 34% at 30 years. The risk of cancer in patients with disease confined to the left colon is less than in patients with pancolitis and tends to increase after 15 years of symptoms.

To detect colon cancer early in its course, it is currently recommended that all patients with extensive ulcerative colitis of 10 years or greater duration be colonoscoped to search for mass lesions and to obtain random mucosal biopsies. If biopsies do not demonstrate dysplasia, repeat colonoscopy is performed at intervals of 1 to 2 years. Mild dysplasia warrants at least yearly evaluation. If moderate-to-severe dysplasia is found on several biopsies, colectomy is advised because of a 30% risk of cancer.

Most extraintestinal complications respond to local therapy or treatment of the underlying bowel inflammation. The notable exceptions are ankylosing spondylitis, sclerosing cholangitis, and pyoderma gangrenosum. Intra-abdominal abscesses, fistulas, and toxic megacolon have lower mortality rates with current medical and surgical therapy. Complications from corticosteroids can be decreased by keeping dosages as low as possible. Drugs and radiologic procedures should be used with care in women of childbearing age.

Kirsner JB, Shorter RG. Recent developments in "nonspecific" inflammatory bowel disease. Part I. *N Engl J Med* 306:775–785, 1982. Part II. *N Engl J Med* 306:837–848, 1982.

An inclusive update on the epidemiology, pathogenesis, and therapy of inflammatory bowel disease with 391 recent references.

Mekhjian HS, et al. Clinical features and natural history of Crohn's disease. *Gastroenterology* 77:907–913, 1979.

Analysis of the 1084 patients involved in the National Cooperative Crohn's Disease Study, examining the presenting symptoms, complications, and need for surgery.

Sinclair TS, Brunt PW, Monat, NAG. Nonspecific proctocolitis in northern Scotland: A community study. *Gastroenterology* 85:1–11, 1983.

A retrospective study of 537 patients in a stable population. Seventy percent had only distal involvement at diagnosis and only 8% required surgery by 5 years.

Summers RW, et al. National Cooperative Crohn's Disease Study: Results of drug treatment. *Gastroenterology* 77:847–869, 1979.

A carefully controlled double-blind comparison of the therapeutic effects of prednisone, sulfasalazine, azathioprine, and placebo in 569 patients.

Azad Khan AK, et al. Optimum dose of sulfasalazine for maintenance treatment in ulcerative colitis. *Gut* 12:232–240, 1980.

This study demonstrates that the optimum dosage of sulfasalazine to decrease the recurrence rate of ulcerative colitis is 1 gm twice a day indefinitely.

Ursing B, et al. A comparative study of metronidazole and sulfasalazine for active Crohn's disease: The cooperative Crohn's disease study in Sweden. II. Result. *Gastroenterology* 83:550–562, 1982.

A randomized cross-over study showing that metronidazole is at least as effective as sulfasalazine in the treatment of active Crohn's disease.

Butt JH, Lennard-Jones JE, Ritchie JK. A practical approach to the risk of cancer in inflammatory bowel disease. *Med Clin North Am* 64:1203–1220, 1980.

A good synopsis of recent literature in a confusing but promising field.

53. HEMORRHOIDS

C. Glenn Pickard, Jr.

Hemorrhoids, the most common anorectal condition encountered in practice, are protrusions into the anal canal of stretched mucosa and underlying vascular cushions of submucosal tissues. Repeated straining to pass a small, hard stool initially produces a prolapse of rectal mucosa. Continued stretching results in redundant tissue that may prolapse outside the anal orifice with defecation. Accompanying loss of support and dilatation of the submucosal veins produce the hemorrhoidal varices responsible for the bleeding and thrombosis that are features of this condition. Internal hemorrhoids originate immediately above the dentate line, involve veins of the superior hemorrhoidal plexus, and are covered by relatively insensitive rectal mucosa. External hemorrhoids originate below the dentate line, involve the inferior hemorrhoidal venous plexus, and are covered by highly sensitive skin (squamous epithelium). This anatomic difference explains, in large part, the difference in symptoms produced by internal compared to external hemorrhoids. Stretched and redundant epithelium of the lower anal canal and perianal region appears as irregular folds or nubbins called *anal skin tags*.

The primary cause of hemorrhoids is unknown. Dietary factors are thought to be important because hemorrhoids are rare in populations that have a high residue diet, and common in Western cultures, in which the diet is refined and low in residue. The role of heredity as a predisposing factor is difficult to assess accurately because hemorrhoids are so prevalent. The frequent occurrence of hemorrhoids during pregnancy is thought to be related to an increased venous pressure within the hemorrhoidal plexus secondary to the gravid uterus. In the patient with cirrhosis and portal hypertension, varices may develop in the hemorrhoidal venous plexus, which constitutes one of the routes of collateral circulation for the obstructed portal system.

Diagnosis

Internal Hemorrhoids

Painless bright-red bleeding with defecation is usually the first complaint of patients with internal hemorrhoids. Bleeding results from abrasion and excoriation of the hemorrhoids by passage of a hard stool or when undue straining occurs with defecation. Blood may streak the stool or drip from the anus in an amount sufficient to discolor the toilet bowel water. A lesser degree of bleeding may be detected as streaks of fresh blood on the toilet tissue or as small blood stains on underclothing. Anemia may result from recurrent hemorrhoidal bleeding over many months; however, hemorrhoidal bleeding should not be accepted as a cause of anemia until other potentially more serious causes of gastrointestinal blood loss have been excluded by appropriate diagnostic tests.

Prolapse of tissue with defecation may occur with hemorrhoids. Initially the prolapsed tissue retracts spontaneously when straining with defecation ceases. At a later stage, the prolapsed hemorrhoids may not spontaneously reduce and digital replacement by the patient is required. With long-standing disease, prolapse may occur with coughing, sneezing, lifting, or prolonged walking or standing until ultimately the prolapse becomes permanent. Such a constant prolapse of rectal mucosa is associated with a chronic mucus discharge, producing wetness and irritation of perianal skin and soiling of clothing.

Pain with internal hemorrhoids is uncommon; when present, it usually is not severe unless irreducible prolapse of internal hemorrhoids with venous congestion, thrombosis, and inflammation has occurred.

Internal hemorrhoids are not visible unless prolapsed and usually are not palpable on digital examination unless thrombosed. Their presence is determined by anoscopic examination. When the anoscope is introduced to its full length and slowly withdrawn, one or more variably sized reddish purple masses of tissue bulge or project into the anal canal. Rectal mucosa covering internal hemorrhoids is distinctly different in appearance from the skin lining the anal canal. The degree of prolapse can be determined by asking the patient to bear down as the anoscope is removed.

An acute irreducible (incarcerated) prolapse of internal hemorrhoids may occur following defecation or straining. Usually there is a past history of symptomatic hemorrhoids. The acutely inflamed, plum-colored protruding mass cannot be reduced because of engorgement and edema from venous congestion and thrombosis and produces an agonizingly painful condition. Inspection reveals an edematous, moist, reddish purple, often excoriated mass protruding from the anus. Attempts at manual reduction should be avoided because the swollen mass of tissue does not remain reduced and manipulation causes additional discomfort for the patient.

External Hemorrhoids

In contrast to internal hemorrhoids, external hemorrhoids frequently present with itching, burning, or pain that may be quite severe with acute thrombosis. In some patients, however, external hemorrhoids are relatively asymptomatic, and bleeding may be the only clue to their presence. The bleeding, however, is rarely as profuse as that encountered with internal hemorrhoids.

External hemorrhoids are visible on inspection without the use of an anoscope. They often are accompanied by skin tags, which may become quite extensive with resultant irritation, itching, and soiling.

Acute thrombosis of an external hemorrhoidal vein produces the sudden appearance of a painful, tender mass at the anal opening. Varying from several millimeters to several centimeters in diameter, this tense, tender swelling often contains a readily visible bluish clot beneath overlying stretched and edematous skin. Anal thrombosis usually follows a sudden episode of straining with coughing, sneezing, heavy lifting, vigorous athletic activity, defecation, or parturition. It commonly occurs in young and otherwise healthy adults and probably is related to a sudden increase in hemorrhoidal venous pressure. Although anal thrombosis may develop in patients with symptomatic hemorrhoidal disease, it is not necessarily related to internal hemorrhoids or other anal abnormalities. The key feature in diagnosis is recognition that the swelling is covered by skin and not by rectal mucosa. This observation differentiates anal thrombosis from internal hemorrhoidal prolapse.

Differential Diagnosis

Other causes for rectal bleeding include colorectal carcinoma, polyps, inflammatory bowel disease, colonic diverticulosis, and anal fissure. Sigmoidoscopy is an important part of the routine examination for hemorrhoids, and barium contrast study of the colon is a frequently indicated additional diagnostic test. Other anorectal conditions that require differentiation from hemorrhoids are rectal prolapse, condyloma acuminatum of the anal canal and perianal area, anal neoplasms, and prolapsed pedunculated rectal polyps. A prominent anal skin tag may indicate an adjacent anal fissure, which usually is located in the posterior midline.

Treatment

Asymptomatic hemorrhoids require no treatment. Regulation of bowel habit and avoidance of constipation by the use of psyllium-containing bulk-forming agents such as Metamucil, Effersyllium, or Hydrocil Instant may relieve hemorrhoidal symptoms and result in regression of early pathologic changes in some instances. Bleeding from internal hemorrhoids often may be controlled simply by softening the stool. Reading while sitting on the toilet should be avoided. Prolonged sitting in this manner with the anus unsupported, coupled with increased intra-abdominal pressure from the elbows-on-knees posture and repeated straining at defecation, produces venous engorgement of the hemorrhoidal plexuses and can aggravate existing hemorrhoidal disease. Hemorrhoids characteristically are intermittently symptomatic; lengthy periods of remission are common, with exacerbations often triggered by constipation or diarrhea. During symptomatic periods, anesthetic-, steroid-, and astringent-containing suppositories such as Anusol-HC and Wyanoid HC are of value.

Pain with acute thrombosis of an external hemorrhoidal vein is most intense at the outset and gradually diminishes over several days as acute inflammation subsides. Discomfort may be alleviated by warm sitz baths and local application of a topical anesthetic ointment. Shortly after the onset of acute symptoms, prompt pain relief can be obtained by evacuation of the clot under local anesthesia.

Reasons for Referral

Patients with acute thrombosis of an external hemorrhoidal vein should be referred for consideration of clot evacuation or complete excision under local anesthesia. Surgical consultation should be obtained in managing the patient with irreducible (incarcerated) prolapse of internal hemorrhoids, even though operative treatment is not advisable for the acute condition.

Patients who have recurring bleeding from internal hemorrhoids and/or extensive and bothersome prolapse should be referred for consideration of rubber band ligation, injection therapy, or hemorrhoidectomy. Rubber band ligation and injection therapy are effective treatments for mild-to-moderate instances of internal hemorrhoids. Both procedures are most frequently done on an outpatient basis and usually produce only minor discomfort for several days with little time lost from work. Surgical hemorrhoidectomy, in contrast, should be reserved for large, far-advanced hemorrhoids. Patients are usually hospitalized for 4 to 5 days and the procedure is most often done under spinal or general anesthesia. The period of limited activity following surgery is usually 3 to 4 weeks.

Buls JG, Goldberg SM. Modern management of hemorrhoids. *Surg Clin North Am* 58:469–478, 1978.
  An excellent general review including pathophysiology, diagnosis, and medical and surgical management.
Tagart REB. Haemorrhoids and palpable ano-rectal lesions. *Practitioner* 212:221–238, 1974.
  Another excellent general review.
Thomson, WHF. The nature of haemorrhoids. *Br J Surg* 62:542–552, 1975.
  Primarily concerned with the pathogenesis of hemorrhoids. Emphasizes the role of the submucosal "cushions."
Burkitt, DP. Varicose veins, deep vein thrombosis, and haemorrhoids: epidemiology and suggested aetiology. *Br Med J* 2:556–561, 1972.
  Gives evidence for the role of low-residue diet as a causal factor in hemorrhoids.
MacLeod, JH. Rational approach to treatment of hemorrhoids based on a theory of etiology. *Arch Surg* 118:29–32, 1983.
  Subscribes to Thomson's theory of causation (see ref., above) and presents a logical argument for more conservative management.
Thomson, H. Rectal disease: Nonsurgical treatment of haemorrhoids. *Br J Hosp Med* 24:298–301, 1980.
  An excellent brief review of clinical features and a thoughtful review of nonsurgical therapy.

54. ANAL FISSURES

C. Glenn Pickard, Jr.

An anal fissure (fissure in ano) is a superficial, longitudinal laceration or ulceration of the modified skin (squamous epithelium) that lines the anal canal just below the dentate line. Because the skin of the lower anal canal is richly innervated by sensory fibers, anal fissures are quite painful. An acute anal fissure is a laceration or tear produced most commonly by passage of a hard bolus of feces. With each defecation, the laceration is stretched again, causing severe pain that may continue for several hours. As a consequence, the patient may resist defecation, become more constipated, and experience excruciating pain with the next bowel movement.

The problem tends to be cyclic, with healing and periods of remission. Constipation initiates a new episode, with the healed fissure split open again by passage of hard feces. A chronic fissure results after several months from this process of healing and recurrent injury; it appears as an elliptic or round ulcer having an edematous and scarred base.

Evaluation

The diagnosis should be suspected from the history of pain during and following defecation. The onset of acute symptoms may be recalled as having been associated with passage of a particularly hard stool. Pain typically is severe and is characterized as cutting, tearing, or burning. Following defecation, pain may become more intense from reflex anal sphincter spasm. Bleeding may be present as a secondary complaint and usually is noted as a small amount of fresh blood on the toilet tissues.

There is usually a single anal fissure located characteristically in the posterior midline of the anal canal (except in postpartum women, in whom the fissure may be in the anterior midline). Severity of pain and tenderness and degree of sphincter spasm associated with an acute fissure often make examination traumatic and extremely painful. Because of its position in the distal portion of the anal canal, the fissure can be seen readily on external examination if traction is placed on the perianal skin to evert the anal opening gently. Because the acute fissure usually can be seen by this maneuver, anoscopic examination should be deferred until treatment makes the procedure comfortable for the patient. Digital examination is very painful and needs to be done only if the diagnosis is unclear. Digital examination usually can be accomplished after application of a topical anesthetic, with careful introduction of the gloved finger by gentle pressure on the anal verge opposite the fissure. Palpation can determine tenderness at the site of the fissure and the degree of sphincter spasm.

A chronic anal fissure commonly presents the diagnostic triad of a distal sentinel pile, a chronic ulcer in the anal canal, and a proximal hypertrophied anal papilla at the dentate level. Gentle traction on the sentinel pile—a fibrotic and edematous skin tag—everts the anus to disclose the distal portion of the chronic fissure. Topical anesthesia facilitates anoscopic examination to further visualize the fissure and the proximal hypertrophied papilla. Long-standing disease may produce enough scarring and fibrosis to result in induration and stenosis of the anal canal.

Differential Diagnosis

Other anal ulcerations that must be differentiated from anal fissure include carcinoma, chancre, ulcerations associated with blood dyscrasias, and fissures associated with granulomatous enterocolitis (Crohn's disease). These diseases have characteristic symptoms and signs, and anal ulceration associated with them should not be confused with an anal fissure. Fissures located laterally or anteriorly in men and fissures located laterally in women should arouse suspicion of another underlying disease. Anal fissures may occur concomitantly with hemorrhoids and may be overlooked if not searched for carefully.

Treatment

An acute fissure with a short history usually heals rapidly and satisfactorily with medical treatment. Pain relief can be achieved by local application of a topical anesthetic ointment before and after bowel movements and as needed otherwise for comfort. Warm sitz baths for 15 to 20 minutes following each stool provide additional symptomatic relief, resolve associated reflex anal sphincter spasm, and facilitate anal hygiene. Local application of a topical steroid cream may enhance healing. Unless an analgesic-and steroid-containing suppository is placed and held in the anal canal until it dissolves, the suppository slides immediately into the rectum where it has no influence on the fissure. Because it is practically impossible to hold a suppository in this manner, it is rarely prescribed in the treatment of fissures. Relief of constipation is essential in successful treatment of anal fissure. Proper diet, a regular bowel habit, and use of stool softeners are important features in correcting constipation.

Medical treatment is much less successful with a chronic anal fissure, although a trial of therapy is warranted. A chronic fissure may heal temporarily, only to recur several weeks or months later.

Reasons for Referral

An anal fissure that does not heal after 3 to 4 weeks of therapy, a chronic fissure with sentinel pile and hypertrophied anal papilla, and a fissure associated with anal stenosis should be referred for surgical treatment. Any fissure that is atypically located or that displays unusual features should be referred for additional diagnostic tests and appropriate therapy.

Crapp AR, Alexander-Williams J. Fissure-in-ano and anal stenosis. *Clin Gastroenterol* 4:619–628, 1975.
An excellent general review.

Shub HA, Salvati EP, Rubin RJ. Conservative treatment of anal fissure: An unselected, restrospective, and continuous study. *Dis Colon Rectum* 21:582–583, 1978.
An excellent discussion of conservative management based on a series of 393 patients.

Ferguson JA, MacKeigan JM. Hemorrhoids, fistulas, and fissures: Office and hospital management. A critical review. *Adv Surg* 12:111–153, 1978.
An excellent review including pathophysiology, diagnosis, and treatment. An extensive bibliography.

55. ACUTE DIARRHEA

C. Glenn Pickard, Jr.

Acute diarrhea is defined as diarrhea of less than a week's duration, occurring in a previously healthy patient. In the United States, acute diarrhea is the second leading cause of morbidity and loss of time from work. Even though most patients with diarrhea do not visit a physician, diarrhea remains one of the most frequent diagnoses made in ambulatory care.

Acute diarrhea usually results from one of several well-known causes that present as clinically recognizable syndromes. The observations that enable one to separate the syndromes clinically are emphasized in Table 55-1.

Evaluation

The majority of patients with acute diarrhea present with a syndrome that resembles viral gastroenteritis. This syndrome is characterized by the abrupt onset of diarrhea, usually associated with nausea, vomiting, and crampy abdominal pain. It is more common in children and young adults and often occurs in epidemic form. The fever is usually low grade and the diarrheal stools are loose and watery without mucus or blood.

Because diarrhea from other causes, including bacteria, parasites, and ulcerative colitis, may initially present with symptoms similar to those of viral gastroenteritis, the practitioner must decide whether to pursue any studies beyond the history and physical examination at the initial encounter. For the great majority of patients, the answer would seem to be *no*, for the following reasons: Most instances of acute diarrhea prove to be self-limited and resolve within several days from the time of onset. Few patients with acute diarrhea, regardless of the cause, are adversely affected by simple supportive treatment and observation during this initial period. Furthermore, even in those instances of known bacterial cause, current recommendations are to withhold antibacterial therapy in most mild cases.

When clinical presentation (see Table 55-1) strongly suggests a bacterial pathogen (e.g., a common-source epidemic following a community picnic, or patients presenting with high fever and bloody diarrhea), additional investigation is indicated. This includes cultures of patients' stools and foods that are the likely source, both as an adjunct to clinical management of the patient and as a public health measure to discover the source of the epidemic.

Fecal Leukocyte Examination

For some patients, the clinical history does not point clearly to the cause, or it seems unwise simply to treat supportively and observe the patient. In these circumstances, the fecal leukocyte smear provides a simple, inexpensive, immediately available source of useful data to help distinguish between inflammatory diarrhea (mostly invasive bacterial infection and ulcerative colitis) and viral infection. Fecal leukocyte smears are positive in approximately 90% of patients with bacterial diarrhea and negative in about 95% of patients with viral gastroenteritis (Table 55-2).

To examine the stool for leukocytes, one or two drops of Löffler's methylene blue are

Table 55-1. Features of diarrhea

Agent	Source	Mode of transmission	Incubation period
Staph. aureus (preformed toxin)	Inadequately refrigerated food contaminated with *Staph.*	Ingestion of food containing preformed toxin	1–6 hours
Toxigenic *E. coli* (noninvasive)	Common cause of travelers' diarrhea; exact source unknown	Ingestion of contaminated water or uncooked fruits or vegetables	2–3 days
Shigella	Frequently found in institutional settings with poor sanitation and hygiene	Fecal-oral	1–2 days
Salmonella (nontyphoidal)	Contaminated food or water, powdered eggs, milk, poultry, pet turtles	Ingestion of contaminated food or water	8–48 hours
Campylobacter	Extensive reservoir in animals; human carriers exist	Contaminated water, contact with infected animals. Probable fecal-oral human-to-human transmission	3–5 days
"Norwalk-like" viruses	Other infected patients	Probably fecal-oral	18–48 hours
Rotavirus	Other infected patients	Probably fecal-oral	48 hours

Key: + + + + = almost always occurs; + + + = usually occurs; + + = occasionally occurs; + = rarely occurs; ± = may or may not occur; − = does not occur.

added to a small fleck of mucus or stool on a clean dry slide. After thorough mixing, a cover slip is placed over the specimen, and it is examined as a "wet mount" preparation. The methylene blue stains white blood cells and enables identification of the motile trophozoites of *Giardia lamblia* and the eggs or larvae of other parasitic infestations. Although there is not complete agreement on the definition of a positive slide, one commonly used definition is 10 to 15 white blood cells per high-power field on five or more fields. Because patients with known bacterial enteritis occasionally have negative cultures, "false-positive" results (i.e., the presence of leukocytes on a smear with a negative culture) may be caused in part by problems with culture techniques. Stained smears obtained from cup specimens give a much higher percentage of positive results (95%) than do smears obtained from diapers or cotton swabs (47%).

Table 55-1 (continued)

			Clinical features		
Age of patient	Onset	Vomiting	Abdominal pain	Fever	Characteristics of diarrhea
Any age	Abrupt	+ + + +	±	Absent	Profuse, watery, no blood or mucus
Young adults and infants	Gradual	+	+ + +	Low-grade	Profuse, watery, no blood or mucus
6 mo to 6 yr; sporadically in other age groups	Abrupt	−	±	High	Frequently bloody mucoid
Any age	Abrupt	+ + + +		−	Variable	Watery, occasionally mucoid
Any age	Gradual	±	+ + + +	High	Bloody mucus stool not uncommon
School children and young adults	Abrupt	+ + + +	+ + +	Low-grade	Watery
Children younger than 3; occ. older	Abrupt	+ + + +	+ + +	Moderate	Watery

Table 55-2. Positive fetal leukocyte smears

Organism	Stools Positive for Fecal Leukocytes (%)
Shigella	69–100
Salmonella	36–80
Invasive *E. coli*	82–100
Virus	0–6

Treatment

Fluid and Electrolytes
Management of all patients should include careful assessment of hydration and appropriate intervention with oral or parenteral fluids. Recent studies, primarily in patients with cholera, have shown that oral fluid replacement with glucose-electrolyte solutions can effectively restore hydration in most patients even when the diarrhea continues. This is possible because the intestinal absorption capacity often remains intact at some sites in the bowel even when there is fluid secretion into the intestinal lumen at other sites.

The composition of the fluid recommended by the World Health Organization (WHO) for treating diarrhea in all age groups is 2% glucose in a solution containing sodium (90 mEq/L), chloride (75 mEq/L), potassium (15 mEq/L), and bicarbonate (30 mEq/L). However, most patients with acute diarrhea in this country do not experience the massive fluid and electrolyte loss associated with cholera, and strict adherence to this formula is unnecessary for them. Table 55-3 gives the composition of many commonly available fluids. Those indicated with an asterisk more nearly approximate the WHO formulation and are recommended for severe instances. For milder illness, fluids such as Coca-Cola and ginger ale are adequate; it is usually recommended that carbonated drinks be "defizzed" before administration, although there is no strong evidence to support the practice. Kool-Aid, which is commonly used for children, has very low concentrations of Na^+ and K^+. On the other hand, bouillon has a very high Na^+ content and can produce hypernatremia when used as fluid replacement in children.

It is recommended that milk and milk products be avoided; some patient with diarrhea have a transient disaccharidase (including lactase) deficiency. Similarly, fats and large meals are avoided because of the clinical impression that they increase cramps and diarrhea, perhaps through gastrocolic reflex and malabsorption. There are no controlled clinical trials to support these measures, but they appear to do no harm and may well be helpful.

When fluid and electrolyte losses are severe, and particularly when they are complicated by nausea and vomiting, IV fluid replacement is necessary.

Antidiarrheal Drugs
Patients often request symptomatic relief from diarrhea. Many pharmacologic agents are available, but their use is controversial.

Absorbents such as kaolin and pectin (Kaopectate) have been used for years, despite the fact that their efficacy has not been established by clinical trials. However, they rarely if ever cause harm and are thus the least controversial alternative.

Pepto-Bismol, another commonly used proprietary agent, has recently been shown to

Table 55-3. Sodium and potassium content of oral liquids

Liquid	Na^+	mEq/liter K^+
Apple juice	1.7	26.0
Coca-Cola	1.0	0.4
Gatorade*	23.0	2.5
Ginger ale*	3.5	0.1
Jell-O (half strength)	15.0	0.15
Lytren	25.0	25.0
Orange juice	0.2	49.0
Pedialyte	30.0	20.0
Pepsi	0	0.6
7-up	5.0	0.3

*The electrolyte values for this product may vary slightly depending on the electrolyte content of local water supplies.

Source: R.G. Pietrusko Drug therapy reviews: Pharmacotherapy of diarrhea. *Am J Hosp Pharm* 36:757–767, 1979.

e an effective prophylactic against travelers' diarrhea. There is speculation that the effectiveness is from the antiprostaglandin effect of salicylates.

The greatest controversy exists regarding opiates and similar synthetic antidiarrheals. There is no doubt that these agents can decrease the frequency of stooling. It is less certain whether this is ultimately beneficial or harmful, and, if helpful, which is the superior agent. The potential for antidiarrheals to do harm is believed to be greater in children. The magnitude of effective fluid loss may be masked by decreasing the frequency of stooling without decreasing fluid loss into the intestinal lumen. It is also contended that "toxicity" may be increased and bacterial diarrhea may become more severe and prolonged. The evidence that these adverse effects occur in adults is less convincing.

The potential for drug toxicity from opiates and synthetic antidiarrheals is also a serious concern, particularly in children. Central nervous system depression resulting in death was reported in a two-year-old child who ingested only six diphenoxylate-atropine tablets. Dyphenoxylate-atropine (Lomotil) has produced hepatic coma when given to adults with chronic liver disease. The potential for abuse of the opiates, such as paregoric or deodorized tincture of opium (DTO), is minor.

For certain patients, the advantages of using an antidiarrheal may outweigh the risks. A short course of an antidiarrheal often curtails the diarrhea at minimal risk. Dosages of the commonly used agents are as follows.

Loperamide (Imodium): 4 mg (two capsules) initially, followed by 2 mg (one capsule) after each loose stool, not to exceed 16 mg (eight capsules) in 24 hours.

Diphenoxylate-atropine (Lomotil): two tablets initially, followed by one tablet after each loose stool, not to exceed eight tablets in 24 hours.

Paregoric: One or two teaspoons orally every 4 hours.

DTO (deodorized tincture of opium): 8 to 10 drops in a glass of water every 4 hours.

The synthetic preparations, diphenoxylate-atropine and loperamide, are not pharmacologically superior to the opiates. However, many patients prefer them because of convenience of dosing. There is evidence suggesting that loperamide may be more effective and less toxic than diphenoxylate-atropine. *Antibiotics are contraindicated* in the great majority of instances of acute diarrhea. There is little evidence to suggest that the course of bacterial diarrhea in mild cases is shortened by antibiotics, and there is evidence that the shedding of *Salmonella* is prolonged in antibiotic-treated patients. Antibiotics also favor the development of antibiotic-resistant bacteria. There is no rationale for the use of antibiotics in viral diarrhea.

Antibiotics may be indicated for severely ill patients in whom a bacterial cause is strongly suspected. Stool culture and sensitivities are necessary because no single antibiotic is certain to be effective against the various pathogens. If antibiotics are begun before culture results are available, common choices are ampicillin, which covers many *Salmonella* and *Shigella* species; doxycycline, which covers many *Campylobacter* species and *Escherichia coli;* and trimethoprim-sulfamethoxazole (Septra), which covers most *Salmonella* species and enterotoxic *E. coli.*

Clinical Course

The majority of patients with acute diarrhea respond to symptomatic and supportive care and become asymptomatic in a week or less. In those instances in which diarrhea persists, other causes should be considered. Cultures for enteric pathogens and special cultures for *Campylobacter* should be obtained. Intestinal parasites, inflammatory bowel disease, and irritable bowel syndrome also must be considered. Malabsorption caused by pancreatic insufficiency or intrinsic bowel disease is also a consideration and usually is suspected on the basis of classic malabsorptive stools; however, in other instances the diagnosis is not suspected until a full investigation is performed, including qualitative and quantitative evaluations of fecal fat content and other studies for malabsorption. Finally, one must always consider gastrointestinal cancers as a possible cause of diarrhea—either because of obstructing lesions causing constipation followed by diarrhea, or rarely, because of secreting villous adenomas.

Koreniowski OM, Rouse JD, Guerrant RL. Value of examination for fecal leukocytes in the early diagnosis of shigellosis. *Am J Trop Med Hyg* 28:1031–1035, 1979.

An excellent study of the role of the fecal leukocyte examination in the diagnosis of shigellosis. Includes a good brief review of previous studies.

Harris JC, DuPont HL, Hornic RB. Fecal leukocytes in diarrheal illness. *Ann Intern Med* 76:697–703, 1972.

An extensive study of fecal leukocyte testing in 55 patients with naturally acquired disease and 114 volunteers who ingested known enteric pathogens.

Pietrusko RG. Drug therapy reviews: Pharmacotherapy of diarrhea. *Am J Hosp Pharm* 36:757–767, 1979.

A superb review of the entire subject of diarrhea. Major emphasis is on therapy, but it also includes an extensive review of pathophysiology and diagnosis. Includes 170 references.

Aserkoff B, Bennett JV. Effect of antibiotic therapy in acute salmonellosis on the fecal excretion of salmonellae. *N Engl J Med* 281:636–640, 1969.

An intriguing article describing a natural experiment in which approximately 1900 persons developed Salmonella enteritis as a result of contaminated turkey at a picnic. One hundred eighty-five patients treated with antibiotics are compared to a similar number of untreated subjects.

Plotkin GR, Kluge RM, Waldman, RH. Gastroenteritis: Etiology, pathophysiology, and clinical manifestations. *Medicine* 58:95–114, 1979.

An extensive review of all aspects of the subject except treatment. Includes 262 references.

Fekety, R. Recent advances in management of bacterial diarrhea. *Rev Infect Dis* 5:246–257, 1983.

An excellent comprehensive review of recently recognized causes of bacterial diarrhea, including pathophysiology, clinical evaluation, and treatment.

Satterwhite TK, KuPont HL. Infectious diarrhea in office practice. *Med Clin North Am* 67:203–220, 1983.

An excellent general review of all infectious causes of diarrhea, including evaluation and treatment.

56. CONSTIPATION
R. Balfour Sartor

Constipation is a symptom that has widely different meanings for both patients and physicians. It is most precisely defined as the passage of less than 35 gm of fecal matter per day. In the clinical setting, a more practical definition is passage of fewer than three stools per week and/or the sensation of incomplete evacuation or straining. Because constipation is frequently the subject of myths and home remedies, the physician's advice is often neither sought nor accepted until an intractable pattern of constipation with periodic purging develops, leading to laxative abuse and dependence. Although the prevalence of constipation is not known, it is common enough to account for a $250 million laxative market in the United States. In a British survey (Connell 1965) it was found that 16% of people 10 to 59 years of age and 50% of those over 60 years old use laxatives.

Predisposing factors for constipation appear to be advancing age, immobility, drug use, and, most important, a low-fiber diet. The habit of ignoring the urge to defecate (a temporary impulse produced by stool distending the rectal ampulla) also may contribute to constipation; it results in decreased responsiveness of this reflex arc, increased volume of stool in the distal colon with subsequent rectosigmoid dilatation, and increased stool desiccation. For unclear reasons, constipation is more frequent in women than in men.

Simple constipation is frequently asymptomatic; the symptoms of cramping abdominal pain, nausea, and fullness are often produced by laxatives used for perceived "irregularity," rather than by the accumulation of fecal matter within the left colon. However, long-standing constipation, usually in conjunction with laxative use, has been strongly associated with colonic diverticulosis and hemorrhoids and weakly associated with hiatal hernias. The colonic dilatation of chronic constipation predisposes patients to sigmoid volvulus.

Long-standing use of certain laxatives can produce "cathartic colon," a motility disturbance manifested by decreased propulsive activity of the right colon. Agents incriminated in this syndrome include cascara, senna, castor and croton oil, and phenolphthalein. In extreme situations, frequent purging can result in electrolyte and renal disturbances, particularly hypokalemia and hyperaldosteronism.

Evaluation

Once it has been determined that constipation is present, the goals of evaluation include detecting intrinsic gastrointestinal pathology (particularly of colonic origin), diagnosing systemic diseases presenting as constipation, and finding easily remediable causes, such as constipating drugs or poor dietary habits.

History

The history is the most important element in evaluating the constipated patient; it should focus on when and under what circumstances constipation first became a problem. The recent onset of constipation dictates a search for gastrointestinal disorders, especially carcinoma of the colon in the middle-aged or elderly patient. In contrast, a long-standing history of constipation beginning in adolescence or early adulthood without a recent abrupt change in bowel function is more compatible with a functional disorder. Many patients with short-segment Hirschsprung's disease are not diagnosed until early adulthood; these young patients have the onset of severe constipation during infancy. The history of anal surgery suggests a possible anal stricture, and laparotomies predispose to obstructing intra-abdominal adhesions. Rectal bleeding, abdominal distention, weight loss, pain, and vomiting suggest intrinsic intestinal disease with partial obstruction. Systemic medical conditions that may produce or exacerbate constipation include hypothyroidism, diabetes with autonomic neuropathy, uremia, hypokalemia, hypercalcemia, and pregnancy. A meticulous drug history of both prescribed and over-the-counter formulations should emphasize laxative use and drugs known to induce constipation. Such drugs include opiates; psychotherapeutics, including antidepressants; aluminum and calcium antacids; anticholinergics; and certain antihypertensive agents. Frequently the patient is reluctant to admit the extent of laxative use or to mention the number of agents, including "home remedies," being used.

A family history may be helpful in determining the patient's attitudes toward constipation and laxative use and in identifying the rare patient with familial pseudoobstruction.

Finally, the dietary patterns of each patient should be carefully outlined. This information helps in establishing a cause for constipation, in planning therapy through dietary manipulation, and in emphasizing to the patient the importance of dietary factors in the pathogenesis of constipation.

Physical Examination

The physical examination should be directed at identifying patients with systemic or gastrointestinal diseases that produce constipation. A careful rectal examination should include evaluation of anal sphincter tone, perianal sensory fibers, anal stricture, amount and consistency of stool in the rectal vault, rectal dilation, and the presence of a fecal impaction. The stool should be tested for occult blood. A proctosigmoidoscopy is essential to search for constricting carcinomas of the lower colon, rectal distention, and melanosis coli. Melanosis coli is an apparently benign darkening of the colonic mucosa produced by pigment-engorged macrophages in the lamina propria of patients who chronically use anthraquinone laxatives (senna and cascara). Patients with large amounts of stool in the rectum on digital examination can be most thoroughly evaluated after a Fleet enema. The stool should be saved for examination.

Laboratory and X-ray

The extent of laboratory or radiographic evaluation depends on the degree of clinical suspicion that an associated disorder is present. All patients should have three separate stools evaluated for occult blood. Serum calcium, glucose, and potassium; thyroid function; and BUN determinations, although not routinely indicated, are useful in patients with suspected systemic disease. Barium enemas are not universally indicated but should be performed in all patients with a recent onset or abrupt worsening of constipation, weight loss, stools positive for occult blood, suggestion of bowel obstruction, or onset of constipation within the first decade of life. Radiographic abnormalities of the "cathartic colon" are usually confined to the right side and include lack of normal haustration (that mimicks chronic ulcerative colitis) and bizarre contractions. Rectal manometry is useful only in the small number of patients whose constipation began in infancy or in those with fecal incontinence not related to impaction or obvious neurologic abnormalities.

Treatment
The main components of therapy are patient re-education, a high-fiber diet, and cessation of laxatives.

Patient Re-education
The wide variation in normal stool frequency should be emphasized, as well as the fact that a stool each day is not essential for health. Life-style changes, such as increasing fluid intake and exercise, may be necessary for long-term benefits. The importance of responding to the urge to defecate at the time it first occurs should be stressed. The potential complications of laxatives should be outlined to reiterate the reasons for stopping these drugs. The benefits of a high-fiber diet should be touted, mentioning its possible preventive role in the pathogenesis of diverticular disease, hemorrhoids, hiatal hernia, and carcinoma of the colon.

High-fiber Diets
High-fiber diets have been demonstrated in numerous studies of constipated patients, including the immobile geriatric population, to increase stool frequency, bulk, water content, and dry weight, and to decrease intestinal transit time. Many patients with mild constipation of short duration respond to dietary manipulation alone, but those whose chronic constipation is complicated by laxative dependence usually require supplemental bulk agents in dosages ranging from 10 to 20 gm of dietary fiber per day. The fiber contents of common foods and supplemental bulk products, with suggestions for their use, are discussed in Chapter 143. Nearly all patients experience temporary sensations of gaseousness, abdominal distention, and cramping during the first few weeks of fiber supplementation. The physician must explain these side effects to patients before initiating therapy, or they will discontinue the diet before beneficial results are obtained. The beneficial effects of bran are lasting and frequently are obtained with less supplementation as the colon is gradually "retrained" over a period of months.

Laxative Cessation
Most patients can stop the use of all laxative agents when the high-fiber diet is initiated. For it to be effective, laxatives should be banned on the first visit. During the 1- to 2-week adjustment period, when the high-fiber diet may not yet be completely effective, the patient will probably experience some discomfort and pass stools irregularly. During this period, Fleet or saline enemas or suppositories can be used to induce a bowel movement if none has occurred in 3 days and the patient is symptomatic. This regimen has the advantage of stimulating the rectal distention reflex while avoiding cathartics. With continued retraining and adaptation, the use of enemas and suppositories should not be necessary for the majority of patients. Some patients, especially those who are institutionalized or immobile, have unresponsive aganglionic colons from protracted laxative abuse, or have neurologic disease, do not respond to increased fiber alone. These patients may require a mild laxative with few side effects, such as milk of magnesia or lactulose (Chronulac), or occasional suppositories or enemas. Such patients should be checked regularly for fecal impactions. Numerous studies have shown decreased use of laxatives in institutionalized geriatric patients using bran therapy alone. Certain laxatives that should *not* be used chronically because of potentially serious side effects include senna (Senokot), which can cause the degeneration of the colonic myenteric plexus leading to irreversible cathartic colon syndrome or melanosis coli; mineral oil, which can cause malabsorption of fat-soluble vitamins or aspiration producing lipoid pneumonia; dioctyl sulfosuccinate (Colace, Dialose), which can cause increased absorption of concurrently administered drugs; and those producing

the cathartic colon, including cascara, castor oil, and phenolphthalein. Soapsuds enemas should never be used because of their irritant effect and the occasional production of hemorrhagic colitis.

Prevention

Prevention of constipation is easier than treatment. The relatively simple act of increasing fiber in the diet probably decreases the incidence of constipation, although experimental data have not yet been collected. There is some evidence that ingrained attitudes are beginning to change, with increased attention to dietary fiber and less fixation on bowel function. It is hoped that these attitudinal changes result in more physiologic norms in bowel function.

Bockus HL. Simple Constipation. In HL Bockus (Ed.), *Gastroenterology* (3rd ed.). Philadelphia: Saunders, 1976. Vol. 2.
A well-written, concise chapter on the pathophysiology and treatment of constipation.
Connell AM, et al. Variation of bowel habit in two population samples. *Br Med J* 2:1095–1099, 1965.
A British survey of 1055 factory workers and 400 patients of a general medical practice, quantitating frequency of bowel movements and laxative use.
Oster JR, Materson BJ, Rogers AI. Laxative abuse syndrome. *Am J Gastroenterol* 74:451–458, 1980.
A review article outlining the physiologic disturbances of this psychiatric illness.
Graham DY, Moser SE, Estes MK. The effect of bran on bowel function in constipation. *Am J Gastroenterol* 77:599–603, 1982.
Twenty grams of either wheat or corn bran added to the diet of constipated women increased the stool weight and frequency, and decreased the transit time by 50%. Six of 10 subjects noted improvement in constipation.
Anderson H, et al. Transit time in constipated geriatric patients during treatment with a bulk laxative and bran: A comparison. *Scand J Gastroenterol* 14:821–826, 1979.
A long-term comparison of transit time and serum calcium and iron levels between patients taking bran and those taking a commercial bulk laxative in a geriatric institutional setting. Bran decreased transit time more than psyllium; its main effect was to increase passage through the rectosigmoid colon.
Hull C, Greco RS, Brooks DL. Alleviation of constipation in the elderly by dietary fiber supplementation. *J Am Geriatr Soc* 28:410–414, 1980.
The addition of bran to the diet of an institutionalized geriatric population prevented constipation and laxative use in 60%, with a saving of $44,000 in laxative expense per year.
Fingl E, Freston JW. Antidiarrheal Agents and Laxatives: Changing Concepts. In JW Freston (Ed.), *Clinics in Gastroenterology*. Philadelphia: Saunders, 1979. Vol. 8, No 1.
A comprehensive review of the mechanisms of action and side effects of different classes of laxatives.
Southgate DA, et al. A guide to calculating intakes of dietary fibre. *J Hum Nutr* 30:303–313, 1976.
A listing of relative amounts of dietary fiber in representative foods of all major food groups.

57. HEMATOCHEZIA AND OCCULT GASTROINTESTINAL BLEEDING

Sidney L. Levinson

Hematochezia

Hematochezia, or visible bleeding from the rectum, can originate from lesions throughout the gastrointestinal tract. The most common cause is local anal disease, usually hemorrhoids or anal fissures. Less often, bleeding is from a more proximal source, such as cancers, polyps, angiodysplasia, or diverticula.

Bleeding usually occurs with a bowel movement, although oozing and subsequent spotting of undergarments sometimes occur. Local anal bleeding frequently follows physical activities or straining at stool. The patient notes streaking or coating of the stools with fresh blood, or blood on the toilet tissue. Occasionally, blood spurts into the toilet bowl at the beginning or end of a bowel movement. Because blood can reflux proximal to the anus from oozing internal hemorrhoids, blood mixed with stool is compatible with local anal disease. The passage of blood alone or blood mixed with mucus usually represents bleeding from a more proximal source, particularly colitis.

Evaluation

Although the initial evaluation must include questioning about upper gastrointestinal problems, the history and physical examination should be concentrated on the colon and rectum. Symptoms may suggest the cause of bleeding. Patients with hemorrhoidal bleeding usually have burning, itching, or aching as a result of inflammation, although hemorrhoidal bleeding can be painless. Cramping or bloating with a change in stool caliber suggests colon carcinoma or a prolapsed polyp. Bleeding from a more proximal source is usually painless. History should include a family history of inflammatory bowel disease, colonic polyps, or cancer, and in particular, familial polyposis syndromes.

In the general physical examination one should look for extraintestinal signs of inflammatory bowel disease, such as iritis, erythema nodosum, or pyoderma gangrenosum. Telangiectases or subcutaneous cysts may be associated with hereditary hemorrhagic telangiectasia or one of the familial polyposis syndromes (e.g., Peutz-Jeghers, Cronkhite-Canada).

The anorectal region must be inspected carefully for fistulas, induration, external skin tags, or prolapsed hemorrhoids. The digital rectal examination may disclose tenderness, induration, or nodularity indicating inflammation of local anal tissues or anorectal fissures. Rarely, a squamous carcinoma is palpable.

After digital examination, the physician should proceed with proctosigmoidoscopy. It is reasonable to use rigid sigmoidoscopy because routine use of the flexible sigmoidoscope is costly and requires skills that are not routinely taught. The availability of a relatively inexpensive, short (30-cm), flexible sigmoidoscope may alter this approach. After passage of the sigmoidoscope, anoscopy should be performed in the left lateral decubitus position with the patient performing a Valsalva maneuver. This assures distention of hemorrhoids that might not appear significant with the patient not straining and in the knee-chest position.

If no source of bleeding is found after proctosigmoidoscopy, most physicians proceed with barium enema, using air contrast to identify polyps. If the barium enema shows only diverticula, or no lesions at all, colonoscopy is indicated. In up to 40% of such patients, colonoscopy uncovers potential sources of bleeding, including carcinomas, colitis, polyps, and angiodysplasia.

Because barium enema can miss up to 36% of cancers and 65% of polyps, and cannot detect angiodysplasia, many physicians advocate bypassing it and proceeding directly to colonoscopy. They argue that if the barium enema suggests a neoplastic lesion, colonoscopy is necessary for additional evaluation; therefore, colonoscopy must be performed whether the barium enema is positive or negative. Also, colonoscopy can detect some angiodysplastic lesions.

If no source of bleeding is found after colonoscopy, it may be prudent to defer additional evaluation, provided bleeding has ceased. Other studies that may be useful include arteriography, to look for an arteriovenous malformation or tumor blush in the small bowel; technetium scans, to look for Meckel's diverticula; and upper gastrointestinal and small bowel series. Arteriography in general should be reserved for patients with rapid, potentially life-threatening bleeding; on occasion, arteriography is done electively in patients who present repeatedly with limited bleeding that requires blood replacement. It is the best clinical test for diagnosing angiodysplasia of the right colon.

Occult Gastrointestinal Bleeding

The test for occult blood has become an important part of the general checkup, both in patients with complaints referable to the gastrointestinal tract and in asymptomatic patients, for whom a stool examination is part of a screening examination.

Occult gastrointestinal bleeding can come from anywhere in the GI tract. In young people, erosive acid-peptic disease is the most frequent cause and arteriovenous malformations, polyps, and cancer are much less frequent. In older patients, polyps of the colon are the most frequent cause, and erosive acid-peptic disease is relatively less frequent. Colorectal cancer is relatively common. Approximately 1 in 20 North Americans develops this cancer; 95 percent of these develop the disease after age 45, and 60% after age 65. Vascular lesions, particularly angiodysplasia of the colon, may bleed intermittently in small quantities and can be recognized only by testing for occult blood. Diverticulosis is not a common cause of occult bleeding and should not be considered an adequate explanation if occult bleeding is found.

Testing for occult blood, in the absence of symptoms, is mainly useful for detecting early cancers or polyps that may develop into cancers. In people with occult bleeding, up to 50% have colonic adenomas or cancers. Identifying colon cancers at a localized or asymptomatic stage increases survival rates. Ten-year survival is 43% for cancers that have spread, 71% for localized tumors, and 90% in asymptomatic patients. It is currently believed, based on indirect evidence, that adenomatous polyps progress to carcinoma. For this reason, it is considered worthwhile to detect polyps when they are asymptomatic and remove them by colonoscopy.

Detection

Most evaluations of the tests for occult blood endorse Hemoccult II slides. Both Hematest and guaiac tests have high false-positive rates and are therefore inadequate for screening. Testing two specimens per day for 3 days increases the detection of occult carcinoma and polyps by almost 50% over the yield of a single test. A stool test must be obtained in the absence of active or incited bleeding (traumatic rectal examination, enema preparation for sigmoidoscopy). Meat and some vegetables can cause false-positive results. Laxatives and iron decrease the frequency of both false positives and false negatives, whereas prolonged storage (> 4 days) or lack of dietary roughage and vitamin C can increase false negatives. Unfortunately, Hemoccult testing alone does not detect all polyps; according to one estimate, sensitivity is approximately 80%.

A single positive stool warrants investigation. The yield increases from age 45. In one study, 12% of patients over age 63 with positive stools were found to have cancer and 35% to have polyps; in patients under the age of 63 with one or more positive stools, 5% had cancer and 26% had polyps. The evaluation of patients with positive stools for occult blood is partly determined by the accompanying symptoms or signs. If suspicion of an upper gastrointestinal lesion is high, an upper gastrointestinal series is indicated. Symptoms of abdominal distention or obstruction warrant barium studies of the colon and subsequently of the stomach and small bowel.

Testing in Asymptomatic People

It is generaly recommended that testing for occult gastrointestinal bleeding be part of the periodic health examination in people over 50 years old. The test is ordinarily repeated yearly; there are no substantial data to support this recommended frequency. Specimens can be collected by patients and mailed. However, compliance with this approach is not good; in one study, only one-third of the people involved returned at least one slide.

Depending on the method used, 1 to 4% of specimens are positive. About half the positive results represent colonic cancer or adenomatous polyps.

The asymptomatic patient in whom occult blood is found on a screening examination should undergo careful sigmoidoscopy as the first step. However, only approximately 25% of sigmoid polyps are found by this method, because most lesions occur in the hard-to-examine 16- to 25-cm range. Therefore, a negative sigmoidoscopic examination should be followed either by a barium enema with air contrast or by colonoscopy. Up to 40% of patients who have a barium enema that is normal or positive only for diverticula have clinically important lesions, including polyps, cancers, vascular dysplasia, and inflammatory bowel disease. Colonoscopy should be performed in all patients in whom the diagnosis is not clear from barium enema. A negative colonoscopic result may be followed by upper gastrointestinal and small bowel x-rays. In selected patients with repeatedly positive stools, upper endoscopy may be performed as well.

High-risk Patients

Patients at high risk for colon cancer include those with a positive family history for polyps or cancer (particularly in first-degree relatives); patients known to have polyposis, previous colon cancers, adenomas, or female genital cancers; and patients with ulcerative colitis of greater than 7 years' duration. These patients require thorough evaluation for a single positive stool for blood.

High-risk patients who have also had long-standing and frequently bleeding hemorrhoids are likely to ignore recurrent bleeding even though it can come from neoplastic lesions. The physician should consider screening with sigmoidoscopy and periodic barium enema or colonoscopy to find superimposed neoplastic lesions.

Follow-up
Those patients in whom no source of bleeding is found require careful follow-up, with repeated barium enema or colonoscopy within 1 to 2 years for repeatedly positive stools.

Levinson SL, et al. A current approach to rectal bleeding. *J Clin Gastroenterol* 3(Suppl. 1):9–16, 1981.
A review of causes of and approach to diagnosis and treatment of rectal bleeding.
Winawer SJ. Screening for colorectal cancer: An overview. *Cancer* 45(March suppl):1093–1098, 1980.
A critical review of costs and benefits.
Tedesco FJ, et al. Colonoscopic evaluation of rectal bleeding: A study of 304 patients. *Ann Intern Med* 89:907–909, 1978.
Describes the yield of colonoscopy in patients with negative proctosigmoidoscopic results and single-contrast barium enemas that were negative or showed diverticula only.
Gilbertsen VA, et al. The early detection of colorectal cancers: A preliminary report of the results of the occult blood study. *Cancer* 45:2899–2901, 1980.
From 873 persons aged 50 to 80 found to have occult GI bleeding, 77 cancers (9%) were detected.
Winawer SJ, et al. Progress report on controlled trial of fecal occult blood testing for the detection of colorectal neoplasia. *Cancer* 45:2959–2964, 1980.
Among men and women aged 40 or older, 1 to 4% of Hemoccult slides were positive.
Winawer SJ. Fecal occult blood testing. *Am J Dig Dis* 21(10):885–888, 1976.
A review of the causes of false-positive and false-negative reactions.
Fletcher SW, Dauphinee WD. Should colorectal carcinoma be sought in periodic health examinations? An approach to the evidence. *Clin Invest Med* 4:23–31, 1981.
A review of the evidence favoring screening for asymptomatic colon cancer.
Winawer SJ, Fleisher M, Sherlock P. Sensitivity of fecal occult blood testing for adenomas. *Gastroenterology* 1982; 83:1136–38.
Hemoccult tests detect polyps better if they are > 2 cm or in the left colon.

58. GALLSTONES AND CHOLESTASIS
C. Thomas Nuzum

Approximately twenty million United States citizens have gallstones. The prevalence of gallstones increases with age, exceeding 25% among persons over 60 years old; women are affected earlier than men. Risk factors for cholesterol stones, the kind found in 80% of patients, include obesity, fecundity, use of oral contraceptives, hypertriglyceridemia (type IV), use of clofibrate, ileal dysfunction, and Native American ancestry. Pigment stones are associated with chronic hemolysis, alcoholic cirrhosis, and duct anomalies impeding bile flow. Long-term studies indicate that 11 to 40% of patients with gallstones undergo gallbladder surgery. Most remain asymptomatic.

Complications
Biliary colic results from transient cystic or common-bile-duct obstruction. Cholecystitis, induced by stasis and infection, or, rarely, by ischemia, presents as an acute syndrome when inflammation reaches the serosa; empyema and pericholecystic abscess occasionally ensue. Chronic cholecystitis is discernible grossly and histologically in most stone-bearing gallbladders, but corresponds to no definite illness. Uncommonly,

stones perforate the gallbladder, entering the abdominal cavity (bile peritonitis) or gut (gallstone ileus).

Whereas gallstones confined to the gallbladder and cystic duct cause focal complications, those lodged in the common duct have more systemic effects: jaundice and maldigestion from cholestasis, and/or septicemia from cholangitis. Choledocholithiasis is the main cause of pancreatitis in nonalcoholics, of liver abscesses in the elderly, and of secondary biliary cirrhosis. Most gallbladder cancers are associated with gallstones, but the annual incidence of this cancer (20 per 100,000 adults) is low.

Common Syndromes

Acute Syndromes

The 2-year National Cooperative Gallstone Study found that most patients without previous symptoms remained asymptomatic, but "a history of biliary tract pain . . . is highly predictive of future biliary tract pain." Although *biliary colic* is often epigastric, lateralization to the right may be elicited by palpation or fist percussion. Radiation to the back is typical. The pain precludes routine activities; over-the-counter analgesics seldom relieve it. The pain lasts 30 minutes to several hours and does not wax and wane as frequently as intestinal colic. Restlessness and nausea are common. A typical attack leaves the patient unwell for half a day or longer. Protracted pain, vomiting, fever, and localizing signs of peritoneal irritation imply *cholecystitis,* particularly if accompanied by polymorphonuclear leukocytosis. Jaundice, septicemia, or pancreatitis suggests that stones are entering the common bile duct (choledocholithiasis). Cholecystectomy reduces, but does not eliminate, the risk of choledocholithiasis; at least 10% of patients undergoing common duct exploration later suffer from retained or recurrent stones.

Chronic Cholecystitis

Discrete severe attacks distinguish biliary colic and cholecystitis from dyspepsia, bloating, and food intolerance, which have no significance regarding gallstones. The distinction is important because "chronic cholecystitis" is a concept without firm clinical criteria, and its complaints are seldom relieved by cholecystectomy. An internist can safely save several hours a month by avoiding discussion of fatty and fried food except in reference to steatorrhea or hyperlipidemia. Patients subjected to gallbladder surgery for symptoms less specific than biliary pain, with objective findings of stones only, are the main sufferers of another ill-defined disorder—the "postcholecystectomy syndrome."

Cholestasis

Mild icterus sometimes accompanies uncomplicated cholecystitis, but jaundice with pruritus, pale stools, and elevated alkaline phosphatase implies cholestasis. The differential diagnosis ranges from drug or hormonal disruption of hepatic bile secretion to gross lesions impinging on the common bile duct. Gallstones and the strictures induced by biliary surgery are the most frequent benign causes of bile duct obstruction. Pancreatitis and pseudocysts also can impede bile flow. Sclerosing cholangitis affecting intrahepatic and extrahepatic ducts is increasingly recognized in association with inflammatory bowel disease. Obstructing cancers arise frequently from the pancreas, occasionally from the bile duct, and rarely from the duodenum. Most malignant lesions cause unremitting, progressive jaundice and acholic stools, but cancers of the ampulla of Vater, like papillomas and stones, can cause variable cholestasis. Malignant extrahepatic obstruction produces more gallbladder dilatation (Courvoisier's law) and less infection than choledocholithiasis.

Finding Stones

Diagnosis of these syndromes depends on locating stones or another lesion in the biliary tract. Because less than 25% of gallstones contain enough calcium to be identified on plain films, other imaging techniques are necessary. Real-time ultrasonography has become the primary test of choice, matching the oral cholecystogram in accuracy and exceeding it in simplicity and diagnostic range.

Oral cholecystography was the conventional method of demonstrating stones in the gallbladder. Under strictly defined conditions, failure to visualize the gallbladder is indirect evidence of disease. For the examination to be interpretable, the patient should be anicteric and must swallow the tablets on 2 successive days while avoiding dietary fat. Opacification occasionally occurs despite a serum bilirubin as high as 4 mg per dl, but diagnosis of cholelithiasis on the basis of nonvisualization only is reliable in the presence of normal liver function.

Ultrasonography is more sensitive than (98%) and as specific as (95%) oral cholecystography, and avoids radiation exposure. Liver disease, vomiting, and malabsorption do not interfere, but obesity and intestinal gas do. Ultrasonography requires no preparation but is most useful after a brief fast, which lets the gallbladder dilate. The technique also provides information about bile ducts, liver texture, portal vein, and pancreas. Although stones in the common duct are less easily identified than stones in the gallbladder, the width of the common and hepatic ducts is an indirect measure of obstruction.

Radioisotopic scans may assist in the diagnosis of acute cholecystitis, but their reliability is uncertain. An injectable iminodiacetic acid derivative (IDA) is excreted by the liver into bile. Nonscintillation of the gallbladder for 2 hours implies cystic duct obstruction, provided the common bile duct appears.

In summary, ultrasound is usually the first method to look for stones. Questionable findings are occasionally elucidated by oral cholecystography or, in the acutely ill, by IDA scan. The simplicity and safety of ultrasonography, plus the definition obtainable by retrograde or transhepatic cholangiography, leave little role for intravenous cholangiography. Computed tomography (CT) is more useful for evaluating masses in and around the liver, bile ducts, and pancreas than for detecting gallbladder disease.

Evaluating Cholestasis

Many algorithms have been devised for distinguishing between medical and surgical causes of cholestasis. A recent study (O'Connor et al., 1984) affirmed that clinical assessment, based on history, physical examination, and routine laboratory tests, remains the most sensitive screening approach. Imaging techniques are very reliable when they indicate extrahepatic obstruction, but are less reliable for negative conclusions, particularly in mild jaundice. Therefore, the triage proposed in Figure 58-1 should only be followed in the light of conventional clinical judgment.

Ultrasound is the best adjunct to initial assessment. When cancer is strongly suspected, CT may be substituted. If the duct system does not appear dilated, liver biopsy is considered next. If, despite normal duct images, a biliary lesion is strongly suspected, or if biopsy is contraindicated, endoscopic retrograde cholangiopancreatography (ERCP) follows. If imaging shows dilated ducts, the choice between transhepatic and retrograde cholangiography depends on the skills available and the treatment contemplated. Percutaneous transhepatic cholangiography (PTC) is often chosen in the presence of complete obstruction, because the anatomy upstream determines possibilities of surgical bypass. ERCP is usually preferable when obstruction is incomplete and evaluation of the pancreas is pertinent. ERCP is feasible when coagulopathy, peritonitis, or pleural disease makes PTC hazardous. In general, PTC is selected for lesions thought to be at or above the cystic duct, and ERCP is preferred in evaluating periampullary lesions, which may yield positive cytologic results. Although CT-guided needle cytology can prove malignancy of a mass, cholangiography is usually performed to provide a road map for drainage.

Management

Biliary colic is managed with analgesics, including opiates as needed; immediate hospitalization is seldom necessary. The current management of symptomatic stones is surgical, but without signs of peritoneal irritation or cholestasis, spontaneous resolution is usual and the timing of surgery is elective.

Newly available medical treatment with bile acid supplements expands the bile acid pool, facilitating dissolution of cholesterol stones by reducing biliary secretion of cholesterol. The process takes too long for patients with major complications, must be renewed for recurrences, and is ineffective with pigment stones and calcified cholesterol stones. Although 25% of stone-bearers qualify for bile acid supplementation, only 5% dissolve their stones. Undetectable calcification is blamed for the high failure rate. Most "successes" do not truly benefit because they would never have developed complications. Nevertheless, the high prevalence of gallstones implies that 200,000 persons

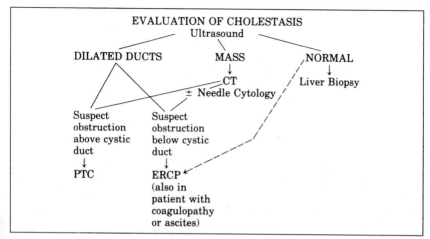

Fig. 58-1. Evaluation of cholestasis: an algorithm whose utility depends on the perspective obtained by history, physical examination, and conventional liver function tests.

in this country would benefit. The issue is patient selection. Oral chenodeoxycholic acid 150 mg/day or ursodeoxycholic acid 600 mg/day may be optimal therapy for thin females with a large operative risk and small radiolucent stones. The side effects are mild diarrhea and minimal liver dysfunction.

Acute cholecystitis and its complications require hospitalization for stabilization and early surgery, as does cholangitis or pancreatitis from common duct stones.

Cholestasis caused by large duct lesions, such as stones and tumors, requires intervention to prevent sepsis and cirrhosis. Endoscopic papillotomy, to drain stagnant bile and stones, is beginning to supplant conventional surgery for choledocholithiasis and ampullary stenosis. Some common duct stones can be reached by retrograde and anterograde cannulation. ERCP and PTC techniques also allow installation of catheters for palliative drainage of malignant obstruction.

Procedural mishaps, discomforts, and expenses* are unconscionable when incurred by overlooking common causes of jaundice not amenable to surgery. These causes include drugs, alcohol and virus. Invasive procedures may be deferred several weeks, as long as the patient is not septic or obviously deteriorating, the ultrasound screening is negative, and the overall impression favors intrahepatic cholestasis.

Asymptomatic gallstones, frequently discovered by ultrasound, do not necessarily call for cholecystectomy. It has been argued that elective surgery prevents carcinoma of the gallbladder and avoids the risk associated with emergency surgery or a complication of gallstones later in life. Despite assuming a relatively high incidence of complications from initially silent stones, Fitzpatrick and colleagues (see references) project life expectancies of operated and unoperated patients that differ little regardless of age, sex, and surgical risk categories. A recent study by Gracie and Ransohoff (see references) shows lower complication rates than those that Fitzpatrick and colleagues assumed. Stones found on screening 123 university faculty members (110 men, 13 women; average age 54) were observed for up to 24 years. The cumulative chances of developing symptoms were 10% by 5 years, 15% by 10 years, and 18% by 15 years; none of the 35 persons at risk over 15 years had symptoms.

For patients with symptoms not clearly related to their stones, an initial period of observation is advisable. Elective cholecystectomy has little mortality among young good-risk patients and is justified when their course fails to dissociate symptoms from stones. The case fatality rate for cholecystectomy rises from 0.2% under age 50 to 6%

*Charges for ultrasound, scintiscan, and liver biopsy are $100 to $200, approximately one-third of the charges for CT, ERCP, and PTC.

over age 70. Older age and cardiopulmonary risk factors favor restraint in response to an equivocal history.

Operations for complications (acute cholecystitis, choledocholithiasis) increase mortality approximately 3-fold in most age and risk groups. There is evidence that common duct exploration increases the hazards of cholecystectomy equally in good-risk and poor-risk patients. These data weaken the argument that the patient with emphysema and asymptomatic stones ought to undergo elective cholecystectomy because a more urgent procedure would subject him or her to *undue* danger. The data do not undermine the counterargument that, because the gallstone complication rate is modest and not increased by lung disease, this patient, facing greater mortality in any surgery, should be treated more conservatively than a comparable subject with normal pulmonary function.

Diabetes is one disorder that may require cholecystectomy for asymptomatic or minimally symptomatic stones. Perhaps neuropathy allows complications of stones to develop more silently in diabetics than in the nondiabetic population. According to uncontrolled studies diabetics with cholecystitis are particularly prone to infections and vascular accidents. These increase disproportionately the hazards of emergency operations. The risks of elective biliary surgery in diabetics appear similar to those of the nondiabetic population.

Gunn A, Keddie N. Some clinical observations on patients with gallstones. *Lancet* 2:239–241, 1972.
  The epigastrium predominated slightly over the right upper quadrant as a primary site of pain from gallstones; the midthoracic spine and right subscapular area were equally frequent referral sites.
Koch JP, Donaldson RM Jr. A survey of food intolerances in hospitalized patients. *N Engl J Med* 271:657–660, 1964.
  Food intolerance investigated in 655 patients did not discriminate between those with and those without gastrointestinal diseases. Of the 390 patients with GI diseases, 30.4% had fatty food intolerance, but of the 120 with GI symptoms and normal x-rays, 30.8% had fatty food intolerance. Among the 145 without prominent GI symptoms, 15.2% acknowledged fatty food intolerance.
Price WH. Gallbladder dyspepsia. *Br Med J* 2:138–141, 1963.
  A prospective study of women aged 50 to 70 in a general medical practice elicited histories of chronic dyspepsia in 12 of 24 who proved to have gallstones, and in 63 of 118 with no stones. The symptom complex did not differ between groups except that fat intolerance was seven times more prevalent among those without stones.
Cooperberg PL, Burhenne HJ. Real-time ultrasonography: Diagnostic technique of choice in calculous gallbladder disease. *N Engl J Med* 302:1277–1279, 1980.
  In 313 patients later proved to have gallstones, the accuracy of real-time ultrasonography was 96%. In prospective comparison, ultrasound revealed stones missed by oral cholecystography (OCG) in 5 of 124 patients, whereas OCG revealed no stones undetected by ultrasound.
Wenckert A, Robertson B. The natural course of gallstone disease: Eleven-year review of 781 nonoperated cases. *Gastroenterology* 50:376–381, 1966.
  The cumulative probability of symptoms was estimated at 6% per year, with major complications at 2% per year.
Lund J. Surgical indications in cholelithiasis: Prophylactic cholecystectomy elucidated on the basis of long-term follow-up on 526 nonoperated cases. *Ann Surg* 151:153–162, 1960.
  This and the preceding reference are widely quoted in support of cholecystectomy for asymptomatic gallstones.
Fitzpatrick GF, Neutra R, Gilbert J. Asymptomatic Gallstones. In WT Branch (Ed.), *Office Practice of Medicine.* Philadelphia: Saunders, 1982. Pp. 703–715.
  Decision analyses based on past data, including the two preceding references, controvert an aggressive approach. The conclusions are reinforced by the following three references.
Gracie WA, Ransohoff DF. The natural history of silent gallstones: The innocent gallstone is not a myth. *N Engl J Med* 307:798–800, 1982.
Ransohoff DF, et al. Prophylactic cholecystectomy vs. expectant management for persons with silent gallstones: A decision analysis to assess survival. *Gastroenterology* 82:1155, 1982.

Thistle JL, et al. The natural history of untreated cholelithiasis during the National Cooperative Gallstone Study. *Gastroenterology* 82:1197, 1982.

O'Connor KW, Snodgrass PJ, et al. A blinded prospective study comparing four current noninvasive approaches in the differential diagnosis of medical vs. surgical jaundice. *Gastroenterology* 84:1498–1504, 1984.

Clinical evaluation is still the most sensitive screening procedure and is more accurate (84%) than ultrasound (78%), computed tomography (81%), or cholescintigraphy (68%). Imaging techniques are more specific and are highly reliable when they indicate extrahepatic obstruction.

Scharachmidt et al. Approach to the patient with cholestatic jaundice. *N Engl J Med* 308:1515–1519, 1983.

Coordinated clinical and cost criteria govern the art in its most lucid form.

59. VIRAL HEPATITIS
Bernard Lo

It is important to distinguish among the several viruses that cause acute viral hepatitis because of differences in patient prognosis and indications for prophylactic treatment of contacts.

Hepatitis A, formerly called infectious hepatitis, is spread by fecal-oral transmission. Fecal excretion of virus starts about 2 weeks before the onset of jaundice and usually ceases by the second week of illness. Hepatitis A is not spread by blood or other body secretions. Transmission is usually person-to-person and sporadic; common-source outbreaks can occur, however, traceable to contaminated water or food and to day-care centers caring for children in diapers. Sexually active male homosexuals are also at increased risk. The illness is self-limited and there is no resulting carrier state or chronic liver disease. In the United States approximately 50% of middle-aged people from a middle-class background have serologic evidence of prior hepatitis A infection.

Hepatitis B, formerly called serum hepatitis, is transmitted by blood, other secretions, contaminated needles and from mother to infant. It is additionally distinguished from hepatitis A by an asymptomatic carrier state and potential sequelae, including chronic persistent or chronic active hepatitis, cirrhosis, and hepatocellular carcinoma. Groups at increased risk for hepatitis B are shown in Table 59-1.

Non-A, non-B hepatitis, the main posttransfusion hepatitis, is caused by several as yet unidentified viruses. It is transmitted by blood, by contaminated needles, and from mother to infant. A chronic carrier state or chronic liver disease may occur. Other viruses, such as Epstein-Barr virus and cytomegalovirus, also may cause acute hepatitis; the liver disease is mild and overshadowed by other clinical features.

Although infection confers immunity to the responsible agent, multiple episodes of acute hepatitis with different viruses are possible. For example, a chronic hepatitis B carrier may develop hepatitis A or non-A, non-B.

Diagnosis

Clinical Evaluation
The history and physical examination help establish the cause and severity of the illness. The classic presentation of acute viral hepatitis is malaise, followed by anorexia, nausea, and right-upper-quadrant discomfort. In icteric patients, jaundice and dark urine occur. The spectrum of disease ranges from asymptomatic and anicteric infections to fulminant hepatitis with coma and death.

History should include the use of all drugs (prescribed, illicit, over-the-counter, and intravenous), as well as transfusions and contact with hepatitis patients. Hepatitis A tends to have a more acute, influenza-like onset and a milder clinical course. Prodromal symptoms of serum-sickness (fever, rash, and arthritis) preceding jaundice suggest hepatitis B.

Nonviral causes of acute hepatitis must be considered in the differential diagnosis:

Table 59-1. High risk groups for hepatitis B infection

	Prevalence of serologic markers of HBV infection	
	HB$_s$Ag (%)	All markers (%)
High risk		
Immigrants/refugees from areas of high HBV endemicity	13	70–85
Users of parenteral drugs	7	60–80
Homosexually active males	6	35–80
Household contacts of HBV carriers	3–6	30–60
Patients of hemodialysis units	3–10	20–80
Intermediate risk		
Prisoners (male)	1–8	10–80
Health care workers with frequent blood contact	1–2	15–30
Low risk		
Health care workers without frequent blood contact	0.3	3–10
Healthy adults (first-time volunteer blood donors)	0.1	3–5

alcohol, drugs (aspirin, acetaminophen, isoniazid, rifampin, methyldopa, and halothane), toxins (paraquat, *Amanita* mushrooms), and infections (syphilis, bacterial sepsis, leptospirosis, and Q fever).

Laboratory Evaluation
Liver function tests show dramatic elevations of transaminases but only moderate elevations of alkaline phosphatase. Elevations of bilirubin are variable; many patients are anicteric, with a bilirubin below 2.5 mg/dl. The degree of elevation of these liver function tests does not indicate the severity of the disease. A better indicator is an abnormal prothrombin time that is not corrected by vitamin K; this finding reflects impaired synthesis of clotting factors. The hemoglobin and white count are usually normal.

Serologic tests are necessary to establish the specific agent responsible for viral hepatitis. IgM anti–hepatitis A virus antibody (anti-HAV) is detectable at the time of clinical illness and is specific for acute hepatitis A. However, IgG anti-HAV is not helpful in the diagnosis of acute infection because it persists for years and may be present from a previous infection.

Serologic tests for hepatitis B include hepatitis B surface antigen (HB$_s$Ag), hepatitis B surface antibody (anti-HB$_s$), hepatitis B core antibody (anti-HB$_c$), and e antigen (HB$_e$Ag). The time course of appearance of these abnormalities is illustrated in Figure 59-1.

HB$_s$Ag is the earliest and most useful marker. In 10% of instances, however, it is never detectable, and in others, it disappears before the patient visits the physician. Moreover, Hb$_s$Ag is not specific for acute hepatitis and may denote chronic rather than acute infection.

Anti-HB$_c$ is found in acute, chronic, or previous infection. IgM anti-HB$_c$ may become a reliable test that is specific for acute infection. Unlike anti-HB$_s$, anti-HB$_c$ does not confer immunity.

The presence of HB$_s$Ab indicates immunity to infection from hepatitis B, although a few cases have been reported of infection in patients with HB$_s$Ab. Such rare patients may have very low titers of HB$_s$Ab, a falsely positive test for HB$_s$Ab, or infection with a different subtype of HB$_s$Ag.

HB$_e$Ag is found only in patients who are positive for HB$_s$Ag. In chronic carriers, patients with chronic HB$_s$Ag hepatitis, and HB$_s$Ag-positive "needlestick donors," it indicates greater infectivity.

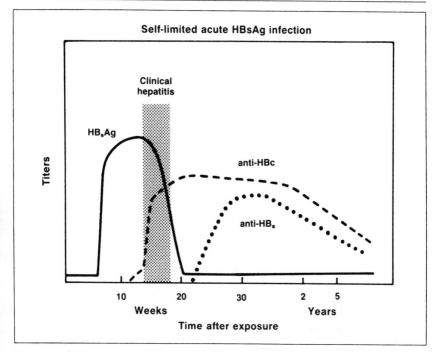

Fig. 59-1. Time course for the appearance of hepatitis B abnormalities.

There are no serologic tests to identify non-A, non-B hepatitis; it remains a diagnosis of exclusion.

Routinely ordering a complete panel of serologic tests in acute hepatitis is costly and unnecessary. In most instances, IgM anti-HAV and HB$_s$Ag are sufficient (Table 59-2). In a few cases, serologic tests do not distinguish acute from chronic hepatitis B infection.

Management

The treatment of all forms of acute hepatitis involves supportive care and avoidance of potential hepatotoxins. For most patients, the disease is self-limited and can be managed on an outpatient basis. Indications for hospitalization are inability to maintain adequate oral intake, insufficient care at home, and fulminant hepatitis (often manifested by encephalopathy and coagulopathy). Activities should be limited mainly by patient symptoms; enforced bed rest in young, otherwise healthy, patients has been shown not to be helpful. Alcohol and drugs that are not essential are usually discontinued because of the fear of additional, drug-induced hepatic damage. However, there is no definitive evidence establishing the danger of drugs. Similarly, there is no evidence that special diets alter the course of the disease.

No medications have been shown to alter the course of acute viral hepatitis. Controlled trials have shown corticosteroids to be of no benefit; they may indeed be detrimental in patients who are Hb$_s$Ag-positive. Vitamin K may correct a prolonged prothrombin time. Sedatives are contraindicated, especially in a patient with agitation or altered mental status, because they can mask or precipitate fulminant hepatitis. If an antiemetic is considered, phenothiazines should be avoided because of the risk of cholestasis as an idiosyncratic reaction.

Liver biopsy is rarely indicated in acute hepatitis. Occasionally it may be used to distinguish viral from alcoholic or drug-related hepatitis. The biopsy results do not alter the treatment, however; also, histologic findings early in acute viral hepatitis do not establish prognosis.

Follow-up of the patient should ensure clinical and biochemical resolution. In hepa-

Table 59-2. Serologic tests in acute viral hepatitis

HB$_s$Ag	IgM anti-HAV	Etiology
−	+	Acute hepatitis A
+	+	Acute hepatitis A in chronic hepatitis B carrier
+	−	Acute hepatitis B or acute non-A, non-B hepatitis in chronic hepatitis B carrier[a]
−	−	Acute hepatitis B or acute non-A, non-B hepatitis[b]

[a]Anti-HB$_c$ would not be useful in distinguishing these possibilities.
[b]Anti-HB$_c$ would distinguish these possibilities; it is positive in acute hepatitis B when HB$_s$Ag is negative, and it is negative in hepatitis non-A, non-B.

titis B, 5 to 10% of patients remain positive for HB$_s$Ag for longer than 6 months. In non-A, non-B hepatitis not related to transfusions, chronic liver disease is rare. Fluctuations in or worsening of liver function test results is common during acute non-A, non-B hepatitis and does not necessarily signify chronic hepatitis. In some patients with chronic infection, liver biopsy may be indicated to provide prognostic information or to guide therapeutic decisions.

Management of Contacts
Household contacts of patients with hepatitis A are at risk; virus shedding has been documented for as long as 2 weeks after the appearance of jaundice, although in most instances it ceases at about 1 week. This risk can be reduced by careful hand washing by the patient after defecation and by administering immune serum globulin (ISG) to household contacts. For adults, 2 cc of ISG administered intramuscularly reduces the incidence of hepatitis in contacts by 70%. Although many adults already have immunity to hepatitis A, screening is unnecessary because ISG is inexpensive and safe.

ISG prophylaxis is not required after casual contact at school or work. It should, however, be considered in two special situations. In day care centers, staff and children exposed to a child in diapers with hepatitis A may be given ISG. Also, because a food handler with hepatitis A may cause a common-source outbreak, ISG should be considered for patrons and other employees of a restaurant.

Because hepatitis B is spread by blood, saliva, and semen, intimate and sexual contacts of the patient are at risk; casual contacts, however, such as colleagues at work, are not at risk. Kissing, sexual intercourse, and sharing eating utensils, razors, toothbrushes, and intravenous needles should be discontinued until the patient no longer has HB$_s$Ag. In most patients, HB$_s$Ag disappears by a few weeks after the resolution of clinical illness.

Hepatitis B immune globulin (HBIG), which contains high titers of anti-HB$_s$, may be effective prophylaxis for sexual contacts. In one study, HBIG reduced the incidence of clinical hepatitis in sexual partners to 4% from 27% in controls given ISG with no detectable titers of HB$_s$Ag but did not benefit household contacts. In another study, 19% of contacts receiving one dose of HBIG (titers of HB$_s$Ab greater than 1:65,000) developed serologic evidence of infection, compared to 15% of contacts receiving recently manufactured ISG with 1:128 titers of HB$_s$Ab and 11% of contacts receiving ISG with 1:16 titers of HB$_s$Ab. Although these differences were not statistically significant, the small sample precluded finding a statistically significant result. Based on these limited data, the Centers for Disease Control (CDC) now recommends one 5 cc dose of HBIG for sexual contacts. HBIG is probably ineffective if given later than 14 days after the last contact. Screening the contact for susceptibility is reasonable if it will not delay the administration of HBIG and if the contact is likely to be already positive for HB$_s$Ag or HB$_s$Ab. Homosexual contacts should receive hepatitis B vaccine with HBIG. Heterosexual contacts should receive a second dose of HBIG if the index case is still positive for HB$_s$Ag three months later.

Management of Hb$_s$Ag Carriers

HB$_s$Ag carriers comprise about 0.2% of the general population and up to 10% of the high-risk groups outlined in Table 59-1. The evaluation of carriers should include a careful history and physical examination, and liver function tests. Symptoms of liver disease (jaundice, malaise, anorexia, and weight loss) and a history of intravenous drug use or exposure to blood should be sought. If this evaluation is negative, liver biopsy is not indicated, because it shows serious disease (chronic active hepatitis, cirrhosis, or hepatocellular carcinoma) in fewer than 5% of patients. Although a liver biopsy may give diagnostic or prognostic information, it unfortunately does not lead to effective therapy.

Sexual and household contacts of HB$_s$Ag carriers are at risk for developing hepatitis B. Carriers positive for HB$_e$Ag are especially contagious; serologic evidence of infection develops in 78% of their sexual contacts, compared to only 25% of contacts of patients who are HB$_e$Ag-negative. However, testing for HB$_e$Ag is not clinically useful because patients who are negative may still be contagious. The presence of HB$_e$Ag does not increase the risk for nonsexual household contacts.

HBIG is not effective prophylaxis for contacts of carriers because of its short-term effect. However, hepatitis B vaccine probably will prove effective.

Prevention of Hepatitis B

Vaccine
Inactivated hepatitis B vaccine is over 90% effective in reducing subsequent hepatitis B in male homosexuals and in dialysis patients and staff. It will probably be shown effective for other high-risk groups: household contacts of HB$_s$Ag carriers, cancer patients, drug addicts, patients and staff in institutions for the mentally retarded, health-care workers with frequent blood contact, and children of HB$_s$Ag-positive mothers. Adults who are not in these high-risk groups do not require vaccination.

Vaccination is unnecessary in people who are immune (positive for anti-HB$_s$) or who are carriers of HB$_s$Ag. Screening is cost-effective before vaccination when the expected prevalence of serologic markers and the attack rate are high, as in male homosexuals. One decision analysis recommended vaccination without screening when the prevalence of serologic markers is low but the annual attack rate is high, as in surgical house staff. However, this recommendation is controversial; when indirect costs such as worry about the long-term effects of the vaccine and patient time are considered, screening before vaccination becomes a reasonable approach for surgery house staff.

The best screening test before vaccination is anti-HB$_s$, which indicates immunity. Screening with anti-HB$_c$ has been suggested because this test is positive in almost all HB$_s$Ag carriers and in most patients with anti-HB$_s$. However, as many as 22% of patients positive for anti-HB$_c$ are negative for anti-HB$_s$. Such patients would be incorrectly classified as immune by anti-HB$_c$ screening because anti-HB$_c$ is not protective.

Immunization requires three doses, with the second and third doses given after 1 and 6 months. Immediate side effects are no greater than with placebo. The long-term risks are unknown, but none have been detected in up to 5 years. Anti-HB$_s$ is induced in over 90% of healthy recipients and lasts for at least 5 years. Giving the vaccine to patients who are already positive for Hb$_s$Ag or anti-HB$_s$ appears safe.

Indications for vaccination and guidelines for screening undoubtedly will change as more information is available and as costs are reduced.

PASSIVE-ACTIVE IMMUNIZATION. Giving both HBIG and vaccine induces both immediate and long-term protection against infection. The simultaneous administration of HBIG does not reduce the effectiveness of the vaccine. Studies on infants of mothers positive for HB$_s$Ag have shown that passive-active immunization is 90% effective. Generalizing from this neonatal data, the CDC now recommends combined passive-active immunization for needlestick, ocular, or mucous-membrane exposure to HB$_s$Ag positive blood, even though no clinical studies of passive-active immunization have been carried out in these settings.

NEEDLESTICK EXPOSURE. Accidental innoculation with blood of hepatitis patients is a hazard for some health care workers. Because of cost, prophylaxis with HBIG or vaccine is given only when "donor" blood is proved positive for HB$_s$Ag. Donors who have acute hepatitis or who are in the high-risk groups (see Table 59-1) should be tested for HB$_s$Ag. A single dose of ISG may be given while awaiting results. If the donor is positive for HB$_s$Ag, one dose of HBIG and the first dose of vaccine are given to the recipient as soon as possible after exposure. The remaining two doses of vaccine are given as usual 1 and 6 months later. A second dose of HBIG is not necessary.

Alternatively, HBIG alone without vaccine can be given after exposure. The first dose of HBIG is given as soon as possible, a second dose is given one month later. In one study, HBIG reduced the incidence of abnormal serum transaminases from 5.9% to 1.4% in this setting.

If the "donor" is unlikely to be positive for HB_sAg (e.g., a hospitalized patient without liver disease), testing for HB_sAg and administering HBIG are not cost-effective and are not recommended. In such low-risk situations and in situations in which the "donor" cannot be identified, ISG is often given as prophylaxis, although there is no evidence that it is effective.

Dienstag JL, Szmuness W, Stevens CE, Purcell RH. Hepatitis A virus infection: New insights from seroepidemiologic studies. *J Infect Dis* 137:328–340, 1978.
Epidemiologic and clinical review of hepatitis A.

Hoofnagle JH. Serologic markers of hepatitis B virus infection. *Ann Rev Med* 32:1–11, 1981.
Concise review of hepatitis B serology.

Dienstag JL. Hepatitis non-A, non-B. *Gastroenterology* 85:639–652, 1983.
Thorough clinical review of non-A, non-B hepatitis.

Immune globulins for protection against viral hepatitis. *Ann Intern Med* 96:193–197, 1982.
Recommendations of the Centers for Disease Control for ISG and HBIG.

Seeff LB, Hoofnagle JH. Immunoprophylaxis of viral hepatitis. *Gastroenterology* 77:161–182, 1979.
Extensive review of evidence for usefulness of ISG and HBIG, together with authors' recommendations.

Inactivated hepatitis B virus vaccine. *Ann Intern Med* 97:379–383, 1982.
Review of hepatitis vaccine and recommendations of the Centers for Disease Control.

Mulley AG, Silverstein MD, Dienstag JL. Indications for use of hepatitis B vaccine, based on cost-effectiveness analysis. *N Engl J Med* 307:644–652, 1982.
Decision analysis of different strategies for screening and vaccination for hepatitis B.

Postexposure prophylaxis of hepatitis B. *Ann Intern Med* 101:351–354, 1984.
New recommendations for passive-active immunization after needlestick exposure and for HBIG in sexual contacts of patients with acute hepatitis B.

Perrillo RP, Campbell CR, Strang S et al. Immune globulin and hepatitis B immune globulin. *Arch Intern Med* 144:81–85, 1984.
A single dose of recently manufactured ISG was as effective as one dose of HBIG. However, because of the small sample size, a type II error is likely.

Seeff LB, Koff RS. Passive and active immunoprophylaxis of hepatitis B. *Gastroenterology* 86:958–81, 1984.
Recent comprehensive, thoughtful review.

IX. URINARY PROBLEMS

Axalla J. Hoole

Lower urinary tract infections are common in females; infections in males occur much less frequently and have a more serious connotation. The symptoms of lower-tract infections—dysuria and urinary frequency—are the presenting complaints in 5 to 10% of patients in a primary care practice. Of these patients, 50 to 75% have either a first-time or recurrent bacterial infection (predominantly cystitis). The remainder have either the urethral syndrome (symptoms of cystitis without identifiable bacteria) or vaginitis (up to 10% in some series).

Infection is traditionally established by urine cultures of greater than 100,000 colony-forming units per milliliter of urine. Unfortunately, this definition was established by comparing patients with pyelonephritis to asymptomatic controls. When this criterion is applied to an ambulatory population, no more than 50% of patients with dysuria have bacterial infection. In recent studies of symptomatic patients, urine specimens obtained by suprapubic aspiration frequently grew a single species of coliform bacteria in concentrations of less than 100,000 colonies per milliliter. These data suggest that in symptomatic patients colony counts of less than 10^5 may be associated with cystitis; these data also increase from 50% to nearly 75% the proportion of women with dysuria who may have bacterial cystitis.

Causes

Bacteria enter the urinary tract from the vaginal introitus, which under normal conditions does not harbor pathogenic bacteria. However, colonization of the introitus by pathogenic bacteria has been shown to precede infection. A group of women has been identified in whom introital colonization readily occurs because of a property of the vaginal mucosal cell that allows pathogenic bacteria to adhere. Although these patients have more infections than their matched cohorts, the clinical application of this observation is not clear.

The conditions under which pathogenic bacteria from the vaginal introitus enter the bladder are uncertain. There are few studies that have examined the relation between intercourse and infection, but the available evidence suggests that it is possible for bacteria to be introduced into the bladder during intercourse, presumably by mechanical milking of the urethra. That the bacteria so introduced lead to infection has not been shown, but the frequency of "honeymoon cystitis" supports this conclusion. Other studies suggest that women who resist the urge to urinate have more infections than those who urinate on demand.

Organisms

Escherichia coli is identified in 80 to 90% of nonhospitalized women with bacterial infection. *Staphylococus saprophyticus,* the second most frequently identified bacterium, is often discarded by laboratories as a contaminant. However, *S. saprophyticus* has been obtained by suprapubic aspiration from symptomatic patients and should not be ignored. Other gram-negative species, such as *Klebsiella* species and *Proteus* species, are infrequently found in ambulatory patients.

In those patients in whom no bacteria are found and who are said to have the urethral syndrome, the cause of symptoms is much more difficult to establish. Viruses, fungi, and mycobacteria have rarely been found; however, *Chlamydia trachomatis* has recently been identified in many of these patients. In addition to microbial agents, allergies or reactions to chemicals, soaps, and deodorants, and, rarely, cancer of the bladder, should be considered.

Evaluation

There are several problems which must be considered when evaluating patients with symptoms of cystitis: identification of infection, location of infection (upper or lower tract), and distinguishing between reinfection and relapse when there are recurrences. Evaluation begins by identifying patients with vaginitis or overt pyelonephritis. A history of vaginal discharge and external urethral burning rather than internal dysuria suggests vaginitis; temperature greater than 99.5°F, systemic complaints, or flank pain suggests pyelonephritis. Patients with a history of urinary tract stones or anatomic abnormalities, diabetes, or immunologic diseases may have complicated infections that need to be treated more vigorously than cystitis.

The history also may help separate relapse from reinfection. Reinfection is a sporadic event with no clear temporal relation to previous infections; relapse frequently recurs within weeks of a previous infection or the cessation of treatment. However, there is no absolute number of infections or number per year that means relapse and demands that urologic investigation be undertaken.

Previous culture results also aid in separating reinfection from relapse. With reinfections, the results of cultures change with each episode, whereas in relapse the causal bacteria usually remain the same from episode to episode and retain the same antibiotic sensitivities.

Laboratory Tests
Examination of urine is used at the time of the patient's visit to make the tentative diagnosis of infection, and a urine culture with antibiotic sensitivities has been recommended to confirm the diagnosis and direct therapy. There is no convenient and specific test for outpatient use that can separate upper- from lower-tract disease.

Urinalysis
Obtaining a proper specimen is often a problem. In-and-out catheterization and suprapubic aspiration of the bladder provide the most reliably uncontaminated urine but are impractical on a routine basis. Therefore, every effort should be made to collect a clean, mid-voided bladder urine sample, even if collection as well as instruction must be done by a nurse. This specimen if properly obtained correlates well with samples obtained by catheterization. Except in patients with long-standing bladder irritation, squamous epithelial cells usually denote an improperly collected specimen.

Bacteriuria
An unspun specimen and sediment from 10 cc of spun urine should be stained and examined for bacteria. A Gram's-stained slide is preferred; however, methylene blue, which highlights bacteria and WBCs, may be substituted. In an unspun specimen, it is generally accepted that the presence of two bacteria per high-powered field (HPF) has a good correlation with colony counts of 10^5 per milliliter. In a urine sediment, at least 10 bacteria are usually present when there is a culture of 100,000 colonies or more, but even small numbers of bacteria in a sediment should correlate well with low colony counts.

Pyuria
Pyuria has not been considered a sensitive test for infection; 20 WBCs per HPF of sediment has less than a 50% correlation with 10^5 colonies. In symptomatic patients, however, pyuria is a more sensitive indicator of infection when low colony counts are considered significant. In a recent study, urine was obtained by suprapubic aspiration from patients with symptoms of cystitis. Pyuria, defined in this study as eight or more WBCs per cubic millimeter of unspun urine, was present in almost all patients with bacterial counts greater than or equal to 10^2 or with positive chlamydial cultures.

Urine Culture
The urine culture has been used routinely to verify infection, but treatment is almost always begun before the results of cultures are known. Also, practice surveys have shown that culture results are thereafter rarely incorporated into management of routine cases. Because bacteriuria and pyuria appear sensitive enough for identifying infection, and clinical findings can indicate those patients with lower-tract disease (see Therapeutic Trial), ritual cultures seem expensive and unnecessary in most ambulatory patients in whom resistant organisms are unusual. Instances in which resistant or unusual organisms might be found and cultures would be indicated would be marked by recurrence or other features, such as recent hospitalization, previous stones, or diabetes.

Antibody Coating of Bacteria

Parenchymal infection of the kidney, unlike superficial infections of the lower urinary tract, is frequently associated with the production of antibodies. Therefore, evaluation of bacteria for antibody coating (ABC) should separate upper-tract from lower-tract infection. Unfortunately, the sensitivity and specificity of this test are not high. Among the difficulties are false-negative results in early pyelonephritis and false-positive results in long-standing cystitis. Also, this test is rarely available on the day of evaluation. These problems reduce the usefulness of the ABC in ambulatory care.

Therapeutic Trial

Another method for separating upper- from lower-tract disease, the therapeutic trial, combines treatment with diagnosis. Acute cystitis, because it is a superficial infection of the mucosa, should respond to almost any antibiotic that reaches a high urine concentration. Recently, a number of drugs have been evaluated in single-dose regimens. In virtually 100% of patients who were ABC-negative, a single high dose of an antibiotic was effective in treating the lower-tract disease. Those who were ABC-positive were treated in the conventional manner, and there was a 25 to 40% recurrence of infection. This observation suggests a clinical method for separating lower- and upper-tract disease. Those who respond to single-dose therapy have lower-tract disease; those who do not respond or relapse within a few days need to be re-evaluated.

Treatment

Because of concern that patients with lower-tract symptoms may have upper-tract disease, protocols for management of cystitis have traditionally involved identification and treatment of potential upper-tract infection. These protocols, which require culture, 2 weeks of therapy, and several follow-up cultures, are expensive and impractical for outpatient management of cystitis and have not been followed by many patients or physicians.

Current evidence suggests that infection can be identified by urinalysis, and the location of infection predicted by response to single-dose therapy. The proportion of ambulatory patients who are ABC-negative and most susceptible to single-dose therapy has varied from 8% in one clinic setting to 60% in another. The one variable that is significantly related to the number of ABC-positive tests is the duration of symptoms before the patient seeks medical attention. Delay of longer than 3 days generally results in increased numbers of positive tests and corresponding failures of single-dose treatment.

In a recent study, patients with symptoms of cystitis were randomly treated with amoxicillin with either single-dose or 14-day therapy, based only on the clinical diagnosis. Treatment was begun before culture results were known and without antibody coating. There was no difference between the results of the two groups.

The number of studies using single-dose therapy is still small. However, the practicality of treating appropriate patients with short courses of antibiotics without routine cultures makes the method compelling. Advantages cited are the lower expense, fewer side effects, and better compliance.

Patients with cystitis may be started on single dose antibiotics without culture if:

1. Symptoms have persisted less than 3 days
2. Vaginitis or overt upper-tract infection is not present
3. No complicating factors exist, such as diabetes, urinary tract stones, anatomic abnormalities, pregnancy, or frequent recurrences
4. The patient can be relied on to return for follow-up visits

Single-Dose Regimens

Successful single-dose regimens include amoxicillin, 3.0 gm, or four tablets of trimethoprim-sulfamethoxazole combination, each containing 80 mg of trimethoprim and 400 mg of sulfamethoxazole. The necessity of follow-up should be emphasized to the patient. Most authorities suggest that a culture is necessary after completion of therapy. Patients who relapse within several days or weeks should be cultured, treated with conventional therapy for at least 2 weeks, and additionally evaluated if necessary.

Conventional Drug Regimens
The most practical regimen has been sulfamethoxazole, 500 mg four times a day for 10 to 14 days. This is one of the cheapest drugs available and is effective against most of the bacteria seen in ambulatory practice. However, many patients who ordinarily would be treated with this regimen are candidates for short-term therapy.

Treatment of Urethral Syndrome
In many instances in which WBCs are present in a urinary sediment but no bacteria are found, *Chlamydia trachomatis* has been identified. For these patients a more effective regimen might be tetracycline, 500 mg four times a day for at least 7 days.

Occasionally, dysuria occurs without bacteriuria or pyuria. This symptom may occur with many diseases or with emotional problems. These patients may be given phenazopyridine (Pyridium) and followed while problems are evaluated.

Prevention of Recurrences
Recurrence of infection may occur because medicine was not taken, a resistant organism was present, or there is relapse from an inadequately treated focus. Usually recurrence comes from reinfection from below, rather than from a relapse of an incompletely treated infection, in the presence of a lesion such as a kidney stone or calyceal diverticulum.

Several studies clearly show that the frequency of recurrent attacks can be decreased by trimethroprim (40 mg)–sulfamethoxazole (160 mg) combination, one-half tablet per day. Other agents, such as methenamine mandelate (Mandelamine), nitrofurantoin, and sulfamethoxazole alone, are less effective but better than placebo.

In those women in whom recurrences are clearly related to sexual activity, a postcoital dose of 500 mg of sulfamethoxazole decreases the number of infections.

Fang LST, et al. Efficacy of single-dose and conventional amoxicillin therapy in urinary tract infection localized by the antibody-coated bacteria technique. *N Engl J Med*, 298:413–416, 1978.
An essay report on the effectiveness of single-dose therapy.
Stamm WE. Single-dose treatment of cystitis. *JAMA* 244(6):591, 1980. (Editorial).
A good review.
Thomas VL, Forland M. Antibody-coated bacteria in urinary tract infections. *Int Soc Nephrol* 21(1982):1–7, 1981.
An excellent, up-to-date review.
Kunin CM. Duration of treatment of urinary tract infections. *Am J Med* 71:849–851, 1981.
An excellent, up-to-date review.
Savard-Fenton M, et al. Single-dose amoxicillin therapy with follow-up urine culture. *Am J Med* 73:808–813, 1982.
Patients were randomly assigned to groups that were treated with either single-dose or conventional therapy. There was no significant difference in the outcomes.
Stamm WE, et al. Causes of urethral syndrome in women. *N Engl J Med* 303:409–415, 1980.
Presentation of evidence suggesting Chlamydia trachomatis *and bacteria with low colony counts as causes of dysuria.*
Komaroff AL. Acute dysuria in women. *N Engl J Med* 310:368–375, 1984.
A review of evaluation and management of lower urinary tract infections.

61. PROSTATITIS

Axalla J. Hoole

The prostate gland is frequently the site of painful and inflammatory problems in postpubescent men. Infections are common, but because of difficulties in obtaining cultures, syndromes that appear to be of infectious origin are often associated with urine and prostatic secretions that are sterile. Lack of clear delineation has resulted in the development of several competing classifications for prostate problems. Recently, the following convention for painful diseases of the prostate was considered.

Acute prostatitis is a systemic, febrile disease, invariably associated with a tender prostate. There is frequently low back and perineal pain as well as dysuria and obstructive symptoms. Although prostatic secretions may contain many leukocytes and bacteria, prostatic massage is not advisable because bacteremia and sepsis may result.

Chronic bacterial prostatitis usually presents with low back or perineal pain that sometimes radiates into the anterior thighs, inguinal region, or testes. There also may be pain associated with bowel movements. Occasionally, symptoms of urinary obstruction and nonpurulent early-morning urethral discharge are present. On physical examination, the prostate is tender and boggy, and usually, somewhat enlarged. Often the pain from massage mimics the original pain, even referring to the same areas. Prostatic secretions contain greater than 10 to 20 WBCs per HPF, and bacteria on smear or culture.

Chronic nonbacterial prostatitis has symptoms similar to those of chronic bacterial prostatitis and is differentiated from it by examination of prostatic fluid, which contains greater than 10 to 20 WBCs per HBF but no bacteria.

Prostatodynia is associated with painful symptoms like those of chronic prostatitis, but neither WBCs nor bacteria are found on examination of prostatic secretions.

With this classification, other terms, such as *prostatosis* and *pelvic floor myalgia*, have been discouraged.

Pathogenesis

Prostate infection can occur in all males but is unusual both before sexual activity and during continued celibacy. Infections are distributed through the decades, with an increase in the later years. Acute prostatits may occur without previous evidence of urinary tract disease in young males; however, in older men acute prostatitis often occurs in association with symptoms of chronic obstruction and may be superimposed on benign prostatic hypertrophy. In fact, in the elderly small areas of inflammation and infection can be found in virtually all glands.

Bacteria in almost all instances ascend to the prostate through the urethra. However, there is no agreement on the bacteria that are causal. In some studies grampositive bacteria (predominantly *Staphylococcus epidermidis*) have been identified in a large number of patients. Many investigators believe that these organisms have not been shown not to be contaminants. The usual gram-negative urinary pathogens (predominantly *Escherichia coli*) are thought by many to be the primary bacterial pathogens. With increasing age, the percentage of gram-negative pathogens increases. *Chlamydia trachomatis* and *Myoplasma hominis* have been identified, but *Trichomonas vaginalis* and viruses have not. Although unusual genitorectal infections are being reported in male homosexuals, there are few cases of prostatitis among them.

Using localization techniques, bacteria have been found in only 10 to 50% of patients with symptoms of chronic prostatitis. Because only small areas of the gland may be infected, obtaining bacteria by massage or biopsy is unreliable. Also, prostatic secretions contain an antibacterial factor recently identified as zinc salts. Prostatic fluid may therefore have an unpredictable inhibitory effect in bacterial cultures. Additionally, chronic prostatitis may be caused by fastidious organisms that are difficult to identify by the usual culture techniques. Prostatodynia and chronic nonbacterial prostatitis are thus diagnoses of exclusion and may represent limitations of our ability to investigate the prostate. As newer techniques are employed, it is probable that fewer patients will be diagnosed as having these problems.

Diagnosis

Acute disease can be identified by the history, physical examination, and presence of WBCs and bacteria in urinalysis and urine culture.

Because the chronic painful prostate diseases all present with the same symptoms, diagnosis depends on collection of expressed prostatic fluid or urine that contains prostatic fluid. This can be accomplished by obtaining and saving the following specimens: (1) the first 10 ml of urine (containing urethral bacteria), (2) a midstream (bladder bacteria) specimen, (3) any prostatic secretions obtained from prostatic massage, and (4) a postmassage urine (containing prostatic bacteria) if no prostatic discharge is initially obtained. Bacterial growth in the prostatic secretions or postmassage urine is most significant when compared to cultures of early or midstream urine.

Because secretions may not be readily produced by massage, a midstream urine sample should be collected before examining the patient, and the patient should be asked to retain a few milliliters of urine in the bladder. If prostatic examination and massage do not produce sufficient fluid, the patient should empty his bladder. This urine should contain bacteria that have been expressed into the prostatic urethra, and can be compared to urethral or bladder urine obtained earlier. If there is an obvious infection, cultures need not be done, but they should be obtained if the patient has a complicated or persistent problem.

Zinc and pH levels in prostatic fluid have been suggested as markers for infection; however, neither of these has been used successfully as a diagnostic test for chronic prostatitis.

Treatment

Patients with *acute prostatitis* are usually treated as outpatients. Hospitalization may be required if sepsis, nausea and vomiting, urinary retention, or other medical problems such as diabetes are present. Antibiotic therapy is begun immediately and changed according to sensitivity patterns. In acute prostatitis, most antibiotics penetrate the prostate well. Any antibiotic to which the usual bacterial pathogens are susceptible may be used. Ampicillin, cephalosporins, and tetracycline are most frequently recommended.

In *chronic prostatitis,* the treatment, like the diagnosis, is not straightforward. Oral antibiotics should be used in those in whom bacteria can be identified. However, because of the difficulty in isolating bacteria or the possible presence of other agents such as *Chlamydia* or *M. hominis,* antibiotics are frequently started on the basis of greater than 10 WBC per HPF in prostatic fluid.

The choice of antibiotics is limited because of poor penetration into prostatic fluid. Among the tetracyclines, which in general have poor penetrance, doxycycline has been shown to have adequate lipid solubility to appear in prostatic secretions. Erythromycin, which also achieves therapeutic levels in the prostate, is effective against gram-positive bacteria. Both are effective against pathogens associated with nonbacterial prostatitis. A combination of trimethroprim and sulfamethoxazole is useful in managing some infections, but penetration into prostatic fluid is very sensitive to prostatic fluid pH, and the drug frequently does not reach therapeutic levels in the infected prostate.

Doxycycline is the drug of first choice because it is effective against both gram-negative urinary pathogens and *C. trachomatis,* and other agents associated with nonbacterial prostatitis. Although there are few data supporting the optimum duration of antibiotic therapy, most authors have empirically chosen 6 weeks for prospective trials.

Other therapeutic maneuvers, such as prostatic massage, sitz baths, and antispasmodics, are mentioned in reviews but are supported by few data other than anecdotes testifying to their effectiveness. One study did show that massage decreased the size of the prostate gland, but no mention was made of change in symptoms. Practical experience suggests that massage is useful in prostatodynia but should be avoided when infection is present. Because prostatic inflammation may be associated with periurethral spasm, a variety of antispasmodics have been used. However, evidence for their efficacy is usually anecdotal. Similarly, sitz baths are a reasonable, but unproven, recommendation.

Neither alcohol nor sexual activity is contraindicated. Excretion of alcohol may burn the inflamed urethra, but sexual activity may decrease prostatic congestion and decrease pain in patients who have prostatodynia. On ejaculation, contraction of the prostatic urethra may provide internal massage.

In patients who relapse after 6 weeks of therapy, a second course of antibiotics may be tried. Many patients continue to have relapses. Recurrences may be suppressed by daily antibiotic therapy. If obstruction and infection persist after adequate medical treatment, surgery may be necessary.

Surgical treatment in chronic prostatitis is controversial. If the prostate is the cause of obstructive symptoms and changes, such as nocturia, decreased stream, large postvoid residual urines (> 50 cc), or bladder trabeculation, then surgical removal of the obstructive tissue (adenoma or benign prostatic hyperplasia) may be curative. In the absence of the symptoms and bladder changes of obstruction, surgical therapy is less likely to be beneficial. Some patients with debilitating chronic prostatitis have had total prostatectomy. This treatment causes impotence and sometimes incontinence. Clearly, potential benefit has to be weighed against these complications. The use of lesser procedures, such as transurethral resection of the prostate for chronic prostatitis, in the absence of obstruction, benefits only about one patient in four. The remaining patients are unchanged or become symptomatically worse.

Management of *prostatodynia* remains difficult. Despite the fact that patients with these symptoms can not be shown to be infected. The symptoms are consistent with prostate disease. Urologic evaluation may reveal decreased urinary flow rates and increased internal sphincter tone. Frequently, however, no lesion is identified. Prostatodynia also may be part of a complex psychosexual problem. For many patients, reassurance is all that is needed; in others, diazepam, 2 mg three to four times a day, may help relieve muscle spasm, or sitz baths and massage may alleviate symptoms. However, an occasional patient may require psychiatric counseling.

Drach GW, et al. Classification of benign diseases associated with prostatic pain: Prostatitis or prostatodynia? *Urol* 120:266, 1978 (Letter to the Editor).
   A letter establishing a workable classification system for painful prostatic disease.
Drach GW. Prostatitis: Man's hidden infection. *Urol Clin North Am* 2(3):499–520, 1975.
   An excellent review of the problem; however, it came from the early trimethoprim era and needs updating.
Drach GW. Prostatitis and prostatodynia. *Urol Clin North Am* 7(1):79–88, 1980.
   A short, but helpful update of the preceding reference.
Fair W. A reappraisal of treatment in chronic bacterial prostatitis. *J Urol* 121:437–441, 1979.
   A discussion of the failure of trimethoprim to live up to its billing.
Fair W. Prostatic antibacterial factor. *Urology* 7(2):169–177, 1976.
   The author suggests an identity for this substance.
Meares EM. Bacteriological localization patterns in bacterial prostatitis and urethritis. *Invest Urol* 5(5):492–516, 1968.
   A report of research on the development of a technique for localizing bacteria from the prostate.
Ristuccia M, Cunha A. Current concepts of antimicrobial therapy of prostatitis. *Urology* 20(3):338–345, 1982.
   An excellent discussion of factors controlling antibiotic penetration into prostatic fluid and a review of current recommendations.

62. BENIGN PROSTATIC HYPERPLASIA
J. Pack Hindsley, Jr.

Benign prostatic hyperplasia (BPH), often called benign prostatic hypertrophy, is the growth of a benign adenoma of periurethral glands that may cause obstruction to the outflow of urine in older men. BPH is uncommon before 40 years of age, but increases in frequency rapidly over the next several decades. The overall prevalence in men over 40 is 80%, increasing to 95% in men 80 and older. Gross obstruction from BPH occurs in 20% of men aged 50 to 60, 30% of men 60 to 70, and 50% of men over 80 years of age.

Etiology
The cause of BPH is unknown, but several observations suggest that normal testes are a necessary condition for its occurrence. Eunuchs do not develop BPH, and there is regression of BPH after castration. The adenoma accumulates much higher levels of dihydrotestosterone than does normal prostatic tissue. These observations suggest that adenomatous tissues use androgenic hormones differently from normal tissue, but the intracellular changes that may result are unknown.

Under the influence of androgenic hormones, and possibly also estrogenic hormones, the periurethral glands of the mature prostate gradually undergo hyperplasia. The adenoma gradually displaces the "true" prostate peripherally and encroaches on the central prostatic urethra, causing obstruction. The fully developed prostatic adenoma is analogous to an orange; the adenoma represents the fleshy part of the orange, and the true prostate represents the rind.

The hyperplastic prostatic adenoma may be composed of any proportion or combination of glandular, fibrous, and muscular tissues. If glandular elements predominate, the adenoma is likely to be mobile and pushed aside by the force of the urinary stream. It therefore may become quite large before severe obstructive symptoms occur. If fibrous or muscular elements predominate, the prostatic urethra is not nearly as distensible, and a much smaller adenoma can cause severe obstruction. Thus, the size of the prostate is not as important as the architecture.

The bladder compensates for obstruction in BPH by increasing the force of contraction to expel the stored urine. As the bladder wall becomes more hypertrophic, it becomes less distensible, and a sensation of fullness occurs more quickly. The bladder also may be unable to generate sufficient pressure to expel the last quantity of stored urine, leading to postvoid residual urine. If the bladder is required to generate increasingly high voiding pressures over a long period of time, the muscle bundles may separate and the inner and mucosal layers herniate outward, resulting in bladder diverticula. Thus, when the bladder contracts, urine is forced into the diverticulum, and when the bladder relaxes, urine drains back into the bladder as postvoid residual urine. The symptoms of bladder outlet obstruction, such as frequency, decreased caliber and force of urinary stream, hesitancy, and nocturia, are readily explained by the secondary compensatory changes to outlet obstruction.

Evaluation

History

The symptoms of outlet obstruction are much more reliable indicators of the need for a surgical procedure than is the size of the prostate gland. The most reliable symptoms are hesitancy and nocturia. Hesitancy implies slow or delayed starting of the urinary stream. The patient may well have to use his abdominal muscles and strain to generate enough pressure to force open the prostatic urethra.

Nocturia, or nighttime voiding, in which the patient is awakened by the need to void 2 or 3 times at night, is a moderately severe symptom and usually indicates the need for a surgical procedure. Nocturia indicates short intervals before the sensation to void is again elicited, which implies inelasticity of the bladder wall with inadequate storage capacity and/or postvoid residual urine.

Physical Examination

The size of the gland does not always correlate with the degree of obstruction. Small fibrous glands or glands with growth medially may be more obstructive than larger, boggy glands.

Postvoid Residual

Measurement of postvoid residual urine by catheterizing the bladder is not now routinely used for evaluation of bladder function in patients with suspected BPH. Traumatic catheterization may cause lacerations, hematuria, and edema sufficient to produce urinary retention. Urinary instrumentation may also introduce infection into an otherwise uninfected bladder.

Intravenous Pyelogram

When history and physical examination findings suggests outlet obstruction, an excretory urogram, or intravenous pyelogram (IVP), is the next logical step. Findings such as hydronephrosis, bladder diverticula, and large postvoid residual suggest that decompensation of the bladder is severe and are indications for surgery. Findings such as "J hooking" of the ureters, trabeculation of the bladder wall, and moderate postvoid residual urine are relative indications for surgery. Patients with only moderate bladder decompensation are more likely to recover normal urinary function than those with severe decompensation. If the IVP demonstrates normal kidneys and good bladder emptying on postvoid films, surgery is not indicated. Some authors recommend routine cystometrograms for all patients being evaluated for bladder outlet obstruction. In patients who have no suspected neurologic diseases, the yield is quite low, and the recommendation results in excessive and unnecessary examinations.

Cystoscopy

Before surgery a cystoscopy is usually performed to rule out other pathology, such as strictures and bladder tumors, and to evaluate the size and configuration of the prostate to determine which type of operation is most appropriate. Because cystoscopy may cause hematuria, infection, or acute urinary retention in patients with BPH, it is usually reserved until it is evident that surgery is necessary.

Treatment

There is no appropriate proven medical therapy in the treatment of BPH. Several studies have shown partial resolution of outlet obstructive symptoms with administration of exogenous estrogens and antiandrogens in some, but not all, patients. These treatments cause impotence, decreased libido, and gynecomastia. Estrogen therapy also increases the risks of myocardial infarction, stroke, and thrombophlebitis. All procedures for removal of the adenoma depend on identifying the dissection plane between the adenoma and the true prostate, which is compressed into an outer rim often called the "surgical capsule." A "prostatectomy" for benign disease is an adenomectomy with the surgical capsule left in place.

Transurethral resection of the prostate (TURP) is the most frequently employed surgical procedure for relief of BPH. Modern resectoscopes have adequate lighting, good visualization, and powerful electrical coagulating and cutting currents. Many patients are now managed by TURP who would have required an open surgical procedure in years past. The major advantage of TURP is that the operation does not require an incision, which may become infected and which may compromise the accessory respiratory muscles in patients with pulmonary diseases. The major problems come from the irrigating solutions used to wash blood and debris from the operative field during resections. During the resection, veins are unroofed that absorb the irrigant, because the irrigating pressure is higher than the venous pressure. Electrolyte solutions cannot be used because of electroconductivity, which would preclude electrical resection currents, and because sterile water causes intravascular hemolysis. Therefore, isotonic, nonelectrolyte solutions of sorbitol or glycine are used. These solutions may cause dilutional electrolyte abnormalities and intravascular fluid overload. In general, these complications do not occur if the resection is carried on for no longer than 1 hour. If a gland is larger than can be resected in an hour, an open surgical procedure is indicated.

Open surgical procedures frequently employed are suprapubic prostatectomy and retropubic prostatectomy. The difference between these procedures is that in the suprapubic operation the prostate is approached through the bladder, whereas in the retropubic operation the prostate is enucleated through the anterior capsule of the prostate. Either operation can be done through a small midline or transverse incision. The perineal prostatectomy has generally been abandoned because impotence usually occurs. The impotence rate with the other operations for BPH is usually reported to be 5% or less.

After a patient has had a procedure for benign prostatic disease, it is important to continue rectal examinations for the subsequent development of nodularity suggestive of cancer in the true prostate or surgical capsule that remains. Depending on the amount of tissue removed by TURP, a patient may expect at least 10 to 15 years before there is regrowth and recurrence of obstruction.

Acute Urinary Retention

If a patient has long-standing BPH and has had a gradual increase of symptoms, he may have the acute onset of inability to void. This is caused by either the inability of the bladder to generate pressures sufficient for voiding or the rapid increase of obstruction at the prostatic level.

The most commmon cause of loss of bladder muscle tone is overdistention of the bladder, frequently seen after long trips in which the patient has failed to void for a period of time. Similar events may occur in the patient who has had excessive oral fluid intake before bedtime. Medications such as anticholinergics and antidepressants also may decrease muscle contractility.

An acute increase of outlet obstruction may be initiated by prostatic edema, infection, rectal pain, or medications that increase the tone of the bladder neck and prostatic urethra. Treatment of the underlying process, such as infection, is the treatment of choice.

Pain following hernia surgery, perirectal abscess, or rectal trauma may cause urinary retention spasm of the pelvic floor muscle. This may respond to warm sitz baths, pain medication, or resolution of the initiating insult.

Certain medications, especially decongestants and over-the-counter cold remedies, contain alpha-adrenergic agents that stimulate the periprostatic muscles, bladder neck, and sphincter, and thereby cause urinary retention. Almost all patients return to their premedication status with discontinuation of the drug.

Treatment of acute urinary retention is best instituted under the supervision and observation of a urologist. Close observation is necessary. It may be possible to "in-and-out" catheterize some patients, whereas others may need short-term indwelling catheters. In one group of patients with acute retention, 46% had resolution of the acute problem and did not require surgery. Most of these patients will probably require surgery eventually, because acute retention usually is an exacerbation of underlying pathology.

Randall A. *Surgical Pathology of Prostatic Obstructions*. Baltimore: Williams and Wilkins, 1981.
  A demonstration of the development and pathogenesis of prostatic obstruction.
Siiteri PK, Wilson JD. Dihydrotestosterone in prostatic hypertrophy. *J Clin Invest* 49:1737–1745, 1970.
  Quantitation of hormone levels in the prostate.
Walsh PC. Benign Prostatic Hypertrophy. In JH Harrison et al., *Campbell's Urology* (4th ed.). Philadelphia: Saunders, 1979. Pp. 949–964.
  A clinical and experimental review of BPH.
Culp DA. Benign prostatic hyperplasia. *Urol Clin North Am* 2:1, 29–41, 1975.
  A review article on the recognition and management of benign prostatic hyperplasia.

63. CHRONIC RENAL FAILURE

William D. Mattern

It is not unusual in ambulatory care to discover that a patient's renal function is abnormal—that is, the overall glomerular filtration rate (GFR) is reduced enough to elevate the BUN and serum creatinine concentrations. Because there may be no history to suggest the presence of underlying renal disease, and the patient may be asymptomatic, the discovery of abnormal renal function is often a surprise to both the patient and physician. Chronic renal failure (CRF) does not usually result in symptoms until the GFR is reduced below 15 ml per minute, a GFR that would be reflected in a normal-sized adult male by a serum creatinine concentration above 8 mg/dl and a BUN above 100 mg/dl. Uremic symptoms develop gradually as the GFR falls below this level. Because of a combination of individual adaptive changes in residual functioning nephrons, the volume and electrolyte composition of the extracellular fluid (ECF) are remarkably well preserved even beyond this point, usually until the GFR declines to below 10% of normal.

Once the abnormality in renal function is noted, the physician is faced with several questions: (1) What is the cause of the renal insufficiency? (2) Is it acute or chronic? (3) Is there a reversible component requiring prompt detection and treatment? (4) At what point should the patient be seen in consultation? (5) What should the patient be told?

Causes

The most common causes of CRF are hypertension nephrosclerosis, glomerulonephritis, diabetic nephropathy, and interstitial nephritis. A less common cause, polycystic kidney disease, also should be kept in mind.

Hypertension nephrosclerosis is suggested by a long-standing history of hypertension, especially with evidence of inadequate control or poor compliance, together with an unremarkable urine sediment and a 24-hour protein excretion in the range of 1 gm.

Chronic glomerulonephritis is suggested by a past history of acute nephritis or of the nephrotic syndrome, along with mild-to-moderate hypertension and a 24-hour protein excretion in excess of 2 gm.

Diabetic nephropathy typically is accompanied by a long-standing history of diabetes mellitus, along with a more recent history of proteinuria, a 24-hour protein excretion in excess of 2 gm, and mild-to-moderate hypertension.

Interstitial nephritis can be caused by (1) analgesic excess (phenacetin); (2) other drugs, such as the nonsteroidal anti-inflammatory drugs; (3) lead exposure, as occurs with the ingestion of moonshine whiskey; (4) urinary reflux during childhood, usually with a history of recurrent urinary tract infections; and (5) hereditary nephritis (Alport's syndrome), usually with a positive family history, with males more severely affected than females. Regardless of cause, chronic interstitial nephritis may present with an unremarkable urine sediment, a 24-hour urine protein excretion in the range of 1 gm, and mild-to-moderate hypertension. It may be presumed mistakenly to be hypertensive nephrosclerosis unless a careful history is taken.

Polycystic kidney disease is inherited as an autosomal dominant trait. The greatly enlarged cystic kidneys are usually palpable. History and physical examination are thus critical in diagnosis.

Evaluation

Patients with a severe abnormality, or whose prior renal function is unknown, or who have had a rapid change in function should be thoroughly evaluated. Elderly patients with diabetes or hypertension who have a modest elevation of serum creatinine compatible with the serum BUN may require no additional evaluation.

The basic components of the evaluation of chronic renal failure, in addition to data from the history, are the urine sediment, the 24-hour urinary protein excretion, and the evaluation of renal size. It is also essential to rule out acute renal failure.

Urine Sediment

The finding of broad, waxy casts in the urine sediment is typical in all patients with chronic renal failure. Striking abnormalities of the urine sediment suggest acute renal parenchymal disease of vascular, interstitial, glomerular, or tubular origin. For example, the acute necrotizing renal vasculitis of malignant hypertension or polyarteritis presents with gross or microscopic hematuria, as does the acute interstitial nephritis induced by certain drugs and the acute glomerulonephritis following streptococcal and other types of bacterial and viral infections. The finding of numerous pigmented granular casts and renal tubular cells in the urine sediment suggests acute tubular necrosis (ATN).

The 24-Hour Urinary Protein Excretion

The measure varies depending on the cause of the chronic renal failure. Usually, patients with vascular disease (nephrosclerosis) and tubular-interstitial disease excrete 1 to 2 gm of protein per day, whereas patients with chronic glomerulonephritis and diabetic nephropathy excrete more than 3 gm of protein per day.

Renal Size

Although documenting reduced renal size establishes that renal failure is chronic, renal size is not reduced in all forms of chronic renal failure. Renal size is reduced in chronic interstitial nephritis and chronic glomerulonephritis, and is usually reduced in nephrosclerosis. It is often normal in diabetic nephropathy, and is greatly increased in polycystic kidney disease. Sometimes a simple x-ray of the abdomen suffices to document renal size, but if the renal outlines are not visualized, a renal ultrasound study or an intravenous pyelogram (IVP) should be obtained.

Intravenous Pyelogram

The IVP provides an indication of renal function and size. When renal function is adequate it defines renal anatomy, particularly the anatomy of the upper collecting system (the renal calyces). However, adequate visualization is usually not possible when the GFR falls below 25% of normal or the serum creatinine concentration is greater than 8 mg/dl. Furthermore, IVP dye can cause acute tubular necrosis in older patients, patients with multiple myeloma, and patients with diabetic nephropathy. Diabetic patients are particularly at risk for this complication, and IVP dye should be avoided if at all possible.

Acute renal failure should always be considered in the patient who presents with abnormal renal function, particularly if the duration of the renal insufficiency is uncertain. Acute renal failure is suggested by (1) a BUN that is increased out of proportion to the increase in the serum creatinine concentration, (2) an "active" urine sediment, and (3) particular clinical settings. If the BUN–serum creatinine ratio is greater than 15 to 1, two possibilities should be considered: (1) prerenal azotemia, from causes such as severe congestive heart failure or acute intravascular volume depletion (e.g., caused by diuretic therapy or bleeding), and (2) urinary tract obstruction, from causes such as prostatic hypertrophy in older men or neurogenic bladder in patients with diabetes.

Although ATN is uncommon in ambulatory patients, it has been increasingly recognized in two situations: (1) following x-ray contrast exposure in high-risk patients, such as those with long-standing diabetes and preexisting renal insufficiency, and (2) following intense effort in the heat, typically among young athletes in training, military recruits, or construction workers. These patients may develop rhabdomyolysis with myoglobinuria, marked by a history of dark urine and a urine dipstick that is positive for blood in the absence of gross or microscopic hematuria.

Even in the patient with established CRF, it is important to consider superimposed acute renal failure, especially from readily reversible causes such as diuretic-induced intravascular volume depletion, lower-urinary-tract obstruction, or urinary tract infection.

Management

There are three important goals in the long-term management of the patient with mild-to-moderate CRF: (1) to reduce as much as possible the rate of progression of the renal disease; (2) to treat, as necessary, the disturbances in body fluid and electrolyte composition that develop as renal function is lost; and (3) to establish a relationship with the patient that provides reassurance during the initial stages and a therapeutic alliance as end-stage renal disease (ESRD) approaches.

Slowing the Rate of Progression

The most useful index of the rate of progression of CRF is the serum creatinine concentration; roughly speaking, it doubles each time the GFR is reduced by one-half. Thus, if the serum creatinine is 1 mg/dl at a normal GFR of 120 ml per minute, a value of 2 would be expected at a GFR of 60, of 4 at a GFR of 30, and of 8 at a GFR of 15. This relation assumes a constant rate of production of creatinine by muscle, and virtually no renal tubular resorption or secretion of creatinine. However, as CRF progresses, the serum creatinine may be lower than expected because muscle creatinine production declines and renal tubular creatinine secretion increases. Nevertheless, sequential changes in the serum creatinine concentration provide a convenient and reasonably reliable estimate of the rate of change in the GFR.

The rate of progression of CRF can be reduced in several ways. In patients with drug-induced chronic interstitial nephritis, the offending drug can be discontinued. In patients with diabetic nephropathy, "tight control" of the blood sugar may contribute to the preservation of renal function. More generally, the correction of three abnormalities—hypertension, hyperphosphatemia, and azotemia—may slow the rate of progression. It recently has been postulated that all of these abnormalities may induce glomerular sclerosis in the chronically damaged kidney. An end point of "control" in each might include, respectively, a blood pressure of 145/95 or less, a serum phosphorus concentration of 5.0 mg/dl or less, and a BUN of 90 mg/dl or less. Lower levels might provide still better preservation of renal function. However, most patients would have difficulty in complying with the necessary medical regimen, which would include large amounts of phosphate-binding antacids, multiple antihypertensive medications, and a low-protein diet.

Hypertension

Hypertension is a problem in most patients with CRF throughout the course of their disease. The "stepped-care" approach applies to these patients just as it does to those with normal renal function. Diuretic drugs remain the cornerstone of therapy. The thiazides are not generally effective when the GFR falls below 25 ml per minute (i.e., serum creatinine > 4.0 mg/dl). The "loop diuretics," such as furosemide or ethacrynic acid, are effective at GFRs below this level. The diuretic response is dose-dependent, and the dose can be varied over a wide range as needed to obtain a response.

Sodium Balance

The management of diuretic dose and dietary sodium intake requires careful attention in patients with CRF. In patients with normal renal function, the kidney can maintain sodium balance over a wide range of sodium intakes, and sodium can be eliminated from the urine when the intake approaches zero. In patients with CRF, the adaptive changes in tubular function permit sodium balance to be maintained only when sodium intake is in the normal range. Urinary sodium excretion cannot be reduced below 20 to 80 mEq per day, and, as a result, aggressive diuretic therapy or dietary salt restriction can lead to acute intravascular volume depletion and prerenal azotemia. On the other hand, acute oral salt loads above the normal range of intake cannot be excreted promptly. Most antihypertensive agents have a tendency to cause salt retention, and administration without adequate simultaneous diuretic therapy can lead to progressive expansion of ECF volume and edema formation, with resulting exacerbation of hypertension or precipitation of congestive heart failure.

Hypokalemia

Hypokalemia is less likely to occur as a complication of diuretic therapy in patients with CRF than in patients with normal renal function. Oral potassium supplements and potassium-sparing diuretics, such as triamterene and spironolactone (Aldactone), should be avoided because acute hyperkalemia may result.

Hyperphosphatemia

Hyperphosphatemia, a relatively late complication in the course of CRF, does not usually occur until the GFR declines below 25 ml per minute. Treatment consists of the administration of aluminum-containing antacids, such as Amphojel and Basaljel, in doses titrated to maintain the serum phosphate concentration at or below 5 mg/dl. These antacids are given immediately after meals; they bind phosphate in the upper intestinal tract, preventing its absorption. The liquid forms are more effective than the tablets or capsules, but frequently are difficult for patients to take because they are not palatable or cause nausea. Constipation is a universal complication of the phosphate-binding antacids but can usually be effectively treated with sorbitol. Magnesium-containing antacids should be avoided because magnesium is absorbed, and there is reduced renal excretion. Hypermagnesemia may result.

Azotemia

Azotemia develops gradually throughout the course of CRF, in parallel with the reduction in GFR. It does not require treatment until late in the course, when the BUN has exceeded 100 to 125 mg/dl. At this point patients usually experience uremic symptoms, including weakness, malaise, and morning nausea. Reduction of the BUN by dietary protein restriction is associated with marked improvement in these symptoms. Most patients are able to adapt to a 40-gm protein-restricted diet, which is recommended when early symptoms of uremia develop. When the BUN exceeds 100 mg/dl and uremic symptoms recur on this diet, plans for chronic dialysis should be made.

Hypocalcemia

Hypocalcemia occurs early in the course of CRF. The major contributing factor is a negative calcium balance from a decrease in the renal production of the active metabolite of vitamin D, $1,25\ (OH)_2D_3$. Oral calcium supplements improve the calcium balance and are routinely given as long as the serum phosphate concentration is below 6 mg/dl. A typical dosage is 500 mg twice a day, given before meals to promote absorption.

Metabolic Acidosis
Metabolic acidosis develops in all patients with chronic renal failure, but it is usually mild and does not reqiure specific treatment unless the plasma bicarbonate concentration falls below 15 mEq/L. In such instances, alkali supplements may be given, in the form of sodium bicarbonate tablets or as Shohl's solution—a combination of sodium citrate and citric acid that contains 1 mEq of bicarbonate alkali—equivalent and 1 mEq of sodium per milliliter. In most patients the plasma bicarbonate concentration can be maintained at or above 15 mEq/L with 30 to 60 mEq of alkali supplement per day.

Anemia
Anemia, usually normocytic, also may develop relatively early in the course of CRF because of decreased renal production of erythropoietin. There is no specific treatment for the anemia, which generally is well tolerated. Transfusions should be avoided unless there is a specific indication, such as hematocrit-dependent angina. Superimposed anemia from folic acid or iron deficiency is suspected when the mean corpuscular volume is abnormal.

Referral
Initial consultation with a nephrologist, although not always essential, can be helpful to verify that reversible contributing causes have been properly excluded and to establish personal contact in the event that subsequent referral for ESRD evaluation is needed. Continuing contact with the primary physician can provide valuable reassurance to the patient with CRF. This relationship may become vital as the patient begins to come to terms with the irreversible and progressive nature of the renal disease, and as referral for ESRD therapy is being considered.

Referral should be considered, in general, when the GFR falls below 25 ml per minute and the serum creatinine concentration rises above 4 to 5 mg/dl. Beyond this point, the rate of loss of function is quite variable. In patients with diabetic nephropathy, progression to ESRD may occur rapidly, often within 6 months. If during this time the patient is followed by a nephrologist, arrangements for dialysis and transplantation can be initiated. Current data suggest that early initiation of ESRD therapy may be particularly beneficial in this subset of patients.

Bourgoignie JJ, et al. Water electrolyte and acid-base abnormalities in chronic renal failure. *Semin Nephrol* 1:91–111, 1981.
An excellent overview of electrolyte and acid-base abnormalities and their management.
Friedman E. Diabetic nephropathy: Strategies in prevention and management. *Kidney Int* 21:780–791, 1982.
The best single statement on the management of diabetic nephropathy, including chronic renal failure, dialysis, and transplantation.
Harkonen S, Kjellstrand CM. Exacerbation of diabetic renal failure following intravenous pyelography. *Am J Med* 63:939–946, 1977.
A careful study highlighting the risk of IVP dye in diabetic patients with renal insufficiency.
Grossman RA, et al. Nontraumatic rhabdomyolysis and acute renal failure. *N Engl J Med* 291:807–811, 1974.
A good clinical description of this condition.
Schreiner GE, McAnally JF, Winchester JF. Clinical analgesic nephropathy. *Arch Intern Med* 141:349–357, 1981.
A good clinical description of this condition.
Torres VE. Present and future of the nonsteroidal anti-inflammatory drugs in nephrology. *Mayo Clin Proc* 57:389–393, 1982.
Good background information on the mechanism of action of these drugs and their multiple potential adverse effects on kidney function.
Brenner BM, Meyer TW, Hostetter TH. Dietary protein intake and the progressive nature of kidney disease. *N Engl J Med* 307:652–659, 1982.

*The best recent article explaining how dietary protein intake may contribute to hyper-
filtration and loss of renal function in diseased and normal kidneys as part of the
aging process. The role of hyperglycemia as a contributing factor to hyperfiltration
and loss of function in the diabetic kidney is also discussed.*
Bricker NS. Sodium homeostasis in chronic renal disease. *Kidney Int* 21:886–897,
1982.
*A good review of sodium balance in chronic renal disease and its importance in rela-
tion to dietary sodium intake and the use of diuretics.*

64. RENAL STONES

Romulo E. Colindres

From 1 to 6% of the population of the United States has or has had renal stones.
Approximately 75% of renal stones are composed predominantly of calcium oxalate
(pure calcium oxalate or a mixture of calcium oxalate and calcium phosphate), 5 to
10% of stones are composed predominantly of uric acid, and 8 to 10% are composed of
magnesium and ammonium phosphate (struvite or infection stones). The remaining
stones are composed of cystine or other constituents.

Conditions that predispose to stone formation include habitually low fluid intake,
prolonged immobilization, a positive family history, associated diseases (gout, primary
hyperparathyroidism, small bowel disease, urinary tract obstruction, and infection),
and use of certain drugs (vitamin D, acetazolamide [Diamox], absorbable antacids).
Inflammatory and other bowel diseases are frequently associated with the formation of
uric acid and calcium oxalate stones as a consequence of fluid and bicarbonate losses,
leading to the production of a persistently concentrated and acid urine. Furthermore,
if malabsorption occurs, calcium is bound by fat in the lumen of the bowel and the
unbound oxalate is absorbed in increased amounts by the colon, which is rendered
more permeable to this compound by the action of unresorbed bile acids. This sequence
of events produces hyperoxaluria—hence the excretion of calcium oxalate, a poorly
soluble calcium salt.

Clinical Manifestations

Renal stones are usually first detected in the fourth decade of life. The occurrence of
stones before that time suggests that the patient has a hereditary condition, such as
primary hyperoxaluria, cystinuria, or renal tubular acidosis. Renal stone disease, especially the idiopathic type, is more common in men. Renal stones caused by primary
hyperparathyroidism and renal tubular acidosis are more common among women.

Renal stones first become manifest in one of the following ways:

Asymptomatic renal stones discovered fortuitously on a plain x-ray of the abdomen or
   on an intravenous urogram
Asymptomatic hematuria
Repeated bouts of urinary infection with or without loss of renal parenchyma
Ureteral obstruction, partial or total, associated with severe pain (see Chap. 65)
Passage of cloudy urine or gravel

Nephrolithiasis is said to be "metabolically active" when there is evidence of new
stone formation, stone growth, or passage of gravel in the past year; all of these conditions are manifestations of crystalluria and supersaturation of the urine with the
mineral constituents of the stones. Metabolically active disease should be investigated
for possible predisposing causes and treated vigorously. Stones are said to be "surgically active" when there is a history of renal colic, urinary obstruction, or infection in
the past year. The presence of surgically active disease need not imply metabolically
active disease, becuase the surgical episodes may have occurred as a consequence of
stones formed in the past.

Pathogenesis

Calcium Stones
Certain metabolic disorders are common in patients with calcium nephrolithiasis. Table 64-1 shows the disorders found in 460 consecutive calcium stone–forming patients. Idiopathic hypercalciuria is the most common metabolic disorder; hypercalciuria, hyperuricosuria, or a combination of both is found in approximately 60% of patients who form calcium stones.

Idiopathic hypercalciuria can be caused by increased absorption of calcium from the gut (absorptive hypercalciuria), impairment of renal tubular resorption of calcium (renal hypercalciuria), or an increased filtered load of calcium as a consequence of hypercalcemia, as seen in primary hyperparathyroidism. Other conditions that can lead to oversaturation of the urine with calcium include acquired or congenital hyperoxaluria; a decreased excretion of citrate (as seen during acidosis), which under normal conditions forms soluble complexes with calcium; a persistently low urine volume; and a decrease in the concentration of ill-defined chemical inhibitors of crystal growth and aggregation in urine. In patients with hyperuricosuria, uric acid may serve as a nidus for the growth and aggregation of calcium crystals.

Uric Acid Stones
The mechanisms that promote formation of uric acid stones include the excretion of increased amounts of uric acid, the excretion of urine that has a persistently low pH, and the excretion of a perennially low urine volume as a result of low fluid intake, diseases of the bowel, or excessive losses of fluid. Hyperuricosuria or hyperuricemia is found in only 50% of patients who form uric acid stones. Conversely, only 25% of patients with gout form uric acid stones. Thus, in the majority of patients, the presence of uric acid stones can be attributed to the chronic excretion of a concentrated and acid urine or to a structural abnormality of the urinary tract. Because the pK of uric acid is 5.47, at a urine pH of 5 or less the less soluble uric acid is excreted in excess of urate salts.

Table 64-1. Metabolic and clinical disorders in 460 consecutive calcium stone–forming patients

Disorder	Patients	
	No.	%
Idiopathic hypercalciuria	95	20.7
Marginal hypercalciuria[a]	53	11.5
Hyperuricosuria	67	14.6
Hypercalciuria and hyperuricosuria[b]	54	11.7
Hyperuricemia	26	5.7
Primary hyperparathyroidism	24	5.2
Renal tubular acidosis[c]	17	3.7
Inflammatory bowel disease[d]	21	4.6
Medullary sponge kidney	7	1.5
Sarcoidosis	3	0.7
No disorder found	93	20.2
Total	460	

Source: From FL Coe, Treated and untreated recurrent calcium nephrolithiasis in patients with idiopathic hypercalciuria, hyperuricosuria, or no metabolic disorder. *Ann Intern Med* 87:405, 1977.
[a]Urine calcium, 140 mg/gm creatinine.
[b]Marginal hypercalciuria not included.
[c]Distal, hereditary form.
[d]Regional enteritis, ulcerative colitis, granulomatous ileocolitis.

Uric acid stones are characteristically radiolucent on intravenous urography. As a result, they can be misdiagnosed as tumors or polyps.

Struvite, or Infection, Stones

Calcium, magnesium, and ammonium phosphate stones, or struvite stones, are formed in the presence of a high concentration of ammonium in a urine having a persistently alkaline pH (7.5 or higher). Under normal circumstances, alkaline urine has a low concentration of NH_4^+. However, in patients suffering from urinary tract infections caused by urea-splitting organisms, particularly of the *Proteus* species, the bacterial urease hydrolyzes urea to form ammonia and HCO_3^-; the resulting urine has an alkaline pH and is supersaturated with calcium phosphate. The high NH_4^+ concentration in urine leads to the formation of magnesium and ammonium phosphate crystals, which grow, aggregate, and become stones that block the movement of bacteria, making treatment of the infection very difficult. Hypercalciuria and the excretion of a small volume of very concentrated urine can contribute to the pathogenesis of struvite stones.

These stones are usually radiopaque and have the configuration of staghorn calculi. Surgical removal is frequently necessary, and the associated infection should be vigorously treated. Recurrence is common, and gradual loss of renal function often occurs.

Cystine Stones

Cystine stones form in children and young adults whose kidney tubules lack the ability to resorb cystine normally. Cystine excretion often exceeds the limit of its solubility (300 mg/L), and growth and aggregation of crystals lead to stone formation. Excretion of an acid and concentrated urine increases the propensity for stone formation.

Cystine stones are pale yellow and slightly radiopaque because of their sulfur content. The stones may be passed into the urine, leading to the clinical picture of renal colic, or they may develop into staghorn calculi. Patients with cystinuria frequently have urinary tract infections. Loss of renal function in this type of stone disease is almost invariable.

Evaluation

The evaluation of patients with nephrolithiasis should proceed as follows:

1. Confirm the diagnosis in patients who have a history of renal colic and/or hematuria but who have not passed stones or gravel in the urine. Occasionally, very radiopaque stones can be seen on a plain film of the abdomen. However, an intravenous urogram is usually done to identify less opaque stones; to determine the number, configuration, and characteristics of the stones more precisely; and to exclude structural abnormalities.

2. Take a careful history to detect any factors that may have contributed to the formation of stones, or to the surgical and metabolic activity of the disease.

3. Whenever possible, determine the composition of stones. The pathogenesis, clinical manifestations, radiographic findings, and, to some extent, treatment are dependent on the type of stones present.

4. If the patient has many stones or metabolically active disease, a detailed evaluation should be done to detect any clinical or metabolic disorder that might be causing the formation of stones. Additional studies may not be needed if the patient has passed a stone for the first time and if no other stones are seen on the intravenous urogram.

Detailed evaluation includes a measurement of the excretion of calcium, uric acid, and creatinine in a 24-hour sample of urine (Fig. 64-1). Urine calcium excretion can be interpreted if the patient is eating normal amounts of calcium, as determined by an easily obtainable dietary history. Hypercalciuria has been defined as the excretion of more than 300 mg of calcium per day in men, and 250 mg per day in women, on a normal calcium intake; or the excretion of more than 140 mg of calcium per gm of creatinine per day; or the excretion of more than 4 mg/kg body weight per 24 hours, in both sexes. The normal excretion of uric acid is less than 800 mg/24 hours in men, and less than 750 mg/24 hours in women.

The initial evaluation of patients with active nephrolithiasis or hypercalciuria should include a measurement of serum calcium concentration. This usually requires three or four measurements, because the difference between normal and abnormal val-

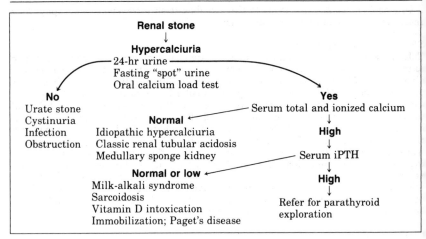

Fig. 64-1. Suggested scheme for approach to diagnosis in renal stone disease, based on presence or absence of hypercalciuria, hypercalcemia, and serum parathyroid (iPTH) elevation. (Reprinted from *Kidney International* Vol. 16: pp. 638–648, 1979 with permission.)

ues may be of the order of 0.1 to 0.2 mg/dl. Subtle elevations of the serum calcium concentration may be important and merit investigation. The initial evaluation also should include measurement of the serum concentrations of sodium, chloride, bicarbonate, potassium, creatinine, uric acid, and phosphorus. A urinalysis should be done of an early morning specimen to look for crystals and to measure pH to detect any defect in urinary acidification. A urine culture should be done to exclude associated infection.

Treatment Principles
If possible, any underlying or predisposing abnormalities such as hypercalciuria, urinary obstruction, or renal tubular acidosis should be corrected. Patients with metabolically or surgically active stone disease should be treated by increasing their urinary volume, reducing the urinary excretion of stone constituents, and increasing the solubility of the constituents. Patients with inactive stone disease, normal calcium excretion, and no associated abnormality may need no treatment beyond that necessary to ensure a urine volume of 2½ L per day.

Treatment Modalities

Fluid Intake
Patients with severe stone disease should be encouraged to drink between 3 and 5 L of fluid every day to ensure a urine volume of at least 2½ L per day. Urinary dilution reduces the propensity for crystallization of calcium and urate salts in urine by lowering the urinary saturation of the constituents of such stones, and increases the minimal supersaturation needed to produce spontaneous nucleation of calcium oxalate.

Reduction of Urinary Excretion of Stone Constituents
Thiazide diuretics, in dosages equivalent to 50 to 100 mg of hydrochlorothiazide per day, decrease the urinary excretion of calcium by 40 to 50% in both renal and absorptive hypercalciuria and reduce the formation or passage of new stones in 80 to 90% of hypercalciuric patients. The thiazide diuretics exert this hypocalciuric effect by increasing the resorption of calcium in the distal convolution of the nephron. A high salt intake must be avoided because extracellular fluid volume expansion may negate the hypocalciuric effect of the diuretic. Thiazide diuretics also may be useful in patients without demonstrated hypercalciuria.

Patients with absorptive hypercalciuria should avoid a high-calcium diet. However, a low-calcium diet may be unnecessary in such patients if they are treated with diuretics. In fact, a low-calcium diet may lead to increased intestinal absorption of non-calcium-containing oxalate salts, thus producing hyperoxaluria.

Cellulose phosphate, an agent that binds calcium in the gut, has been used as an experimental drug for several years and will soon be approved for use in the treatment of absorptive hypercalciuria.

Increasing the Solubility of Stone Constituents

Uric acid and cystine are more soluble in alkaline than in acid urine. The limit of uric acid solubility in urine is about 15 mg/dl at a pH of 5.0 and 200 mg/dl at a pH of 7.0. Similarly, the solubility of cystine in urine increases two- to threefold at a pH above 7.5. A urine pH of 6.5 to 7.0 in a person eating a normal diet can be achieved by giving 1 mEq of bicarbonate per kilogram body weight per day divided in three or four doses. Approximately 2 mEq/kg body weight of bicarbonate is necessary to achieve a sustained urine pH of 7.5. Bicarbonate can be given as tablets (1 gm = 12 mEq) or as Shohl's solution (sodium citrate and citric acid, 1 cc = 1 mEq). A carbonic anhydrase inhibitor such as acetazolamide (Diamox), 250 mg, can be given at bedtime. Patients should be instructed to measure their urine pH with a dipstick to document the adequacy of the chosen dosage of bicarbonate.

Patients with cystinuria can be treated with D-penicillamine, which forms soluble complexes with cystine. This drug is very toxic and should be used only after other measures have failed.

Inhibitors of Crystal Growth and Aggregation

Organic phosphate, prescribed as neutral phosphate at a dosage of 2 to 2.5 gm per day, has been an effective form of treatment for some patients with active stone disease and a normal calcium excretion or in patients with hypercalciuria who do not respond to thiazide diuretics.

Follow-up

The recurrence rate of calcium stones is 15% at 1 years and 66% at 9 years. Patients with renal stones should be followed at least at yearly intervals to evaluate the metabolic and surgical activity of their disease. Patients who have complications such as infections, renal colic, or loss of renal function and those being treated with drugs should be seen at closer intervals. Follow-up studies may include, as appropriate, intravenous urography; measurements of 24-hour urinary excretion of calcium, oxalate, or uric acid; measurement of creatinine clearance; and urine cultures.

Coe FL, Brenner BM, Stein JH (Eds.), *Nephrolithiasis*, Vol. 5 (Contemporary Issues in Nephrology Series). New York: Churchill Livingstone, 1980.

This book contains 11 chapters written by acknowledged experts in the field and deals with the pathogenesis, natural history, clinical presentations, and treatment of the various forms of nephrolithiasis.

Smith LH. Urolithiasis. In LE Earley and CW Gottschalk (Eds.), *Strauss and Welt's Diseases of the Kidney* (3rd ed.). Boston: Little, Brown, 1979. Pp. 893–931.

An excellent, concise, well-written, and thorough review of the topic by one of the most experienced workers in the field.

Coe FL. Treated and untreated recurrent calcium nephrolithiasis in patients with idiopathic hypercalciuria, hyperuricosuria, or no metabolic disorder. *Ann Intern Med* 87:404–410, 1977.

The author reviews the metabolic and clinical disorders found in 460 consecutive calcium stone–forming patients. He demonstrates convincingly that treatment with thiazide diuretics and allopurinol is an effective way to prevent recurrence of calcium oxalate stones in patients with hypercalciuria and hyperuricosuria, respectively.

Pak CYC, et al. Ambulatory evaluation of nephrolithiasis: Classification, clinical presentations, and diagnostic criteria. *Am J Med* 69:19–30, 1980.

The authors employ a simple ambulatory protocol to evaluate 241 patients with nephrolithiasis. They find that only 10.8% of such patients have no metabolic abnormality. The most common abnormalities in these patients are absorptive hypercalciuria, which occurs in 54.3% of the patients, and renal hypercalciuria, which occurs in 8.3%.

Muldowney FP. Diagnostic approach to hypercalciuria. *Kidney Int* 16:637–648, 1979.

The author proposes a reasonable approach to the diagnostic evaluation of patients with nephrolithiasis based on demonstration of the presence or absence of hypercalciuria and on the serum calcium concentration.

Lemann JL, Adams ND, Gray RW. Urinary calcium excretion in human beings. *N Engl J Med* 301:535–541, 1979.

A very thorough discussion of the many factors that influence urinary calcium excretion in humans.

Lemann JL. Idiopathic Hypercalciuria. In FL Coe, BM Brenner, JH Stein (Eds.), *Nephrolithiasis*, Vol. 5 (Contemporary Issues in Nephrology Series). New York: Churchill Livingstone, 1980. Pp. 86–115.

An outstanding discussion of the syndrome of idiopathic hypercalciuria. The author discusses the definition of hypercalciuria, the source of extra urinary calcium in the condition, and its treatment.

Griffith DP. Struvite stones. *Kidney Int* 13:372–283, 1978.

A very comprehensive and well-written review of the pathogenesis, clinical manifestations, and treatment of stones caused by urea-splitting organisms.

Yendt ER, Cohanim M. Prevention of calcium stones with thiazides. *Kidney Int* 13:397–409, 1978.

The authors find that 90% of patients with calcium nephrolithiasis treated with low doses of thiazides show improvement of their renal stone disease whether or not hypercalciuria is present. They suggest that thiazide diuretics may decrease stone formation by several mechanisms, including some that are independent of their hypocalciuric effect.

Pak CYC, et al. Evidence justifying a high fluid intake in treatment of nephrolithiasis. *Ann Intern Med* 93:36–39, 1980.

The authors provide experimental evidence demonstrating that dilution of the urine reduces the state of saturation of calcium phosphate, calcium oxalate, and monosodium urate. These results provide objective evidence for the beneficial effect of increased fluid intake in the treatment of nephrolithiasis.

65. ACUTE RENAL COLIC
C. Richard Morris

The peak incidence of renal colic occurs in the third to fifth decades. Only 10% of patients experience their initial episode before age 30, and fewer than 7% present after the age of 60 years. Whites are more often affected than blacks, and the frequency in men is three times that in women.

Severe flank pain (colic) occurs when stones produce obstruction as they descend through the collecting system. They may traverse the ureter without producing symptoms, but obstruction often occurs at one of four sites along the course of the ureter: the ureteropelvic junction, the point of entry into the bony pelvis, the posterior pelvis (near the broad ligament in women), and the ureterovesical junction.

Evaluation

History

Colic is abrupt in onset and typically occurs in the early morning hours in patients who are sedentary or at rest. The pain crescendos over 20 to 60 minutes and may last for hours. It is incredibly severe and is often associated with nausea and vomiting. Spontaneous resolution is gradual over minutes to hours. Stones in the proximal and midureter cause flank pain that radiates to the abdomen. As stones enter the distal ureter, pain radiates to the groin and testicle in men and to the labia majora in women. Stones in the intramural segment of the vesical ureter produce symptoms of bladder irritation. Impaction of the stone at any point in the ureter results in intense local inflammation and intense pain in the area of impaction.

Physical Examination
Other than demonstrating costovertebral angle tenderness, the examination is unremarkable. Impaction may produce localized, deep tenderness over the area of inflammation and tenderness elicited on percussion over the obstructed kidney.

Laboratory Tests
Microscopic hematuria is nearly invariable (75–100%), and gross hematuria occurs in 18% of patients. Infection must be sought. Pyuria is common, even in the absence of infection.

X-ray
Radiographic evaluation is necessary to confirm the diagnosis, to assess stone size and number, and to determine the degree of obstruction. Although this should be deferred until the patient is comfortable and circumstances permit optimal studies, undue delay severely limits their usefulness. Stones are nearly invariably radiopaque (92%). Most (40–80%) are seen on plain films of the abdomen and pelvis, but identification can be improved by evacuating the bowel, obtaining lateral and oblique views, and inspecting common points of obstruction. Intravenous pyelography permits the most accurate assessment of obstruction, but the technique should be modified to include delayed exposures.

Delay in the contrast appearance is the first indication of obstruction. Radiolucent stones should be suspected when filling defects are present at a point of obstruction. If radiographic studies are normal, other causes of pain and hematuria should be sought.

Assessment
Ninety percent of stones less than 5 mm in diameter pass spontaneously, but it is impossible to predict which will not. Patients can usually be managed with analgesics and observed as outpatients. Indications for surgical consultation include concurrent infection, severe or increasing obstruction, deterioration in renal function, persistent pain, and severe gross hematuria. The extent of recovery in renal function is inversely related to the duration and severity of obstruction. In experimental animals, recovery is usually complete if obstruction is limited to 1 to 2 weeks. Little or no function returns after 6 weeks. Limited data from humans suggest incomplete recovery after 30 to 60 days of complete obstruction.

Assessment of the cause of stone formation depends on the stone type and the activity of the disease. During the passage of a stone, the urine should be filtered through a gauze, and stone analysis should be performed. The activity of disease must be assessed historically and by serial radiographic studies. It is clear that some patients have only a single stone, whereas others have frequent recurrences. Differences in causation do not appear to determine stone frequency. The probability of recurrence after a single stone is 50% in 5 years. In those in whom there is recurrence, chronicity is the rule. The extent of evaluation after a single stone is controversial. When new stones appear or existing stones increase in size, one should seek specific causes that can be treated effectively. Initial studies should exclude infection, cystinuria, hypercalciuria, and hyperuricosuria.

Wilson DR. Nephrolithiasis: Diagnosis and medical management. *Compr Ther* 7:31–39, 1981.
   A good summary article.
Strauss AL, Coe FL, Parks JH. Formation of a single calcium stone of renal origin. *Arch Intern Med* 142:504–507, 1982.
   Discusses the implications of having a single stone.
Silverman DE, Stamey TA. Management of infection stones: The Stanford experience. *Medicine* 62:44–51, 1983.
   Discusses a therapeutic approach to stones associated with infection.

66. PROTEINURIA
Katherine A. Huffman

Normally the urine contains 150 mg or less of protein per 24 hours, composed of albumin (40%), immunoglobulins and other plasma proteins (20%), and protein of uroepithelial origin—Tamm-Horsfall protein—(40%).

Pathophysiology
Proteinuria occurs as a result of one of three major abnormalities: impaired function of the glomerular capillary wall, overproduction of, or decreased tubular resorption of, freely filterable protein. The glomerular capillary wall acts as a molecular sieve that retards the passage of large proteins such as albumin. Therefore, albuminuria reflects increased permeability of the capillary wall. Smaller proteins (e.g., myoglobin and lysozyme) are filtered across the capillary wall and resorbed by the tubule or excreted in the urine. Overproduction proteinuria results from an increased excretion of a normally filterable protein, exemplified by excretion of myoglobin or light chains. Tubular proteinuria, which is rare, occurs when the tubules have an impaired ability to reabsorb low molecular weight proteins. This discussion focuses on albuminuria, the most common type of proteinuria.

Detection of Proteinuria
There are two commonly used laboratory methods to detect proteinuria. The dipstick test is convenient and specific but does not detect light chains or protein at a concentration of less than 30 mg/dl. False-positive reactions are uncommon but may occur with decomposed or alkaline urine. The protein precipitation test, using 5% sulfosalicylic acid, is exquisitely sensitive, although less convenient, and gives false-positive reactions with radiographic contrast agents, tolbutamide, penicillins, and sulfisoxazole. The major advantage of the sulfosalicylic acid test is its ability to detect light-chain proteins. For routine screening in a physician's office, the dipstick method is adequate and efficient, and does not give confusing, false-positive reactions. Because the test depends on concentration, however, unusually concentrated or dilute urine gives misleading results. If clinical suspicion for light-chain proteinuria is high, the sulfosalicylic precipitation test should be used.

Diagnostic Evaluation
Proteinuria is abnormal and requires additional evaluation, except when the urine is highly concentrated or when the patient has an intercurrent acute illness or urinary tract infection, or has been exercising heavily. In the latter instances the urinalysis should be repeated after resolution of the illness or before exercise. The initial diagnostic step is quantification of the protein lost per 24 hours and careful examination of the urine sediment. Proteinuria coupled with hematuria or pyuria represents different renal disease processes and is evaluated differently from isolated proteinuria. When cellular elements or casts are present, the patient should be referred to a nephrologist for consideration of a renal biopsy.

If the 24-hour protein excretion exceeds 150 mg and there are no other urine sediment abnormalities, the following steps should be undertaken to establish a diagnosis:

Take history and physical examination, noting any family history of renal disease and any evidence for collagen vascular or other systemic illness.

Repeat quantification of urine protein, particularly if the first sample was collected when the patient was clinically ill (febrile, severely hypertensive, or in congestive heart failure).

Evaluate for orthostatic proteinuria (see Isolated Nonnephrotic Proteinuria); if orthostatic proteinuria is diagnosed, a serum urea and creatinine should be obtained, but an extensive renal evaluation is not necessary.

Order laboratory studies, including CBC, serum urea, creatinine, glucose, total protein, albumin, 24-hour creatinine clearance, and urine culture.

If the patient has nephrotic-range proteinuria ($\geq$ 3.5 gm/24 hr), obtain a serum cholesterol, antinuclear and syphilis serology antibody. Referral to a nephrologist should be made for consideration of a renal biopsy.

If polycystic kidney disease is suspected, renal ultrasound should be performed.

If paraproteinemia is suspected, serum protein electrophoresis and urinary immunoelectrophoresis are necessary.

Isolated Nonnephrotic Proteinuria

Isolated proteinuria is defined as urinary protein in excess of 150 mg per 24 hours in the absence of any other urine sediment abnormalities. It is helpful and important to distinguish isolated nonnephrotic from nephrotic-range proteinuria. The former category includes functional, orthostatic, and constant proteinuria.

Functional proteinuria is defined as transient low-grade proteinuria in the absence of apparent renal disease. Congestive heart failure, fever, seizures, heavy exercise, emotional stress, hypertension, and infusion of albumin or epinephrine can cause proteinuria that resolves when the stimulus is removed. In a recent report of 313 emergency medical admissions with no known renal disease, 30 (9.5%) had proteinuria greater than 1 + on admission, which had resolved by the ninth hospital day. The major diagnoses in these patients were congestive heart failure, seizures, pneumonia, and fever. When isolated proteinuria is detected in a patient who is acutely ill, the first step is to reconfirm the presence of proteinuria after the acute stress subsides.

Orthostatic (postural) proteinuria is characterized by the appearance of proteinuria in the upright position and its disappearance in the recumbent position. The total amount of protein excreted is usually less than 1.5 gm/24 hours. It typically occurs in otherwise healthy, asymptomatic people and is detected incidentally during a routine examination. Because the prognosis and need for additional evaluation differ between orthostatic and nonorthostatic (constant) proteinuria, differentiation is important.

A quantitative method to detect the presence of orthostatic proteinuria has been established. On arising at 7 AM, the patient voids and discards the urine. Thereafter, all urine is collected in a single container until 10 PM, when the patient voids into the same bottle and immediately assumes a recumbent position. At 7 AM on the following morning (immediately on arising), the patient voids into a second bottle. If the patient has orthostatic proteinuria, the recumbent collection should contain 75 mg of protein or less, and the sum contents of both specimens should be 1,500 mg or less. Alternatively, a qualitative test using sulfosalicylic acid can be used; the recumbent specimen should be negative, and the upright specimen should be positive.

The mechanism by which an upright posture causes proteinuria is not well understood. The appearance of proteinuria may reflect altered glomerular capillary-wall permeability, which is manifested when coupled with the hemodynamic consequences of an upright position (e.g., decreased renal blood flow). Renal histologic results from men with orthostatic proteinuria showed that 8% of patients had unequivocal evidence of renal disease, 45% had subtle but definite alterations of the glomerulus, and 47% appeared normal. Ten years after the time of diagnosis, 49% of all of these individuals had proteinuria, yet none had impairment of renal function. Therefore, the prognosis of patients with orthostatic proteinuria appears to be excellent. A renal biopsy is not indicated unless there are changes in the patient's clinical picture, such as alterations in the urine sediment, serum creatinine, or amount of proteinuria. Yearly follow-up examinations are advised, including repeat urinalysis.

Constant proteinuria is an arbitrary category that includes patients whose proteinuria persists during recumbency but does not fall into the category of nephrotic-range proteinuria because less than 3.5 gm of protein per 24 hours is excreted. This group is generally regarded with concern, although data on the importance and prognosis of constant proteinuria are scarce. A 40-year follow-up study of university students with proteinuria on entrance physical examinations found that the mortality rate was increased only in those who had constant proteinuria or clinically obvious renal disease. Those who had intermittent proteinuria had the same mortality rate as persons with no renal abnormalities.

If the patient has normal creatinine clearance and no other urine sediment abnormalities, there is no reason to perform a renal biopsy. As long as there is no clue to underlying renal disease, clinical follow-up at 3-month intervals is advised initially. If renal function and urine sediment remain unchanged, less frequent clinic visits are appropriate. The appearance of hematuria, an increase in proteinuria, or a decrease in creatinine clearance wa:·rants additional evaluation, with consideration of a renal biopsy.

Nephrotic Syndrome

Protein excretion in excess of 3.5 gm per 24 hours is termed *nephrotic-range proteinuria*. The nephrotic syndrome is defined as nephrotic-range proteinuria together with its consequences: hypoalbuminemia, hyperlipidemia, and edema.

Initial evaluation of the nephrotic syndrome should include determinations of 24-hour protein and creatinine clearance. Unless the nephrotic syndrome is clearly caused by an associated systemic illness (e.g., diabetes mellitus), referral to a nephrologist for kidney biopsy is in order.

The nephrotic syndrome can be divided into two groups by cause: idiopathic and secondary. The idiopathic nephrotic syndrome is additionally classified by glomerular histopathology. Of the primary glomerulopathies, only minimal-change disease clearly responds to steroid therapy. The rate of rise of serum creatine may be retarded by the use of corticosteroids in membranous glomerulopathy. The importance of making a histopathologic diagnosis is not only in detecting treatable disease but also in providing the patient and clinician with an appreciation for the clinical patterns and prognoses that characterize different lesions. The nephrotic syndrome may be associated with a variety of infections, malignancies, drugs, allergies, systemic diseases, and inherited disorders. If the underlying disease can be treated successfully, or if it spontaneously remits, the nephrotic syndrome also may resolve.

Reuben DB, et al. Transient proteinuria in emergency medical admissions. *N Engl J Med* 306:1031–1033, 1982.
Nine and one-half percent of emergency medical admissions had transient proteinuria that disappeared by the ninth hospital day.

Robinson RR. Isolated proteinuria in asymptomatic patients. *Kidney Int* 18:395–406, 1980.
A very lucid and concise review of the mechanisms, clinical importance, and prognosis of nonnephrotic proteinuria in the asymptomatic patient.

Rytanf DA, Spreiter S. Prognosis in postural (orthostatic) proteinuria. *N Engl J Med* 305:618–621, 1981.
A 42- to 50-year follow-up of six patients diagnosed by Thomas Addis. None developed renal disease or died of a renal cause.

Levitt JI. The prognostic significance of proteinuria in young college students. *Ann Intern Med* 66:685–696, 1967.
A retrospective study with a 37- to 45-year follow-up showing that persons with intermittent proteinuria have no increase in mortality, whereas those with constant proteinuria or clinically apparent renal disease have a definite increase in mortality.

Earley LM, Gottschalk CW. *Strauss and Welt's Diseases of the Kidney* (3rd ed.). Boston: Little, Brown, 1979. Pp. 62–71, 765–813.
A good textbook approach to proteinuria and an in-depth discussion of the nephrotic syndrome.

Glassock RJ, et al. Primary Glomerular Diseases. In BM Brenner and FC Rector (Eds.), *The Kidney* (2nd ed.). Philadelphia: Saunders, 1981.
A detailed, complete review of primary glomerular disease.

Brenner BM, Hostetter TH, Humes HD. Molecular basis of proteinuria of glomerular origin. *N Engl J Med* 298:826–833, 1978.
A review of the properties of the glomerular capillary wall that impart to it the ability to retard the passage of protein and other macromolecules.

Collaborative study of adult idiopathic nephrotic syndrome. A controlled study of short-term prednisone treatment in adults with membranous nephropathy. *N Engl J Med* 301:1301–1306, 1979.
The most often-quoted reference to support treating membranous nephropathy with prednisone. The treated group had a less rapid rate of rise in serum creatinine.

67. URINARY INCONTINENCE IN THE ELDERLY
Mark E. Williams

Approximately 10% of elderly men and 15% of elderly women living in the community have urinary incontinence; in the institutional setting, the prevalence approaches 50%. Urinary incontinence can result in substantial psychological, social, medical, and economic problems. If not effectively treated, it increases social isolation, frequently results in a loss of independence through institutionalization, and predisposes to infections and skin breakdown.

Normal Physiology
To maintain urinary continence, intravesicular pressure must be less than intraurethral pressure. Intravesicular pressure is related to intra-abdominal pressure, the amount of urine contained in the bladder, and the contractile state of the detrusor muscle. Destrusor tone is augmented by decreased central nervous system inhibition, cholinergic stimulation, and increased afferent stimulation; it is diminished by cholinergic inhibition, muscle relaxants, and decreased afferent stimulation.

Intraurethral pressure is maintained through periurethral striated muscle, smooth muscle of the urethra and bladder neck, and the urethral mucosal thickness. The external urethral sphincter, which allows voluntary cessation of urine flow, is not necessary for continence.

Smooth muscle tone of the urethra and bladder neck is an important determinant of intraurethral pressure and thus bladder outlet resistance. Factors that increase tone include prostatic hypertrophy and alpha-sympathetic stimulation. Tone is weakened by sympathetic blockade; muscle relaxants, such as diazepam; bladder prolapse, which decreases the sphincter's mechanical advantage; and the consequences of surgical manipulation of the pelvis, bladder, or urethra. Thickness of the urethral mucosa in women is maintained by estrogens and decreases in estrogen deficiency.

The following neurologic pathways are involved in maintaining continence. Stretch receptors in the bladder wall communicate the volume status to the brain. When a critical degree of bladder distention is reached, detrusor contractions occur, which must be inhibited by higher cortical centers to avoid abrupt bladder emptying. Voluntary voiding is accomplished in part by increasing intra-abdominal pressure through contractions of the abdominal muscles and diaphragm, synchronized with relaxation of the urethral sphincter.

Pathophysiology
Five basic causes of incontinence are detrusor instability, overflow incontinence, sphincter insufficiency, functional illness, and iatrogenic factors. Although any of the mechanisms may predominate, combinations often occur.

Detrusor instability is the most common type of incontinence, occurring in up to 70% in some series. Synonyms include *unstable bladder, spastic bladder,* and *uninhibited bladder.* The essential lesion is uninhibited bladder contractions sufficient to overcome urethral resistance. Three basic mechanisms can cause this instability: (1) defects in CNS inhibitory mechanisms, such as in frontal lobe lesions; (2) hyperexcitability of afferent sensory pathways, such as in acute cystitis, small bladder capacity, bladder wall hypertrophy, and fecal impaction; and (3) deconditioned voiding reflexes.

Deconditioned reflexes may affect CNS inhibition and afferent stimulation by altering micturition patterns. For example, chronic frequent low-volume voiding results in decreased bladder capacity, increased detrusor tone, and increased bladder wall thickness. These events can establish a vicious cycle of incontinence, anxiety, frequent voiding to avoid another accident, increased bladder tone, increased likelihood of incontinence, anxiety, frequent voiding to avoid another accident, increased bladder tone, and so on.

Clinical features of detrusor instability are generally nonspecific. There are no characteristic findings on physical examination. On cystometrogram the classic finding is a bladder that begins to show spontaneous contractions at very low volumes.

Overflow incontinence occurs when intravesicular pressure exceeds intraurethral pressure only at high bladder volumes. Causes are (1) bladder outlet obstruction, such as by prostatic hypertrophy, calculi, or carcinoma; (2) detrusor inadequacy, also called *atonic bladder* and *neurogenic bladder*, which may occur in Parkinsons's disease, diabetic autonomic neuropathy, or lumbosacral spinal cord disease; and (3) impaired afferent sensation, a form of atonic or neurogenic bladder, such as in diabetes mellitus. Clinical features include a palpable or percussible bladder, often with suprapubic tenderness. A cystometrogram reveals no bladder contractions despite high pressures (greater than 20 cm H_2O) and high volumes (more than 400 cc).

Sphincter insufficiency, or stress incontinence, is common in elderly women. The probable causes are postmenopausal changes in the urethral mucosa, related to the decline of estrogens, combined with weakness of the pelvic muscles that comes with aging and multiparity. In addition, urinary tract infections can precipitate stress incontinence. The prevalence of symptomatic stress incontinence depends on the definition; as many as 50% of young nulliparous women admit occasional minor "leakage." Stress incontinence in men usually occurs only with urinary tract infection, after surgery, or as a result of severe neurologic disease.

Clinical features include incontinence following coughing, laughing, straining, or other conditions that cause an abrupt increase in intra-abdominal pressure. Patients are often dry at night, and there are no symptoms of detrusor instability. Physical examination may demonstrate visible leakage of urine on coughing or during abdominal palpation (to increase intra-abdominal pressure). Pelvic examination may reveal a reddened vulva or periurethral tissue (secondary to decreased estrogen), or relaxed pelvic musculature. Palpable funneling of the urethra may be demonstrated by placing the tips of the first two fingers on each side of the urethra and extending them only 1 or 2 cm into the vagina. If an impact is felt against the fingertips when the patient coughs, then funneling is present. Laboratory studies may disclose signs of urinary tract infection.

Functional incontinence is suggested by a history of accidents on the way to the toilet or early in the morning. Musculoskeletal limitations may prevent an otherwise continent person from reaching the toilet in time.

Patients occasionally become incontinent to command more attention. Usually an element of depression, hostility, or anger is present. This "spiteful" incontinence is intermittent, usually does not occur at night, and can be a difficult management problem.

Iatrogenic incontinence may aggravate or unmask any of the above problems. The use of potent, fast-acting diuretics or physical restraints may make it difficult for elderly people to be continent. Psychoactive medications such as sedatives, hypnotics, or antipsychotics may create a loss of attention to bladder cues. Sphincter weakness may be precipitated by muscle relaxants, sympathetic blockers, or other agents that affect the autonomic balance in the central nervous system.

Evaluation

No one of the diagnostic tests ordinarily used is good enough to be considered definitive. For example, a cystometrogram in continent people, especially elderly women, may show the same kinds of abnormalities seen in incontinent people.

The history should include the onset, duration, and pattern of incontinence (e.g., intermittent, continuous, morning, night); the amount of urine lost; any neurologic symptoms; coexistent medical problems, such as diabetes mellitus, Parkinson's disease, or multiple sclerosis; and all medications being used.

The physical examination should include a complete neurologic evaluation and a careful pelvic and rectal examination, including a vaginal smear for epithelial maturation, which is an estrogen effect. Special studies include serum glucose, calcium, electrolytes, and BUN to exclude polyuric syndromes; urinalysis; and, when indicated, cystometrogram and cystoscopy.

The diagnosis may be simplified if the following points are kept in mind: (1) a palpable or percussible bladder usually signifies overflow incontinence; (2) the absence of signs of overflow or stress incontinence suggests detrusor instability; (3) if stress incontinence is present, particularly in older women, it may be the only lesion, or it may be mixed with detrusor instability; cystometric studies are indicated, therefore, to differentiate the two.

Treatment
More than 75% of ambulatory patients can expect resolution of incontinence with optimal management. Consequently, an optimistic and supportive outlook is appropriate. A correct diagnosis is the prerequisite to effective treatment. Iatrogenic causes and occult urinary tract infection should be ruled out. Behavioral strategies are complementary to pharmacologic approaches.

Detrusor Instability
Medications are used to decrease detrusor contractions. Imipramine, a tricyclic antidepressant with coexistent anticholinergic and alpha-sympathetic activity, is the current treatment of choice. The usual starting dosage is 25 mg at bedtime, but higher dosages are frequently required. Complications of this regimen include (1) increased residual volume or acute urinary retention; (2) mental status changes, such as confusion or "sundowning"; and (3) cardiovascular effects, such as orthostatic hypotension and the precipitation of arrhythmias or heart block (the presence of these factors before treatment does not contraindicate therapy).

Anticholinergic or antispasmodic medications, such as propantheline or flavoxate, are second-line drugs, and there is no evidence that one group of drugs is superior to the other. The dosage must be titrated, especially in elderly people.

Overflow Incontinence
Pharmacologic interventions attempt to increase detrusor contractions or decrease bladder outlet resistance. Cholinomimetic agents such as bethanechol serve the former purpose, whereas alpha-adrenergic blocking agents such as phenoxybenzamine, or skeletal muscle relaxants like diazepam, dantrolene, or baclofen, decrease outlet resistance.

A nonpharmacologic strategy is frequently the treatment of choice in overflow incontinence. Surgery is preferred in instances of mechanical outlet obstruction, such as prostatic hypertrophy, calculi, or carcinoma. In extreme instances, an artificial sphincter can be implanted surgically.

Intermittent self-catheterization is sometimes indicated. Infection is less likely than with continuous indwelling catheterization, and it can be done by family members with minimal training if the patient is unable to perform the procedure.

Sphincter Insufficiency
Sphincter insufficiency can be treated pharmacologically by alpha-adrenergic agonists such as phenylpropanolamine, which increase urethral tone. In addition, oral or topical estrogens can improve stress incontinence in estrogen-deficient women by restoring the thickness of the urethral mucosa. Exercises to strengthen pelvic muscles, and increased ambulation, which augments the perception of bladder filling, can be helpful. In resistant situations, surgical procedures to support a prolapsed bladder are usually effective.

Functional Incontinence
Functional incontinence is best managed by a behavioral approach. To avoid paradoxically conditioning the patient toward incontinent behavior, it is important to avoid unpleasant stimuli such as bed pans, low or cold toilet seats, toileting at fixed intervals, or toileting immediately after an episode of incontinence. Successful toileting should be positively reinforced. Bladder content can be estimated by keeping an incontinence chart to record the micturition pattern. The patient is checked every 2 hours for 48 hours, and a record is kept of whether the patient is wet or dry. The pattern obtained establishes the optimal toileting program for that patient.

Palliative Measures
Palliative measures supplement more specific treatments. These must be socially acceptable (i.e., they must control the smell but not be excessively bulky under the clothing), and they must keep the patient dry. Strategies meeting these requirements are the use of rubber or plastic pants with absorbent pads or superabsorbent chemicals, intermittent self-catheterization as discussed above, and collection devices. Indwelling catheters and collecting systems are used only as a last resort.

Williams ME, Pannill FC. Urinary incontinence in the elderly: A review of physiology, pathophysiology, diagnosis and treatment. *Ann Intern Med* 97:895–907, 1982.
An extensively referenced review summarizing the relevant literature on urinary incontinence, which expands on the material in this chapter.

Krane RJ, Siroky MB (Eds.). *Clinical Neuro-Urology.* Boston: Little, Brown, 1979.
An excellent general reference.

Willington FL (Ed.). *Incontinence in the Elderly.* London: Academic, 1979.
This book, by a British expert, provides useful summaries of areas underemphasized by other authors.

Bradley WE. Innervation of the male urinary bladder. *Urol Clin North Am* 5:279–293, 1978.

Kuru M. Nervous control of micturition. *Physiol Rev* 45:425–449, 1965.
Excellent Reviews of the neurologic control of micturition.

Newman JL. Old folks in wet beds. *Br Med J* 1:1824–27, 1962.
A personal view of the psychological effects of incontinence and how health providers often have an inaccurate perspective of the problem.

Raz S. Pharmacological treatment of lower urinary tract dysfunction. *Urol Clin North Am* 5:323–334, 1978.

Westmore DD. Urinary incontinence: Which drugs to use. *Drugs* 17:418–422, 1979.
Useful reviews of the pharmologic treatment of incontinence.

Castleden CM, Duffin HM. Guidelines for controlling urinary incontinence without drugs or catheters. *Age Ageing* 10:186–190, 1981.
An excellent review of behavioral treatments of incontinence.

68. URINARY CATHETERS

J. Pack Hindsley, Jr.

Urinary catheters are used in numerous settings and for many different indications. Types commonly available include (1) those without inflatable balloons, (2) Foley catheters for long-term use, and (3) three-way catheters for irrigation. The adult male urethra should readily accept a #16 or #18 (circumference in millimeters) French catheter. Size is not frequently a limiting factor in women.

Drainage Systems

In the *open system*, the catheter drainage bag is frequently disconnected from the catheter. Indications for open drainage systems—massive hematuria, conditions requiring bladder irrigation, and instillation of medications—are unusual in routine medical practice. With open catheter drainage, nearly half of all patients are infected within 72 hours and 100% within 7 days.

In the *closed system*, the catheter or drainage bag is never opened to external contamination, and retrograde infection is thereby delayed by several weeks compared to an open system. Only 2 to 3% of patients are infected in 2 days, and it takes approximately 4 weeks for all to be infected. To maintain sterility in closed systems, the following rules should be followed:

1. The catheter must be inserted under sterile conditions after the urethral meatus and the skin surrounding the urethra are carefully cleansed with surgical cleansing agents such as iodophor or Hibiclens. The catheter bag is attached to the catheter and is never disconnected until the catheter is removed.
2. The catheter bag should be drained approximately every 8 hours with care not to contaminate the spigot.
3. The bag should be hung below the patient and never inverted.

It is assumed that infection nearly always reaches the bladder from the catheter bag; bacteria are carried along the interface between air bubbles and the urine as bubbles ascend the catheter into the bladder. If a closed system is maintained, infections in the drainage bag almost always precede bacteriuria. Clinical trials placing formalin, hydrogen peroxide, and antibacterial agents in the drainage have all shown a resulting decrease in bacteriuria. For long-term drainage, antiseptics such as 30 cc of hydrogen peroxide should be added to the drainage bag with each emptying. The use of prophylactic systemic antibiotics to suppress or prevent bacteriuria while a catheter is in place is condemned. It has been shown that long-term use of suppressive antibiotics results in infection with resistant organisms.

Care of the urethral meatus is frequently recommended, but a recent report comparing povidone-iodine (Betadine) ointment, green soap, and no care showed that the patient receiving no care had fewer infections than the other two groups. One explanation for this is that natural defenses are broken down by detergents.

Most authors recommend treating bacteriuria found at the time of removal of a urinary catheter with appropriate antibiotics. Although most physicians think this recommendation is appropriate, it is not clear that it is necessary.

Three-way catheters, designed in the early 1960s to replace the standard Foley catheter, have a channel for urine, a second channel to the balloon, and a third channel for irrigating substances. Studies comparing "open" urinary systems to three-way irrigation systems showed that urinary tract infections can be delayed by irrigation of the bladder with an antiseptic or antibiotic solution through the irrigating channel. Since the advent of the closed drainage system, however, the routine use of the three-way irrigating system has not been necessary.

Use of Catheters

In-and-out catheterization implies insertion of a urethral catheter into the bladder, with removal of the catheter immediately after drainage of urine. This is most frequently done with a simple rubber or plastic catheter, without any balloon or other device for maintaining the catheter in the bladder.

In women, in-and-out catheterization is frequently the best means of obtaining an adequate specimen for culture. If the patient is uninfected before catheterization, the risk of infection from in-and-out catheterization is approximately 4%.

In men, in-and-out catheterization may be performed to relieve acute urinary retention caused by overdistention or medications. (See Chap. 62, Benign Prostatic Hyperplasia.)

Intermittent catheterization (IC) refers to frequent in-and-out catheterizations in patients who are unable to void. Used for any length of time, IC generally is safer than indwelling catheterization. The greatest problem with IC is that it often is done incorrectly. The most frequent mistakes are (1) improper cleansing techniques, (2) teaching catheter use only in bed with mirrors rather than with a touch technique, which allows catheterization in bathrooms or a sitting position, (3) improper use of fluids, such as allowing drinking before bed or trips, (4) advising catheterization at rigid, specific intervals rather than letting patients find their own frequency.

Training of patients and families is best done in the hospital, under the supervision of a urologist or nurse well trained in IC techniques. IC must be taught in a systematic manner, with the problems outlined and the techniques supervised. Properly taught and applied, IC can be a superior technique for managing a compromised urinary system in paraplegics and patients with neurogenic bladders or other neurologic disorders.

Short-term catheterization is indicated for acute urinary retention caused by trauma, medication, urinary stones, or blockage of the urinary outlets by prostatitis, benign prostatic hyperplasia, or strictures. Catheterization also may be necessary for the management of surgical and medical illnesses that require close monitoring of urinary output, such as massive trauma, burns, congestive heart failure, and fluid and electrolyte disturbances. One test of the appropriateness of catheterization is that the catheter not be used for the convenience of the physician or medical personnel.

Long-term catheterization may be arbitrarily defined as catheterization lasting longer than 30 days. Patients may undergo years of catheter drainage of the urinary system. Long-term catheterization has the potential for causing serious infections, bladder stones, and fistulas. Talbot in 1959 reported on 59 patients who had catheters for 1 to 14 years (see references). All patients had bacteriuria, but 72% had no evidence of renal damage. However, the goals of rehabilitation for all patients should include the eventual removal of indwelling urinary catheters.

There are no studies on proper care of long-term catheters. Most urologists feel that long-term catheters should be changed every month to 6 weeks, because they may become encrusted with salts precipitated in the urine. Patients with continuing problems with encrustation of the catheter may be instructed to irrigate the catheter periodically with tap water. Bacteriuria is a constant problem with long-term indwelling catheters. However, antibiotics are not recommended except for acute symptomatic infections. Public health nurses, and sometimes, family members, can be trained in catheter changing and care, but the physician in charge must not abandon the patient with an indwelling catheter.

Problems with Catheters

Difficulty passing the catheter is most frequently caused by inadequate lubrication. Lubricant applied to the tip of a catheter is almost always wiped off in passage through the first several centimeters of the urethra. If a catheter-tipped syringe is filled with 5 to 10 cc of water-soluble lubricant and the lubricant *gently* introduced into the urethra, adequate lubrication for easy catheter passage is almost always obtained.

If the catheter cannot be passed because obstruction is met, the physician must try to determine the cause. If prostatic cancer or urethral stricture is suspected, the urethra should be lubricated as described above, which may allow a small #12 or #14 French catheter to pass through the nondistensible portion of the urethra. However, if prostatic hypertrophy is encountered, a larger catheter (#20 or #22 French) may push aside the obstructing lobes and pass into the bladder. Excessive force and rigid instruments should always be avoided. Once a catheter is placed, the balloon should not be expanded until a free flow of urine is obtained. If a patient complains of discomfort when the balloon is blown up, the fluid should be let out of the balloon immediately and the catheter repositioned; otherwise, urethral lacerations may result.

There have been recommendations to limit the quantity of urine released by catheterization to avoid shock from rapid bladder decompression. There is no scientific basis for this. Pressure in the bladder returns to normal levels after the first 10 to 15% of the urine escapes. Postobstructive diuresis is an unrelated problem. An alert patient is able to replace the fluid loss adequately by oral fluid intake. If the patient is not alert or conscious, intravenous fluids are necessary. Close monitoring of BUN, creatinine, and electrolytes is mandatory. Rarely, a person is left with a concentrating defect similar to nephrogenic diabetes insipidus.

After a Foley catheter is withdrawn, swelling at the prostatic urethra or bladder neck, with or without infection, may occasionally cause obstruction. This problem is best managed by antibiotic therapy and intermittent catheterization.

Cox CE, Hinman F. Incidence of bacteriuria with indwelling catheter in normal bladders. *JAMA* 178:919–921, 1961.
   Spontaneous clearing of bacteriuria from normal bladders.
Burke JP, et al. Prevention of catheter-associated urinary tract infections. *Am J Med* 70:655–658, 1981.
   A modern article explaining the use of urinary catheters.
Kunin CM, McCormack RC. Prevention of catheter-induced urinary tract infections by sterile closed drainage. *N Engl J Med* 274:1155–1161, 1966.
   An important study of closed urinary drainage systems.
Talbot HS, Mahoney EM, Jaffe SR. The effects of prolonged urethral catheterization: 1. Persistence of normal renal structure and function. *J Urol* 81:138–156, 1959.
   Prolonged catheter usage in a paraplegic population.

X. MUSCULOSKELETAL PROBLEMS

Osteoarthritis, also called *osteoarthrosis* and *hypertrophic* or *degenerative joint disease,* is a generally noninflammatory arthritis seen radiographically in 90% of adults over the age of 50. It is the most common form of chronic arthritis and is responsible for pain and limitation of motion in approximately one-quarter of the adult population.

Primary osteoarthritis accounts for 90% of patients with osteoarthritis in an unselected practice. The most commonly involved joints are the distal interphalangeals (DIPs), proximal interphalangeals (PIPs), hip, knee, first metatarsal phalangeal joint (MTP), and cervical and lumbosacral spine. Some degree of degenerative change in articular cartilage is universal with increasing age, but onset, rate of progression, and severity vary greatly. If a joint is maligned or has been traumatized or inflamed, the changes appear more rapidly. Secondary osteoarthritis results from mechanical incongruity and/or of cartilage destruction, which may be caused by congenital defects, joint infection or inflammation, trauma, or endocrine-metabolic disease.

Clinical Presentation

The most common presenting symptoms in patients with osteoarthritis are pain, stiffness, joint enlargement, and limitation of joint motion. The pain of osteoarthritis begins insidiously; patients describe an aching or nagging discomfort. Morning stiffness or stiffness after prolonged immobility generally lasts less than 30 minutes. Early in the course, joint pain occurs after vigorous activity, but with deterioration pain may occur after modest or minimal activity, and eventually, even at rest. For most patients with early osteoarthritis, flares of symptoms are self-limited. It is not clear whether this is the natural course of the disease, whether the pain is caused by synovitis from hydroxyapatite crystals, or whether pain leads to resting of the joint and resolution of symptoms.

Joint enlargement results from osteophyte formation and feels hard in comparison to the spongy feel of synovial proliferation. Deformity and subluxation result from bony overgrowth, loss of cartilage, and collapsed subchondral bone and cysts. Limitation of motion results from joint surface incongruity, muscle spasm, capsular contracture, and structural blockage from osteophytes or loose bodies.

Diagnostic Evaluation

The diagnosis of osteoarthritis is based on characteristic symptoms and physical findings. X-ray evaluation is extremely helpful in the diagnosis of osteoarthritis of weight-bearing joints and the spine. The four cardinal radiologic features that must be present to make a definite diagnosis include (1) unequal loss of joint space (an early finding), (2) osteophytes, (3) eburnation (juxta-articular sclerosis), and (4) subchondral bone cysts. However, the severity of pain in osteoarthritis correlates poorly with the radiologic appearance of the joint. Because the radiographic findings of osteoarthritis are extremely common, the clinician should always consider another diagnosis, especially if the following are present: (1) the complaint is in an uncommon joint for osteoarthritis, such as the glenohumeral joint; (2) signs and symptoms of systemic illness exist; (3) neuromotor or vascular symptoms are present; (4) symptoms have been present for less than a month or are of acute onset; (5) there is objective evidence of synovitis, which is unusual in osteoarthritis.

Laboratory tests are normal in primary osteoarthritis, and therefore are useful only when a diagnosis other than osteoarthritis is suggested by clinical findings.

The approach to osteoarthritis varies somewhat according to the site of involvement.

Hand

Involvement of the hand is characterized by bony proliferation and the absence of objective synovitis in the small joints of the fingers: Heberden's (DIP joints) and Bouchard's (PIP joints) nodes. Early symptoms usually include aching, discomfort, and stiffness, increased by heavy finger use. Metacarpophalangeal joints are rarely involved, except for the first MCP (the base of the thumb), which produces pain increased by gripping and twisting movements of the hands. X-ray evaluation of Heberden's and Bouchard's nodes is unnecessary.

Hip

Approximately 60% of patients with osteoarthritis of the hip complain of pain in the area of the greater trochanter and, less frequently, pain in the groin, back of the thigh, low back, or referred to the knee. The pain and stiffness associated with early osteoarthritis of the hip usually follow immobility and periods of excessive weight bearing.

The hip is relatively inaccessible to examination by observation or palpation. The earliest abnormality is reduced internal rotation (normal internal rotation is 35–45°) and abduction (normal is 45–50°). With progression of disease, hip motion is restricted in all directions, and the hip is flexed and foreshortened.

Important negative findings include absence of abnormality in other joints and a normal neuromuscular and vascular examination. Areas about the hip should be palpated for discrete tenderness secondary to bursitis, tendinitis, or muscle spasm. If the pain is referred to the area of the greater trochanter, trochanteric bursitis may be the cause of the pain.

Unequal leg length may be a cause of osteoarthritis of the hip; a difference greater than 2 inches, measured from the symphysis pubis to the medial malleolus, can cause hip pain by placing stress on the abductor muscles of the longer leg. Because the leg on the involved side is generally shortened by disease, the finding of a longer leg on the symptomatic side suggests that greater disparity existed before the onset of disease.

The earliest x-ray finding of osteoarthritis of the hip is unequal narrowing of the joint space. Minor narrowing may be detected if there is a difference in width of greater than 1 mm between the joint spaces of the normal and affected sides. If bilateral narrowing is present, unequivocal narrowing must be present before the diagnosis can be made with confidence. The joint space is probably abnormal if it is less than 4 mm in patients under age 70 or less than 3 mm in patients over 70. Osteophytes alone are not diagnostic of osteoarthritis, nor is there a relation between the presence of osteophytes and clinical symptoms.

Primary osteoarthritis of the hip may be classified into two prognostic groups by radiologic picture: superolateral and medial. With superolateral disease, persistent unilateral involvement and progressive symptoms are the rule. In the medial form of osteoarthritis, involvement is usually bilateral initially or with time, and progression is variable.

Knee

Osteoarthritis of the knee produces pain after weight bearing, particularly climbing, descending stairs, and rising from a sitting position. The diagnosis is made by (1) eliminating other possible causes of knee pain such as pes anserinus or patellar bursitis, tendinitis, internal derangement, inflammatory joint disease, joint instability, and hip disorders; and (2) finding specific clinical and x-ray evidence of osteoarthritis. A weight-bearing film of both knees provides the most sensitive method of looking for cartilage loss and assessing the amount of varus or valgus deformity. Both AP and lateral views are necessary. Both knees should be included in the x-rays to evaluate the importance of radiologic changes.

Spine

Virtually everyone has pathologic evidence of osteoarthritis of the spine by age 70, occurring in the vertebrae or posterior diarthrodial joints. The most commonly involved areas are the lower cervical spine (C6–7) and the lower lumbar spine (L3–5, S1). Osteoarthritis of the spine produces poorly localized pain, which may radiate along the paraspinal areas and extend to the buttocks. Nerve root encroachment by an osteophyte or irritation by synovitis may produce neurologic symptoms. If the spinal cord is compressed, upper motor neuron symptoms may develop. Stiffness and decreased range of motion are common symptoms as well. On examination, stiffness, crepitus, local pain and tenderness, and muscle spasm may be present. In the neck, lateral flexion, rotation, and extension are usually more limited than forward flexion. Two very common syndromes occur in the cervical spine: compression of the 6th cervical nerve and compression of the 7th cervical nerve. In the former, one may note weakness in the biceps on shoulder flexion and in the wrist extensors by testing wrist extension against resistance. There is diminished biceps deep tendon reflex and diminished sensation to the thumb and index finger. In compression of the 7th cervical nerve, one notes weakness of the triceps by testing extension against resistance, a diminished triceps deep tendon reflex, and diminished sensation to the index and middle fingers.

In the lumbar spine, L4–5 and L5–S1 are most commonly involved. Acute symptoms may be superimposed on chronic mechanical low back pain. Severe loss of spinal mobility usually does not occur until late in the disease.

Involvement of the spine requires AP and lateral and oblique x-ray views. Diagnostic findings include straightening or reversal of lordosis; narrowing of the intervertebral disc spaces with anterior and posterior osteophytes; laterally situated osteophytes on the vertebral bodies; deformity of the vertebral bodies; sclerosis; and encroachment on the intervertebral foramina by osteophytes and malaligned vertebral bodies.

Treatment

In the medical management of osteoarthritis, the natural history of the disease must be kept in mind. For example, osteoarthritis of the fingers is generally not progressive and does not lead to crippling or loss of function. Although osteoarthritis of the weight-bearing joints, especially unilateral disease, is more likely to progress, one-third of cases do not.

Preservation of function and reduction in pain are the major goals of management. The therapeutic plan should begin with an evaluation of the effect of the disease on the patient's life. What necessary activities can't the patient do? Does the pain interfere with work, play, or sleep, and how much discomfort is experienced with these activities? Treatable components of joint symptoms such as bursitis and tendinitis should be identified, and biomechanical factors, which may exacerbate the degenerative process, should be reduced.

Biomechanical Factors

Early treatment in osteoarthritis of the hip or knee should be directed at correction of biomechanical problems that accelerate the degenerative process. If a discrepancy in leg length exists, a trial of therapy with a heel wedge of equivalent height may reduce symptoms considerably. Appliances such as canes and crutches are very helpful. For example, a static force of 385 pounds on one hip may be reduced to 66 pounds with a downward push of 38 pounds. Quadriceps-strengthening exercises in osteoarthritis of the knee are useful in providing additional support to the joint. Weight reduction should be recommended, although it is often difficult to achieve. In normal gait, three to five times the body weight is distributed across the knee or hip, and even a modest weight loss can reduce this force considerably.

Osteoarthritis of the cervical or lumbosacral spine may be painful because of nerve entrapment, muscle spasm, and/or joint inflammation. General measures include a cervical collar and cervical traction for cervical spine pain. For lumbosacral spine pain, useful general measures include instructions on techniques to reduce stresses on the back, isometric exercises for the abdominal muscles, and stretching of the hip flexors. A custom-made corset, available through physical therapy departments, is helpful. In acute pain, muscle spasm, or nerve entrapment, the mainstays of treatment are bed rest and analgesics.

Local Measures

In general, cold is likely to be useful in acute musculoskeletal pain and heat in subacute pain. There is no proof that deep heat is better than superficial heat. There is no advantage of one type of superficial heat over another (moist heat, hot packs, hot soaks, paraffin, hot mud). Heating pads should be discouraged because patients may fall asleep during the application and suffer first-degree burns. Relative contraindications to heat include sensory neuropathies and circulatory impairment.

In patients with osteoarthritis of the hands, avoiding excessive finger use, such as in crocheting, is sometimes all that is required for symptomatic relief. Local symptomatic relief may be achieved by soaking the hands in warm water in the morning and using nylon spandex stretch gloves at night. Osteoarthritis of the first carpal-metacarpal joint responds well to thumb splinting. Rarely is surgery necessary, but persons with refractory pain may be considered for joint osteoplasty or arthrodesis. Neither is ideal, and both require lengthy treatment. In patients with Heberden's and Bouchard's nodes occasionally one joint is symptomatic out of proportion to the others, and local steroid injection into the joint or mucinous cyst may offer temporary benefit.

Steroid Injections

A careful search for pes anserinus, trochanteric bursitis, or tendinitis is useful, because these conditions respond to local steroid injection. Intra-articular steroids usually have little role in osteoarthritis of the hip or knee, but can be tried if there is clinical evidence of synovitis (caused by intra-articular debris), or if the onset is abrupt. Steroid injection of the hip is a difficult procedure and should be undertaken only by a skilled rheumatologist or orthopedic surgeon. Steroid injections should not be done more than six times in the life of a joint and not within 6 weeks before joint surgery.

Drug Therapy

Anti-inflammatory medication is often useful in osteoarthritis for symptoms such as swelling, stiffness, and warmth. Aspirin and most nonsteroidal anti-inflammatory drugs (NSAIDs) are comparable in their effects and should be used intermittently. Recent evidence suggests that prolonged use of NSAIDs may accelerate cartilage degeneration. All the NSAIDs have similar side effects, which include gastrointestinal intolerance, fluid retention, platelet abnormalities, and hepatic and renal dysfunction (see Chap. 70). Both patient tolerance to side effects and individual therapeutic response may vary from one preparation to another. Therefore, one may be effective when others fail, and, if necessary, several alternatives should be tried. For the majority of patients, flares of symptoms with inflammation are self-limited, and aggressive medication is rarely necessary. Patients should be educated to use aspirin and NSAIDs in a way that best enables them to function with their disease.

Surgery

When joint destruction is advanced and pain or disability is refractory to conservative treatment, total joint replacement should be considered. An "end-stage" joint is likely when the patient is prevented from sleep or minimal weight bearing by pain, requires narcotics for pain, or has an unacceptable functional limitation. Other considerations include whether the damaged joint is the primary limiting condition, whether the total joint replacement will outlive the patient, and whether there are other treatment options. In the young patient with medial compartment narrowing and varus deformity of the knee, osteotomy may be recommended as a procedure to postpone total joint replacement. Contraindications to total joint replacement include youth (great physical activity may hasten loosening, requiring revision surgery), lack of motivation (recovery after total joint replacement requires vigorous physical therapy), the presence of active infection or severe neurosensory deficits, and inadequate "bone stock."

Pain relief is achieved in more than 90% of patients who undergo total joint replacement of the knee and hip. Clinical failure requiring revision surgery occurs in approximately 2% of patients. Operative mortality ranges from 0.5 to 1.9%; facilities treating 50 patients per year or fewer have a higher mortality. Morbidity is less than 2%, and complications include loosening of the prosthesis with time, deep or superficial infection, and dislocation.

For total joint replacement to be successful, the patient must have a clear understanding of goals. Physical activity is not completely normal after total joint replacement, and patients often must modify habits that place the prosthetic hip or knee at risk of dislocation. The best results in total joint replacement require careful patient selection, medical follow-up, patient education, and rehabilitation management.

Bland JH, Stulberg SD. Osteoarthritis: Pathology and Clinical Patterns. In WN Kelly et al. (Eds.), *Textbook of Rheumatology*. Philadelphia: Saunders, 1981. Pp. 1471–1490.
  A good general discussion of pathology.
Sheon RP, Moskowitz RW, Goldberg VM. Soft Tissue Rheumatic Pain: Recognition Management, Prevention. Philadelphia: Lea & Febiger, 1982. Pp. 172–202.
  A good discussion on examination and diagnosis of soft-tissue symptoms associated with osteoarthritis.
Gofton JP. Studies in osteoarthritis of the hip. Part I. Classification. *Can Med Assoc J* 104:679–683, 791–799, 911–915, 1007–1011, 1971.

A lengthy treatise, which includes a definition and classification of primary OA of the hips, an x-ray method for determination of leg-length inequality, and analysis of biomechanical factors.

Liang MH, Cullen KE, Poss R. Primary total hip or knee replacement: Evaluation of patients. *Ann Intern Med* 97:735–739, 1982.

A review of outcomes in total joint replacement and suggested evaluation of patients.

Jubb R. Nonsteroidal anti-inflammatory drugs and articular cartilage. *Curr Med Lit (Rheumatol)* 3:1, 6–8, 1984.

A review of basic research on the effects of ASA and NSAIDs on articular cartilage.

Altman RD. An approach to developing criteria for the clinical diagnosis and classification of osteoarthritis. *J Rheumatol* 10:2:180–183, 1983.

Uses a mathematical model to develop 13 useful criteria for diagnosing OA.

Forman MD. A survey of OA of the knee in the elderly. *J Rheumatol* 10:2:282–287, 1983.

An epidemiologic survey of selected symptoms and signs of OA of the knee in a population over age 60.

70. MANAGEMENT OF RHEUMATOID ARTHRITIS

Suzanne V. Sauter

Rheumatoid arthritis (RA) is a chronic inflammatory disease of unknown cause that may affect any synovial joint and associated tendon sheath. There is no one typical presentation. It may begin as a symmetric subacute polyarthritis or as an acute asymmetric oligoarthritis or monoarthritis. Morning stiffness lasting several hours is a prominent symptom, as are pain and easy fatigability. Pain cannot always be related to the magnitude of synovitis or deformity, nor can functional impairment be assessed by degree of deformity. Fatigability may be related to the mild-to-moderate anemia that often occurs. Many organ systems may be involved, including the lacrimal and salivary glands, pericardium, lungs, spleen, and bone marrow.

The course of the disease is highly variable. Approximately 30 percent of patients have a mild course characterized by months to years of complete or partial remissions between periods of flares and little if any deformity. Another 10 percent have a single period of active arthritis lasting 6 to 12 months, followed by a long clinical remission with only occasional flares. About half the patients have a progressive disease. Only a small minority—approximately 3% of patients—have a progressive, erosive, destructive arthritis that is resistant to therapy.

A poor prognosis has been associated with insidious onset with involvement of large proximal joints, presence of rheumatoid factor, development of rheumatoid nodules, and extra-articular manifestations of the disease.

The variable course of rheumatoid arthritis means that therapy must be tailored to the patient and may last from months to years. Comprehensive management must include drug, physical, and occupational therapy.

Drug Therapy

Strategy

Drug therapy is usually instituted in three steps. The first line of drug therapy, to which up to 80% of patients respond, includes aspirin and other nonsteroidal anti-inflammatory drugs. The second line, effective in an additional 15 to 20%, includes gold, penicillamine, and antimalarials. The third line of therapy, the immunosuppressives, is needed in only a few patients. These drugs, primarily prednisone, azathioprine (Imuran), and methotrexate, are used only after consultation with a rheumatologist.

A first-line drug is used to control pain and decrease inflammation; it does not retard progression of disease. A second-line drug is used only after 6 months of adequate first-line therapy in patients who have evidence of progressive disease, especially the development of marginal erosions. A third line of therapy is required only in those who do not respond to second-line drugs and have unrelenting disease.

First-Line Drugs

Aspirin is the drug of first choice and the standard to which all other drugs are compared. During the past 10 years, there has been a proliferation of nonsteroidal anti-inflammatory drugs (NSAIDs); however, in large trials none has been shown to be superior to aspirin in all parameters. All are more expensive, and the long-term toxicities are not as well characterized.

Aspirin is well absorbed from the small intestine. Because its absorption is reduced by elevation in intraluminal pH, concomitant use of antacids decreases serum salicylate levels, and intermittent use results in fluctuating salicylate levels. If aspirin is given regularly in anti-inflammatory doses, a small increase or decrease in dose may result in significantly higher or lower drug levels in vivo.

The anti-inflammatory dosage of aspirin is 3.5 gm a day or more; up to 7.8 gm a day may be needed to obtain a response. The therapeutic serum level is about 20 to 25 mg/dl. Tinnitus and decreasing acuity, symptoms of salicylate toxicity, may occur at lower serum levels. Salicylate levels are helpful in older people, who may not report tinnitus or loss of acuity; in assesing compliance; and in identifying patients who have tinnitus at low dosages.

Aspirin is available in many forms: enteric-coated, microencapsulated, dispersed in a matrix, buffered, condensed, substituted, and mixed with other analgesics (Table 70-1). Enteric-coated and matrix preparations appear to reduce gastrointestinal blood loss, slow absorption, and increase plasma half-life. Condensed aspirin, or salicylsalicylic acid (Disalcid), may also cause less dyspepsia and gastrointestinal toxicity. Substituted salicylates generally are better tolerated by people with dyspepsia and other symptoms related to aspirin.

There is little to recommend one of the substituted salicylates over another. There is no evidence that substituted salicylates are less effective than aspirin.

Diflunisal (Dolobid), a drug structurally similar to aspirin, is not metabolized to salicylate, but its clinical pharmacology is similar to that of aspirin.

Nonsteroidal anti-inflammatory drugs (NSAIDs) are summarized in Table 70-2.

The response to aspirin and the newer NSAIDs varies widely from patient to patient. Aspirin should be used first and a switch to another first-line drug made only after there has been no response to aspirin given at therapeutic levels for several weeks to months. Choosing one of the newer drugs is often based on cost, patient tolerance, ease of dosing (NSAIDs now can be given one to four times a day), and specific toxicities. If a patient does not respond to one of the newer drugs, it is preferable to switch to a drug in another class rather than to another drug in the same class. Combinations of two or more NSAIDs or NSAIDs and aspirin appear to be irrational, except as mentioned in Table 70-2. Because these drugs are highly protein bound, use of two drugs decreases plasma levels and increases excretion. Because of this protein binding, drug interactions occur, particularly with anticoagulants. Therefore, care must be used when adding aspirin or a NSAID to other medications.

TOXICITY OF ASPIRIN AND NSAIDs. Aspirin and NSAID drugs share similar side effects as well as mode of action. All can cause peptic ulceration, gastritis, bleeding, and other gastrointestinal problems. The frequency of peptic ulceration is about 1 to 5% for all drugs. Constipation is common; occasionally diarrhea occurs, especially with meclofenamate.

The use of aspirin in pregnancy is controversial. Although it is apparently not teratogenic, it can cause small birth weight, delayed labor, and bleeding in the mother and newborn child. The newer nonsteroidal drugs generally are not used during pregnancy.

Aspirin acetylates the platelet membrane and can prolong bleeding for the life of the platelet, or 7 to 10 days. NSAIDs inactivate cyclo-oxygenase and can prolong bleeding time, usually for 24 hours or less.

All the NSAIDs and aspirin can cause a decrease in glomerular filtration rate (GFR), possibly because they are prostaglandin inhibitors. Acute reversible renal failure, prerenal azotemia, and hyperkalemia may occur. Reversible azotemia has been described with all NSAIDs except sulindac. People with underlying renal disease, heart failure, cirrhosis, or sodium depletion from diuretics seem to be at particular risk. These anti-inflammatory drugs should not be used for patients with severe renal impairment. Acute interstitial nephritis has been reported with the propionic acid derivatives, es-

Table 70-1. Selected salicylate preparations

Type	Dosage	Comments
Plain aspirin	3.5–7.0 gm/day in divided doses, 325-, 500-, or 1000-mg tablets	Should be taken with meals. Do not use with anticoagulants. Use of antacids decreases serum levels. Tinnitus at > 35 mg/dl. Allergic reactions include vasomotor rhinitis, bronchospasm, nasal polyps, angioneurotic edema, urticaria
Enteric-coated		
Ecotrin	3.5–6.0 gm/day in divided doses, 325- or 500-mg tablets	
Enseals	3.5–6.0 gm/day in divided doses, 325-mg tablets	
Easprin	2.9–3.8 gm/day in divided doses; may be increased to 6.0 gm; 975-mg tablets	
Matrix		
Zorprin	3.2–6.0 gm/day bid, 800-mg capsules	
Substituted		
Choline salicylate (Arthropan)	3.2–6.0 gm/day in divided doses, liquid 870 mg/5 ml	
Magnesium salicylate	1.8–4.8 gm/day in divided doses, 600- or 650-mg tablets	Hypermagnesemia may occur
Magnesium choline (Trilisate)	1.5–3.0 gm/day in once- or twice-a-day dose, 500- or 750-mg tablets	
Buffered aspirin	3.5–6.0 gm/day in divided doses	Buffers are magnesium and aluminum hydroxide or magnesium carbonate and aluminum glycinate. Salicylate levels are lower
Condensed		
Disalcid	3.0–5.0 gm/day in divided doses, 500-mg tablets	May have lower salicylate level

Table 70-2. Nonsteroidal anti-inflammatory drugs

Drug	Dosage	Half-life	Selected toxicities and side effects	Comments	Cost
Aspirin	3.0–6.0 gm qd divided into 3–4 doses for therapeutic serum levels of 20–25 mg/dl	Varies widely from 30 min to 8–10 hrs	Allergic reactions: vasomotor rhinitis, bronchospasm, nasal polyps, urticaria	Patients who have allergic reaction to aspirin should not receive other nonsteroidals. Do not use with anticoagulants	0.18–0.20/qd no dispensing fee charged
Propionic acid derivatives				The following do not include dispensing fee	
Ibuprofen (Motrin, Rufen)	400–600 mg tid or qid (anti-inflammatory ≥ 1600 mg/day)	4–6 hrs	Hepatic toxicity: hepatitis and cholestatic jaundice	All similar in effectiveness; difference is in cost and ease of scheduling	
Fenoprofen (Nalfon)	300–600 mg qid	4–7 hrs			0.45–0.60 qd
Naproxen (Naprosyn)	250–500 mg bid	12–15 hrs		Aspirin added to naproxen has resulted in subjective improvement in symptoms above naproxen alone	0.64 qd
Indoleacetic acid derivatives					
Pyrrolealkanoic acid					
Indomethacin (Indocin)	25–50 mg tid; Indocin SR can be given qd		Hepatic toxicities	For relief of morning stiffness, indomethacin has been effective as a nighttime dose (75 mg Indocin SR) in combination with	0.50–0.90 qd

Drug	Dosage	Pharmacokinetics	Side effects	Notes	Cost
Sulindac (Clinoril)	150–200 mg bid	16–18 hrs; metabolized by liver to active form	Sulindac associated with diarrhea; fewer CNS side effects than indomethacin but associated with pancreatitis	aspirin. Tolmetin causes positive sulfosalicylate test for urinary protein. Sulindac may have less nephrotoxicity	0.60 qd
Tolmetin (Tolectin)	400 mg tid–qid				0.60–0.80 qd
Fenamates					
Meclofenamate (Meclomen)	100 mg tid	2 hrs	Diarrhea in 10–33%; nausea, 11%; hepatitis, 4%	Do not use with anticoagulants	0.90 qd
Enolic acid derivatives					
Piroxicam (Feldene)	20 mg qd	Rapidly absorbed but half-life of 45 hrs	Side effects similar to those of other nonsteroidals		0.80 qd
Isoxicam (Maxicam)	300–400 mg qd				0.60 qd
Phenylbutazone (Butazolidin)	300 mg qd (usually in divided doses of 100 tid)	80 hrs		Not recommended for long-term therapy	0.20–0.25 qd generic
Oxyphenbutazone (Tandearil)	200–300 mg qd in divided doses	80 hrs	Aplastic anemia; side effects have diminished its usefulness compared to others	Active metabolite of phenylbutazone Do not use with anticoagulants	0.44–0.66 qd

pecially fenoprofen (Nalfon). Acute papillary necrosis can occur. Both are apparently rare and occur after weeks to months of therapy.

The NSAIDs block the natriuretic effect of thiazide diuretics. They compete with aldosterone for the mineralocorticoid receptors. Impaired sodium excretion occurs and fluid overload can result. Therefore, these drugs must be used with extreme care in patients with hypertension and those at risk for congestive heart failure.

Agranulocytosis, aplastic anemia, and thrombocytopenia occur very rarely with indomethacin (Indocin), phenylbutazone (Butazolidin), oxyphenbutazone (Tandearil), and the propionic acid derivatives, tolmetin (Tolectin) and piroxicam (Feldene).

Dermatologic side effects, especially rash, urticaria, Stevens-Johnson syndrome, and toxic epidermal necrolysis, are very rare but can occur. Tinnitus and loss of auditory acuity usually accompany salicylate toxicity. Otherwise, CNS side effects are also very uncommon; the elderly seem to be especially susceptible. Confusion, apathy, delirium, hallucinations, headaches, depersonalization, and depression have been reported with aspirin and indomethacin (Indocin), but probably occur with all NSAIDs.

Second-Line Drugs

None of the NSAIDs has been shown to slow the disease process in patients with progressive, destructive, erosive, polyarticular disease. In patients who have not responded after at least 6 months of adequate first-line drug therapy and who have evidence of progressive disease (especially the development of marginal erosions), a second-line drug—gold, penicillamine, or an antimalarial—is indicated. There is equivocal radiographic evidence that gold halts joint destruction in patients with early disease. Both gold and penicillamine can improve subjective and objective disease activity, such as morning stiffness, grip strength, and number of swollen and tender joints. Sedimentation rates and titers of rheumatoid factors also are reduced. Although hydroxychloroquine can reduce the symptoms of rheumatoid arthritis, there is no evidence that it can halt disease progression. All second-line drugs can improve or normalize hemoglobin and improve the subjective sense of well-being.

Gold therapy is often used before penicillamine or antimalarial drugs. There is no evidence to suggest that gold is more effective; however, gold is an older drug with better characterized benefits and toxicities.

Although gold is indicated in active disease, it is ineffective in patients with destructive disease without synovitis, except perhaps in Felty's syndrome. Contraindications include pregnancy, history of gold toxicity, and renal insufficiency.

Two parenteral gold preparations, gold sodium thiomalate (Myochrysine) and gold thioglucose (Solganal), are most widely used. An oral gold preparation, auranofin, is under investigation. Usually gold is given in two test doses of 10 mg and 25 mg intramuscularly before beginning a trial of 50 mg intramuscularly each week for 20 weeks. Because gold is a slow-acting drug, a 1-gm trial is necessary to assess efficacy. If gold is effective after 20 weeks, it is then administered every other week until a total dosage of 1.5 gm is given, followed by 50 mg every 3 to 4 weeks. There are no clear guidelines to the cessation of therapy if the arthritis is inactive. Often the gold is continued for years or until it is no longer effective.

Side effects to gold have been reported in up to 75% of patients, and proteinuria in up to 25%. Because of the wide range of toxicities, one must be very familiar with the drug before prescribing it. Toxicities include rash, stomatitis, alopecia, proteinuria, hematuria, nephrotic syndrome, eosinophilia, thrombocytopenia, leukopenia, aplastic anemia, flushing, pulmonary infiltrates, myalgias, arthralgias, diarrhea, and metallic taste.

Policies for monitoring gold therapy vary considerably. Some centers obtain a blood count, including platelet count, and a urinalysis before each injection; others obtain these before every other injection. In either situation, the patient always should be queried before each injection about rash, itching, oral lesions, and metallic taste.

If a patient does not respond to gold or develops a toxicity, *penicillamine* can be used. Penicillamine is begun after the gold toxicity resolves; the two are not given concurrently. Penicillamine is well absorbed from the gastrointestinal tract but must be given on an empty stomach.

The toxicity of penicillamine has been minimized by a "go slow, go low" regimen. The initial dosage of 250 mg per day is increased by 125- to 250-mg increments every

3 months, to a maximum dosage of 1000 mg per day. Usually 2 to 3 months are needed after initiation or change in therapy before its effect can be assessed.

Penicillamine has a high incidence of toxic effects and should be used with great care. Side effects include leukopenia, thrombocytopenia, aplastic anemia, membranous glomerulonephritis with proteinuria and nephrotic syndrome, hematuria, rash, dysgeusia, stomatitis, and induction of autoimmune syndromes such as myasthenia gravis and systemic lupus erythematosus. The incidence of nephrotoxicity may be increased if there has been prevous nephrotoxicity to gold. The appearance of dysgeusia, the most frequent side effect, does not necessitate stopping therapy. Often supplementation of the diet with oral zinc corrects the change in taste. Mild proteinuria ($< 1-2$ gm/24 hrs) may be corrected by reduction in the dosage. Penicillamine can block vitamin B_6, (or pyridoxine) metabolism, and supplementation may be necessary if the diet is inadequate.

Evaluation for side effects includes blood count, platelet count, and urine analysis. These tests are commonly done once every 2 weeks during the first 6 months of therapy and monthly thereafter.

Hydroxychloroquine is usually reserved for patients who have not benefited from therapy with gold or penicillamine. Hydroxychloroquine (Plaquenil) appears to be about as effective as gold in reducing signs and symptoms. The incidence of toxic side effects is probably lower than that of gold or penicillamine. Hydroxychloroquine is given orally at a maximum dosage of 400 mg per day. If the patient responds, the dosage should be reduced after approximately 8 weeks of therapy to the minimum needed to control symptoms.

The most important side effects occur in the eye: pigmentation around the macula, retinal edema, and scotomata, resulting in decreased color vision and visual acuity. Fortunately, decreasing acuity is rare—approximately 1 per 1000 patients a year— and blindness is very rare. Other side effects include rash, leukopenia, agranulocytosis, heartburn, nausea, diarrhea, and CNS problems.

Third-Line Drugs

CORTICOSTEROIDS. Steroids are indicated for rheumatoid vasculitis, but the indications for steroids in rheumatoid synovitis are unclear. Few side effects occur when steroids are used for only 1 to 2 weeks. Before beginning prednisone, all other regimens, such as nonsteroidal drugs, rest, and joint protection, should be maximal.

Prednisone is commonly used because of its short duration of action. It should be used at the lowest possible dosage, usually less than 10 mg per day, and preferably in an alternate-day schedule. Once a corticosteroid is started, it is often very difficult to stop because of flares of arthritis after withdrawal of the drug. The benefit of steroids must be weighed against the long-term consequences, which include cataracts, hypertension, diabetes mellitus, myopathy, osteoporosis, cushingoid habitus, and hyperlipoproteinemia. Intra-articular steroid injections have been widely used, but there are few studies of their efficacy. Benefits from a single injection of a long-acting agent such as triamcinolone hexacetonide (Aristospan) may last from a few days to months. To use repeated injections, each with only short-term benefit, is illogical, if not dangerous. There is no indication for ACTH or parenteral steroid preparations in the management of rheumatoid arthritis.

Immunosuppressive Agents

Azathioprine (Imuran), which is approved for use for rheumatoid arthritis, should be used only under the supervision of a rheumatologist. An oral dose of 1 to 2 mg per kilogram is given daily. The major toxic reaction is leukopenia, but allergic hepatitis can occur. There is a risk for increasing lymphoreticular and epithelial malignancies. Methotrexate has been used experimentally for rheumatoid arthritis.

Supportive Care

Drug therapy is only one part of the management of rheumatoid arthritis. Other forms of care, such as physical and occupational therapy and surgery, are often necessary to decrease pain and maintain function.

Physical Therapy
Physical therapy includes the application of heat and cold, splints, ambulatory aids, and exercises. It is important for the maintenance of range of motion, strengthening weakened muscles, and protection of joints. It is not known how much deformity can be prevented, but there is some evidence that overuse or misuse of inflamed joints may hasten deformity.

Referral to a physical therapist experienced in the treatment of arthritis is helpful when tailoring supportive programs. Referral should occur early in the disease as well as when there has been a major change in disease activity. A physical therapist can outline an exercise and rest program as well as instruct in the use of heat, cold, ultrasound (deep heat), paraffin, and contrast (heat, followed by cold) for the control of pain. The therapist also can provide gait analysis and prescribe correct footwear.

Rest
During periods of acute synovitis, rest of joints decreases swelling and pain, Patients may feel more fatigued and require limited bed rest. Usually 8 to 10 hours at night and 1 to 2 hours during the day are sufficient. If only a single joint, such as a wrist, is inflamed, it can be maintained in a functional position with a lightweight plastic splint. After periods of rest, active range-of-motion exercises are necessary to prevent atrophy. With chronic inflammation, pain and swelling contribute to disuse and atrophy of muscles and flexion contractures.

Heat and Cooling
Cooling is used to decrease pain during acute flares, and heat is used for chronic disease. Use of heat and cooling should be discussed with a therapist because they can be applied in several ways. Indiscriminate use of heat can cause burns, and improper use of ice can cause skin necrosis. Neither should be used if a sensory neuropathy is present. Heat can be applied by the therapist in the form of ultrasound or hot packs, or in a Hubbard tank. A patient can be taught the use of mineral oil–paraffin baths for hands and other joints. Most patients obtain considerable pain relief from hot showers, a heating pad, or an electric blanket.

Exercise
Range-of-motion exercises are done twice a day, preferably during a time of minimal stiffness such as following a hot shower. Strengthening exercises require increasing the number of repetitions. Weights are seldom used in exercises for rheumatoid arthritis. In general, isometric exercises are preferable to isotonic exercises because there is less stress on joints. During a flare, the number of repetitions is reduced, but the exercise program, especially the range-of-motion exercises, is not stopped.

Gait Analysis
If the hips are painful or knee deformities are present, a therapist can help in choosing the appropriate cane, crutch, or walker needed to improve gait and protect the damaged joint.

Footwear
Rheumatoid arthritis commonly causes severe foot deformities, such as subluxation of metatarsophalangeal joints, hallux valgus deformities, cock-up or claw toes, widened forefoot, flat feet, inversion of the ankle, or development of high longitudinal arch with weight bearing over the lateral foot. With these deformities, calluses can develop over the points of bony protrusion or painful bunions may form over a hallux valgus. A physical therapist may provide information on appropriate footwear, such as extra-depth shoes, or make appropriate modifications, such as use of molded, closed-cell foam innersoles. In general, shoes should be wide and deep enough to accommodate the wider forefoot and cock-up toe deformities. The shoe should have soft and pliable material, a strong heel counter, and rubber or crepe soles. For painful metatarsal heads, a metatarsal bar can be added to the rubber sole of a shoe just behind the metatarsal heads. With severe foot deformities, a prosthetist-orthotist can design shoes to accommodate the deformity.

Occupational Therapy

Occupational therapists experienced in the treatment of patients with RA can advise patients concerning the use of lightweight splints and adaptive and assistive devices; they also can assess activities of daily living. Referral should be made early in the disease, to teach joint protection and energy conservation before joint deformities occur. Although some splints, such as molded plastic resting splints and gauntlet-type wrist splints, are available commercially, it is advisable to have an occupational therapist check them for proper application. Often therapists can construct either static (resting) or dynamic splints to prevent or correct mild deformities. A wide variety of assistive and adaptive equipment can be made or purchased, such as raised toilet seat, grab bar, long-handled shoe horn, and adapted bath sponge, eating utensils, combs, and button hooks. A therapist can make an analysis of daily activities and provide advice on appropriate equipment to improve function and reduce stress on inflamed joints.

The occupational therapist may need to work with a vocational rehabilitation counselor to assess employment opportunities or modifications in the current job, or to assist in job training or retraining. Educational and social support groups are sometimes available to provide information and support for arthritic patients. Some communities have resource directories for recreational opportunities and other resources for those with arthritis.

Disability

Patients who have severe functional disability from rheumatoid arthritis may be eligible for disability insurance (SSDI) if they have contributed to Social Security. Disability is defined by statute as "the inability to engage in any substantial gainful activity by reason of any medically determinable physical or mental impairment which can be expected to result in death or which has lasted or can be expected to last for a continuous period of not less than 12 months." "Substantial gainful activity" was defined as the ability to earn $300 a month in 1982.

The specific medical disability criteria for active rheumatoid arthritis include a "history of persistent joint pain, swelling, and tenderness involving multiple major joints with signs of joint inflammation on current examination despite prescribed therapy for at least 3 months, resulting in significant restriction of function of the affected joints and clinical activity expected to last at least 12 months." To this information about the clinical presentation must be added documentation of the diagnosis: "positive serologic test for rheumatoid factor, or antinuclear antibodies, or elevated sedimentation rate, or characteristic biopsy changes."

The disability determination team needs objective evidence about functional impairments. This can be provided in part by carefully kept records of physical, radiographic, and laboratory findings.

If medical criteria are insufficient to determine disability, the judgment is based on "functional residual capacity"—that is, the ability to perform basic work activities, such as sitting, standing, walking, lifting, pushing, pulling, and carrying, and activities that require fine dexterity. Finally, some estimate is made of the ability to perform any work. Factors included in this step are age, education, and previous work experience. No consideration is given to availability of work. For a detailed description of the evaluation process, disability determination, and review process, see the reference by Meenan and colleagues.

Surgery

A large number of surgical interventions are now available for correcting the deformities of RA. Therefore, consultation with an orthopedic surgeon is necessary for the management of crippling arthritis. Because there are few absolute indications for surgery, the patient, surgeon, and primary physician must work together. Most surgery is undertaken for a combination of objective deformity or joint destruction and subjective pain or inability to function.

For some hand deformities, such as tendon tear, soft-tissue surgery can be helpful. For persistent synovitis of one or two joints (e.g., elbow or knee) that have failed to respond to medical therapy, a synovectomy may be helpful; it does not slow the disease process but can relieve pain and decrease swelling for several years. Soft-tissue surgery is indicated for nerve entrapment that has not responded to conservative therapy; it is usually done for carpal tunnel syndrome when synovitis has compressed the median nerve.

Arthroscopic surgery is done for some knee problems such as meniscal tears. Arthroplasty, or total joint replacement, is now well established for hip, knee, and metacarpophalangeal joints. Arthrodesis, or joint fusion, is still used to stabilize unstable ankles, thumbs, or proximal interphalangeal joints.

Simon LS, Mills JA. Nonsteroidal anti-inflammatory drugs. *N Engl J Med* 302:1170–1185, 1237–1243, 1980.
  A somewhat outdated but otherwise excellent review of pharmacology, indications, and side effects of the NSAIDs.
Dromgoole SH, Furst DE, Paulus HE. Rational approaches to the use of salicylates in rheumatoid arthritis. *Semin Arthritis Rheum* 11:257–283, 1981.
  A lengthy discussion of the pharmacology and clinical usefulness of salicylates forms the central part of the paper. Side effects, toxicities, and individual preparations are discussed in detail.
Kimberly RP, et al. Reduction of renal function by newer nonsteroidal anti-inflammatory drugs. *Am J Med* 64:804–810, 1978.
  A review of renal toxicity of the NSAIDs.
Bunning RD, Barth WF. Sulindac: A potentially renal-sparing nonsteroidal anti-inflammatory drug. *JAMA* 248:2864–2867, 1982.
  Information on possible renal-sparing effects of sulindac.
Ward JR, et al. Comparison of auranofin gold sodium thiomalate and placebo in the treatment of rheumatoid arthritis: A controlled clinical trial. *Arthritis Rheum* 26:1303–1315, 1983.
  Recent study of parenteral and oral gold preparations. It references all the classic controlled drug trials showing efficacy of parenteral gold as well as those that have suggested that gold is a remittive agent in RA.
Multi-Center Trial Group. Controlled trial of D-penicillamine in severe rheumatoid arthritis. *Lancet* 1:275–280, 1973.
  First major report of the use of penicillamine in the treatment of rheumatoid arthritis with objective benefit. High dose was associated with excess number of side effects. Compare with the following reference.
Dixon AS, et al. Synthetic D-penicillamine in rheumatoid arthritis. Double-blind controlled study of a high- and low-dosage regimen. *Ann Rheum Dis* 34:416–421, 1975.
Yelin E, et al. Work disability in rheumatoid arthritis: Effects of disease, social and work factors. *Ann Intern Med* 93:551-556, 1980.
  A study of 180 persons in Massachusetts and California explored factors that influenced work disabiity from RA. Factors that affected employment included length of illness, severity of disease, education, and autonomy at work place.
Meenan RF, Liang NH, Hadler NM. Disability Task Force of the Arthritis Foundation. Social security disability and the arthritis patient. *Bull Rheum Dis* 33:1–7, 1983.
  A summary of the eligibility criteria for Social Security disability and the process for disability determination. The article includes information on the medical disability criteria, the appeals process, and the process of re-evaluation. There are also suggestions on the physician's role in the process of disability determination.

---

71. GOUT

Bernard Lo

Precipitation of sodium urate or uric acid causes gouty arthritis, tophi, renal stones, and gouty nephropathy. Gout is much less common in women because before menopause they have lower serum urate levels than men.

Clinical Presentation

Gouty Arthritis
The classic gouty attack is podagra; about half of first attacks involve the big toe, and about 90% of patients with gout eventually experience podagra. Other attacks usually involve a single joint in the legs, with distal joints involved most frequently. Polyarticular attacks may occur, with asymmetric involvement of joints in the legs, sometimes sparing the foot. Attacks may be triggered by alcohol ingestion (especially if the patient is fasting), trauma, and surgery. Drugs that raise the serum urate level (most diuretics, low-dose aspirin) or lower it (allopurinol, probenecid) also may provoke attacks.

The acute attack resolves completely after several days or weeks even if untreated. After the first attack, 62% of patients have a second attack within 1 year, and 78% have one within 2 years. However, 7% do not experience another gouty attack in more than 10 years.

Tophaceous deposits of urate have become increasingly rare following the widespread use of hypouricemic drugs and almost always are preceded by gouty arthritis in primary gout. Common locations of tophi are the ear, hand, forearm, olecranon bursa, and feet.

Renal Stones
Between 20 and 25% of patients with gouty arthritis have renal stones; the stones precede arthritis in 40% of patients. The risk of stones is 1 per 114 patients with gouty arthritis per year, approximately eight times the risk in patients without hyperuricemia. The risk rises with increasing urinary uric acid excretion. Other risk factors for uric acid stone formation are decreased fluid intake, uricosuric drugs, and ingestion of purine-rich foods.

Gouty Nephropathy
Interstitial deposits of sodium urate may result in decreased concentrating ability, proteinuria, or azotemia, although decreased renal function in patients with gout is uncommon and usually mild. In gouty men treated with drugs to lower the serum urate level, a serum creatinine level of greater than 1.6 mg/dl developed in 3.1% in 10 years, compared to 0.5% of controls. Most of the azotemia was attributed to concurrent diabetes, hypertension, or atherosclerosis. There is no conclusive evidence that lowering the serum urate level prevents azotemia.

Diagnostic Evaluation

The arthritis caused by primary gout may be diagnosed by clinical criteria, which include maximum inflammation within 1 day, redness, involvement of the first metatarsophalangeal (MTP) joint, unilateral MTP attack, unilateral tarsal joint attack, oligoarthritis attack, asymmetric swelling, tophus, complete termination of attack, more than one acute attack of arthritis, and hyperuricemia. If six criteria are present, gouty arthritis can be diagnosed with 85% sensitivity and 93% specificity, compared to the clinical diagnoses of rheumatologists specializing in gout.

Obtaining a serum urate level supplements information from the history and physical examination. However, the serum urate level is normal in 8% of patients with acute gouty arthritis, often because of drugs. On the other hand, between 9 and 18% of patients with other types of arthritis have elevated serum urate levels.

Joint aspiration is helpful if the diagnosis is uncertain, for example during first attacks or if septic arthritis is suspected. Fluid is sent for Gram's stain, culture, and examination for crystals. Urate crystals are needle-like, and negatively birefringent under a polarizing microscope. False negative aspirations occur in 5% of instances because of aspiration of the wrong site when swelling is diffuse, inexpert search for crystals, or dissolution of crystals late in an attack.

Colchicine is sometimes given as a therapeutic trial to establish the diagnosis of gouty arthritis. However, other forms of arthritis occasionally respond to colchicine.

The clinician also should consider whether the gout is secondary to other diseases (e.g., myeloproliferative disorders) or drugs (alcohol, moonshine whiskey, diuretics, and aspirin). In addition, the patient should be evaluated for tophi, stones, and gouty nephropathy.

Treatment

Acute Gouty Arthritis
Nonsteroidal anti-inflammatory agents are effective in reducing inflammation and pain. Indomethacin is given, 50 mg every 6 hours for 1 or 2 days, and tapered over the next 2 to 3 days. Common side effects are headache, nausea, and abdominal discomfort. Dizziness, confusion, peptic ulcer disease, gastrointestinal bleeding, and fluid retention also may occur.

Phenylbutazone is an effective alternative to indomethacin. However, because of a higher frequency of gastrointestinal side effects and the rare occurrence of bone marrow toxicity, many physicians are reluctant to use phenylbutazone in gout. The experience with other nonsteroidal agents is less extensive. Naproxen may be given as a 750-mg loading dose, followed by 250 mg tid. There is no definitive evidence that any one nonsteroidal agent is superior.

Colchicine terminates most acute attacks. Oral dosage is 0.5 mg every hour until relief of pain or side effects occur. Unfortunately, up to 50% to 80% of patients cannot tolerate oral colchicine because of diarrhea, cramps, or vomiting. Many clinicians prefer intravenous administration of colchicine, which avoids gastrointestinal side effects. The dose is 2 mg diluted in 20 cc saline and injected into an intravenous line, since sclerosis of the vein and extravasation may be painful. A dose of 1 mg may be repeated every 6 to 12 hours if needed. Because of possible bone marrow toxicity, no more than 5 mg should be given during a single attack, and less should be given to patients on maintenance colchicine or with liver or renal disease.

Intra-articular injections of steroids are useful in patients who cannot tolerate other drugs. Systemic steroids may be effective, but also may cause rebound attacks.

With many effective drugs available for acute gout, physicians will wish to individualize treatment based on their own experience, the patient's clinical situation, and response in previous attacks. Both nonsteroidal anti-inflammatory agents and colchicine are more effective if given at the beginning of an attack.

Recurrent attacks of gouty arthritis may be prevented by colchicine 0.5 mg 1 to 3 times daily. Recurrent attacks also may be an indication for drugs to lower the serum urate level. These agents, however, should not be started during an acute attack, because they can exacerbate or prolong the attack.

Lowering Serum Urate Levels
The appropriate use of hypouricemic drugs is controversial. Some experts recommend starting them after one severe attack of arthritis or one renal stone. However, many patients with infrequent attacks or stones may prefer not to take daily medication. As in any chronic disease, patient understanding and consent are essential. Taking urate-lowering drugs irregularly may precipitate gouty attacks.

Serum urate can be lowered by either uricosuric agents, such as probenecid or sulfinpyrazone, or by allopurinol, which decreases production of uric acid. There are no good studies comparing these two approaches. For most patients, *uricosuric agents* are preferred, because life-threatening side effects with allopurinol, although rare, are being recognized more frequently.

Uricosuric drugs should be started at low doses and fluid intake increased to prevent uric acid stones. Probenecid is started at 250 mg bid and increased to 500 mg bid 3 to 4 days later. Subsequently, the daily dosage is increased by 500 mg every 1 to 2 weeks until the serum urate level is normal. Usually 1 to 2 gm daily are needed. Side effects are gastrointestinal problems, skin rashes, and hypersensitivity reactions. The effect of penicillin, cephalosporins, indomethacin, and heparin is increased.

Sulfinpyrazone is started at 50 mg bid and increased by 100 mg daily in the same manner as probenecid. Usually 300 to 400 mg are needed, given in three or four divided doses. Toxicity is gastrointestinal and hematologic.

About 25% of patients do not attain normal serum urate levels on uricosuric agents, usually because of azotemia or the concomitant use of low doses of aspirin.

Allopurinol should be used in patients with renal stones, tophi, renal failure, and myeloproliferative diseases and in patients who have not improved with uricosuric agents or cannot tolerate them. Allopurinol also has been recommended in the 10 to 20% of patients with primary gout who are "overproducers" and therefore overexcretors of uric acid, as determined clinically by a 24-hour excretion of uric acid greater than 600 mg per day for men on a purine-free diet and 700 mg per day for a moderately restricted purine diet. Such diets are impractical in outpatients; on an unrestricted diet, the extrapolated upper limit of normal is 800 mg per day. The rationale for using allopurinol in such patients is that uricosuric agents would additionally increase urinary uric acid excretion and might cause renal stones. However, the risk of stones may be overemphasized in patients without previous renal stones, tophi, renal failure, and myeloproliferative disease. A series reporting a 16% incidence of stones included patients with tophi and previous stones, and the authors did not follow the precautions discussed for the use of uricosuric drugs. Moreover, in patients without tophi, the excess uric acid pool is excreted in a few days, after which urinary excretion, and presumably the risk of stones, returns to the original steady-state level.

A single daily dose of 300 mg of allopurinol usually lowers serum urate levels to normal. In a few patients, larger doses are needed. Gastrointestinal intolerance has been reported in 0.4% to 16% of patients, and skin rashes in 1.8% to 10%. Life-threatening hypersensitivity reactions involving skin, liver, and kidney were reported in 2 of 1835 patients; such reactions are fatal in 26% of cases. Adverse effects are more common in patients on thiazides or with renal failure. Rashes are more common if ampicillin or amoxicillin is given concurrently. By inhibiting hepatic microsomal enzymes, allopurinol potentiates the effect of sodium warfarin (Coumadin), azathioprine, and mercaptopurine.

When a uricosuric agent of allopurinol is started, 0.5 mg of colchicine bid also should be given to prevent gouty attacks. After the serum urate has been normal for 6 to 12 months, colchicine can be discontinued. Avoiding excessive alcohol and purine-rich foods (such as organ meats, anchovies, sardines, and yeast) and losing weight may reduce symptoms in some patients. Rapid weight loss should be avoided, however, because ketosis may precipitate attacks of gouty arthritis.

A common problem is recurrent gouty attacks in patients taking diuretics. Reasonable approaches are to discontinue the diuretic, such as by using a beta-blocker alone for hypertension; to substitute spironolactone or triamterene, which do not increase serum urate; or to add a uricosuric agent.

Wyngaarden JB, Kelley WN. *Gout and Hyperuricemia.* New York: Grune & Stratton, 1976.
A comprehensive monograph.
Huskisson EC, Balme HW. Pseudopodagra. *Lancet* 2:269–271, 1972.
A review of disorders that mimic gouty arthritis of the big toe.
Wallace SL, et al. Preliminary criteria for the classification of the acute arthritis of primary gout. *Arthritis and Rheum* 20:895–900, 1977.
A discussion of the sensitivity and specificity of clinical criteria for gouty arthritis. The "gold standard" for the diagnosis of gout was the clinical diagnosis of a rheumatologist specializing in gout. Because the instances of gout and other specified types of arthritis were solicited from specialists, the sensitivity and specificity of the criteria in other populations may be different.
Hadler NM, et al. Acute polyarticular gout. *Am J Med* 56:715–719, 1974.
Attacks usually involved asymmetric polyarthritis of joints in the legs, sparing the foot in one-third of cases.
Wallace SL, Bernstein D, Diamond H. Diagnostic value of the colchicine therapeutic trial. *JAMA* 199:93–96, 1967.
Seventy-six percent of patients with acute gouty arthritis responded to colchicine, as did one patient with erythema nodosum and arthritis (not sarcoid) and two patients with undiagnosed monoarticular arthritis of the knee. Of 44 patients with rheumatoid arthritis and 6 patients with sarcoid, none responded.
Wortman RL, Fox IH. Limited value of uric acid to creatinine ratios in estimating uric acid excretion. *Ann Intern Med* 93:822–825, 1980.
Ratios based on spot urine and serum measurements of uric acid generally do not correlate with 24 hour urine uric acid excretion.
Lupton GP, Odom RB. The allopurinol hypersensitivity syndrome. *J Am Acad Dermatol* 1:365–374, 1979.
Severe reactions characterized by fever, skin lesions, eosinophilia, and abnormal hepatic and renal function were fatal in 26% of patients. Most patients had preexisting

renal disease and were taking thiazides. Two-thirds were being treated for asymptomatic hyperuricemia.

McInnes GT, Lawson DH, Jick H. Acute adverse reactions attributed to allopurinol in hospitalized patients. *Ann Rheum Dis* 40:245–249, 1981.

Skin reactions occurred in 1.8% of hospitalized patients taking allopurinol, gastrointestinal reactions in 0.4%, and life-threatening hypersensitivity reactions in 0.1%.

Yu TF. The efficacy of colchicine prophylaxis in articular gout—a reappraisal after 20 years. *Semin Arthritis Rheum* 12:256–264, 1983.

Review of usefulness of colchicine in preventing acute gouty attacks.

72. OSTEOPOROSIS
Philip D. Sloane

Osteoporosis is a common condition that leads to considerable pain and disability and contributes to thousands of deaths annually in the elderly. Osteoporosis-related fractures primarily involve the hip, spine, and wrist, and cost over one billion dollars a year in acute medical services alone.

Osteopenia is a general term for demineralized bones of whatever cause. The term *osteoporosis* refers to a variety of conditions all characterized by a decrease in bone mass with an otherwise normal structural matrix. The majority of cases are idiopathic, most commonly in the elderly (involutional osteoporosis). Approximately 15% of instances are secondary to identifiable factors such as hyperthyroidism, use of exogenous corticosteroids, Cushing's disease, malabsorption, or renal tubular acidosis.

Causes

Osteoporosis of the elderly can be considered simply part of normal aging. For both men and women, skeletal mass reaches a peak by age 30, is maintained until approximately age 45, and then begins to decline. The rate of decline averages about 1% per year and is up to three times as rapid in postmenopausal women than in men. Because women generally begin with a smaller bone mass and have accelerated bone loss for several years after the menopause, they are more prone to developing osteoporosis.

The causes of osteoporosis in the elderly are not well understood. Probably several factors interact. The amount of bone present in early adulthood appears important. Blacks have less osteoporosis than whites, primarily because their peak bone mass is greater. Similarly, obese, large-framed people are less likely to suffer from osteoporosis than those who are thin. It has been suggested that several aspects of diet play a role, including low calcium intake, mild vitamin D deficiency, and excessive acid intake from diets high in meat and carbonated beverages. Finally, hormonal factors—estrogens, androgens, calcitonin, parathyroid hormone, glucocorticoids, and thyroxine—maybe important. Estrogen deficiency, particularly with an early, surgical menopause, has been linked to bone demineralization. Other possible causes of osteoporosis include habitual inactivity or immobility and a familial predisposition, possibly related to body build. Osteoporosis is also associated with certain diseases such as rheumatoid arthritis, diabetes, chronic obstructive pulmonary disease, and alcoholism.

Diagnosis

Differential Diagnosis

Osteopenia also results from osteomalacia, an abnormally slow rate of bone matrix calcification caused by vitamin D deficiency or, rarely, tissue insensitivity to vitamin D. Although pure osteomalacia is rare in the elderly, it can coexist with osteoporosis. The distinction is important because osteomalacia can be treated with vitamin D. Osteomalacia can be detected by decreased levels of serum $1,25(OH)_2$ vitamin D.

Other conditions associated with osteopenia that can mimic osteoporosis include hyperparathyroidism, multiple myeloma, neoplasms with or without metastases to bone, and renal tubular acidosis.

Presentation
Osteoporosis often is first suspected when a relative demineralization (osteopenia) of bone is noted on x-rays taken for an unrelated reason. Symptoms such as back pain or pathologic fractures develop late in the course of osteoporosis, often after 20 to 25 years of net bone loss. Back pain occurs when there are compression fractures and is exacerbated by new fractures usually located in the mid-to-low thoracic or lumbar region and often occurring during minor activity such as walking, making a bed, or tugging open a window. Multiple compression fractures of the thoracic spine lead to chronic backache, disability, and a thoracic kyphosis. In addition to the spine, the wrist, hip, and rib bones are most commonly affected by fracture—often with very mild trauma.

History
Often the history identifies risk factors for osteoporosis long before the onset of symptoms. Patients at risk for osteomalacia can also be identified because of malabsorption; previous gastrectomy; dietary vitamin D deficiency; prolonged ingestion of phenytoin, phenobarbital, or glutethimide; renal tubular acidosis; and severe chronic renal disease.

Physical Examination
There may be no specific findings on physical examination unless an acute fracture is present. Height loss of up to 5 inches is found in severe cases because of vertebral compression fractures. The "dowager's hump," a thoracic kyphosis developing in middle age, may also be noted.

X-rays
X-rays are not helpful in the early identification of patients at risk. Osteopenia is not evident on x-ray until bone mass is reduced by 25 to 35%, and spontaneous fractures frequently develop with this degree of osteopenia. More sensitive techniques to assess bone mineral content, such as photon beam absorptiometry and neutron activation analysis, are available, but they are experimental and expensive, and therefore not suited for routine medical practice.
    Although limited as screening tools, x-rays are valuable in the diagnosis of symptomatic osteoporosis. Patients with a relatively atraumatic fracture or a history of multiple fractures should have lateral x-rays of the spine. If generalized osteopenia is absent, a pathologic fracture should be suspected. Pseudofractures suggest osteomalacia. The major x-ray signs of osteoporosis are anterior wedging of the thoracic vertebral bodies; biconcavity and "codfish" appearance of lumbar vertebral bodies; widening of the intervertebral spaces; cortical thinning, often into a "pencil-thin line"; and accentuation of vertical trabeculae from loss of horizontal trabeculae.

Laboratory Tests
There are no laboratory findings diagnostic of osteoporosis; however, the laboratory is used to exclude other causes of osteopenia. The following tests are recommended for all older patients with generalized osteopenia: calcium, phosphorus, and alkaline phosphatase (all of which are normal in most instances of osteoporosis, and abnormal in osteomalacia); albumin (to allow interpretation of serum calcium); serum and urine protein electrophoresis (to rule out multiple myeloma); T_4 (to screen for hyperthyroidism); and BUN-creatinine (to rule out chronic renal disease). If other causes of secondary osteoporosis are suspected, such as Cushing's disease, alcoholism, or cirrhosis, additional laboratory studies are needed.

Treatment
Treatment of established osteoporosis with fractures should be individualized, with consideration to the patient's age, severity of disease, and other health problems. Patients with acute symptoms, such as back pain secondary to a compression fracture, require rest, analgesia, external support, heat, and stool softeners. Immobilization, including use of an appliance such as a back brace, should be minimized because it aggravates demineralization. Although acute pain usually subsides in about 4 to 6 weeks, it can take a great deal longer.
    In one trial of treatment for postmenopausal women with generalized osteoporosis and one or more (usually, several) nontraumatic vertebral fractures, patients treated with a combination of calcium (1500–2500 mg $CaCO_3$/day), conjugated estrogen

(0.625–2.5 mg/day), and fluoride (50–60 mg/day) had only one-twentieth the rate of subsequent fractures of patients not specifically treated. The addition of vitamin D to the regimen produced no additional benefit and was associated with hypercalcemia in some patients.

For all patients, rehabilitation is important. Retraining in the instrumental activities of daily living, and practice using ancillary equipment, such as a long-handled shoehorn, can be extremely useful.

Prevention

Because osteoporosis has a 15- to 20-year asymptomatic phase and is usually far advanced by the time it is diagnosed, strategies begun earlier in life may prevent or delay the disease. During childhood, physical exercise, adequate intake of calcium and vitamin D, and possibly, fluoridation of drinking water provide maximum accumulation of skeletal mass. In adulthood, all persons should be encouraged to exercise.

Of the many therapeutic agents that have been given to prevent osteoporosis, only a few decrease the rate of demineralization and probably diminish the rate of subsequent fractures as well. These include the following.

Calcium alone appears to retard bone demineralization in osteoporosis. Men and premenopausal women require at least 1 gm and postmenopausal women at least 1.5 gm of elemental calcium daily to avoid having a negative calcium balance. Dietary sources of calcium include sardines (560 mg of calcium/100 gm), green vegetables (100–200 mg/100 gm), cheeses (up to 1200 mg/100 gm), and skim milk (1.2 gm per quart, with absorption diminished by high phosphate content). Simple calcium supplements include TUMS antacids (6 tablets = 1200 gm calcium) and bone meal.

Estrogens apparently reduce the rate of fractures by one-half to two-thirds. They appear to be most effective in the few years immediately following menopause, the time at which bone demineralization is most rapid. To minimize the risk of endometrial cancer (see Chap. 86), it is generally recommended that estrogens be given in a low dosage, accompanied by a progestin given daily during the last 5 to 10 days of estrogen therapy each month. Many authors recommend yearly endometrial biopsies for patients receiving estrogen therapy, but the appropriate frequency is not yet known.

There is little evidence that *vitamin D* supplementation at any dosage level improves the course of osteoporosis. When given alone, high dosages (10,000–50,000 IU/day) of vitamin D appear to worsen osteoporosis. Use of a low-dosage supplement, such as one multivitamin tablet per day, is reasonable, to ensure that intake exceeds the recommended dietary allowance of 400 IU, because mild osteomalacia may coexist with osteoporosis.

High-dosage *fluoride,* combined with calcium and vitamin D, has been shown to increase bone density in osteoporosis. It is uncertain, however, whether the newly mineralized bone is as strong as normal bone. Side effects include severe joint pain and gastrointestinal symptoms. Although promising, this treatment remains experimental.

Calcitonin use is currently experimental; there is little evidence that it is of value in the treatment of osteoporosis.

Marx JL. Osteoporosis: New help for thinning bones. *Science* 207:628–630, 1980.
   A highly readable narrative review of current concepts of the pathophysiology of osteoporosis.
Nachtigall LD, et al. Estrogen replacement therapy. 1. A 10-year prospective study in the relationship to osteoporosis. *Obstet Gynecol* 53:3, 1979.
   A study demonstrating the effects of estrogen replacement on the development of osteoporosis in women.
Nordin BEC, et al. Treatment of spinal osteoporosis in postmenopausal women. *Br. Med J* 1:451–454, 1980.
   Compares the effect on bone density of six treatment regimens for symptomatic osteoporosis.
Riggs BL, et al. Effect of the fluoride/calcium regimen on vertebral fracture occurrence in postmenopausal osteoporosis. *N Engl J Med* 306:445–450, 1982.
   Provides evidence that fluoride, calcium, and estrogen improve the clinical course of symptomatic osteoporosis.
Avioli LV. What to do with "postmenopausal osteoporosis"? (editorial). *Am J Med* 65:881–884, 1978.
   An editorial providing a cautious appraisal of treatment options.

Thomson DL, Frame B. Involutional osteopenia: Current concepts. *Ann Intern Med* 85:789–803, 1976.
An extensive review that focuses on the pathogenesis and treatment of osteoporosis.
Bruber HE, Baylin DJ. The diagnosis of osteoporosis. *J Am Geriatr Soc* 29:490–497, 1981.
A clinical review describing a systematic approach to elderly patients with spinal compression fractures.

73. NONARTICULAR RHEUMATISM
Robert S. Lawrence

The majority of patients presenting with aches and pains in the regions of the body close to diarthrodial joints suffer from "nonarticular rheumatism," commonly categorized as bursitis, tenosynovitis, and fibrositis. Bursitis and tenosynovitis also contribute to much of the morbidity associated with generalized inflammatory disorders such as rheumatoid arthritis, gout, gonorrhea, systemic lupus erythematosus, and dermatomyositis.

Bursitis
More than 150 bursae are distributed throughout the body and serve to reduce friction between moving structures (tendons, ligaments, muscles, bones, and skin). Considerable anatomic variation exists. Bursitis occurs when the synovial membrane lining a bursal sac becomes inflamed. Known causes include trauma, infection, and inflammation either as part of a systemic disease such as rheumatoid arthritis or from microcrystals (e.g., gout and pseudogout).

Bursitis occurs most commonly in middle and old age. Typically, patients experience the abrupt onset of pain, aggravated by movement, after an episode of trauma or unaccustomed repetitive use of the part. If the bursitis is superficial, there may be local tenderness, swelling, and erythema. Fever may be present; if there is fever in association with inflammation of a superficial bursa (e.g., olecranon or prepatellar), the likelihood of septic bursitis is increased. Whenever a fluctuant swelling exists in the region of a bursa, it should be aspirated and the fluid sent for culture and analysis, including WBC/RCB count, protein, glucose, crystals, and mucin clot quality. Deep bursitis may only produce limitation of movement and some regional tenderness. Aspiration of deep bursae requires detailed knowledge of surrounding anatomic structures and usually should be left to an orthopedist or rheumatologist.

Analysis of the aspirated fluid can be used to guide the choice of therapy. Typically, with trauma there are red cells and a good-to-intermediate clot; with bacterial infection there are a large number of WBCs (e.g., 10,000–20,000), decreased glucose, and poor clot; with inflammatory (e.g., rheumatoid) arthritis, there is moderate leukocytosis (1000–20,000) and poor clot; and with microcrystalline bursitis, crystals are present and can be identified by using a polarizing microscope.

If the bursitis is traumatic, the part is splinted, heat is applied for 30 minutes tid or qid, and aspirin or one of the nonsteroidal anti-inflammatory drugs (e.g., naproxen 250 mg bid or tid) is given for about a week. If symptoms persist or fluid reaccumulates, the bursa can be injected with a long-acting corticosteroid. If septic fluid is aspirated, the patient should be hospitalized for parenteral antibiotics and repeated aspirations of the bursa. Surgical drainage may be required. Fluid consistent with gout or rheumatoid disease requires appropriate drug therapy of the primary disease.

The diagnosis and management of bursitis in specific anatomic regions are discussed in chapters devoted to the neck, shoulder, and knee (see Chaps. 74, 75, and 77, respectively).

Tenosynovitis
The tendon sheaths surrounding long tendons are essentially tubular bursae; therefore, many of the preceding comments apply to tenosynovitis. Irritation by trauma or repetitive use of a poorly conditioned part is the usual cause of tenosynovitis. When such a

history is absent, the diagnosis of tenosynovitis should alert the clinician to the possibility of a systemic disease such as gonorrhea, gout, or systemic lupus erythematosus.

The long tendons of the hand and wrist are most commonly involved. The extensor pollicis longus is particularly susceptible to trauma as it passes over the radial styloid. When a nodular thickening of the tendon develops or a stenosis of the tendon sheath forms, the condition is called de Quervain's disease. The first step is injection of the sheath (and nodule, if present) using a mixture of 1 to 2% lidocaine (Xylocaine) and depocorticosteroid, but surgical release is often necessary. Involvement of the flexor tendons of the hand may produce "trigger" fingers, which also require steroid injection or surgical release. In the absence of repeated trauma, trigger fingers may be a complication of rheumatoid arthritis, myxedema, or amyloidosis.

Fibrositis

Fibrositis is the usual name given to an ill-defined syndrome of generalized aching and stiffness. The name itself is misleading because in fact the syndrome is not associated with demonstrable pathologic changes in connective tissues. Of all patients complaining of musculoskeletal pain that does not come from the local joints, none are more baffling or difficult to treat than those with fibrositis.

Diagnosis

Fibrositis usually occurs in middle-aged or elderly people. They complain of diffuse aching pain and stiffness affecting many joints and muscles. The symptoms are usually present each day, the stiffness may be worse in the morning, and the aching often is more severe in colder weather. A careful history reveals a disturbed sleep pattern that in recent studies has been identified as a disorder of non-REM sleep.

On examination the patient has marked tissue tenderness. Typically there are localized areas of tenderness, described as trigger points.* There is also skin-fold tenderness over the scapula. There are no objective signs of inflammation of joints or soft tissues. Some physicians include palpable muscle spasm as part of the syndrome.

Typically, laboratory examination for rheumatic diseases—erythrocyte sedimentation rate, antinuclear antibody, tests for rheumatoid arthritis—is completely normal. Sleep EEG often reveals a characteristic pattern of both delta (1 cps) and alpha (8–10 cps) activity during non-REM sleep, rather than the normal predominance of delta waves. The fibrositis syndrome has been experimentally induced in healthy volunteers by depriving them of stage-4 slow-wave non-REM sleep but not by depriving them of REM sleep alone.

Treatment

Administration of chlorpromazine, amitriptyline (25 mg), or doxepin (25 mg) several hours before bedtime often alleviates the symptoms in some patients, perhaps by correction of the sleep disorder.

The following comprehensive therapeutic regimen has been proposed by Smythe (see references), based on clinical experience.

1. Reassurance. The disease is not crippling or serious, but pain is real and follows a typical pattern.
2. Explanation of origin of pain. In greater or less detail, depending on their needs, patients should be told that
   a. Pain of deep origin is necessarily referred
   b. Referred tenderness is at constant, predictable sites
   c. Exaggerated reflex hyperemia indicates tissue hyperreactivity
   d. The condition is aggravated by cold, sleep disturbance, tension, and depression

---

*Trigger points are most frequently found in one or more of the following locations: (1) midpoint of upper fold of trapezius and area just anterior to trapezius on right and left sides, (2) second costochondral junction, (3) along L4–S1 interspinous ligaments, (4) origin of supraspinatus muscle near medial border of scapula, (5) lateral epicondyle just distal to the radial head, (6) upper outer quadrant of buttocks, and (7) medial collateral ligament of the knee proximal to the joint line and anterior to the semimembranosus tendon.

3. Relief of mechanical stresses in neck and low back (probably the primary source of referred pain and tenderness)
   a. Because the neck is vulnerable to mechanical stresses during sleep, the arch of the neck should be supported by a folded pillow.
   b. Because the low back is vulnerable in hyperextension, there is a need for strong abdominal muscles to maintain the low back in a flexed position. Abdominal support and an unsagging mattress may help.
4. Medical therapy
   a. Salicylates or other simple analgesics may break chronic pain cycles. The patient must be compliant and persistent. Anti-inflammatory drugs are not helpful.
   b. Heat, massage, liniments, or other counterirritant and relaxation therapies are helpful.
   c. Amitriptyline or doxepin is useful for sleep disturbance.
5. Attitudes and expectations. Patients should be encouraged to
   a. Recognize perfectionistic impatience
   b. See that challenges give life meaning, and to accept their condition within limitations
   c. Pursue fitness even if there is some increase in symptoms
   d. Break tension with rest, diversion, exercise, or escape

If the patient remains skeptical of the diagnosis or becomes dissatisfied with the treatment plan, the judicious use of a rheumatologic consultation can be very helpful to persuade the patient that his or her primary care physician is doing the right thing.

When pain is particularly severe at a trigger point, injection with lidocaine (Xylocaine) or with a mixture of lidocaine and depocorticosteroid regularly produces relief of symptoms. The effect may last as long as a few weeks, but symptoms usually recur. Because relief is transient and fibrositis is a chronic disease, injection should at most play only a small role in the usual, long-term management of fibrositis.

Kelly G. Bursitis, Tenosynovitis, and Fibrositis. In LR Barker, JR Burton, and PD Zieve (Eds.), *Principles of Ambulatory Medicine*. Baltimore: Williams & Wilkins, 1982. Pp. 613–619.
   A succinct chapter on the subject with useful tables summarizing techniques of aspiration of bursae, analysis of bursal fluid, treatment methods, and methods of injection of bursae or joints.
Swartout R, Compere EL. Ischiogluteal bursitis: The pain in the arse. *JAMA* 227:551–552, 1974.
   The colorful title is a sample of the breezy style of this report of 18 patients with ischiogluteal bursitis. The data were collected over 20 months after one of the authors himself suffered this "exquisite, relentless, all-dominating pain in the buttock."
Younghusband OZ, Black JD. De Quervain's disease: Stenosing tenovaginitis at the radial styloid process. *Can Med Assoc J* 89:508–512, 1963.
   A review of 12 cases with detailed description of the anatomy, diagnostic signs, and therapy. Written by surgeons, the emphasis is on moving rapidly to surgical intervention if medical management is not successful.
Smythe HA. Nonarticular Rheumatism and Psychogenic Musculoskeletal Syndromes. In DJ McCarty Jr (Ed.), *Arthritis and Allied Conditions*. Philadelphia: Lea & Febiger, 1979. Pp. 8811–8891.
   A comprehensive review of the fibrositis syndrome with extensive references and several useful tables and figures.
Calkins E. Rheumatic disease in the elderly: Finding a way through the maze. *Primary Care* 9:181–195, 1982.
   A general review of the diagnosis and management of articular and nonarticular rheumatism in the elderly, with many useful suggestions about treatment.
Webber JB. Common pain syndromes: Upper extremities. *Geriatrics* 36:59–69, 1981.
   A detailed discussion of the causes of pain in the upper extremity in the elderly with emphasis on inflammatory disorders of capsules, ligaments, and tendons and compression neuropathies.
Ganda OP, Caplan HI. Rheumatoid disease without joint involvement. *JAMA* 228:338–339, 1974.

An interesting case study of an elderly patient who over 5 years had no severe arthritis yet had multiple subcutaneous rheumatoid nodules, rheumatoid pleuritis with effusion, nodular scleritis, and a high titer of rheumatoid factor.

74. NECK PAIN
Peter Curtis

The two major symptoms associated with neck diseases are pain and limited motion. The pain may be in the neck only or may radiate to the shoulder and down the arm. The most common cause, considering all age groups as a whole, is myofascitis. With increasing age, degenerative change of cervical vertebrae (spondylosis) is almost ubiquitous, but it is associated with pain in only a small number of patients. Although neck injury may lead to changes at an earlier age, spondylosis as a cause of painful neck disease is usually found in older patients. Neck pain also may be a symptom of problems located in the arm or shoulder, notably carpal tunnel and outlet compression syndromes. Other causes of neck pain include lymphadenitis and infection (particularly in young patients), systemic diseases (e.g., ankylosing spondylitis and other inflammatory diseases), or metastases to the cervical vertebrae. Trauma, particularly motor vehicle accidents, can lead to whiplash and other neck injuries. Sedentary occupations, desk work, and driving of motor vehicles are often associated with pain, but the precise anatomic cause of pain is uncertain in many instances.

Evaluation

The *history* should be sufficient to identify patients in whom systemic or metastatic disease is likely. Other information that helps identify the cause includes the onset of pain (sudden or gradual); the main focus (arm, shoulder, back); and the character of pain or motions that cause pain. Myofascial pain may occur suddenly, often in association with new activity or mild trauma. The most common areas of pain are the lower pole of the scapula and the posterior aspect of the shoulder, radiating into the neck. Pain from nerve root compression may be aching and/or lancinating, depending on which portion of the root is affected—motor or sensory. If upper cervical roots are involved, pain may appear as an occipital headache; other roots may refer into the shoulder, arm, or thorax according to the level of involvement.

Physical examination should include detailed evaluation of the arm, shoulder, and thorax as well as the neck. Inspection may indicate differences in position, swelling, or spasm. Palpation determines if bone or muscle is involved. In myofascial syndromes the bellies of muscles are tender, and trigger points may be identified. In radiculopathy, typical radiation of pain may be demonstrated by moving the neck through a normal range of motion. Tapping on the vertebral body is a very nonspecific test. A positive Adson's maneuver suggests a thoracic outlet syndrome. With the patient's hand placed palm up in the lap, the radial pulse is palpated. The head is rotated first to the affected side and then to the other, with a Valsalva maneuver performed in each position; obliteration of the pulse in either position is considered a positive test. The specificity of this test is poor. Muscular weakness, atrophy, and diminished deep tendon reflexes suggest nerve root involvement. Lesions at the C4–C5 interspace (C4 root) cause weakness of shoulder abductors; at C5–C6 (C5 root), weakness of elbow flexors and diminished biceps and brachioradialis reflexes; at C6–C7 (C7 root), decreased elbow extensors and diminished or extinguished triceps reflexes (C7 is the primary innervation of the triceps). Occasionally, central spinal cord compression affects descending tracts, causing upper motor neuron findings. In this case, there is spasticity and increased muscle tone instead of flaccidity, and heightened rather than decreased deep tendon reflexes.

Laboratory studies are indicated only as suggested by the history. X-rays may be useful in identifying spondylosis if neurologic deficits are noted; however, the findings are often nonspecific because at age 50, 50% of patients have radiographic evidence of cervical spondylosis, and at 65, 85%. Bony metastases, Paget's disease, myeloma, or ankylosing spondylitis also can be identified by x-ray. X-ray findings are helpful only when there is precise association between x-ray and clinical findings. An electromyogram is necessary if entrapment neuropathy (e.g., carpal tunnel syndrome) is suspected but rarely useful in evaluating cervical spondylosis.

Management

Once organic disease has been excluded by history and clinical examination, acute or chronic neck pain can be managed by simple measures, such as ice or heat, analgesics, and rest, as well as the specific therapies listed below. Usually a specialist is consulted about patients with neurologic deficits.

Management of myofascial pain is discussed in Chapter 75. Several therapeutic modalities are used to manage pain from spondylosis. Because the most common conditions are osteoarthrosis of the cervical spine and mechanical derangements (e.g., apophyseal joint injury, or nerve root or soft-tissue irritation), therapy is directed toward reassuring and supporting the patient, relieving pain, reducing mechanical stresses, and relieving muscle spasm. Clinical studies have not definitively ascribed benefit to one therapeutic modality over another. Unfortunately, one is left to try out various approaches and make empirical choices based in part on what is most economical and simple to implement.

Drugs

A variety of drugs have been used. Aspirin or acetaminophen (Tylenol) is usually sufficient for pain relief; however, for severe disease a narcotic may be necessary, particularly at night. Any of the nonsteroidal anti-inflammatory drugs may be tried and in some instances may be effective. Muscle relaxants are usually of no benefit beyond their sedative effects.

Supportive Management

Moist heat, usually provided by warm baths (15–20 minutes) taken just before bedtime, can be helpful in promoting muscle relaxation. Other forms of heat include a heating pad and hydrocollator pack. A soft collar, positioned to produce the least pain, allows the cervical muscles to relax. The collar is designed to relieve strain on the cervical muscles and to restrict flexion-extension movements. At night, the collar can be discarded and the patient advised to use one pillow only. The pillow should be thin at the center and thickened at the ends, and is tucked carefully around the neck. When undertaking activities such as typing or reading, patients should position objects to avoid flexion of the neck. Also, hyperextension of the neck for a prolonged period of time, as when working overhead, can cause neck pain. Patients with chronic severe neck pain may need to use a molded plastic collar for approximately 3 to 4 months.

Traction

Mild or chronic neck pain can be treated in outpatients by intermittent traction either in the physical therapy department, or, more economically, using a home traction kit obtainable from the local drugstore. Home traction may be done either sitting in a doorway, with the apparatus suspended from the door frame, or in bed. Traction pull should be at least equivalent to the weight of the head, about 7 pounds. Usually traction is ordered with weights of between 7 and 15 pounds. In a few patients, traction makes the pain worse and should be discontinued after a brief trial. Continuous traction is rarely indicated but is given to some patients suffering from intractable pain. This must be done in the hospital, and then only for a period of 3 to 4 days.

Physical Therapy

Mobilization and manipulation are being used increasingly in physical therapy units for chronic neck pain and as a useful preventive measure. Mobilization involves careful and gentle movement of the neck through the range of motion, often using gentle traction with the hands. It can be taught to one of the patient's family members. Manipulation is performed by many different kinds of health providers, especially osteopaths and chiropractors, and often seems successful, although its efficacy is not supported by controlled studies. Neurologic symptoms following a manipulation are a rare event but can affect older people, particularly as a result of injury to the vertebrobasilar arteries. Exercises are also helpful, particularly in the late recovery phase and to prevent recurrences.

Injection Therapy

Injection therapy is based on the unproven theory that pain originates in apophyseal joints and can be eradicated by injection with local anesthetic and/or corticosteroid. The procedure is undertaken with the patient prone and the neck flexed; 1 to 2 cc of 1% lidocaine (Xylocaine) is used, often with the addition of a crystalline suspension of steroid. A long (3-cm) needle is inserted 1 inch lateral to the spinous process (midline) and pushed down through the posterior ligament into the joint area. The mixture is injected at several points around the joint.

Surgery

A small number of patients with intractable pain or progressing neurologic deficits may be considered for surgery. This is usually considered after a failure of medical management.

Whiplash injuries are hyperextension injuries of the neck usually resulting from a road traffic accident. Anterior cervical structures (muscles, larynx, esophagus, temporomandibular joint, ligaments) are stretched and sometimes torn. In mild-to-moderate instances, the victim may be unaware of injury until a few hours later, when muscles become painful or the patient develops a "wry" neck. It is important to carry out a detailed neurologic examination and to obtain an appropriate x-ray of the cervical spine to look for fracture or dislocation. A CT scan is becoming increasingly used to detect damage to the cervical spine.

Therapy includes rest (using a soft cervical collar), analgesics, and local ice/heat treatments. Occasionally symptoms secondary to mild whiplash injury are improved by gentle cervical manipulation. Injection of local anesthetic into trigger points may be helpful. If the symptoms persist for more than 4 weeks, gentle cervical traction (7–10 lb) may help relieve pain. If root signs and symptoms appear, myelography may be indicated to exclude a lacerated cervical disk. At this stage, particularly if litigation is involved, the clinical picture frequently becomes confused by "trauma neurosis." Severe cases of whiplash should be admitted to the hospital for evaluation and referred to the neurologist or neurosurgeon, since there is danger of neurologic damage.

Cloward RB. Acute cervical spine injuries. *CIBA Clin Symp* 32:1–32, 1980.
   Good illustrated review of the emergency management of acute cervical spine injuries.
Kelsey JL. Epidemiology of the radiculopathies. *Adv Neurol* 19:386–398, 1978.
   Useful discussion of the epidemiology of radiculopathies, particularly nerve root problems and neuritis related to cervical disc disease.
Grieve GP. *Common Vertebral Joint Problems.* New York: Churchill Livingstone, 1981.
   An excellent book giving comprehensive guidance on physical examination, mobilization, and manipulation techniques, and a critical look at a wide range of therapeutic modalities used in joint disease—over 1300 references.
Buerges PU. Myofascial pain syndromes. *Postgrad Med* 53:161–168, 1973.
   Useful review of the common sites of myofascial pain syndromes and their management.
Murray-Leslie CV, Wright V. Carpal tunnel syndrome, humeral epicondylitis, and the cervical spine: A study of clinical and dimensional relations. *Br Med J* 1:1439–1442, 1976.
   An article describing the clinical relationships between cervical spine disease and other soft tissue syndromes.
Poser CM. The frustrating problem of neck pain. *Consultant* 8:156–162, 1980.
   Short review article dealing with chronic nonspecific neck pain.
Kraus H. *Clinical Treatment of Back and Neck Pain.* New York: McGraw-Hill, 1970.
   Comprehensive textbook on the management of back and neck pain.
Krueger BR, Okazaki H. Vertebral-basilar distribution infarction following chiropractic cervical manipulation. *Mayo Clin Proc* 55:322–332, 1980.
   Article indicating dangers of chiropractic manipulation with some useful references.
Saunders RL, Wilson DH. The surgery of cervical disk disease. *Clin Orthop* 146:119–127, 1980.
   Review of indications and methods of surgical management of cervical disk diseases.

75. SHOULDER PAIN
Peter Curtis

Pain in the shoulder is often associated with limited movement. Because the symptoms are often intermittent, many patients seek help only after recurrences or if the problem becomes chronic. In a population survey of rheumatic disorders, neck-shoulder-brachial pain was found in 9% of men and 12% of women over the age of 15.

Anatomy
The shoulder joint consists of two functioning joints (the glenohumeral and acromioclavicular) and three gliding surfaces (long head of biceps, subacromial bursa, and musculotendinous cuff). The musculotendinous or rotator cuff strengthens the capsule of the joint through the insertion into its substances of five muscles: supraspinatus, infraspinatus, teres minor, subscapularis, and long head of the triceps.

Shoulder pain may arise from structures outside the shoulder such as cervical vertebrae, heart, lungs, or diaphragm; however, musculoskeletal disorders of the shoulder are responsible for the majority of instances. Although many specific conditions are described in orthopedic texts, most musculoskeletal problems are either the "myofascial syndrome" (fibrositis-myofibrositis, or scapulothoracic muscular syndrome) or one of a continuum of interrelated traumatic or degenerative soft-tissue processes—bursitis, tendinitis, or rotator cuff syndrome. Less frequently, well-defined conditions can be identified, such as rotator cuff tears, calcific tendinitis, or adhesive capsulitis.

General Evaluation
A *history* of pain and/or decreased mobility is the usual complaint; less frequently, swelling in or about the shoulder is noted. In myofascial disorders, the patient complains of pain to the touch or tenderness over the posterior aspect of the shoulder girdle. This pain may radiate to the neck or arm.

The earliest and often most intense pain is felt over the deltoid muscle and may spread to the entire shoulder or radiate downward into the lateral or anterior aspect of the arm. Pain from any of the structures of the shoulder joint except the acromioclavicular (A-C) joint is referred along the same dermatome (C5), which includes the shoulder and the lateral surface of the arm to the hand. Pain from the A-C joint, which is innervated by C4, is felt directly over the A-C joint. Patients with degenerative diseases often have a slow and gradual increase in the pain; pain occurring suddenly should suggest other causes. With degenerative processes, some joint mobility usually is preserved, and the patient complains more about movement of the shoulder in a specific direction. However, with infection, blood in the joint, or severe calcific tendinitis, movement in any direction is excruciating. Fever is not associated with degenerative processes and suggests other causes. Although multiple painful joints usually suggest systemic disease, often several degenerative processes, such as bursitis or tendinitis, occur simultaneously.

The *physical examination* includes examination of the neck, arm, lungs, and thorax with careful neurologic testing for cervical disease. The shoulder is inspected for swelling and position. The patient is asked to abduct the arms (the painful arc test) to help delineate rotator cuff problems, and the shoulder is palpated to pinpoint areas of tenderness, such as muscles (in the myofascial syndrome), the insertions of the rotator cuff muscles over the humeral tuberosities, the biceps insertion through the bicipital groove, or the A-C joint. Not uncommonly, there is diffuse tenderness over several structures, which prevents specific anatomic diagnosis. The patient is asked to try to move the shoulder actively in a full range of motion. Typically, some motion is possible in degenerative problems, and limitation of motion can be improved with gentle and slow assistance. With acute inflammatory processes or intra-articular bleeding and infection, limited motion (usually in all planes) is not improved by assistance. After assessing the passive range of motion, specific muscles are tested against resistance. The most frequently affected are the supraspinatus and biceps tendon.

Laboratory evaluation is not usually indicated unless specific extrinsic causes of shoulder pain are being considered. X-rays are usually not helpful in patients suspected of having degenerative disease of the shoulder; in selected patients with new shoulder pain, however, x-rays are done to search for calcium deposits and bony lesions.

Evaluation for Specific Conditions

Myofascial Syndrome
Fibrositis myofibrositis is the most common shoulder problem seen in ambulatory care. The cause is unknown. Often there are "trigger points" along the upper pole of the scapula where pressure stimulates referred pain. Small, tender nodules may be palpable in this area; these nodules show no specific histologic characteristics. Other findings include "scapulocostal grating" on moving the scapula or, sometimes, a "snapping" scapula caused by flicking of an osseous spur on the vertebral margin of the bone against muscle.

Bursitis, Tendinitis, and Rotator Cuff Syndrome
This process begins in the supraspinatus or bicipital tendons, which have relatively poor blood supply and are under stress. With time, the tendinous insertions about the shoulder become frayed and inflamed. As the degeneration advances, inflammation involves other tendons and bursae and, ultimately, the entire capsule and acromioclavicular joint. Depending on the distribution, patients may present with complaints of any of these structures. It is often difficult to make an exact anatomic diagnosis, but testing of specific structures may make a precise diagnosis possible. These degenerative conditions occur most frequently in patients between 50 and 60 years and are more common in women and in the winter months. The disease process is unilateral in 75% of patients. Bursitis is often precipitated by minor trauma and is associated with other soft-tissue disorders. The onset is often slow, and the condition may persist with exacerbations and remissions for up to 2 years. Improvement is slow.

The patient usually presents with aching in the shoulder, limited abduction of the arm with a painful arc of motion between 45° and 120° (positive painful arc test), and loss of function of affected structures. Between about 45° and 120°, the rotator cuff tendons move under the coracoacromial arch. If these tendons are swollen and inflamed, they become impinged under the arch, and pain occurs. (From 120°–180°, the A-C joint is used for elevation; therefore, pain that occurs only after 120° abduction suggests A-C joint involvement.) There may be tenderness over the deltoid insertion in the upper arm, and the patient may complain of tingling down the arm. X-ray of the shoulder may show calcification in the rotator cuff, calcium deposits in the supraspinatus tendon, and sclerosis and cystic changes in the head of the humerus.

Rotator Cuff Rupture
Close to 25% of people have some attrition of the rotator cuff by the age of 50. Partial or full tears of the cuff therefore tend to present in middle age following trauma, often a fall on the outstretched arm. The pain is acute, and the patient complains of weakness of the arm, reduced range of motion, and pain at the limits of internal and external rotation. Partial tears are often associated with other inflammatory or degenerative disorders of the shoulder. Arthrograms are useful in confirming the diagnosis if there is no improvement after 6 weeks or if there has been obvious trauma. Early surgical repair of complete tears produces the best outcomes.

Calcific Tendinitis
Calcific deposits are present in the shoulder tissues of most people over the age of 35. Calcific tendinitis occurs in 2.7 to 8% of the population. There are three stages of the condition: (1) an asymptomatic stage, in which calcific deposits are only detected on x-ray, (2) a chronic intermittent phase, and (3) an acute flare-up. The acute condition usually affects a relatively young and active person. The patient complains of excruciating pain, often down the arm. The surrounding muscles are acutely tender and in spasm. There is a painful arc of passive motion from 0° to 60°, and the patient holds the arm splinted. The pain is caused by a calcium deposit "boil," which may subsequently rupture, releasing a toothpaste-like material and relieving the pain. The condition usually subsides within 14 days.

Adhesive Capsulitis (frozen shoulder)
This condition occurs as a result of the marked reduction in volume of the glenohu-meral joint, with tightening and thickening of the joint capsule. The peak incidence occurs between 50 and 70 years of age, and the incidence is higher in women. Adhesive capsulitis is often associated with other clinical conditions, such as myocardial infarc-tion, long-term intravenous infusions, thyroid disease, diabetes, and depression; it also occurs in situations in which there is shoulder immobilization (e.g., hemiplegia, frac-tures). The symptoms include generalized loss of motion, chronic pain, and minimal tenderness. Symptoms develop over a period of several months and last up to 2 years. Recovery is usual. Arthrography shows a marked decrease in joint space, and the hu-meral head may show some osteoporosis.

Treatment
The treatment of musculoskeletal shoulder problems is usually directed to alleviating the pathologic and anatomic cause of the disability or pain. However, because the clin-ical picture may not suggest a specific syndrome, management often involves an em-piric sequence of therapies.

Physical Therapy
Common practice includes cooling, using ice pack applications for 20 to 30 minutes three times daily for the acute stage, and heating, using hot packs for 20 minutes several times a day in the subacute conditions.

Exercises
In the acute phase, it may be necessary to rest the arm in a sling and treat the pain with passive range-of-motion exercises, hot-cold compresses, nonsteroidal anti-inflam-matory agents, or injection of local anesthetics with or without steroids. Subsequently, active exercises are important to increase mobility and maintain muscle bulk and flex-ibility. The affected arm and hand are used as a pendulum; they are swung back and forth, increasing the arc progressively. Other exercises include "wall-walking" with the fingers (gradually abducting the arm by walking the fingers up the wall), circle exer-cises (bending over and making ever-larger circles with the arm), and the use of over-head pulleys. Many patients have associated postural and muscle imbalance problems, and attention should be directed toward improving posture and providing suitable pil-lows or mattresses for support during rest. Exercises should be undertaken for about 5 minutes every hour during the day.

Drugs
Salicylates (600–900 mg every 6 hours) are cheap and effective. Acetaminophen and propoxyphene derivatives relieve acute pain but are not anti-inflammatory. *Nonsteroi-dal anti-inflammatory drugs (NSAIDs)* are used extensively for musculoskeletal shoul-der syndromes, although there are no well-controlled studies that show significant ben-efits except in acute inflammatory conditions. The agents produce both an analgesic and an anti-inflammatory effect and may be given as a therapeutic trial for 1 to 2 weeks. No one agent is established as better than another. Commonly used NSAIDs include ibuprofen (Motrin), sulindac (Clinoril), naproxen (Naprosyn), and indomethacin (Indocin). Because patients may respond better to one NSAID than another, different agents should be tried if there is no initial improvement. The possible side effects of these drugs (indigestion, gastric erosion, skin rash) should be reviewed with patients before prescribing.

Treatment of Specific Conditions
The treatment of *myofascial pain* revolves around identifying triggering factors such as wrong desk or chair height for a sedentary employee, peculiar position of body while sitting in class or movie theater, or an unusual way of doing a repetitive task such as lifting overhead on an assembly line.

This analysis may take time and some imagination to sort out, but mechanical mis-use of arm-neck-shoulder is a major cause of pain.

Other precipitating causes include sleep disturbance and/or depression, endocrinop-athies (particularly diabetes mellitus and hypothyroidism), and other inflammatory forms of arthritis.

If nothing is found, the syndrome should be treated as a use-related musculoskeletal disorder with local heat, massage, active range-of-motion movements, and stretching exercises. Muscle relaxants have not proved effective. If trigger points are found, anesthesia of the area can usually be obtained by injecting 1 to 5 ml of lidocaine (Xylocaine) using a 1½-inch 22-gauge needle. If a first injection does not effect complete relief, a second injection may be used. Some authorities have recommended injecting steroids, but this practice is of questionable benefit. If there is no response to repeated injections, the diagnosis should be reassessed. Other techniques, such as local application of ethyl chloride, have been tried but with less success than local anesthetic injection.

Local steroid injections into periarticular tissue have been shown to produce benefit in *rotator cuff syndrome* if specifically inflamed structures are identified. This can be done by first injecting lidocaine to determine if localization is correct. Because the injection is made into the tendons, one may feel the needle hit bone; otherwise, injection is made into soft tissue and is more readily absorbed systemically. The dosage for periarticular injection has not been precisely defined; however, the equivalent of 40 mg of prednisone is most frequently recommended. The usual method is to mix 1 to 2 ml of 1% lidocaine with the colloidal steroid. Patients should be warned that pain in the shoulder is likely to increase over the 12 hours following an injection. This problem often can be avoided by the use of a longer acting local anesthetic, such as bupivacaine (Marcaine), instead of lidocaine. Repeated injections of steroids into the same site produce atrophy; not more than 2 or 3 injections should be given over a 12-month period.

Calcific Tendinitis is usually managed by orthopedic specialists. Calcific deposits can be "needled" and washed out with saline using a two-needle technique, but the benefit is questionable.

Adhesive capsulitis is treated initially with conservative therapy—heat, exercises analgesics. If there is no response, patients are referred for distention arthrography.

Lawrence JS. *Rheumatism in Populations*. London: Heinemann 1977.
   A good general text describing the epidemiology of various types of arthritis, musculoskeletal symptoms, and back pain.
Cyriax J. *Textbook of Orthopaedic Medicine*. London: Bailliere Tindall, 1976. Vol. 1, pp. 204–243.
   Although the therapeutic portion of this two-volume textbook is somewhat outdated, the section on physical diagnosis of soft-tissue lesions is excellent.
Booth RE, Marvel JP. Differential diagnosis of shoulder pain. *Orthop Clin North Am* 6:353–379, 1975.
   A good general review of the wide range of causes of shoulder pain and their differentiation by clinical laboratory and radiographic methods.
Ramamurth CP. *Orthopedics in Primary Care*. Baltimore: Williams & Wilkins, 1981.
   An excellent and practical small book providing a simple, logical approach to common problems in primary care. Short on references.
Simon WH. Soft-tissue disorders of the shoulder. *Orthop Clin North Am* 6:521–538, 1975.
   A short review article of the diagnostic and surgical approach to the management of frozen shoulder, calcific tendinitis, and bicipital tendinitis.
Anonymous. Frozen shoulder: Adhesive capsulitis. *Brit Med J* 283:1005–1006, 1981 (Editorial).
   A succinct editorial on frozen shoulder with a good list of references.
Neviaser JS. Adhesive capsulitis and the stiff shoulder. *Orthop Clin North Am* 11:327–330, 1980.
   A short review paper on adhesive capsulitis from a symposium issue of Orthopedic Clinics of North America *on disorders of the shoulder.*
Swezey RL. *Arthritis: Rational Therapy and Rehabilitation*. Philadelphia: Saunders, 1978.
   One of the major comprehensive textbooks on physical therapy.
Gray RG, Tenenbaum J, Gottlieb NL. Local corticosteroid injection treatment in rheumatic disorders. *Semin Arthritis Rheum* 10:231–254, 1981:
   An excellent review article on the indications, methods, and side effects of steroid injection therapy.

Bland JH, Merrit JA, Bonsley DR. The painful shoulder. *Semin Arthritis Rheum* 7:21–47, 1977.
A good review paper of the anatomy of the shoulder and causes, differential diagnosis, and management of soft-tissue disorders of the shoulders.

76. LOW BACK PAIN

Nortin M. Hadler

At least 70% of people experience low back pain (LBP) at some time in their lives. LBP is a self-limited disease; approximately 40% of patients remit in 1 week, 60 to 85% in 3 weeks, and 90% in 2 months. Along with remission, LBP is characterized by a striking likelihood of recurrence. The first attack of low back pain is usually the shortest and least severe; recurrences usually last longer. Back symptoms, with equal occurrence in men and women, begin in the third to fourth decade and peak in the 40s to early 50s.

Etiology

The cause of low back pain is unknown in the overwhelming majority of patients. Many structures possess sensory innervation, and several are potential sources for pain that mimics the symptoms of disc herniation. Despite endless speculation on the pathogenesis of nonspecific low back pain, there is no clear-cut way to diagnose fibrositis, myositis, or any other of the causes that have been ascribed to this regional disease. Seldom are we able to ascribe any episode of back illness to a particular back disease.

Structural abnormalities of the disc occur early in life, frequently before 30. In older patients, disintegration is almost ubiquitous. Disc herniation arises in that part of the spine subjected to the heaviest mechanical stresses, usually C5–C6, L4–L5, and L5–S1. Intradiscal pressure measured in various positions has shown that inappropriate standing, lifting, and sitting all increase stresses on intervertebral discs.

Evaluation

History

In evaluating low back pain, we generate a series of questions to separate patients with LBP of systemic cause from the vast majority with self-limited regional disease.

Clinical settings that should greatly increase one's suspicion of systemic disease include (1) back pain in the elderly, accompanied by historical or physical signs of malignancy; pain with metastasis or myeloma tends to be more continuous, progressive, and prominent when the patient is recumbent; (2) back pain along with fever, which suggests infection and requires a more careful and aggressive approach; and (3) back pain with five specific historical features that together are up to 95% sensitive and 85% specific for ankylosing spondylitis. These features are (a) age of onset less than 40 years, (b) insidious onset, (c) duration of at least 3 months, (d) morning stiffness, and (e) improvement with exercise.

Information about the quality of pain, age of patient, and presence of systemic complaints mandates additional consideration before relegating the patient to the diagnostic category of regional musculoskeletal back disease. Tumor, infection, and ankylosing spondylitis do not exhaust the list of diseases that present as backache, but most of the other problems are accompanied by hints that are obvious in the history and physical examination.

Physical Examination

The back and neurologic examination usually determines whether surgical consultation is necessary. Inspection of gait and heel-and-toe walking assesses weakness of the gastrocnemius and tibialis anterior muscles. A change in posture including loss of lumbar lordosis is totally nonspecific, as are pelvic tilt, scoliosis, and degree of kyphosis or lordosis. Measurements of spinal motion are seldom useful in evaluating low back pain, but normal mobility should direct thinking to causes of pain that are other than musculoskeletal. Straight leg raising is a clinical test that is often misinterpreted. To be positive, pain should be present during the early arc of straight leg raising. This suggests to some surgeons a protruding disc in the L5–S1 disc, affecting the 5th lumbar nerve root. Other authors feel that the crossed straight leg raising test (straight leg raise on the unaffected side increases symptoms on the affected side) is an even more specific sign of a herniated nucleus pulposus. Flexion of the knee with the patient prone—the femoral stretch test—is of some use in diagnosing L3 lesions. There are no stretch tests for lesions at L1, L2, S3, or S4. These tests combined with neurologic testing for motor weakness and sensory defects are important in defining the extent of neuromuscular compromise. With minor neurologic abnormalities, one would not seek emergency surgical consultation; referral is triggered by signs and symptoms suggesting the cauda equina syndrome. This syndrome, presenting as acute pain and loss of autonomic function, results from central herniation of a disc below L1 and L2, which in most people is opposite the lower end of the spinal cord. It is imperative to inquire about bladder and bowel dysfunction and to check for saddle anesthesia, rectal tone, and cremasteric reflexes in patients with acute back pain.

X-rays
Disc degeneration is a phenomenon of aging that need not give rise to any symptoms. By age 50, 80 to 95% of adults show evidence at autopsy of lumbar spondylosis (degenerative disc disease with narrowing of disc space, marginal sclerosis, vacuum phenomenon, disc calcification), and 87% of this age group have similar findings by x-ray. By age 60, 95% of asymptomatic patients have radiographic disc disease. Therefore, the mere demonstration of degenerative disc disease on lumbar spine films does not confirm the cause of low back pain; it is so commonly present that it seldom provides definitive causal information. Lumbar spine x-rays are helpful in excluding possibilities such as infection and metastasis but are an unnecessary expense in patients in whom the history and physical examination generate no specific question to be answered by x-ray.

Treatment of Acute Episodes
Approximately 40% of patients with LBP become well within 1 week, 80% within 2 weeks, and 90% within 2 months, regardless of the treatment. Therefore, the initial management of low back pain should be conservative even in the face of mild neurologic abnormalities.

Bed Rest
   The first principle of management is bed rest. Intradiscal pressures are lowest in the supine and prone positions. There is no established rule for how long strict bed rest should be continued, but only a minority of patients require it for more than 1 to 2 weeks. Unfortunately, bed rest may be one of the most difficult prescriptions to write for young active workers for whom total or even limited bed rest may result in a considerable loss of income. This treatment must be tempered by reason and reduced to limited activity as necessary. Lifting, bending, and prolonged sitting should be excluded if possible unless they can be done in short periods with appropriate back and arm support.

Traction
Traction often has been recommended in low back pain. However, with the usually applied weights of only 10 to 15 pounds, neither traction to the spinal segments nor stretch of the paraspinal muscle takes place. Studies have shown that at least 25% of total body weight is required merely to overcome lower body resistance. As presently administered, 50 to 100 pounds of traction would be needed to be effective. There has been one controlled study of lumbar traction in the management of lower back pain. In this study, no differences in outcome were discernible between a group treated with low-weight traction and a group treated with effective traction. The need for hospitalization, the extra expense to carry out the procedure, and the absence of demonstrable benefits in an already self-limited process militate against employing traction.

Drugs

Innumerable analgesic and anti-inflammatory agents, sedatives, hypnotics, and muscle relaxants have been recommended for the immediate relief of low back pain. There is no study demonstrating that any of these agents is more efficacious than salicylate therapy. There have been a few studies demonstrating the efficacy of several drugs compared to placebo, but no drug convincingly demonstrates a greater effect than aspirin. Many agents have not been properly tested, and their efficacy or lack thereof remains unknown. The recommendation for drugs in most patients with low back pain is for simple salicylates or acetaminophen while awaiting the natural progress of events.

Physical Modalities

The benefit of most physical modalities, such as ultrasound, short-wave diathermy, heat, cold, or roentgen therapy, has not been convincingly demonstrated. Any relief is usually transient. There is no evidence to suggest that local heat has any effect on a disc lesion or any lasting effect on a patient's symptoms. However, little is lost with a trial of local heat supplied by heating pad or hot water bottle.

Manipulation

Manipulation is very widely used in both Britain and Canada by physicians and non-physicians, often as an alternative to bed rest. In the United States, manipulation is practiced almost exclusively by chiropractors. The effectiveness of physicians has been compared to that of chiropractors in the management of low back pain; the treatment modalities used were similar except that chiropractors emphasized manipulation instead of medication. No statistical difference could be detected in the outcome of the two groups of patients, although the patients of chiropractors felt significantly more welcome as well as more satisfied with the explanations and treatments. In two reasonably and adequately designed studies, manipulation was not shown to be clinically effective despite the possibility that spinal manipulation may occasionally result in transient reduction of small lumbar disc protrusion.

Corsets and Braces

Although generally recommended for chronic or subacute low back pain, corsets or back braces occasionally are used for acute pain. Corsets are employed in an attempt to decrease intradiscal pressure during normal standing through one of two possible biomechanical mechanisms: (1) unloading vertebral pressure by increasing intra-abdominal pressure, or (2) immobilizing the spine. However, studies have failed to indicate that either mechanism takes place. The usefulness of bracing is tenuous if based on these theoretical grounds.

Exercises

Directed physical therapy and personal exercise programs are nearly universally prescribed for patients with low back pain who have chronic symptoms or are in the resolving phase of an acute episode. There are three basic types of exercises commonly recommended: (1) back hyperextension exercises to strengthen the paravertebral muscles, (2) spinal mobilizing exercises (especially flexion), and (3) isometric spinal flexion with secondary increased intra-abdominal pressure. The goals of recommended regimens vary greatly. Some are aimed at strengthening lumbar extensor or abdominal muscles or increasing overall spinal mobility.

Two controlled studies have examined exercise programs and their effect on chronic low back pain. In both studies, isometric exercises yielded better clinical results than the usual flexion-extension exercises. It has been shown that many of the flexion-extension exercises actually increase interdiscal pressures. It hardly makes sense to advise against bending, lifting, and loading of the lumbar spine while prescribing sets of exercises that mimic such activity. The principle behind the isometric regimen is to eliminate any exaggerated hyperextension of the lumbar spine and encourage isometric contraction of the trunk muscles while standing, walking, sitting, and lying down. Specific exercises are aimed at strengthening weak abdominal muscles. When reclining, patients lie on the back with 2 to 3 pillows in a wedge shape under the head and shoulders and one pillow under the knee. The sequence of active contractions is listed below.

1. Contract the abdominal muscles (pull umbilicus toward spine) as hard as possible Relax.
2. Contract the gluteus. Relax.
3. Combine abdominal and gluteal contractions to produce a pelvic tilt with flexion of the lumbar spine.
4. Contract the hip adductors and pelvic floor.

After the above are mastered, the contractions are held as long as possible (5–15 seconds). Progress should be made by increasing duration and number of performances. These exercises can be performed standing and even while walking.

Surgery

Surgery plays no role in treatment of the vast majority of patients with low back pain. Most episodes of low back pain are self-limited; even most recurrences are. self-limited. For most patients a reasoned conservative approach to management can provide considerable palliation during an acute episode. Improvement may be judged objectively by improved straight leg raising, improved neurologic signs, and increased spinal mobility. Many surgeons claim that refractory cases requiring surgical intervention can be identified by 6 weeks; however, nearly 50% of these patients respond to additional conservative management. Thus surgical series selected in this fashion must improve on the 50% figure before ascribing improvement to surgery.

Signs that suggest the need for immediate surgical attention are the development of new neurologic signs or the progression of motor weakness during conservative therapy. Prolonged paralysis before attempting surgery should be avoided because recovery of function is more complete if surgery is not delayed. Pain is a relative indication; surgery is more effective in eliminating radicular pain than backache. Because the results of surgery improve in the presence of prolapse, the preoperative evaluation should include myelography. One must realize, however, that as many as one-third of normal persons may have an asymptomatic but myelographically demonstrable prolapse. In patients with classic severe sciatica with neurologic signs, approximately 10 to 20% have negative explorations. Those with negative explorations have a poorer prognosis; they are more likely to develop postlaminectomy syndrome. Therefore, in addition to the difficulties involved in improving on the natural history of low back pain by surgery, there is the possibility that the patient will be made worse.

When a prolapsed disc can be identified and removed, patients experience a briefer duration of symptoms than when treated conservatively; after 6 months, however, the results in one well-designed study were nearly identical for conservatively and operatively treated patients. In view of the good results with conservative therapy for lumbar disc prolapse causing sciatica, surgical intervention should be reserved for specific indications such as the cauda equina syndrome and major or progressive paralysis.

Quinet RJ, Hadler NM. Diagnosis and treatment of backache. *Semin Arthritis Rheum* 8:261–287, 1979.
  An exhaustive and thoroughly referenced discussion, from which this chapter is excerpted.

77. KNEE PAIN
Axalla J. Hoole

Knee pain in ambulatory patients can be caused by many mechanical problems and diseases. Younger patients are more likely to have mechanical and developmental problems than systemic or inflammatory disease. With aging development problems are less common, and inflammatory and degenerative problems increase. The young are likely to have a history of recent trauma, and older patients, one of recurrent, but lesser trauma, which has been considered trivial and overlooked.

Evaluation

History

Mechanical problems of the knee, of either intrinsic or extrinsic structures, usually are accompanied by a history of trauma and involve a single joint that is not inflamed. Systemic disease usually involves more than one joint, and the articular problem is accompanied by signs and symptoms of systemic disease as well as inflammatory changes of the joints. Effusion of the knee usually suggests involvement of intrinsic rather than extrinsic structures.

Patients with knee pain also complain of crepitus, swelling, and instability that is expressed in a variety of ways—buckling, giving way, or locking. An accurate history often points to the specific mechanical derangement. Patients with meniscal tears or loose bodies may complain that the knee locks or cannot be straightened. Patients with loose bodies may feel something out of place that can be manipulated to restore function; ligamentous damage may be suggested by buckling.

Physical Examination

Joints other than the knee must be examined, with the physician looking for signs of systemic disease. The leg should be inspected for subtle flexion, which may suggest the leg cannot be fully extended; quadriceps atrophy, which suggests disuse; valgus or varus deformity; and ecchymosis. Swelling may be generalized or local from either fluid or synovial thickening. Large effusions are not difficult to detect, but small effusions must be sought. With the knee in extension, milk the fluid from the medial knee compartment; with pressure to the lateral region a bulge should appear medially. Even with small effusions, this should create a bulge that can be pushed from one side to the other.

By palpating the knee, one can detect specific tender areas or local enlargement or swelling. Anteriorly, there may be swelling of the patellar bursae or tenderness of the patella or the anterior tibia tuberosity. Posteriorly, bulging in the popliteal fossa may represent a Baker's cyst, characteristically found just medial to the midline. Tenderness medial to the midline suggests anserine bursitis. Medially and laterally, tears of the collateral ligaments are associated with tenderness and instability. Following the general examination, there are countless tests that may be performed to elicit signs of ligamentous and meniscal injury. Although most of these tests lie in the realm of the orthopedic specialist, examination of the medial and lateral collateral ligaments and cruciate ligaments (using the "anterior-posterior drawer sign") should be routinely included in the knee examination of the bone.

Laboratory Tests

Laboratory evaluation is indicated only if systemic-inflammatory diseases are suspected. X-rays are usually indicated when effusion is present, particularly following trauma. Aspiration of joint fluid is suggested in all patients who present with knee effusion for the first time, particularly those with fever or signs of inflammation who may be infected or have gout or pseudogout. Thereafter, repeat evaluation depends on changes in the clinical condition.

Management

Identification and management can be simplified by grouping the problems as follows:

1. Single painful knee with little or no swelling or inflammation (patellofemoral pain)
   a. Chondromalacia patellae (younger patients)
   b. Dislocating patella
   c. Degenerative joint disease (patellofemoral osteoarthritis)
   d. Osgood-Schlatter disease (children)
   e. Prepatellar bursitis or infrapatellar bursitis
   f. Reflex sympathetic dystrophy (Sudeck's atrophy)
2. Single swollen knee without inflammation
   a. Osteoarthritis
   b. Baker's cyst (intact or ruptured)

c. Torn ligaments
d. Loose bodies and osteochondritis dissecans
e. Meniscal tears
3. Multiple or single inflamed joint. These problems so often lead to inpatient management that they are not discussed here.
   a. Any inflammatory joint disease (pseudogout characteristically affects the knee rather than more distal joints)
   b. Infection

Single Painful Knee with Little or No Swelling

Chondromalacia patellae is a specific pathologic diagnosis that refers to a common condition in young adults, found more frequently in women than men. Because the diagnosis is difficult to correlate with symptoms, many rheumatologists use patellofemoral disease to refer to the syndrome. Characteristically, there is pain on arising after sitting for several hours with the knee flexed at 90°, when descending stairs, or when squatting. The medial or lateral margin of the patella is tender, and the patella grinding test is positive. (The patella grinding test is performed by pushing the patella distally. When the quadriceps is tightened, crepitation and tenderness are caused by motion of the patella instead of a smooth painless motion.) There should be no effusion. The pain is thought by some to be caused by degeneration and fissuring of the articular surface of the patella; however, this finding is present in asymptomatic patients operated on for other reasons. Also, 50% of asymptomatic students have been found to have a positive patella grinding test. Some authorities now believe that malalignment of the patella, as indicated by an abnormal quadriceps angle, is the important anatomic problem. The quadriceps angle is formed by lines from the center of the patella to the anterior iliac spine and the femoral tubercle. The normal angle is 15°; greater than 20 is considered abnormal. In malalignment, the patella is positioned medially.

Chondromalacia may be difficult to distinguish from patellofemoral osteoarthritis. However, patients with osteoarthritis are usually older (over 45), without a history of recurrent pain as young adults, and with evidence of degenerative changes in other parts of the knee and other joints.

Conservative management is usually sufficient. Patients must be reassured that the condition is benign and usually self-limited. For most, restricting athletic activity, isometric quadriceps exercises, and aspirin result in improvement in 2 to 3 weeks. Those who do not respond should be referred to an orthopedist.

Osgood-Schlatter disease, a problem of adolescents, is a traction apophysitis of the anterior tibial tuberosity. These patients complain of pain over the anterior tibial tuberosity, which is usually slightly enlarged and tender. Curtailing exercises is usually sufficient treatment; persistent pain may require immobilization with a cylinder cast.

Prepatellar bursitis (housemaid's or nun's knee) is found in carpenters, carpet layers, gardeners, and other people who spend time in repeated or prolonged kneeling. The problem appears over a few hours or a few days as a swelling just over the anterior aspect of the knee, usually unaccompanied by joint effusion or signs of severe inflammation. Patients complain of pain and swelling. Septic prepatellar bursitis does occur, usually associated with a laceration, abrasion, or wound over the area. Infected bursae are red, warm, and tender in a localized area over the patella. Examination is sufficient for the diagnosis of prepatellar bursitis. X-rays are not indicated. If inflammation or infection is present, fluid should be aspirated and sent for culture.

Treatment of noninfected bursitis is by aspiration of as much fluid as possible followed by corticosteroid instillation and pressure dressing. Patients with chronically painful bursae may be referred to an orthopedist for excision. Septic bursitis is usually caused by gram-positive organisms, especially *Staphylococcus aureus,* and is usually treated with parenteral antibiotics.

Single Swollen Joint without Inflammation

Osteoarthritis of the knee is extremely common; radiographic changes occur early and can be found in many people by age 40. Before age 45 osteoarthritis is found more often in men; but more often in women thereafter. It is frequently associated with obesity (more so in women than in men) and varus deformity, and less frequently with Baker's cyst and effusions. The pain associated with osteoarthritis characteristically occurs after periods of immobilization and improves with light activity, however, continuous activity may worsen the pain. Pain that occurs primarily at night or when descending steps suggests patellofemoral involvement. Although patients with degenerative joint disease of the knee may have effusion, the presence of instability or locking suggests internal meniscal or cartilage damage. Infrequently, there is synovial thickening, associated with a mild inflammation.

Conservative treatment is sufficient for most patients. This includes weight reduction, exercises to maintain range of motion and quadriceps strength, moist heat, and analgesics. Aspirin or acetaminophen is recommended because they are less expensive than nonsteroidal anti-inflammatory drugs and just as effective. Steroids have been used intra-articularly; some studies have shown benefit, but not greater than that reported from intra-articular injection of saline. Injections are generally not recommended except for larger Baker's cysts associated with osteoarthritis. Patients with constant pain, whose life is altered by the arthritis and who have an articular mechanical derangement, may be considered for surgery, which includes a range of procedures from arthroscopic surgery and irrigation to arthroplasty and joint replacement.

Baker's cysts—cysts within the popliteal fossa—occur more often in older people. The cysts appear to be related to degeneration of the posterior joint capsule and distention of the gastrocnemio-semimembranous bursa. These cysts are most commonly associated with osteoarthritis, meniscal tears, and rheumatoid arthritis. Cysts that enlarge into the calf are usually associated with rheumatoid arthritis.

Symptoms may at first be only tightness or a mechanical impairment to walking. Patients may note that the size of the cyst varies. Large cysts may compress other structures in the popliteal space. Venous compression can lead to venous distention and edema. Impairment of the tibial or common peroneal nerve can occur. Rupture of the popliteal cyst may lead to acute pain and swelling that may suggest deep vein thrombosis or a gastrocnemius tear.

Additional evaluation is not required for asymptomatic cysts. Ultrasonography is the most useful noninvasive test to demonstrate the cyst. A knee arthrogram can be performed to document the size of a cyst, and in patients with possible ruptured Baker's cysts a venogram or Doppler examination may be necessary to distinguish cysts from deep venous thrombosis.

Treatment is necessary only for symptomatic patients. In those patients with tense symptomatic cysts, aspiration of the knee until the cyst can be felt to disappear followed by instillation of the equivalent of 40 mg of prednisone is recommended. Bed rest for several days is beneficial. Symptoms should disappear rapidly.

Meniscal tears and torn ligaments are usually suggested by a history of trauma, and patients with such tears should be referred for treatment.

Hoppenfeld, S. Physical examination of the knee joint complaint. *Orthop Clin North Am* 10:3–20, 1979.
A very useful and understandable review of the examination of the knee.
Noble J. The painful knee. *Br J Hosp Med* 22:169–176, 1979.
Presents a classification and discussion of an approach to knee pain.
Wigley RD. Popliteal cysts: Variations on the theme of Baker cyst. *Semin Arthritis Rheum* 7:1–10, 1982.
An excellent review of this problem.
Gruber MA. The conservative treatment of chondromalacia patellae. *Orthop Clin North Am* 10:105–115, 1979.
A good overview of the disease.
Wilson F.C. Degenerative disease of the knee: Clinical aspects and management. *NC Med J* 39:360–363, 1978.
A very brief but useful overview for initial reference.
Kellgren JH, Lawrence JS. Osteo-arthrosis and disc degeneration in an urban population. *Ann Rheum Dis* 17:388–397, 1958.
Population study from which data on prevalence and associated findings of osteoarthrosis are usually taken.

78. NOCTURNAL LEG CRAMPS
Laurie Dornbrand

Nocturnal leg cramps are common and troublesome, but are almost never associated with serious unsuspected disease. The major issues for the clinician are recognition of the usual presentation, differential diagnosis, and treatment options.

Nocturnal cramps usually occur in the calves, with palpable firmness and bulging of the involved muscle. Episodes may occur more than once a night and are often severe and distressing. The muscles may remain sore and tender for up to several hours. Patients sometimes attain relief by dorsiflexing the involved foot or by getting out of bed and pressing the foot firmly against the floor. Massaging the muscle is usually less effective.

The "restless leg syndrome," although less common, is often discussed along with nocturnal leg cramps. Both occur at night in bed, respond to the same drugs, and have a benign prognosis. In addition to cramps, manifestations of "restless legs" include creeping sensations, jerking, twitching, aching, and numbness.

Nocturnal leg cramps occur most frequently in the elderly; in younger people they are more likely to occur after unaccustomed exercise. Surveys of ambulatory patients have uncovered a history of night cramps in 40 to 50%, with the prevalence increasing to 70% in those aged 50 or over. Of course many do not seek medical attention for this condition.

Diagnosis
The diagnosis is based on a typical history and the exclusion of pathologic conditions associated with cramps. It is especially important to rule out ischemic conditions. Peripheral vascular disease is suggested by symptoms of exercise-related pain, cramps, weakness, numbness or tingling, and the findings of diminished pulses, sensory deficits, and cool or discolored skin. Diabetic neuropathy also is associated with cramps. Patients with ischemia or diabetic neuropathy do not have as good a prognosis or response to drugs as patients with uncomplicated nocturnal leg cramps, and treatment should be directed at the underlying disorder. Other conditions associated with cramps include metabolic disorders (hyponatremia, hypokalemia, uremia, hyper- or hypothyroidism), pregnancy, and partial denervation (as in amyotrophic lateral sclerosis).

There are no specific physical findings or laboratory tests to confirm the diagnosis. Explanations for nocturnal leg cramps are speculative and generally fall into two categories: metabolic and mechanical. Stimulation of leg muscles at night by accumulation of unspecified metabolites has been implicated. It also has been suggested that flaccid muscles, such as those passively plantar flexed, have an increased tendency to recoil into spasm, because there is inadequate muscle tension to limit spontaneous contractions. However, the pathophysiology of the problem remains elusive.

Treatment
Many different treatments have been suggested, including drugs, exercises, alteration in sleeping positions, and even the use of magnets between the mattress and sheet. Because cramps occur at irregular intervals, adequately controlled trials are necessary to evaluate therapies and to distinguish effects of therapy from placebo effect. Most of the reports on treatment of cramps lack controls or have other weaknesses of experimental design.

Quinine, 200 to 300 mg at night, is the classic therapy. It is believed to work by increasing the refractory period and thus stabilizing the muscle membranes. It also decreases the excitability of the motor end-plate by competitively blocking acetylcholine. Relief usually occurs within the first week of treatment. Many patients remain free of cramps when quinine is discontinued and require only occasional doses of the drug thereafter. The major contraindications to its use include pregnancy, a history of quinine hypersensitivity, and G6PD deficiency. Both 200-mg and 300-mg tablets are available over-the-counter, at a cost of 10 to 15 cents per dose. The drug Quinamm, marketed specifically for treatment of nocturnal leg cramps, formerly was a combination of quinine and aminophylline but currently consists of 260 mg of quinine sulfate. It requires a prescription and costs about 35 cents a dose.

Vitamin E has been reported effective in large but uncontrolled series. The usual dosage is 400 IU per day, with the duration of therapy unspecified. It has been suggested that simultaneous administration of inorganic iron may inactivate the vitamin. Conjugated estrogens (Premarin) may counteract the effectiveness. The risks of vitamin E therapy are considered to be minimal, although there have been some anecdotal reports of associated problems including fatigue, hypertension, and thrombophlebitis, usually with dosages of more than 400 IU per day.

Small and uncontrolled series claim success with diphenhydramine (Benadryl), carisoprodol (Soma), methocarbamol (Robaxin), and chloroquine. Although phenytoin (Dilantin) is often mentioned as a therapy, no studies have been published on its effectiveness. There is little evidence to support the use of any of these drugs before quinine or vitamin E.

Calf muscle stretching exercises have been reported to relieve symptoms within 1 to 7 days. The patient stands facing a wall 2 to 3 feet away and leans forward with hands on the wall and heels remaining on the floor until a pulling sensation is felt in the calves. The stretched position should be held for 10 seconds and repeated after a 5-second period of relaxation. It is suggested that this sequence be repeated three times a day until the cramps are gone.

Sleeping positions designed to minimize involuntary plantar flexion of the foot during sleep also have been recommended, based on the theory that nocturnal cramps result from spontaneous contraction of flaccid calf muscles. Patients who sleep on their back should keep the covers loose or use a board or pillow at the foot of the bed. Patients who are prone to cramps should let their feet extend over the end of the mattress. All patients should consciously stretch their legs with feet dorsiflexed rather than plantar flexed.

In the absence of general agreement on the cause of nocturnal leg cramps or controlled studies of therapies, the practitioner may select among the alternatives discussed. Vitamin E is slightly cheaper than quinine but may require administration over a longer period of time for effective control of symptoms. Stretching exercises and modification of sleeping position are free of cost but may require unacceptable changes in habits or life-style for some patients. Happily, these treatments are as free of complications as the condition they are designed to alleviate.

Jones K, Castleden GM. A double-blind comparison of quinine sulfate and placebo in muscle cramps. *Age Ageing* 12:155–158, 1983.

A very small study (9 patients) that supports the effectiveness of quinine.

Ayers S, Mihan R. Nocturnal leg cramps (systremma). *South Med J* 67(11):1308–1312, 1974.

A report of the success of vitamin E in 125 patients.

Daniel HW. Simple cure for nocturnal leg cramps. *N Engl J Med* 301(4):216, 1979.

All patients with frequent nocturnal cramps treated with a simple stretching exercise reported cure within a week.

Weiner LH, Weiner HL. Nocturnal leg muscle cramps. *JAMA* 244(20):2332–2333, 1980.

A mechanical approach to the pathophysiology and treatment.

Brenning R. Motor manifestations in molimina crurum nocturna (including 'restless legs'). *J. Am Geriatr Soc* 19(8):700–708, 1971.

Discusses both nocturnal cramps and restless legs syndrome, with 21 references.

XI. REPRODUCTIVE SYSTEM PROBLEMS

79. VAGINITIS
Jack D. McCue and Laurie Dornbrand

The diagnosis of vaginitis is based on the patient's complaints of itching, burning, dysuria, dyspareunia, and malodorous or unusual discharge, and is supported by microscopic examination of vaginal secretions. Because the character and quantity of "normal" vaginal secretions may vary considerably from one woman to another, and at different times during the menstrual cycle, the presence of a discharge is not in itself abnormal. Symptoms are very nonspecific and determination of cause from clinical findings alone is unreliable. Microscopic evaluation of the discharge is essential and should include potassium hydroxide (KOH) and saline preparations of vaginal secretions; Gram's stains are also useful in some instances. Detection of infection is dependent on the number of organisms present and is impaired by recent douching.

Most of the organisms associated with vaginitis can be found in asymptomatic women, and treatment is usually aimed at the relief of symptoms rather than the eradication of organisms.

Candida Vaginitis
The prevalence of positive cultures for *Candida albicans* in asymptomatic women with normal vaginal secretions is about 20%. Factors that predispose to *Candida* colonization and infection include diabetes, corticosteroid therapy, pregnancy, broad-spectrum antibiotics (including metronidazole), obesity, heat- and moisture-retaining clothing (such as nylon underwear), and high-dose oral contraceptive pills.

Pruritus is the most common complaint associated with *Candida* vaginitis. A history of abrupt onset of symptoms favors the diagnosis but is not very specific. Vulvar inflammation and even edema may be quite pronounced, with resultant dyspareunia and dysuria. A dry, cottage cheese–like discharge is 90% specific for yeast and is present in about 75% of instances. The diagnosis is established by a positive KOH preparation. One or more drops of 10% KOH solution are mixed with a specimen of vaginal discharge, and pseudohyphae or budding yeast forms sought under high-dry microscopic examination. If the preparation is done properly, vaginal epithelial cells and leukocytes are lysed with only their outlines visible. The KOH reagent tends to lose potency on standing, especially when not refrigerated, and should be replenished periodically. The Gram's stain has been reported to be more sensitive than the wet mount in identifying yeast, but most clinicians do not consider it worth the extra trouble to perform. Cultures are not recommended because the growth of yeast may reflect colonization rather than infection.

Occasionally the clinical presentation strongly suggests *Candida* infection, but yeast cannot be demonstrated on smear or even on vaginal cultures. *Candida* can, however, be demonstrated in 55% of such women from vulvar and rectal cultures, suggesting that *Candida* infection may present as a vulvar disease without detectable *Candida* organisms in the vagina. Therefore, it may be justified to treat apparent or suspected *Candida* vulvitis empirically, despite a negative KOH preparation.

Treatment
Effective therapeutic agents and their usual dosages include miconazole 2% (one applicator qd × 7 days), clotrimazole (one applicator of cream or one vaginal tablet qd × 7–14 days), and nystatin (one vaginal tablet qd × 14 days). All are safe in pregnancy. It is recommended that these medications be inserted at bedtime to reduce leakage and prolong contact with the vaginal mucosa; when medication is used during menses, tampons should be avoided because they may absorb the therapeutic agent. A 3-day, double-dose regimen of clotrimazole (two vaginal tablets qd × 3 days) has been reported to be an equally effective regimen in nonpregnant patients. Although several studies have claimed to demonstrate the greater efficacy of miconazole and clotrimazole over nystatin, many used nonstandard dosages and were nonblinded. Studies comparing all three agents suggest that miconazole may be superior for achieving negative cultures and preventing relapses but equivalent in relieving symptoms

Treatment of asymptomatic male sexual partners is not indicated except possibly in some instances of recurrent candidiasis in which it is suspected the man may harbor organisms beneath the foreskin or in the urethra. *Candida* balanitis is treated with topical nystatin.

Recurrent yeast infections are a common and distressing problem. In such instances, predisposing factors should be addressed, including control of diabetes, avoidance of heat- and moisture-retaining nylon undergarments, and reduction of corticosteroid and oral-contraceptive estrogen dosages. Prophylactic treatment for a week before the onset of menses with any of the above-mentioned therapeutic agents has been advocated. In one study, the use of clotrimazole during days 5 through 11 of the menstrual cycle for a period of 4 months controlled symptoms but did not eliminate positive cultures. Despite the strong association of recurrent vaginal candidiasis with positive stool cultures for *Candida,* simultaneous treatment with oral nystatin to eliminate the presumed gut reservoir has not proved clinically effective.

Trichomonas Vaginitis

The prevalence of trichomoniasis varies considerably in different clinical settings, ranging from 13 to 23% in women attending gynecologic clinics, to 75% in prostitutes. The organism is sexually transmitted and is found in the presence of other sexually transmitted diseases, such as gonorrhea. Many women (25–44%) from whom trichomonads are cultured are asymptomatic. The long-term effects of chronic asymptomatic trichomoniasis are not known, although it has been suggested that one-third of asymptomatic women become symptomatic within a few months after positive cultures are obtained. Extragenital or disseminated trichomoniasis is unknown.

In symptomatic patients, pruritus and increased or malodorous discharge are common complaints; dysuria is reported by about 20%. The classic frothy discharge (caused by CO_2 bubbles) is 70% specific for the presence of *Trichomonas* vaginalis but is found in only 10% of instances; usually the discharge is indistinguishable from bacterial vaginitis. The so-called pathognomonic "strawberry cervix" with punctate hemorrhages or telangiectasias is found in only 2 to 3% of instances.

Diagnosis depends on demonstration of the organism, usually by microscopic examination of a specimen of discharge mixed with saline. Pear-shaped, motile organisms (about twice the size of white blood cells) with unipolar flagella are detected in approximately 60 to 70% of infected women. Because the mobility of the organism aids in its identification, the slide should be examined as soon as possible after preparation. The specimen should be taken from the vaginal vault rather than the endocervix, where trichomonads are infrequently found.

Cultures are considerably more sensitive than saline preparations in detecting trichomonads but are not commonly available. In addition, most commercially available media do not yield the sensitivity reported from research settings. Although trichomoniasis is sometimes diagnosed on the basis of endocervical cytologic findings, the reliability of the pap smear as a diagnostic test is quite variable, depending on the way it is performed and the skill of laboratory personnel in interpreting it. Smears made from the cervix alone are less likely to contain organisms than those that include specimens from the vaginal pool. False-positive readings can also occur because of a resemblance between trichomonads and inflammatory cells.

Treatment

Many gynecologists and infectious disease experts advocate treating all patients who have detectable trichomonads. They argue that asymptomatically infected women are likely to become symptomatic and also that they should be treated as a public health measure to reduce the venereal transmission of the organism. Clinicians may prefer to individualize these treatment decisions. Asymptomatic patients with cellular atypia on pap smear should be treated, because the atypia may represent an inflammatory response to the trichomonad, which often resolves with eradication of the organism.

Metronidazole (Flagyl) is the drug of choice: a single 2-gm dose achieves a cure rate of approximately 90%, as does the traditional 1-week regimen of 250 mg three times a day. Spacing the tablets out in a twice-a-day schedule or taking them with food may minimize nausea. Patients should be warned not to consume alcoholic beverages during the course of therapy because they may experience abdominal distress, nausea, vomiting, flushing, or headache. The use of metronidazole is contraindicated during the first trimester of pregnancy and in nursing mothers, although it may be used if breast feeding is suspended for 36 to 48 hours. Several studies suggest that the drug is safe in the last two trimesters of pregnancy. Clotrimazole vaginal suppositories have been suggested for use during the first trimester. A 1-week course of therapy has been reported to relieve symptoms, although it cures only about 20% of patients.

Treatment of male sexual partners of infected women is usually recommended. Most men carrying *Trichomonas* are completely asymptomatic, and the organism is spontaneously eliminated from the male urogenital tract over a period of weeks. However, during this time the organism can be reinoculated into the vagina. The single-dose metronidazole regimen is the one most commonly prescribed for male contacts. Because this often requires the physician to prescribe a drug for an unseen patient, some accompany the prescription with a handout explaining the treatment and its rationale. An alternative approach is for the man to use a condom or abstain from intercourse for several weeks.

Douching with vinegar (2 tablespoons in a quart of water) twice weekly has been suggested as an alternative therapy to inhibit the growth of trichomonads by reducing vaginal pH. The reliability of this method has not been established.

Bacterial Vaginitis ("Nonspecific Vaginitis")

The organism associated with bacterial vaginitis is a short, facultatively anaerobic gram-negative rod previously called *Corynebacterium vaginale* and *Hemophilus vaginalis* and currently known as *Gardnerella vaginalis*. It can be found without infection and frequently persists after clinical cure of vaginitis. Although it may cause infection by itself, it usually participates in a polymicrobial infection along with other anaerobes. Because of confusion about the role of *G. vaginalis,* the less specific term *bacterial vaginitis* may be more appropriate. Symptoms are typically milder than those of *Candida* or *Trichomonas* infections, and there may be little or no observable inflammation of the vagina or vulva.

In practice, bacterial vaginitis is usually diagnosed empirically when candidiasis and trichomoniasis are excluded. However, in a recent study of the cause of bacterial vaginitis, 46 of 53 culture-proven cases had at least three of the following findings: pH greater than 4.5, presence of "clue cells," positive "sniff test," and a "homogeneous" (i.e., nonflocculent) quality of secretions. Clue cells are epithelial cells studded with innumerable small gram-negative rods seen on the saline preparation and sometimes more readily on Gram's stain. The positive "sniff test" refers to a fishy odor released with the addition of KOH reagent to vaginal secretions. Whether these findings are as sensitive in the hands of other clinicians has yet to be demonstrated. Culture is presently a research tool.

Treatment

Metronidazole (500 mg bid × 7) is currently favored as the most effective agent, based on a small study comparing four different therapies. Ampicillin (500 mg qid × 7), which had previously been recommended on the basis of several uncontrolled studies, was less effective but still might be considered as an alternative therapy. Tetracycline (500 mg qid × 7) is also used but has a lower success rate, consistent with the frequent in vivo resistance of the organism to this drug. Topical sulfonamides have not been shown to be effective.

The treatment of sexual partners remains controversial. *G. vaginalis* has been found in the urethra of 79% of male partners of infected women, and treatment with a regimen similar to that used in women has been recommended to prevent reinfection. However, there are no data on the effect of treatment of the consort, and some clinicians prefer to treat sexual partners only when bacterial vaginitis fails to respond or recurs. It is not known whether abstinence or use of condoms affects the rate of treatment failures or recurrence.

Other Conditions

Atrophic vaginitis can cause the same symptoms as infection. On physical examination, changes consistent with estrogen deficiency are noted, including pale and dry vaginal epithelium and thin vulvar skin. Treatment is local estrogen in the form of creams or suppositories (see Chap. 86).

Gonorrhea is an uncommon cause of vaginitis symptoms because it does not cause vulvar inflammation. It can, however, cause discharge and urethritis. The decision to culture for gonorrhea depends on the population of patients served. A Gram's stain is not a reliable test for the presence or absence of gonorrhea.

Other possible causes of vaginitis symptoms include dermatologic conditions such as scabies or neurotic excoriation, trauma, herpesvirus vulvitis, and increased attention to normal vaginal discharge.

Not infrequently, a specific cause cannot be demonstrated for vaginitis. If clinical findings are highly suggestive of *Candida* infection, a trial of antiyeast therapy is warranted despite a negative KOH preparation. If there is no reason to suspect one or another cause, metronidazole may be the most appropriate therapeutic choice. It treats a bacterial vaginitis as well as a clinically similar trichomonal infection that may have been missed because of a falsely negative saline preparation. Measures that increase vaginal acidity also may be considered in this situation, on the theory that acid-tolerant organisms such as *Lactobacillus* survive at the expense of pathogenic ones. Alternative choices include vinegar douches (2–4 tablespoons white vinegar in 1 quart of water), Aci-jel vaginal jelly, or the addition of *Lactobacillus* to the vagina directly by applications of plain yogurt. None has been rigorously evaluated.

McCue JD, et al. Strategies for diagnosing vaginitis. *J Fam Pract* 9:395–402, 1979.
  Predictive values, sensitivities, specificities for signs, symptoms, and laboratory test results for 821 patients with vaginitis are given. Good ideas on approach to diagnosis, but dated treatment recommendations.

Eliot BW, Havat RCL, Mack AE. A comparison between the effects of nystatin, clotrimazole, and miconazole on vaginal candidiasis. *Br J Obstet Gynaecol* 86:572–577, 1979.
  The three drugs were equivalent in curing vaginal candidiasis, but more patients in the nystatin and clotrimazole groups relapsed.

Robertson WH. A concentrated therapeutic regimen for vulvovaginal candidiasis. *JAMA* 244:2549–2550, 1980.
  In a double-blind placebo-controlled study, the 3-day double-dose regimen was as effective as a 7-day single-dose schedule.

Davidson F, Mould RF. Recurrent genital candidiosis in women and the effect of intermittent prophylactic treatment. *Br J Vener Dis* 545:176–183, 1978.
  Intermittent prophylactic treatment kept symptoms below a critical level but did not affect the return of yeasts to the vagina on culture.

Milhe JD, Warnock DW. Effect of simultaneous oral and vaginal treatment on the rate of cure and relapse in vaginal candidiosis. *Br J Vener Dis* 55:362–365, 1979.
  It didn't work.

Rein MF. Trichomoniasis. In GL Mandell, RG Douglas, Jr, and JE Bennet (Eds.), *Principles and Practice of Infectious Diseases.* New York: Wiley, 1979. Pp. 2147–2149.
  A concise but cogent summary including diagnostic techniques applicable to men.

McLennan MT, Smith JM, McLennan CE. Diagnosis of vaginal mycosis and trichomoniasis. Reliability of cytologic smear, wet smear, and culture. *Obstet Gynecol* 40:231–234, 1972.

Hager WD, et al. Metronidazole for vaginal trichomoniasis. Seven-day vs. single-dose regimens. *JAMA* 244:1219–1220, 1980.
  The authors report an 86% cure rate with a 2-gm dose (16% nausea/vomiting) versus 92% with the standard regimen (8% nausea/vomiting).

Spiegel CA, et al. Anaerobic bacteria in nonspecific vaginitis. *N Engl J Med* 303:601–606, 1980.
  Gardnerella vaginalis was the predominant organism in vaginal fluid from most women with nonspecific vaginitis, but concentrations of other anaerobes were also significantly higher. See also editorial in the same issue.

Pheifer TA, et al. Nonspecific vaginitis. Role of *Haemophilus vaginalis* and treatment with metronidazole. N Engl J Med 298:1429–1434, 1978.
  Nonspecific vaginitis is a polymicrobial infection caused by anaerobes and Gardnerella vaginalis. A better cure rate with metronidazole than ampicillin is demonstrated. Topical sulfa was ineffective.

Amsel R, et al. The nonspecific vaginitis: Diagnostic criteria and microbial and epidemiologic associations. *Am J Med* 74:14–22, 1983.
  A clinical description of bacterial vaginitis, with discussion and testing of all the standard diagnostic criteria.

Berg AO, et al. Establishing the cause of genitourinary symptoms in a family practice: Comparison of clinical examination and comprehensive microbiology. *JAMA* 251:620–625, 1984.

Using common office and laboratory procedures, diagnosis could be established for only 34% of women reporting a broad spectrum of genitourinary symptoms. The addition of selected, nonroutine studies raised the proportion of patients diagnosed to 66%.

80. ORAL CONTRACEPTIVES
Axalla J. Hoole

Birth control pills (BCPs) are now taken by millions of women throughout the world. Almost all use combination pills; only a small number take progestogen-only "minipills." Despite this popularity, most birth control is still accomplished by other methods.

The success of the various methods of birth control is expressed as both *method effectiveness*—the idealized effectiveness of the method used properly—and *use effectiveness*—the actual effectiveness found in practice. It is incorrect to compare methods of birth control without using the same system of evaluation. The method effectiveness of condoms is about 98%; however, the use effectiveness varies from 60 to 97% depending on the skill of the group being surveyed. Any method, including coitus interruptus, may work for careful couples, but no method is effective unless practiced by people dedicated to its success (see Table 80-1).

Types of oral contraception include combination pills, progestogen-only pills, and "morning-after pills."

Combination Pills
Combination pills contain estrogen—either mestranol or ethinyl estradiol—and one of several progestogens. The estrogens have approximately equal hormonal potency, but the progestogens vary widely in their hormonal properties. Norethindrone, used in the majority of BCPs, has progestational activity that lies between norgestrel, the most progestogenic, and norethynodrel, the most estrogenic of the progestogens.

Prevention of ovulation by suppression of follicle-stimulating hormone and luteinizing hormone requires both estrogen and progestogen. Progestogen alone can prevent implantation by providing an inhospitable endometrium, but contraception is less certain than with combination pills. For most BCPs the progestogen has the predominant effect on the endometrium. The most commonly used pills and their estrogen and progestogen contents are listed in Table 80-2.

Contraindications
Several large studies have shown that the estrogen component of BCPs is associated with dose-related cardiovascular complications. Risk decreases with decreasing estrogen to 50 mg; below this level, additional decreased risk has been difficult to demon-

Table 80-1. Methods of contraception

Method	Method effectiveness (%)	Use effectiveness (%)
Diaphragm	97–98.5	71.1–98.1
Condom	97–98.5	64.0–97.0
Combination birth control pill	99.6–99.9	90.0–99.3
IUD	97.0–99.0	94.4–99.6
Withdrawal	91.0	75.0–80.0

Source: L.B. Tyrer and L.E. Bradshaw. Barrier methods. *Clinics in Obstetrics and Gynecology.* April 1979.

Table 80-2. Contraceptives available in the United States

Drug[a]	Estrogen (µg)	Progestin[b] (mg)	Progestin potency
Ovulen (Searle)	Mestranol (100)	Ethynodiol diacetate (1)	High
Enovid-E (Searle)	Mestranol (100)	Norethynodrel (2.5)	Medium
Ortho-Novum 2 mg (Ortho)	Mestranol (100)	Norethindrone (2)	Medium
Norinyl 2 mg (Syntex)	Mestranol (100)	Norethindrone (2)	Medium
Ortho-Novum 1/80 (Ortho)	Mestranol (80)	Norethindrone (1)	Low
Norinyl 1 + 80 (Syntex)	Mestranol (80)	Norethindrone (1)	Low
Enovid 5 mg (Searle)	Mestranol (75)	Norethynodrel (5)	Medium
Demulen (Searle)	Ethinyl estradiol (50)	Ethynodiol diacetate (1)	High
Ovral (Wyeth)	Ethinyl estradiol (50)	Norgestrel (0.5)	High
Norlestrin 2.5/50 (Parke-Davis)[c]	Ethinyl estradiol (50)	Norethindrone acetate (2.5)	Medium
Norlestrin 1/50 (Parke-Davis)[c]	Ethinyl estradiol (50)	Norethindrone acetate (1)	Medium
Ovcon-50 (Mead Johnson)	Ethinyl estradiol (50)	Norethindrone (1)	Low
Norinyl 1 + 50 (Syntex)	Mestranol (50)	Norethindrone (1)	Low
Ortho-Novum 1/50 (Ortho)	Mestranol (50)	Norethindrone (1)	Low

Product	Estrogen	Progestin	Androgenic Effect
Demulen 1/35 (Searle)	Ethinyl estradiol (35)	Ethynodiol diacetate (1)	High
Norinyl 1 + 35 (Syntex)	Ethinyl estradiol (35)	Norethindrone (1)	Low
Ortho-Novum 1/35 (Ortho)	Ethinyl estradiol (35)	Norethindrone (1)	Low
Ortho-Novum 10/11 (Ortho)	Ethinyl estradiol (35)	Norethindrone (0.5)	Low
followed by	Ethinyl estradiol (35)	Norethindrone (1)	Low
Brevicon (Syntex)	Ethinyl estradiol (35)	Norethindrone (0.5)	Low
Modicon (Ortho)	Ethinyl estradiol (35)	Norethindrone (0.5)	Low
Ovcon-35 (Mead Johnson)	Ethinyl estradiol (35)	Norethindrone (0.4)	Low
Lo/Ovral (Wyeth)	Ethinyl estradiol (30)	Norgestrel (0.3)	Medium
Loestrin 1.5/30 (Parke-Davis)[c]	Ethinyl estradiol (30)	Norethindrone acetate (1.5)	Medium
Nordette (Wyeth)	Ethinyl estradiol (30)	Levonorgestrel (0.15)	Medium
Loestrin 1/20 (Parke-Davis)[c]	Ethinyl estradiol (20)	Norethindrone acetate (1)	Medium
Ovrette (Wyeth)		Norgestrel (0.075)	Medium
Nor-Q.D. (Syntex)		Norethindrone (0.35)	Low
Micronor (Ortho)		Norethindrone (0.35)	Low

[a]Some available in 21-day regimens or in 28-day regimens with seven placebo tablets.
[b]Norethynodrel has no androgenic effect. Norethindrone, norethindrone acetate, and ethynodiol diacetate have a moderate androgenic effect. Norgestrel has a relatively strong androgenic effect.
[c]Also available with seven iron tablets instead of seven placebo tablets.
Source: *The Medical Letter*, July 22, 1983.

strate. Progestogen-dominant BCPs also may carry a cardiovascular risk. Recently, progestogens have been shown to affect lipoprotein lipid concentrations; progestogen-dominant oral contraceptives were found to be associated with an increase in low-density lipoprotein–cholesterol levels. Because of these findings, it is now thought that estrogens are not the only cause of cardiovascular risk, but that the progestogen-estrogen balance is also important.

A several-fold increase in risk for both thromboembolic disease and stroke, as well as a small increase in risk for myocardial infarction, has been noted in users of birth control pills. The risk for these problems dramatically increases both after age 35 and with cigarette smoking. After age 40, the mortality rate associated with the use of BCPs is greater than that of pregnancy.

Combination pills are contraindicated in women over age 40 who smoke and in women with a past history of thromboembolic or vascular disease. Other contraindications include active liver disease, abnormal liver function tests, undiagnosed breast masses, uterine bleeding of unknown origin, and secondary amenorrhea.

Relative contraindications include smoking and age greater than 35 years, hypertension, migraine headaches, and diabetes mellitus. There is a general consensus that a small percentage of patients taking BCPs develop hypertension, which resolves when the pill is stopped. Some patients with migraine headaches develop an increase in headaches while on BCPs and should thereafter not use hormonal contraception; however, many have no change in migraine pattern. Because it is impossible to predict those in whom headaches will develop, patients with a history of migraine headaches may begin on BCPs. Some workers have found a lowering of glucose tolerance among users of BCPs. Patients with abnormal glucose tolerance may take BCPs if they are aware of the potential change in glucose tolerance. Carcinoma of the endometrium and breast have not been clearly shown to be increased by BCPs; carcinoma of the cervix may be associated with a small risk.

A number of unpleasant symptoms have been reported among BCP users, including depression, change in libido, nausea, and weight gain. However, if these symptoms occur, they are not necessarily caused by the pill; the same symptoms are prevalent among potential BCP users and have been shown to be common among women given placebo BCPs.

The initial evaluation of patients desiring BCPs should include a history to disclose any of the above contraindications and a physical examination that includes blood pressure and breast and pelvic examinations. The only laboratory evaluations necessary are a Papanicolaou smear and measurement of glucose or liver function when indicated.

Selection of Birth Control Pills
Because the major serious side effects are believed to be caused by estrogens and to be dose-related, the primary goal has become the administration of the lowest possible estrogen dose. Attempts to balance the clinical features of individual patients by selecting BCPs with estrogenic or progestogenic progestogens (e.g., giving hirsute women a BCP containing an estrogenic progesterone) have largely been abandoned. Because of the relation between the estrogen-progestogen balance and cardiovascular risk, de-emphasizing the progestogenic component may be inappropriate.

The combination pills most frequently prescribed contain 30 to 50 µg of mestranol or ethinyl estradiol. There are more bleeding complications at 30 µg but possibly less risk of cardiovascular complications. If bleeding occurs at 30 or 35 µg, a 50-µg pill can be substituted. This dose may support regular periods without exposing the patient to greater risk. Because of the breakthrough bleeding that occurs with the low dose (30 to 35 µg of estrogen), many practitioners begin at 50 µg. Patients should be warned that menstrual periods diminish in flow and duration. Even if pills are begun on the first day of the period, alternate contraception is needed and should be used for at least 14 days.

Side Effects
Reductions in the dose of estrogen have greatly decreased both the cardiovascular complications and many side effects. But because of decreased support for the endometrium, breakthrough bleeding and amenorrhea have increased. Other common side effects such as nausea, fatigue, or fluid retention (usually mild) may occur, but with low-

dose pills these too are less bothersome. Acne may occur in patients taking combination pills with a highly progestogenic progesterone, such as norgestrel. In such instances, a pill with a less progestogenic progesterone may be substituted.

Breakthrough bleeding may occur during the first several periods after starting at a low dose, when changing to a lower-dose pill, or sporadically. Bleeding that occurs when starting pills is usually self-limited and often can be managed by reassurance; however, both initial and sporadic bleeding respond to additional estrogen—20 μg of ethinyl estradiol daily for 7 days. Following this therapy, sporadic breakthrough bleeding frequently does not recur. Switching to a pill with more estrogen, 30 to 50 μg, may be effective, but a dose greater than 50 μg exposes patients to increased risk. Doubling the BCP for several days is usually not effective.

Amenorrhea has become a common problem with the use of low-dose pills. It results from insufficient estrogen for withdrawal bleeding and most patients return to normal cycles when the pill is stopped. Pelvic examination and a pregnancy test are recommended after the first missed period. Gynecologists do not recommend stopping BCPs or increasing the estrogen dose, which may needlessly increase risk. Primary care physicians should consult a gynecologic specialist if withdrawal bleeding does not occur for two or more periods.

Follow-up examination for patients taking BCPs is recommended on an annual basis for breast examination and Papanicolaou smear.

Progestogen-Only Pills

"Minipills" are infrequently used in this country. The usual dose of progestogen is either 0.350 mg of norethindrone or 0.075 mg of norgestrel daily, much less than is in the combination pills. Effectiveness is equal to or better than barrier methods used correctly but not as good as combination pills. Breakthrough bleeding is common, and an increased incidence of ectopic pregnancies has been reported. However, there are none of the side effects of estrogens, and there are decreased progestogenic side effects because of the low dose. Advocates of progestogen-only pills suggest their use in breast-feeding mothers (breast feeding does not reliably provide contraception, and progestogen does not affect the volume of breast milk) and in patients who cannot use combination BCPs because of side effects or contraindications.

Postcoital Contraception

The "morning-after pill" is useful for women who have had unprotected intercourse who have compelling reasons for not becoming pregnant (e.g., following rape or when psychiatric problems would follow conception). Therapy must be started within 72 hours and consists of conjugated estrogens, 10 mg orally three times a day for 5 days. Nausea almost always accompanies this high-estrogen dose. Recently a combination pill containing 0.1 mg ethinyl estradiol and 1.0 mg of dl-norgestrel was given in two doses 12 hours apart as soon as possible, but within 72 hours after unprotected intercourse. There were fewer side effects and a failure rate of only 0.16%. Postcoital contraception is usually effective; however, therapeutic abortion is recommended if pregnancy occurs because of possible adverse effects on the fetus from the hormonal therapy.

Ling WY, et al. Mode of action of dl-norgestrel and ethinyl estradiol combination in postcoital contraception. *Fertil steril* 32:297–302, 1979.
  Suggests the mechanism of contraception of postcoital hormones.
Speroff L. Which birth control pill should be prescribed? *Fertil Steril* 27:997–1008, 1976.
  An excellent, practical approach to hormonal contraception.
Andrews WC. Oral contraceptives. *Clin Obstet Gynaecol* 6(1):3–26, 1979.
  A review of risk from oral contraception.
Vessey MP, et al. Mortality among women participating in the Oxford Family Planning Association Contraceptive Study. *Lancet* 2:731–733, 1977.
Mortality among oral-contraceptive users. Royal College of General Practitioners' Oral Contraceptive Study. *Lancet* 2:727–731, 1977.
  Two of the earliest large studies to show the risks for oral contraception.
Wahl P, et al. Effect of estrogen/progestin potency on lipid/lipoprotein cholesterol. *N Engl J Med* 308:862–867, 1983.
  A large multicenter study that shows a relation between progestogenic potency and

LDL-cholesterol. This work suggests a role for progestogens and estrogen/progesto- genic balance in the risk for thromboembolic disease carried by BCPs.

81. ABNORMAL VAGINAL BLEEDING
Lamar E. Ekbladh

Abnormal vaginal bleeding may be defined broadly as any vaginal bleeding occurring at a time or in a pattern different from that of the usual menstrual vaginal bleeding, or bleeding that represents a major change from the woman's usual pattern.

Normal Bleeding
The following are norms for menstrual vaginal bleeding in the United States.

	Range	Mean
Age at menarche	9 to 17 years	12.8 years
Age at menopause	48 to 55 years	51.0 years
Cycle length	21 to 35 days	28 to 29 days
Duration of menstrual blood flow	2 to 8 days	4.6 days
Blood loss	30 to 40 cc/ menstrual cycle	35 cc

During the first gynecologic year (first year after menarche), approximately 55% of cycles are anovulatory, and irregular cycles are quite common. By gynecologic year 8, only about 6% of cycles are anovulatory, and irregular cycles are much less common. Ovulation decreases in frequency with increasing age and become infrequent near the menopause, with an increase in the irregularity of periods.

Patterns of Abnormal Vaginal Bleeding
The following terms are used to describe the various patterns of abnormal bleeding. The patterns do not necessarily suggest a particular cause, but provide a convenient way to describe and record the patient's complaint.

Oligomenorrhea: infrequent, irregular episodes of bleeding, usually occurring at inter- vals greater than 40 days
Metrorrhagia (hypermenorrhea): uterine bleeding excessive in both amount and dura- tion of flow, occurring at regular intervals
Polymenorrhea: frequent but regular episodes of uterine bleeding, usually occurring at intervals of 21 days or less
Hypomenorrhea: uterine bleeding that is regular but decreased in amount
Intermenstrual bleeding: uterine bleeding, usually not excessive, occurring between otherwise regular menstrual periods
Menometrorrhagia: uterine bleeding, usually excessive and prolonged, occurring at fre- quent and irregular intervals
Spotting: vaginal bleeding occurring intermittently and usually not of sufficient quan- tity to require a pad or tampon

Flow
Some estimate of the quantity of flow should be made. There is a great deal of variation in the absorbency of pads and tampons and in the frequency with which women change them; however, the number of pads or tampons used each day remains the best esti- mate of the quantity of vaginal bleeding. A rough estimate of the severity of bleeding is: light—one to two pads or tampons per day; heavy—five pads or more per day. The passage of large numbers of blood clots also usually signifies heavy bleeding.

Causes

The causes of abnormal vaginal bleeding include a vast array of gynecologic and non-gynecologic conditions. These are classified into *organic causes,* in which a specific genital lesion or disease can be shown to be the cause of the bleeding, and *dysfunctional causes,* in which no specific organic lesion of the genital tract is present, and a dysfunction of the neuroendocrine system is responsible for the abnormal bleeding. Dysfunctional bleeding is additionally subdivided into *ovulatory* (cycles during which ovulation is occurring) and *anovulatory* (cycles during which ovulation is not occurring), which is most common in adolescence and near the time of menopause.

Recognized organic causes of abnormal vaginal bleeding are listed in Table 81-1.

Evaluation and Management

History

Information that should be obtained and recorded for all patients includes the interval and regularity of the menstrual cycle, time of intermenstrual bleeding, and duration of unusual bleeding. If the cycles are regular, the interval should be given (e.g., regular q 5 weeks). If the cycles are irregular, the range should be specified (e.g., irregular q 3–6 weeks).

If intermenstrual bleeding occurs, the cycle should be noted as premenstrual (bleeding occurs 5–7 days before the usual period), postmenstrual (bleeding occurs 5–7 days after the period), or midcycle (bleeding occurs within a few days of the midcycle).

Finally, the total duration of unusual bleeding should be recorded (e.g., for the past 6–8 months).

Evaluation begins by determining if a serious problem is likely to exist. In the pubertal patient, the problem may be the patient's or parent's anxiety about the age of onset of menses and/or worry about the irregular periods that frequently occur during the first year or two after menarche. Frequently, counseling and provision of information are all that is required in the otherwise healthy adolescent girl. However, it is better to proceed with an evaluation rather than risk missing a serious disease, such as an ectopic pregnancy.

Once it is decided that evaluation is required, a complete medical history, physical and pelvic examination, and Papanicolaou smear comprise the first step. Particular attention must be paid to systemic illnesses, such as blood dyscrasias, clotting disorders, and thyroid disease, and to the use of medications. Because the statistical probabilities of diagnoses vary greatly from age group to age group, details of evaluation and management are considered by age.

Adolescent Women (under 20 years old)

Even though most patients with abnormal vaginal bleeding in this age group have anovulatory dysfunctional bleeding, pregnancy must be considered and ruled out. Malignancy and other causes are quite rare.

Table 81-1 Organic causes of abnormal vaginal bleeding

Type	Disorder
Organ diseases	
Cervix	Neoplasia, eversion, cervicitis, condylomata, infection
Vulva, vagina	Neoplasia, leiomyomata, infection, foreign body, adhesions, atrophy
Uterus	Neoplasia, leiomyomata, endometritis, pregnancy, polyp, endometriosis, adenomyosis, intrauterine devices
Ovary	Neoplasm (estrogen-producing tumors, such as granulosa cell), pelvic inflammatory disease
Clotting disorders	Idiopathic thrombocytopenic purpura, von Willebrand's
Drugs	Anticoagulants, oral contraceptives, digitalis
Systemic diseases	Systemic lupus erythematosus, chronic renal failure

Anovulatory dysfunctional uterine bleeding results from the failure of ovulation and the continued unopposed secretion of estrogen by the ovarian follicle. In the absence of progesterone, proliferative endometrium continues to develop until it becomes quite hypertrophic, resulting in irregular and excessive bleeding.

Anovulatory bleeding with irregular periods of varying duration and amount of bleeding is normal in the young woman for 1 to 2 years after menarche. Once regular menses are established, however, it is uncommon for serious menometrorrhagia to develop. Anovulatory periods are characterized by irregularity, excessive flow, and relative painlessness compared to normal menses. The pelvic examination in anovulatory dysfunctional bleeding is completely normal. Pregnancy testing and Papanicolaou smears are indicated. There usually is no need for cervical or endometrial biopsy.

Several forms of treatment are considered acceptable and appropriate.

1. For patients with irregular, light-to-moderate bleeding who do not desire pregnancy but do not want any contraception, a progestational agent (Provera, 10 mg; Norlutin, 5 mg; Norlutate, 5 mg) should be given on days 15 to 24 of each cycle for two to five cycles
2. For patients with irregular, moderate-to-heavy bleeding or lack of response to a progestational agent, low-dose oral contraceptives for three cycles should be used, followed by the regimen in #1
3. For patients with massive prolonged bleeding unresponsive to the above regimens, conjugated estrogen (Premarin), 25 mg intravenously every four hours, should be given until bleeding stops (maximum six doses), followed by cyclic low-dose oral contraceptives for 2 to 4 months
4. If all of the above measures fail, a dilatation and curettage is indicated

Women in the Reproductive Years (age 20–40)
Abnormal bleeding in this age group is usually from one of three conditions: pregnancy or its complications; benign tumors of the uterus, such as leiomyomata; or inflammatory disease (endometritis secondary to an IUD, recent delivery, or abortion).

Pregnancy is the most common cause of abnormal bleeding, particularly early pregnancy, either intrauterine or ectopic. The usual symptoms and signs of pregnancy may be absent, particularly early in pregnancy, and one should therefore carry out laboratory pregnancy testing to rule out or confirm pregnancy.

The usual urine slide test is positive in approximately 50% of normal pregnancies at 35 days after the last menstrual period, and positive in 95% at 42 days since the last period. Therefore, the urine slide test is most useful only if it is positive. Because of the significant rate of false-negative urine tests, serum immunoassay for human chorionic gonadotropin (HCG) should be done if the urine test is negative. Serum tests may be positive as soon as 21 days after the last period and are positive in virtually 100% of pregnant women at 42 days. Properly done, a serum test for HCG that is negative 42 days after the period effectively rules out pregnancy.

Endometritis causing abnormal bleeding is usually obvious from the history and physical examination. Recent abortion or childbirth may result in a chronic endometritis with resultant abnormal bleeding. On pelvic examination, the expected finding is a tender uterus that may or may not be enlarged.

The IUD is also a well-recognized cause of abnormal bleeding and endometritis, which is usually treated simply by removal of the IUD.

Fibromyomata are the most common benign tumors of the uterus and are frequent causes of abnormal bleeding. Characteristically, they produce menometrorrhagia, often with increased pain during menses and frequently with the passage of large clots. Most often, the diagnosis can be made by finding on pelvic examination the characteristic irregular, knobby enlargement of the uterus. In this situation, an endometrial biopsy is necessary. Treatment frequently requires hysterectomy, although suppression of ovulation by birth control pills may decrease the bleeding.

Perimenopausal Women
Abnormal bleeding in this age group is commonly organic in origin, and endometrial carcinoma must be ruled out. Dysfunctional bleeding tends to be acyclic and caused by anovulation and/or endometrial hyperplasia. In the perimenopause, cycles may initially become shorter and periods heavier followed by lengthening cycles with scant bleeding. Any intermenstrual bleeding should be evaluated.

Postmenopausal Women

Any bleeding occurring after 6 months of amenorrhea should be considered abnormal, and a full evaluation, including endometrial biopsy, should be undertaken. Although other conditions may cause the bleeding, one must seriously consider endometrial cancer because it is present in a significant percentage of postmenopausal women who present with bleeding. Because a routine examination with cervical Papanicolaou smear detects only about 50% of endometrial cancers, endometrial biopsy must be employed. Recent techniques for office biopsy of the endometrium have been refined, and this procedure, rather than the traditional D and C, is now the procedure of choice. In its favor is low risk of morbidity (<1%), high diagnostic yield (95% accurate for endometrial carcinoma and 80% for endometrial polyps), minimal patient discomfort, and relatively low cost. The D and C has been thought to eliminate additional abnormal bleeding; however, there is little evidence that the therapeutic effect of either the D and C or the endometrial biopsy is other than transient. Any patient with a pathologic diagnosis of hyperplasia (cystic, adenomatous, or atypical) or malignancy should be referred for additional evaluation.

In addition to its use in postmenopausal bleeding, the endometrial biopsy can be recommended as a useful adjunct in many other instances of unexplained abnormal menstrual bleeding. If the diagnosis is not made after a routine history and physical examination, including Papanicolaou smear, then endometrial biopsy should be performed in all instances of unexplained abnormal bleeding *except* in teenagers with a normal examination; women with midcycle spotting (Kleinregel), premenstrual spotting or oligomenorrhea; and patients in whom pregnancy is suspected.

Grimes D. Diagnostic dilation and curettage: A reappraisal. *Am J Obstet Gynecol* 142:1–6, 1982.
   An excellent article that reviews thoroughly the cost-effectiveness and diagnostic accuracy of the endometrial biopsy versus the D and C.
Goldfarb JM, Little AB. Abnormal vaginal bleeding. *N Engl J Med* 302:666–669, 1980.
   A brief but pertinent review of the approach to the patient with abnormal bleeding.
Strickler RC. Dysfunctional uterine bleeding. *Postgrad Med* 66:135–150, 1979.
   A discussion of the causes and management of irregular vaginal bleeding with emphasis on deciding whom and when to treat.
Brenner PF, Subir R, Mishell DR. Ectopic pregnancy. *JAMA* 243:673–676, 1980.
   A very good review of 300 instances of ectopic pregnancy. Signs and symptoms of the ectopic pregnancy and its relation to risk factors such as pelvic infection and previous surgery are discussed. It is important to be familiar with the diagnosis of ectopic pregnancy in the treatment of irregular vaginal bleeding.
Yen SSC. Neuroendocrine regulation of the menstrual cycle. *Hosp Pract* 14:83–102, 1979.
   Careful reading of this excellent description of the menstrual cycle will enable treatment of dysfunctional vaginal bleeding to be more satisfying. The physiology is clearly presented and up-to-date.
Speroff L, et al. *Clinical Gynecologic Endocrinology and Infertility* (2nd ed.). Baltimore: Williams & Wilkins, Chap. 8, Pp. 151–166, 1978.
   A concise, clear, and thorough approach to diagnosis and management of irregular vaginal bleeding.
Dewhurst J. *Integrated Obstetrics and Gynecology for Postgraduates* (3rd ed.). St. Louis: Mosby, 1981.
   An excellent textbook review of dysfunctional bleeding.

82. DYSMENORRHEA

Lamar E. Ekbladh

Dysmenorrhea is painful menstruation considered severe by the patient. The pain consists of lower abdominal cramping that may radiate to the lower back and upper thighs. It may be accompanied by nausea, vomiting, diarrhea, headache, weakness, fatigue, swelling, and even syncope. This complex of symptoms is referred to as the *primary dysmenorrhea syndrome*. It is estimated that 40 to 50% of menstruating women suffer from moderate-to-severe dysmenorrhea at some time, and 10% may be incapacitated, with resulting absences from work or school. In approximately 80% of patients the problem may be defined as *primary dysmenorrhea*, or painful menses without associated pelvic pathology.

The natural history of primary dysmenorrhea has not been fully characterized, but the overall prevalence seems to increase from the first year past menarche and to decrease with age beginning in the 20s. Dysmenorrhea has commonly been observed to lessen after pregnancy, which may explain why the prevalence of the problem declines in the childbearing years.

Recent research into the pathophysiology of primary dysmenorrhea has related it to high-intensity myometrial activity stimulated by prostaglandins. The resulting increase in intrauterine pressure is associated with decreased blood flow and tissue ischemia, which is thought to be the cause of dysmenorrhea. The improvement in dysmenorrhea after childbirth may be related to the permanently increased vascularity of the uterus induced by pregnancy. Prostaglandins also may initiate the associated symptoms of diarrhea, nausea, vomiting, and headache, although their relation to such symptoms as weakness, fatigue, and swelling is more tenuous. Evidence to support the role of prostaglandins includes the finding of elevated prostaglandin F_2 concentrations in secretory compared to proliferative endometrium and in menstrual fluid of women with primary dysmenorrhea compared to women without dysmenorrhea. Symptoms of the primary dysmenorrhea syndrome also have been reproduced with intrauterine or intramuscular injections of prostaglandin F_{2x}. The view that this condition is psychogenic is outmoded and not supported by current evidence.

Evaluation

Although dysmenorrhea is probably the most common gynecologic complaint, many women do not report the problem because of a fatalistic attitude or the belief that there is no cure. With the advent of better understanding of pathogenesis and more successful treatments, it is incumbent on physicians to ask their menstruating patients about dysmenorrhea. Another objective of patient evaluation is to identify women with secondary dysmenorrhea, or painful menses caused by pelvic disease.

A typical history for primary dysmenorrhea includes an onset coinciding with the start of ovulating cycles about 6 to 12 months after menarche, with gradually increasing severity into the childbearing years. Symptoms may last for only a few hours or persist for the entire menses.

Secondary dysmenorrhea should be suspected whenever the problem begins after the age of 20 or pain occurs before the onset of a period or between menses. Occasionally, dysmenorrhea in a young girl results from a uterine or vaginal anomaly causing outflow obstruction. The major causes of secondary dysmenorrhea include endometriosis, intrauterine devices, pelvic inflammatory disease, and, less commonly, myomas and endometrial polyps. Endometriosis is probably the most common of these and should be suspected when rectal pain, dyspareunia on deep penetration, and/or infertility are present. In addition, findings of a fixed retroverted uterus or cul-de-sac nodules should increase suspicion of endometriosis. The intrauterine device is also a very common cause of dysmenorrhea and should be removed if symptoms fail to respond to mild analgesics. Pelvic inflammatory disease or its sequelae are suggested by tender, thickened, adnexal organs, especially when coupled with a history of recurrent pelvic infections. An enlarged irregular uterus suggests a myoma.

Treatment

Antiprostaglandin drugs clearly have become the treatment of choice. Aspirin, a prostaglandin synthetase inhibitor, may be effective for relief of mild dysmenorrhea in usual doses of two to three tablets four times a day. For more severe dysmenorrhea, or when aspirin is ineffective, one of the newer antiprostaglandin drugs may be needed, such as ibuprofen (Motrin), naproxen sodium (Naprosyn), and mefenamic acid (Ponstel). Numerous double-blinded, placebo-controlled studies confirm the efficacy of these agents; although methods of assessing symptomatic relief have varied, considerable or complete relief of pain has been consistently reported in 75 to 95% of patients (slightly less for ibuprofen). Usual doses are one tablet three to four times a day, beginning with the onset of symptoms. Most of the studies involving naproxen sodium have used an initial dose of two tablets, but there is no evidence that such a loading dose is necessary. Some investigators have started medication before the onset of menses, but no difference has been demonstrated in resulting pain relief. Zomepirac sodium (withdrawn from the market because of anaphylactic reactions) is the only agent that has been evaluated specifically for relief of the concomitant symptoms of dysmenorrhea syndrome, but the others are likely to be effective as well. Patients who do not respond to one antiprostaglandin drug occasionally respond to one of the others. Side effects are few and are usually gastrointestinal, as in aspirin.

Oral contraceptives are also very effective in reducing the pain of primary dysmenorrhea. Any of the low-dose cyclic combination pills give relief of pain in 90% of patients. The suggested mechanism is suppression of ovulation and reduction of the bulk of endometrium, which reduces premenstrual and menstrual production of prostaglandins. Oral contraceptives are indicated in teenagers and young women who desire contraception and have no contraindications to hormonal use. Oral contraceptives also may be used when analgesics fail or are needed in excessive quantities.

Calcium channel blockers, specifically nifedipine, have been found to inhibit myometrial activity and relieve pain in primary dysmenorrhea. The clinical role of this drug has not yet been established.

Nonpharmacologic approaches are preferred by some women. Although rigorous data are lacking, a number of remedies are suggested on the basis of anecdotal experience. Calcium and magnesium supplements have been recommended, taken daily in a 2:1 ratio beginning several days before menses is expected. A usual starting dose is 500 mg calcium and 250 mg magnesium. Dolomite, a calcium preparation containing magnesium, may be contaminated with lead or arsenic and should be avoided. Other suggested remedies include rasberry leaf tea, heat, massage, and exercises.

Treatment of secondary dysmenorrhea should be directed at the underlying cause, although the pain itself may respond to the same agents used in primary dysmenorrhea. When endometriosis, chronic pelvic inflammatory disease, or uterine myoma is suspected, patients should be referred for gynecologic evaluation. Dysmenorrhea associated with intrauterine devices usually requires removal of the device; occasionally patients who cannot tolerate one of the larger devices, such as a Lippes loop, may be able to use a Copper 7.

Rosenwaks Z, Seegar-Jones G. Menstrual pain: Its origin and pathogenesis. *J Reprod Med* 25:207, 1980.
   A good review of concepts of the etiology of primary dysmenorrhea and the pharmacology of prostaglandins.
Sobczyk R. Dysmenorrhea: The neglected syndrome. *J Reprod Med* 25:198, 1980.
   A useful article that reviews the total impact of dysmenorrhea on women and society.
Ylikorkala O, Dawood MY. New concepts in dysmenorrhea. *Am J Obstet Gynecol* 130:833, 1978.
   A good review of the entire problem of dysmenorrhea and the early experience with antiprostaglandins.
Dingfelder R. Primary dysmenorrhea treatment with prostaglandin inhibitors: A review. *Am J Obstet Gynecol* 140:874–879, 1981.
   A summary of published reports on the effectiveness of prostaglandin inhibitors.
Budoff PW. Zomepirac sodium in the treatment of primary dysmenorrhea syndrome. *N Engl J Med* 307:714–719, 1982.
   A consideration of the frequency and severity of nine different symptoms of the dysmenorrhea complex, as well as response to zomepirac.
Lundstrom V. Treatment of primary dysmenorrhea with prostaglandin synthetase inhibitors: A promising therapeutic alternative. *Acta Obstet Gynecol Scand* 57:421–428, 1978.
   A comparison of naproxen and indomethacin to placebo, as well as the effect of initiating therapy before or at the beginning of menses; a single, "exceptional" patient responded only when treatment was begun 5 to 6 days before the onset of menses, but otherwise results were similar.
Andersson KE, Ulmsten U. Effects of nifedipine on myometrial activity and lower abdominal pain in women with primary dysmenorrhea. *Br J Obstet Gynaecol* 85:142–148, 1978.

Nifedipine 20 to 40 mg orally reduced myometrial activity and relieved menstrual pain in 10 women, with moderate increase in heart rate and transient facial flushing.

Jessop C. Women's curse: A general internist's approach to common menstrual problems. *West J Med* Jan, 138:76–82, 1983.

Reviews pathophysiology and treatment of primary dysmenorrhea as well as premenstrual syndrome and hypermenorrhea.

83. PREMENSTRUAL SYNDROME

Linn Hatley

Premenstrual syndrome (PMS) is a constellation of symptoms occurring during the luteal phase of the menstrual cycle. Common manifestations include headache, breast swelling and tenderness, abdominal bloating, edema of the extremities, fatigue, depression, irritability or tension, acneiform eruptions, constipation, increased thirst or appetite, and craving for sweet or salty foods. The symptoms begin 2 to 12 days before the onset of the menses and subside with the onset of menstruation. Dysmenorrhea is not part of this syndrome, although many patients suffer from both problems. Some investigators have differentiated PMS into a number of syndromes characterized by clusters of symptoms, such as mood or behavior disturbances, autonomic reactions, water retention, and pain. There has been little consistency or usefulness in such classifications.

The reported prevalence of recurrent premenstrual symptoms has ranged from 25 to 100%, with considerable variation in the operational definition of the syndrome and in the methods used to obtain the information. The consensus of questionnaire data is that 70 to 90% of reproductive-aged women are affected, with as many as 20 to 40% reporting that their symptoms are severe enough to be mentally or physically incapacitating. The costs of absenteeism and work inefficiency are estimated to be considerable, and severe forms of PMS have been linked with accidents, child abuse, marital problems, criminal behavior, and suicide.

Despite the prevalence of this syndrome, little is known about its causes, and there is no consistently effective treatment. Although many causes and therapies have been explored, the evidence is uniformly contradictory and inconclusive. Most of the trials of therapeutic agents have been uncontrolled, and interpretation of the data is additionally complicated by the occurrence of a significant placebo effect. The response rate to placebo has generally been 25 to 40% (with a range of 15 to 88%). It is accepted that a placebo can relieve premenstrual symptoms for several cycles, but few of the available studies have been done in a double-blind controlled fashion over sufficient time to rule out the placebo effect.

Possible Causes

Hormones
Contradictory and inconclusive evidence has supported a number of possible hormonal causes for PMS, including relative estrogen excess, progesterone deficiency, or a reaction to withdrawal from either estrogen or progesterone. Increased activity of the renin-angiotensin-aldosterone system has been found in patients with PMS and correlated with both psychological symptoms (e.g., depression) and physical problems (e.g., weight gain). Elevated luteal-phase prolactin levels have been implicated, but several studies have failed to substantiate this connection.

Neurotransmitters
Cyclic decreases in levels of central nervous system dopamine and serotonin have been blamed for mood disturbance, increases in existing neurotic behavior, and, in extreme cases, psychosis. Because dopamine is known to have a natriuretic effect on the kidney, it is possible that a deficiency is linked to premenstrual fluid retention as well.

Fluid Retention

Symptoms of abdominal discomfort, headache, and mastalgia have been attributed to selective "fluid shifts," presumably as the result of estrogen-mediated sodium retention. However, premenstrual weight gain and fluid retention have not been consistently documented, and the majority of studies have failed to correlate fluid retention with severity of PMS symptoms. The response of these symptoms to diuretics has been unpredictable and often no better than to placebo.

Hypoglycemia

Increased insulin repsonse to an oral carbohydrate level has been found to occur during the luteal phase of the menstrual cycle. It has been proposed that this accounts for symptoms of nervousness, sweating, and craving for sweets. However, PMS symptoms are rarely limited to times when hypoglycemia is likely to be maximal, nor are they reliably relieved by the ingestion of food.

Vitamin Deficiency

Claims that vitamin B_6 deficiency causes estrogen excess, as a result of impaired hormone metabolism, first led to the use of this vitamin in PMS. More recently, it has been suggested that premenstrual estrogens cause a relative deficiency of available vitamin B_6. This vitamin acts as a coenzyme in the biosynthesis of dopamine and serotonin; decreased levels of these neurotransmitters have been linked to PMS symptoms, especially mood disturbances.

Vitamin A also has been thought to alleviate PMS, by either an antiestrogenic or a diuretic effect, but there is little evidence to support these hypotheses.

Psychological Factors

Although psychological and emotional factors may modulate the perception, expression, and severity of PMS symptoms, they cannot explain all the physiologic changes that have been demonstrated in women with the complaint. Tricyclic antidepressants, tranquilizers, and lithium all have been used in the treatment of PMS, but none has been shown to be more effective than placebo.

Treatment Strategy

It is discouraging for both physicians and patients that a better understanding of the causes and treatment of PMS has not emerged. Symptoms may help guide the choice of interventions, but in general it is best to begin with the simplest and safest interventions and proceed to more potentially toxic ones only if necessary. Patients may be reassured to learn that their symptoms are part of a recognized disorder. Reducing sodium and concentrated sweets in the diet may alleviate symptoms related to fluid retention and hypoglycemia. Vitamin B_6 may be more effective than placebo. Promising results were obtained in a small double-blind crossover study using a daily dosage of 500 mg; patients should not exceed this dose because ataxia and sensory neuropathy have been associated with dosages above 2 gm.

Oral contraceptives have been recommended, in part because in a number of surveys premenstrual symptoms were fewer or less severe in users compared to nonusers. Higher progestin doses correlated with fewer depressive symptoms, whereas headache or swelling was unchanged and, in some patients, even worse with oral contraceptive medication. Women who are willing to use oral contraceptives and have no contraindications may respond.

Symptoms related to fluid retention, such as swelling, weight gain, and headaches, may be more likely to improve with a diuretic. Spironolactone may be the most logical choice because it interferes with the action of aldosterone, although there is no evidence it is more effective than thiazides. In a placebo-controlled study, spironolactone, 25 mg four times a day, given on days 18 to 26 of the menstrual cycle, was effective in reducing weight gain and relieving psychological symptoms.

Cyclic mastalgia is a relatively uncommon manifestation of PMS. Treatment is discussed in Chapter 85.

Progesterone therapy is currently in vogue for severe forms of PMS. It has been enthusiastically recommended on the basis of uncontrolled studies but was found to be no better than placebo in two double-blind controlled trials. Synthetic progestogens are not effective and may even worsen the symptoms; the natural hormone is not available in oral forms and must be administered either intramuscularly (50–100 mg, in oil) or by suppository (100–400 mg, rectally or intravaginally) daily, from midcycle to the onset of menstruation. Both alternatives are expensive, and their efficacy is unproved. However, they may be tried in women whose symptoms are disabling.

Clare AW. The treatment of premenstrual symptoms. *Br J Psychiatry* 135:576–579, 1979.

A review of the literature, including oral contraceptives, progesterone, bromocriptine, diuretics, psychoactive drugs, and pyridoxine therapy.

Dalton K. *The Premenstrual Syndrome and Progesterone Therapy.* London: Heinemann, 1977.

Presentation of work supporting progesterone therapy and progesterone deficiency as the cause of PMS.

O'Brien P.M., et al. Treatment of premenstrual syndrome by spironolactone. *Br J Obstet Gynaecol* 86:142–147, 1979.

Use of diuretics in women with PMS. Few articles are available regarding this therapy.

Reid RL, Yen SSC. Premenstrual syndrome. *Am J Obstet Gynecol* 139:85–104, 1981.

Comprehensive review of theories of etiology and therapy with complete reference list. The best review available.

Steiner M, Carroll BJ. The psychobiology of premenstrual dysphoria: Review of theories and treatments. *Psychoneuroendocrinology* 2:321–335, 1977.

A review of theories and therapy of PMS.

Ylostalo P, et al. Premenstrual syndrome. *Obstet Gynecol* 59:292–298, 1982.

A comparison of bromocriptine and a progestational agent in the treatment of PMS. Better results were obtained with bromocriptine.

Abplanalp JM. Psychologic components of the premenstrual syndrome: Evaluating the research and choosing the treatment. *J Reprod Med* 28:517–524, 1983.

A discussion of the methodologic problems that impede the evaluation of PMS, particularly its psychologic components.

84. PELVIC INFLAMMATORY DISEASE

John S. Kizer

Pelvic inflammatory disease (salpingitis, salpingo-oophoritis, and acute adnexitis) refers to an acute or subacute ascending genital tract infection. Although there may be associated endometritis and parametritis, the hallmark of pelvic inflammatory disease (PID) is an acute infectious suppuration of the fallopian tubes and ovaries.

PID is one of the most important sexually transmitted diseases in the United States, for several reasons. The prevalence is high—1% during the childbearing years (2% in women aged 20–24)—and has been increasing over the past decade. The acute symptoms are disabling. Also, there are a variety of chronic complications: pelvic pain, dyspareunia, infertility, and ectopic pregnancies.

Risk factors for PID include sexual promiscuity, the presence of an intrauterine device (IUD), and instrumentation of the cervix (e.g., hysterosalpingography, uterine curettage, or attempted abortion). The increased risk of PID in sexually active teenagers compared to the risk in sexually active adults appears to be related to the greater promiscuity of teenagers rather than to any known physiologic difference between the two groups.

Bacteriology

Classically, *Neisseria gonorrhoeae* has been the organism associated with PID. However, in some series, fewer than one-third of instances of PID verified by laparoscopy appeared causally related to this organism. Moreover, in some patients *N. gonorrhoeae* is obtained from the cervix but not from either the fallopian tubes or peritoneal fluid.

In recent years, Scandinavian studies have suggested that as many as one-half of all instances of PID are secondary to *Chlamydia trachomatis;* in North America *C. trachomatis* has been identified in 10 to 20% of cervical or fallopian-tube cultures. *Mycoplasma hominis* and *Ureaplasma urealyticum* may cause 10 to 15% of cases, but the evidence is less substantial. In the remainder of cases, PID appears to be polymicrobial. Coliforms, anaerobic streptococci, and anaerobic gram-negative bacteria all have been obtained from inflamed fallopian tubes. Tuberculous salpingitis, which was at one time relatively common, is currently a medical rarity.

The microbiologic profile of PID varies according to the clinical situation. For example, gonococcal infection is more common among patients evaluated in emergency departments than in those seen in outpatient departments, presumably because of the more acute clinical symptoms associated with gonococcal infection. Previous surgical instrumentation of the uterine cervix may increase the frequency with which coliforms and anaerobic bacteria are responsible. Organisms other than *N. gonorrhoeae* are more likely to be isolated in second and third infections. The frequency of isolation of the gonococcus diminishes with the age of the patient; this organism is present in only a small proportion of patients aged 30 to 39. It is not known whether acute gonococcal PID causes changes leading to secondary infection with other organisms or whether the failure to observe *N. gonorrhoeae* in later adult life is caused by partial immunity to the gonococcus. It appears that the sequelae of PID are more often related to non-gonococcal organisms, possibly because the course of these infections is relatively indolent, and patients delay evaluation.

Evaluation

Patients suspected of having PID present with a wide range of symptoms, varying from mild lower abdominal pain and tenderness to the acute onset of pelvic pain following menses, with fever and exquisite adnexal tenderness ("classic" PID). Clinical findings provide an unreliable means of diagnosis. For example, in one study patients were laparoscoped if they had lower abdominal pain and two or more of the following complaints: fever, vomiting, menstrual irregularity, proctitis symptoms, tenderness on bimanual examination, probable adnexal mass or swelling, and erythrocyte sedimentation rate (ESR) greater than 15 mm per hour. Of these patients, 65% had visual evidence of salpingitis, 23% had no abnormal findings, and 12% had other problems such as acute appendicitis, pelvic hemorrhage, or endometriosis. The only symptoms that occurred with greater frequency in patients with salpingitis than in those with normal adnexa were fever (49% of the salpingitis group and 19.6% of the negative group) and proctitis symptoms (6.9% versus 2.7%). Patients with abnormal vaginal discharge, increased ESR, tenderness on bimanual examination, and pelvic pain were the most likely to have adnexitis, but this combination was found in only 20% of the patients.

Despite the variability of clinical findings, adnexitis remains a clinical diagnosis. In an attempt to refine the clinical diagnosis of PID, the following criteria have been suggested. All patients should have (1) a history of lower abdominal pain, (2) lower abdominal tenderness (preferably rebound), (3) tenderness with movement of the cervix, and (4) adnexal tenderness. In addition, one or more of the following should be present: (1) fever, (2) leukocytosis, (3) elevated Westergren ESR, (4) inflammatory adnexal mass on sonography, and (5) culdocentesis revealing bacteria and white blood cells in peritoneal fluid.

Laboratory tests are little better than clinical findings in defining the diagnosis. A culture cannot be used to plan therapy on the day of examination, and a Gram's stain of cervical discharge is unreliable. Laparoscopy can be used to make the diagnosis and has been advocated by some as a routine procedure; however, for most clinicians laparoscopy is impractical and should be reserved for uncertain diagnoses and recurrences. Cultures of the endocervix should be taken at the time of the first visit to determine if sexual contacts should be treated for *N. gonorrhoeae* and after treatment to identify treatment failures.

Treatment

The management of adnexitis is directed at treatment of the acute symptoms as well as prevention of long-term sequelae. There is evidence that infertility follows salpingitis less frequently when treatment is started within 2 days of the beginning of symptoms. This suggests that treatment should be started immediately, before culture results are available.

Although the manifestatons of PID might suggest a specific cause, the responsible organism cannot be diagnosed with certainty before the culture results are obtained. Therefore, initial therapy should be broad enough to cover all the most common causes of salpingitis. The Centers for Disease Control have recommended one of the following antibiotics, followed by doxycycline, 100 mg orally twice a day for 10 to 14 days:

1. Procaine penicillin G, 4.8 million units intramuscularly and 1 gm of probenecid by mouth, or
2. Cefoxitin, 2.0 gm intramuscularly, or
3. Amoxicillin, 3.0 gm by mouth, or
4. Ampicillin 3.5 gm by mouth

Oral tetracycline, 500 mg orally four times a day, may be substituted for doxycycline but has the disadvantage of requiring more frequent dosing and not being effective against some anaerobes. In patients with penicillin allergy, spectinomycin, 2 gm, can be substituted for the penicillin derivatives. These recommendations are based on available evidence, which does not include randomized clinical trials.

When PID follows surgical instrumentation of the cervix, there is an increased likelihood that coliform and anaerobic bacteria are responsible and treatment with an aminoglycoside as well as an antibiotic directed against anaerobic organisms (e.g., clindamycin or metronidazole) may be prudent.

Hospitalization is appropriate when the differential diagnosis includes a surgical emergency. The Centers for Disease Control also recommend inpatient therapy for patients with uncertain diagnoses, suspected pelvic abscess, toxicity, pregnancy, inability to tolerate or follow an outpatient regimen, or lack of response to outpatient therapy; it is also recommended if follow-up after 48 to 72 hours cannot be arranged. Hospitalization may also be appropriate for patients with a temperature greater than 38°C or with peritoneal signs. More controversial are recommendations for inpatient therapy for all adolescents and women with an IUD in place. There are no clinical trials of the effects of inpatient versus outpatient management on the acute course and outcome of PID.

Complications

Following PID, chronic pelvic pain and dyspareunia occur in 20 to 25% of patients. In these patients, laparoscopy may reveal dense perigenital adhesions, which are presumed to be the cause of pain; however, in many patients the pelvis is entirely normal. The success of surgery in alleviating these symptoms is disappointing, and the pain often persists in those who have had a technically successful operation.

In women who have had PID, the risk of subsequent ectopic pregnancy is increased tenfold; the cumulative incidence is about 5%. PID is the underlying cause of about 40 to 50% of ectopic pregnancies.

After one bout of PID, 10 to 15% of women are infertile; after three episodes, approximately 75% are infertile. Post-PID damage is thought to be the cause of 30 to 40% of all occurrences of infertility. The infertility results from post-PID scarring and distortion of the adnexa and fallopian tubes. Microsurgery restores fertility in 30 to 60% of carefully selected patients.

St. John RK, Brown ST (Eds.). International Symposium on PID. *Am J Obstet Gyneco* 138:845–1109, 1980.
  More than 40 articles covering current viewpoints on etiology, epidemiology, and sequelae of PID. Little information with respect to treatment and no controlled studies of alternate antibiotic regimens.
Westrom L, Mardit PA. Epidemiology, Etiology, and Prognosis of Acute Salpingitis: A Study of 1,457 Laparoscopically Verified Cases. In D Hobson and KK Holmes (Eds.). *Nongonococcal Urethritis and Related Infections.* Washington, DC: American Society of Microbiology, P. 84.
  A good study of the Swiss experience concerning the causes and long-term sequelae of PID.

Cunningham FG, et al. Evaluation of tetracycline or penicillin and ampicillin for treatment of acute pelvic inflammatory disease. *N Engl J Med* 26:1380–1383, 1977.
No difference was found between the two CDC-recommended regimens.

85. BENIGN BREAST DISEASE
William H. Goodson III and Laurie Dornbrand

Benign breast disease, also often referred to as *fibrocystic disease* or *mammary dysplasia,* is a term used for noncancerous thickening nodularity or lumpiness of the breast. The histologic patterns of this condition include a variety of inconsistently classified abnormalities of breast structure. Other benign conditions may present as breast nodularity including fat necrosis, which results from trauma, and fibroadenomas. The latter are mobile, solid, rubbery nontender lumps that are usually unilateral and represent a proliferation of connective tissue rather than glandular tissue. Intraductal papilloma and duct ectasia are less common and usually present with nipple discharge rather than lumps.

Breast thickening, nodularity, and lumpiness are estimated to occur in 60 to 90% of women by midlife, and there is no precise definition of when such changes become disease. However, it seems reasonable to apply the term *disease* to discrete masses that raise the suspicion of cancer or to lesions that cause major discomfort.

Breast growth is mediated by a number of hormones, primarily estrogen, progesterone, and, indirectly, prolactin. Benign breast disease is considered to be caused, or at least exacerbated, by "hormonal dysfunction," although there is disagreement on which hormones are involved and their precise role in the pathogenesis. Relative estrogen excess or progesterone deficiency during the luteal phase of the menstrual cycle has been blamed because of evidence that benign breast disease improves when estrogens are inhibited pharmacologically, when progesterone is given, or when progesterone is more dominant in a fixed-combination oral contraceptive. Prolactin has been implicated, in part because of therapeutic response to prolactin-lowering agents.

The risk of breast cancer developing in women with benign breast disease has been studied mainly in the subset of women who have had a biopsy. These patients represent only a minority of affected women. The cancer risk has been reported to be two to three times greater than in unaffected women. The risk increases with the more histologically hyperplastic or proliferative forms of the disease. However, only a small proportion of women biopsied for benign conditions subsequently develop cancer, and most breast cancer patients do not have a history of previous biopsy for benign disease.

Clinical Presentation and Evaluation
Benign breast disease occurs most frequently in women 30 to 50 years old. Findings may range from bilateral, ill-defined nodularity to prominent unilateral lumps or even a single dominant lesion. Characteristic lesions are flat and lobulated, with an elastic consistency. The upper outer quadrant of the breast is most frequently involved. Many patients are asymptomatic, but others note dull, aching pain, tenderness, and a feeling of fullness or heaviness in the breasts, which is often worse prior to menses.

Aspiration, using a 10-cc syringe and a 22-gauge needle, is a simple first test for any discrete mass. If fluid is aspirated, and the mass totally disappears leaving no residual, the lesion is defined as a gross cyst, a form of fibrocystic disease. If a gross cyst is incompletely resolved by aspiration, or refills within 6 to 8 weeks, cancer must be suspected (although it is unusual) and excisional biopsy is recommended.

Biopsy is necessary to evaluate persistent solid masses. Excisional biopsy, which can be performed as an office procedure under local anesthesia, is the most definitive procedure. Fine needle aspiration biopsy can also be successful, but requires special training on the part of the surgeon to be sure of obtaining an adequate sample, and special skill on the part of the cytologist for correct interpretation. Core needle biopsy (e.g., Trucut needle) is helpful only when it is positive for cancer. Because there is a possibility of sampling error with both needle tests, negative results may require further evaluation.

When benign breast disease is diagnosed by biopsy, the pathologist may identify the specific features that are associated with increased risk of subsequent cancer. For example, gross cysts in women under 40 years of age and atypical lobular hyperplasia are associated with a threefold or greater risk of subsequent malignancy. A smaller risk is associated with ductal hyperplasia, papillary apocrine change, or cystic disease—a general term for all findings together. There is little or no subsequent risk of cancer with duct ectasia, sclerosing adenosis, or cysts without hyperplasia.

In addition to discrete nodules, clinicians frequently must evaluate areas of solid tissue without discrete edges. These areas may represent cyclic engorgement of breast tissue, which for unclear reasons appears and then frequently disappears during or after the next menstrual cycle. Lesions that are irregular, thickened, and asymmetric compared to the other side, but which are not a discrete mass (or otherwise suggestive of cancer), may be observed to see if they persist after the next menstrual cycle. Sometimes administration of a mild diuretic before menses helps eliminate such areas of nondiscrete palpable thickening, or softens them so that an underlying nodule can be more readily detected. Mammography or ultrasound examination may also be helpful in discerning a discrete mass in the middle of such an area. Discrete or persistently solid masses should be biopsied.

In many patients with nondiscrete thickening or irregularity, no definitive diagnosis can be made immediately. The treating physician must then decide between careful observation and a wide, random biopsy. Careful observation occasionally will miss a small, early cancer. A random fine needle aspiration biopsy may occasionally detect malignancy, even though there is no discrete mass and mammography is negative. However, if all such patients are subjected to biopsy, the number of biopsies performed for removal of irregularities in normal tissue or minimal changes of mammary dysplasia would be unacceptably high. Therefore, the best course still seems to be very careful observation, perhaps at intervals as frequent as every 2 to 3 months.

Treatment

Apart from vigilance in detecting malignancy superimposed on benign breast disease, the most common management problem is treatment of pain and tenderness associated with fibrocystic disease. Most breast symptoms are greatest in the premenstrual period when hormonally mediated increases in blood flow and tissue edema can cause painful stretching of breast tissue. Most treatments are aimed at decreasing tissue engorgement or decreasing the effects of hormones on breast tissue. A firm supporting brassiere, such as one with cotton straps or of the type designed for joggers, may also help by minimizing pulling and tugging from movement of the breast on the chest wall. Sometimes it is even necessary to sleep wearing such a brassiere. Other treatment alternatives follow:

Methylxanthine withdrawal—eliminating consumption of caffeine and other methylxanthines (tea, colas, chocolate, theophylline)—is reported to lead to resolution of breast nodules, pain, and tenderness within 1 to 6 months. A response rate of 65% was reported in one uncontrolled study, but a subsequent controlled study found only a minor reduction in palpable nodules in women advised to abstain from methylxanthine-containing foods. Relief of breast symptoms has not been considered separately, although there is anecdotal evidence to suggest that abstention from caffeine may decrease pain and tenderness. The intervention is benign and may be an appealing first step for women who prefer to avoid medications.

Salt restriction during the 1 or 2 weeks before menses has been recommended to reduce the amount of vascular fluid available for breast engorgement. (To prescribe an effective low-salt diet, see Chap. 141.) Mild diuretics such as hydrochlorothiazide have been used to increase the effect of salt restriction and are usually given for 3 or 4 days before the onset of menses, the time of maximal discomfort. The response rate for this approach has not been reported.

Vitamin E has been reported in an uncontrolled trial to result in reduction of nodules and symptoms in 10 of 12 patients treated for 8 weeks with 800 IU daily. However, a subsequent randomized trial of 600 IU per day for 2 months did not show a benefit.

Danazol, a synthetic androgen that blocks estrogen synthesis, is the only hormonally active drug currently approved by the FDA for use in benign breast disease. Dosages have ranged from 100 to 400 mg every day, and duration of therapy from 3 to 6 months. The response rates, in mostly uncontrolled studies, have ranged from 54 to 90%. Tenderness responded within the first month of therapy, whereas nodules were slower to regress. The benefits of therapy may last for a year or more, but after that symptoms are likely to recur. The usefulness of this drug is limited by its side effects, which include menstrual irregularities or amenorrhea, decreased libido, facial hair, acne, voice changes, headaches, and weight gain. However, danazol may allow women with disabling symptoms to return to normal activity.

Bromocriptine, a dopamine analogue, blocks release of prolactin, which has a permissive effect on breast growth. It has been reported to relieve pain associated with fibrocystic disease in 75% of subjects in two double-blind controlled studies that together had a total of 50 patients. Patients with cyclic premenstrual pain and nodularity responded, but those with noncyclic symptoms did not. The dosages used were 2.5 mg every day during the first week of the menstrual cycle and 2.5 mg twice a day for the remainder, for two to three cycles. The optimal length of treatment and its long-term effects are not known. Side effects include nausea, dizziness, and malaise; in some patients, side effects caused termination of treatment. In one study in which danazol and bromocriptine were used sequentially, patients preferred bromocriptine because they found the side effects less distressing. However, the drug has not been approved in the United States for use in fibrocystic disease.

Other drugs have been less well studied. Vitamin B_6, which promotes hepatic metabolism of estrogens, has been recommended in dosages of 60 to 100 mg per day. Tamoxifen, which blocks estrogen receptors in target tissues, has been reported to relieve pain and cause regression of nodules when given from day 5 to day 25 of the menstrual cycle for a total of 4 months. However, its anti-estrogen side effects of atrophic vaginitis, menstrual irregularity, and hot flashes may be as unacceptable as the breast symptoms being treated, and therefore limit its use. Conflicting reports on a number of synthetic progestogens have appeared in the European literature. Thyroid hormone has been reported to relieve breast pain in euthyroid women with fibrocystic disease. Oral contraceptives are occasionally prescribed, based on epidemiologic association of decreased incidence of proliferative breast disease in oral contraceptive users, but there are no prospective trials to support this approach.

Surgery—mastectomy with breast reconstruction—has occasionally been performed for control of pain associated with fibrocystic disease and "prophylactically" for presumed premalignant lesions. As treatment for pain or other symptoms, it is a very extreme approach, since even severe symptoms wax and wane, and also because hormonally active drugs have become available. The data are inadequate to support prophylactic surgery on the basis of benign biopsies or presumed high-risk mammographic patterns.

Ernster V. The epidemiology of benign breast disease. *Epidemiol Rev* 3:184–202, 1981.
   A comprehensive review of occurrence estimates, associated risk factors, and evidence for association with breast cancer.
London RS, Sundaram GS, Goldstein PJ. Medical management of mammary dysplasia. *Obstet Gynecol* 59:519–523, 1982.
   A recent, well-referenced review of therapeutic options.
Drugs for breast pain (editorial). *Br Med J* 282:505, 1981.
   A brief summary of findings in studies of bromocriptine and danazol.
Montgomery ACV, et al. Treatment of severe cyclic mastalgia. *J Roy Soc Med* 72:489–491, 1979.
   A crossover study comparing bromocriptine and danazol. The response rate was the same (70%) but patients preferred bromocriptine.
Golinger RC. Hormones and the pathophysiology of fibrocystic mastopathy. *Surg Gynecol Obstet* 146:273–285, 1978.
   A review of evidence for hormonal causation/association, with 198 references.
Ernster VL, et al. Effect of caffeine-free diet on benign breast disease: A randomized trial. *Surgery* 91:263–267, 1982.
   Caffeine abstention was found to offer some limited benefit in women with severe benign breast disease.
London R, et al. Mammary dysplasia: Clinical response and urinary excretion of 11-desoxy-17 ketosteroids and pregnanediol following alpha tocopherol therapy. *Breast* 4:19–22, 1978.
   Clinical improvement was related to vitamin E therapy in a small study of 12 patients.

The placebo-treated group did not have demonstrable disease, so they are not true controls.

Ricciardi I, Ianniruberto A. Tamoxifen-induced regression of benign breast lesions. *Obstet Gynecol* 54:80–84, 1979.

A response rate of 71% was observed in an uncontrolled study of 63 patients.

Humphrey LJ. Subcutaneous mastectomy is not a prophylaxis against carcinoma of the breast: Opinion or knowledge? *Am J Surg* 145:311–312, 1983.

Discusses the lack of statistical support for or against subcutaneous mastectomy as cancer prophylaxis.

86. MENOPAUSE

Robert H. Fletcher

Menses cease at an average age of 48 years; the menopause is unusual before age 40 and commonly occurs in the 50s. Ordinarily, menses first diminish in both frequency and amount, then cease altogether. If there is bleeding between periods, if there are heavy periods, or if bleeding resumes after a pause of several months, an underlying disease should be considered. In the United States, roughly 30% of women have hysterectomies before natural menopause. For those who have had oophorectomies as well, the symptoms of menopause (other than bleeding) occur rapidly and are relatively severe unless replacement estrogens are given; the long-term sequelae of menopause, particularly osteoporosis, are also believed to be more common in these women.

Symptoms of Menopause

Only approximately one-third of women associate any symptoms other than change in menses with their menopause. Of these, nearly all describe hot flashes, which ordinarily occur over no longer than a 5-year period.

For a few women, hot flashes can cause considerable morbidity. The following is a description of a severe hot flash.

> The typical episode starts with a kind of aura, with a discomfort in the lower epigastrium, often with a chill followed quickly by an intense hot feeling ascending toward the head. The affected skin, mainly the face, becomes red. This is accompanied by anxiety and unease in the precordium. After a short interval, a variable amount of sweat breaks out. A feeling of exhaustion ends the attack. (Glaveck, 1889.)

There is no sound evidence that symptoms other than hot flashes are specifically related to the menopause. Nonspecific symptoms, such as irritability, nervousness, weakness, tiredness, and headaches, although sometimes attributed to menopause, do not seem to occur more commonly during the age range in which menopause ordinarily occurs (45–54 years old) than in other age groups.

Treatment of Hot Flashes

Estrogen preparations have been used to relieve hot flashes ever since they became available in this century. It has been presumed that hot flashes are the result of estrogen deficiency and thus could be improved by exogenous estrogens; however, it has not been possible to confirm this postulated mechanism. In any case, exogenous estrogens are frequently given to women in the menopause and beyond. Depending on the region of the country and socioeconomic class, from 10 to 40 percent of women in the United States received exogenous estrogens in the mid-1970s; the rates have been falling recently.

Estrogens are usually given in the least expensive preparation—conjugated estrogens (Premarin), 0.625 or 1.25 mg per day. Some gynecologists recommend 10 days a month off the pill, on the theoretical grounds that cyclic estrogen is more physiologic than continuous unopposed estrogen. For the same reason, others recommend giving estrogen throughout the month and adding a progestational agent each month (e.g., Provera, 5 mg qd for 7–10 days). On this regimen, most women spot after the withdrawal of progesterone; spotting at other times in the cycle is abnormal.

Estrogens relieve hot flashes more effectively than do placebos. In a randomized, double-blind, controlled trial with crossover for 30 women complaining of menopausal symptoms, both estrogen-treated and placebo-treated (control) patients improved. However, the patients on active drugs experienced greater improvement and were relieved of virtually all their symptoms. These differences were large and statistically significant despite the small size of the study. Although other symptoms were assessed, most of the changes in symptoms were explained by changes in hot flashes; changes in other symptoms were generally smaller and not statistically significant. The results of this study are supported by the conclusions of other, less sound trials.

When estrogens are given to relieve hot flashes, it is rarely necessary to give them for longer than 5 years, usually the longest interval in which symptoms occur; it is preferable to give estrogens for as short a time as possible. After the first few years, the drug can be discontinued and the patient monitored for return of symptoms. If hot flashes recur, they do so over several weeks. Estrogens can then be reinstituted and nothing lost by the attempt.

Besides estrogens, other drugs that have been touted for menopausal symptoms include antianxiety drugs, opiate antagonists, and parasympatholytic drugs. Evidence supporting their specific value for this purpose is weak.

"Complications" of Menopause

Several chronic diseases of later life—osteoporosis, cardiovascular disease, atrophic vulvovaginitis, and genitourinary atrophy—are believed to result in part from estrogen deficiency following the menopause. Because of this belief, estrogens are frequently given well beyond the time that hot flashes are a problem, and also to women who do not have hot flashes at all, in the hope of preventing disease.

Osteoporosis

Women are more prone to osteoporosis, and consequently fractures (particularly of the hip, spine, and radius), than are men of similar age. Also, early surgical menopause is associated with more severe complications of osteoporosis later in life.

It seems clear that giving exogenous estrogens prevents both osteoporosis and fractures. The usual decline in bone mineral content after the menopause (about 1–3% per year) can be blocked by daily estrogen administration. Available studies show that in general approximately one-third to two-thirds of fractures can be prevented by regular use of exogenous estrogens, beginning about the time of menopause. Protection increases with the duration of drug use but becomes substantial and statistically significant only after 6 years of estrogen administration. One study found a greater reduction in fractures years later when estrogens were begun within 5 years of menopause. Another study found that most of the protective effect was among women who had had an oophorectomy; little could be demonstrated among women with natural menopause. No study has shown differences in effect among the various forms and dosages of estrogen; however, most women studied were taking conjugated estrogens in one of the common daily doses (0.625 and 1.25 mg).

Atrophic Vulvovaginitis

Because genital tissues are estrogen-dependent, all women experience some degree of vulvar atrophy after menopause. The time of onset and severity of this effect is extremely variable, perhaps because of endogenous estrogen production. Atrophy results in thin, dry, easily traumatized genital tissues, which can lead to dyspareunia, cracking, and secondary infections with sexual intercourse. Symptoms are less common in the absence of intercourse. Exogenous estrogens given orally reverse atrophic vulvovaginitis in 4 to 6 weeks. Topical estrogens also have been used for this purpose. Some women find the topical preparations inconvenient; also, estrogens are absorbed through the vaginal mucosa in amounts similar to those absorbed from the orally administered drug. An advantage of topical estrogens, however, is that once atrophy has been reversed it may be possible for women to maintain the effect with infrequent doses (e.g., 1–2 per week), using their own symptoms as a guide.

Genitourinary Atrophy

The urethra and bladder, which are embryologically related to the genital tract and thereby estrogen-dependent, also involute when estrogen is withdrawn; this is said to result in symptoms such as urinary frequency, urgency, and dysuria. There is no sound evidence that these symptoms are in fact more frequent in postmenopausal women or are an independent effect of estrogen withdrawal or respond to treatment with exogenous estrogens. However, some postmenopausal women with genitourinary atrophy and incontinence do seem to have improvement in incontinence when estrogens are given.

Risks from Exogenous Estrogens

Endometrial Cancer
More than a dozen studies have found that women taking estrogens have a risk of endometrial cancer that is between 1.4 and 11.3 times greater than those who do not. Most studies report a four- to sevenfold increase in risk. The studies have been controversial, but disagreement has been over the size of the risk rather than its existence. Risk appears to increase with increasing duration of use; there is some suggestion of risk after just a few years of use, and risk is certainly present after about 5 years. No consistent relation had been found between type of drug or dose and risk. Similarly, the various schedules in which estrogens are given—intermittent, cyclic, and continuous—have not been related to risk. Cancers in estrogen users are, on the average, found at earlier stages; such patients might therefore have a better prognosis and a better opportunity for effective treatment.

Some experts have recommended that women taking exogenous estrogens have endometrial biopsies at 6-month intervals for the early detection of endometrial cancer. Although this advice is logical, the inconvenience and expense would be staggering at the rate estrogens are currently prescribed. The addition of cyclic progesterone may decrease the risk of endometrial cancer associated with exogenous estrogens.

Gallbladder Disease
Based on circumstantial evidence and physiologic arguments, estrogens are suspected of causing gallbladder disease. There is little direct evidence for or against this assertion. The only large study of this possibility found an approximately twofold increase in recognized gallbladder disease among women taking estrogens, but this association could be explained in many ways other than cause and effect.

Breast Cancer
Because breast tissue is estrogen-responsive, and the growth of some breast cancers is estrogen-dependent, exogenous estrogens are suspected of being risk factors for breast cancer. So far, the evidence from clinical studies is inconsistent. Because of the relatively high incidence and severity of breast cancer, however, and the prevalence of estrogen use, the question cannot be dismissed lightly. Presumably, the relative risk, if increased at all, is small.

Uterine Bleeding
Use of exogenous estrogen is associated with an increased frequency of uterine bleeding, estimated to occur in approximately 3 women per 1000 a month. This is a source of additional morbidity and cost from diagnostic evaluation of postmenopausal bleeding.

Benefit Versus Risk of Exogenous Estrogens
Several authoritative groups have reviewed the various benefits and risks of exogenous estrogens and declined to make general recommendations. The incidence of the major long-term risks—fracture and endometrial cancer—and major benefit (decrease in complications of osteoporosis) are of roughly similar magnitude, approximately 0.3 to 3.0 per 1000 a year for hip fracture, depending on age, and 5 to 25 cancers per 1000 a year for women with an intact uterus. The decision for or against estrogens is therefore heavily influenced by the respective importance women and their physicians attach to these two conditions and whether the woman is believed to be at particularly high risk for osteoporosis (Chap. 72).

Two commonly occurring special situations should strongly influence the decision in favor of giving estrogens. First, when estrogens are given only for the relief of hot flashes, they need not be given for long. Because the increased risk of endometrial cancer is relatively minor up to about 5 years, benefit can be had with little risk.

Second, many women have had a hysterectomy by the time of menopause and have no risk of endometrial carcinoma. They are in a position to experience the major benefits of estrogen use without its major risks.

Coope J, Thomson JM, Poller L. Effects of "natural estrogen" replacement therapy on menopausal symptoms and blood clotting. *Br Med J* 2:139–143, 1975.
A randomized, controlled, double-blind crossover trial of estrogens for menopausal symptoms, including 30 patients. The best available reference on this question.

Hulka BS, et al. "Alternative" controls in a case-control study of endometrial cancer and exogenous estrogen. *Am J Epidemiol* 112:376–387, 1980.
One of the most careful and comprehensive of several case-control studies of the risk of estrogens and endometrial cancer.

Weiss NS, et al. Decreased risk of fractures of the hip and lower forearm with postmenopausal use of estrogen. *N Engl J Med* 303:1195–1198, 1980.
A case-control study of protection against fractures, including evidence for a dose-response effect.

Weinstein MC. Estrogen use in postmenopausal women—Costs, risks, and benefits. *N Engl J Med* 303:308–316, 1980.
Applies formal cost-benefit analysis with particular attention to how estimates of years of life are affected by various decisions.

The Menopause Collective, P.O. Box 192, West Somerville, MA 02144.
This group provides a packet of information on menopause, particularly for women who are interested in self-help groups.

Magera BE, Amerson AB, Wilson E. Estrogen therapy of perimenopausal and postmenopausal patients. *Am J Hosp Pharm* 36:1062–1071, 1979.
An excellent review.

Mulley G, Mitchell JRA. Menopausal flushing: Does oestrogen therapy make sense? *Lancet* 1:1397–1399, 1976.
A review of the evidence for and against the presumption that hot flashes are the result of estrogen deficiency.

Estrogen use and postmenopausal women: A National Institutes of Health Consensus Development Conference. *Ann Intern Med* 91:921–922, 1979.
Summary of a consensus of experts.

Boston Collaborative Drug Surveillance Program. Surgically confirmed gallbladder disease, venous thromboembolism, and breast tumors in relation to postmenopausal estrogen therapy. *N Engl J Med* 290:15–19, 1974.
The study providing the main evidence that exogenous estrogens might cause gallstones in humans. Because the finding might have resulted from the use of data that were collected for another purpose, this should be regarded as a hypothesis.

Wood C. Menopausal myths. *Med J Aust* 1:496–499, 1979.
A description of the symptoms of 948 normal women aged 20 to 65 years; no symptoms occurred in excess at the time of menopause.

Hulka BS. Effect of exogenous estrogen on postmenopausal women: The epidemiologic evidence. *Obstet Gynecol Surv* 35:389–411, 1980.
An authoritative review of risks and benefits.

Hulka BS, et al. Breast cancer and estrogen replacement therapy *Am J Obstet Gynecol* 143:638–644, 1982.
The risk for breast cancer among women taking exogenous estrogens, relative to those who did not, was 1.2 to 1.3 and not statistically significant.

87. FEMALE SEXUAL DYSFUNCTION

Cheryl F. McCartney

Female sexual dysfunctions are underreported to physicians. A recent study of 100 "normal" couples revealed that 63% of the women suffered from arousal or orgasmic dysfunctions, yet in a survey of women's attitudes toward gynecologic practices, 72%

of women said they would not discuss sexual concerns with their physicians. Although primary care physicians are not expected to do intensive psychotherapy, they should be able to detect the existence of sexual problems and treat or rule out organic causes. Some women are able to resolve their dysfunctions through their own efforts to learn about their bodies and through their communication with partners, but many require appropriate education and specific suggestions that the physician can provide. Women who do not respond to these measures should be referred to selected mental health professionals.

Types of Dysfunction
The manifestation of any sexual problem usually takes one of three forms: lack of interest, lack of arousal, or lack or orgasm. These correspond to the three distinct but neurologically connected phases of the sexual response cycle. The *desire* phase originates in the brain and is mediated by neurotransmitters. The *excitement* phase in women occurs through reflex dilatation of genital blood vessels, resulting in swelling of genital tissues and vaginal lubrication. The *orgasm* phase involves reflex contractions of muscles surrounding the vaginal introitus. Each phase can be disrupted by organic and/or psychic factors.

In the absence of organic causes, sexual dysfunctions are presently considered psychosomatic disorders—an expression of anxiety through a physiologic disturbance. Contrary to past formulations, the anxiety need not always be deep-rooted and unconscious but can be anywhere on the spectrum, often including superficial, conscious, situation-specific anxiety. Generally, the more severe the anxiety, the earlier in the sexual response cycle the dysfunction occurs. Thus, desire-phase problems often require more complex treatment than orgasm-phase problems.

Detection and Evaluation
Discovery of problems is positively correlated with both physician comfort in discussing sexual matters and routine inclusion of questions about sexual function in the system review. It is important for the physician to initiate questions about sexual function because, in additon to being reticent about introducing the subject, some patients do not recognize the importance of their sexual concerns. Instead, patients with sexual problems may present with vague somatic complaints (e.g., abdominal pains or headaches) or mood disturbances (e.g., anxiety or depression). Once a problem is identified, detailed questioning should pinpoint the phase of the dysfunction (desire, excitement, or orgasm), whether it is secondary (function was normal at one time) or primary (function was never normal), and whether it is general (happens always) or situational (occurs only under specific circumstances). The role of medical problems, such as diabetes, and psychological problems, such as depression or marital conflict, should be assessed. When there is a history of stressful life events, the physician should make specific inquiry about its effect on the patient's sexual adjustment. This should be followed by a physical examination for organic causes. History and treatment are enhanced by a conjoint interview with the patient and her partner. Because some women have female partners, the physician should not always assume the relationship is heterosexual.

Organic Causes of Sexual Dysfunction

Gynecologic Disorders
Lesions of the female genitalia caused by injury, infection, surgery, childbirth, or neoplasm can cause painful intercourse (dyspareunia), leading to a secondary loss of desire. Radical pelvic surgery can disrupt sensory and motor nerves involved in excitement and orgasm. Reduced estrogen levels after oophorectomy (surgical menopause) affect excitement-phase lubrication and swelling unless exogenous hormones are given.

Drugs
Most drugs that affect female sexual function influence the desire phase. Depressant drugs, such as alcohol, sedative-hypnotics, antianxiety agents, narcotics, and antipsychotics, reduce desire. Stimulant drugs, such as cocaine and amphetamines, have been reported to enhance it, although chronic use results in reduced desire. Mixed effects on desire are reported for hallucinogens and marijuana. Androgens stimulate desire. The orgasm phase can be delayed in women taking high doses of antianxiety or antidepressant agents and lost with high doses of cocaine or amphetamines.

Illness
Desire is generally reduced secondary to the weakness, pain, and debilitation of acute or chronic disease, malnutrition, and fatigue. Illnesses that specifically interfere with hormone production or innervation of the genitals have direct effects on sexual function. For example, neuropathy of the sensory nerves of the clitoris can impair orgasm in diabetic women.

Aging
Some elderly women (and their partners) need counseling to adjust their expectations and techniques of lovemaking to the physical effects of aging. Vaginal lubrication occurs more slowly, orgasmic contractions become less vigorous, and erotic sensations become less intense with aging. Estrogen cream or lubricant jelly may be helpful; lubricants should be water-soluble, such as K-Y jelly, rather than petroleum jelly (Vaseline) which is not. Elderly women are able to desire and enjoy sex. Surveys have indicated that 25% of 70-year-old women still masturbate.

Misinformation and Psychological Causes

Ignorance
Sexual problems may be caused by lack of information. For example, couples who do not know that the excitement phase in men is shorter than in women (about 3 minutes for men, 12 minutes for women) will not allow the woman sufficient time to become aroused; she may therefore experience pain on penetration because of insufficient lubrication, and will not have orgasm. If sex is unpleasant for her, she may then avoid it. "Mythology" can be equally damaging. Common examples are the notion that masturbation is abnormal or that orgasm should occur simultaneously in men and women. It also should be noted that coital anorgasmia is not considered a sexual dysfunction; many women require clitoral stimulation in addition to intercourse to achieve orgasm.

Stressful Life Events
Marital or family problems and sexual trauma (e.g., rape and incest) can produce or worsen sexual dysfunction in previously functional women, as may body changes such as in pregnancy, hysterectomy, mastectomy, colostomy, or overweight.

Intervention
Ambulatory care physicians should attempt to treat sexual dysfunctions at their level of expertise. Skills progress in complexity from permission giving, through giving of limited information and specific suggestions, to performing intensive therapy. The decision to treat or refer can be made after an initial evaluation of the patient clarifies the level of therapy needed.

Permission
Some women need only confirmation that they are normal to relieve guilt about erotic thoughts, feelings, fantasies, dreams, and desires. They may need permission to initiate sex, to ask for more time to get aroused, to ask for specific kinds of stimulation, or to refuse sex when they are uninterested. The physician's attitude that a woman is entitled to sexual satisfaction allows her to adopt this attitude herself.

Information
Patients with misconceptions about sexuality can benefit from specific information about sexual anatomy, physiology, and behavior. Such information can be given to the patient during the usual pelvic examination by demonstration of a woman's genital anatomy to her (and her partner) with the aid of a mirror. Patients can be encouraged to educate themselves with recommended reading material and to ask questions at subsequent visits. Suggested references are included at the end of the chapter.

Specific Suggestions
Simple solutions to sexual problems may emerge from the evaluation of the dysfunctional couple, for example, to put a lock on the bedroom door or to leave children with relatives for a short visit to give the couple privacy at home. Women with physical impairments should be encouraged to collaborate with their partners in changing or modifying their usual sexual repertoire. In general, they should allow more time for

arousal to develop. The pleasures of physical closeness rather than the goal-orientation of orgasm should be emphasized. Patients should be encouraged to return to describe the effects of a change in technique. Sometimes the original suggestion does not quite work but a subsequent modification does, or it may become clear that referral for more intensive therapy is needed.

Intensive Therapy
When the above measures seem inadequate, referral for more intensive therapy should be considered. In recent years, brief behavioral techniques have been developed that have proved highly successful in the hands of experienced therapists. Secondary anorgasmia, dyspareunia, and nonorgasmic vaginismus are essentially 100% reversible, and primary anorgasmia is approximately 80% reversible. Qualified therapists have graduate degrees in the medical or behavioral sciences and special training and supervised experience in therapy of sexual dysfunctions. They may be located through local medical schools or physician colleagues. Some are certified by AASECT (American Association of Sex Educators, Counselors, and Therapists). Therapists who engage in intercourse with patients for any reason must be avoided. Their abuse of the power of the professional relationship can cause severe and lasting psychological damage.

Because psychological or marital problems may coexist with sexual dysfunctions, therapists must be skilled in recognizing them and modifying behavioral treatment accordingly. Ambulatory care physicians should not risk harming patients by attempting to use a therapy with which they are unfamiliar. They make a valuable contribution in locating competent therapists and preparing patients to accept and benefit from referral.

For the Patient
Kaplan H, Witkin MH. *Sexuality: Better Homes and Gardens Women's Health and Medical Guide*. Des Moines, Iowa: Meredith Corporation, 1981.
A basic, illustrated introduction to female sexuality and related topics.
Boston Women's Health Book Collective. *Our Bodies, Ourselves* (2nd ed.). New York: Simon and Schuster, 1979.
Clearly written coverage of sexual anatomy, physiology, development, feelings, and fantasies, with a specific discussion of masturbation.
Barbach LG. *For Yourself: The Fulfillment of Female Sexuality. A Guide to Orgasmic Response*. Garden City, NY: Doubleday, 1975.
Details a self-help program for anorgasmic women using masturbation training to achieve orgasm, with a good description of Kegel exercises.

For the Physician

Kaplan HS. *The New Sex Therapy: Active Treatment of Sexual Dysfunctions*. New York: Brunner/Mazel, 1974.
An excellent description of the basic concepts of human sexuality as well as the author's integration of psychoanalytic and sex therapy techniques in treating sexual dysfunctions.
Kaplan HS. *Disorders of Sexual Desire*. New York: Brunner/Mazel, 1979.
Introduces and discusses the more complex sexual dysfunction, desire-phase disorder.
Munjack DJ, Oziel LJ. *Sexual Medicine and Counseling in Office Practice: A Comprehensive Treatment Guide*. Boston: Little, Brown, 1980.
The effects of illnesses, drugs, and body changes on sexuality are related to stages in the life cycle. Sex counseling treatment plans are described.
Marks I. *Review of behavioral psychotherapy. II. Sexual Disorders. Am J Psychiatry* 138:750–756, 1981.
A review of the literature on outcome of behavioral treatment of sexual disorders.
Frank E, Anderson C, Rubinstein D. Frequency of sexual dysfunction in "normal" couples. *N Engl J Med* 299:111–115, 1978.
One hundred couples were surveyed about sexual satisfaction in marriage. Sixty-three percent of women reported arousal or orgasmic dysfunction.
Drugs that cause sexual dysfunction. *Med Lett Drugs Ther* 22:108–110, 1980.
An updated listing of the effects of drugs on sexual function.

Zussman L, et al. Sexual response after hysterectomy-oophorectomy: Recent studies and reconsideration of psychogenesis. *Am J Obstet Gynecol* 140:725–729, 1981.

Audiovisual Material

Renshaw D, Lief H. *Primary Care of Common Sexual Problems: Diagnostic and Therapeutic Guidelines.* American Medical Association, AMA Counsel on Continuing Physician Education, 1981.
A 1-hour videotape that can be rented from the American Medical Association.
Lipsius SH, et al. *Management of Sexual Dysfunction: Common Elements of Sexual Dysfunction Psychotherapies.* Glendale: Audiodigest, 1978.
Basic principles of simple sexual dysfunction therapy.

88. IMPOTENCE

Richard A. Davidson

Impotence, less pejoratively called *erectile dysfunction,* is defined as an inability to maintain an erection adequate for sexual intercourse. Impotence should be distinguished from other male sexual dysfunctions, such as loss of libido, premature ejaculation, and inability to ejaculate.

Most men have at least one episode of erectile dysfunction at some point in their lives. From 8 to 15% of men over the age of 40 have recurrent impotence. Because of embarrassment, the problem is frequently avoided by both patient and clinician; it is more likely to be detected if routine questions about sexual function are included in the primary care physician's review of systems.

The literature concerning impotence is both enriched and confused by contributions from disparate fields. Studies from endocrinology, urology, vascular surgery, psychiatry, psychology, and general medicine reflect the different kinds of patients seen in these fields. Since the 1950s it generally has been believed that the majority of patients with impotence have a functional cause of their problem. This impression recently has been challenged. Diagnostic techniques such as radioimmunoassay and phalloarteriography have uncovered abnormalities in patients thought to have "psychogenic" impotence, although the causal role of these abnormalities has not always been clearly established. Diagnosis is additionally complicated by the interplay between functional and organic problems. Patients with organic disease often have coexisting psychological difficulties such as depression. Differentiating cause from effect in this situation may be quite difficult. In considering how vigorously to pursue the evaluation of impotence, physicians should bear in mind that most occurrences in young men, particularly when sporadic, under stressful sexual situations or after heavy use of alcohol, are psychogenic. Organic causes are more likely to be responsible, alone or in combination with psychogenic causes, in men over 40 years of age.

Organic Causes

Drugs
The most commonly used drugs that may cause impotence are the antihypertensive medications, especially guanethidine, reserpine, clonidine, alpha-methyldopa, and spironolactone. Beta-blocking agents and diuretics are considered much less likely to cause impotence, and vasodilator drugs such as hydralazine and prazosin probably do not. Because it may take 2 or 3 months for the side effects of some antihypertensive drugs to resolve, long trials of alternative agents may be required to recognize and correct the problem. Other drugs frequently associated with impotence are the opiates, amphetamines, barbiturates, antidepressants, phenothiazines, benzodiazepines, anticholinergics, estrogens, and alcohol.

Diabetes
From 30 to 60% of diabetic men are impotent. Impotence has not been correlated with either severity or chronicity of diabetes, and there is debate about the mechanisms. As many as 80% of impotent diabetics have autonomic neuropathy, which may interfere with the sacral parasympathetics controlling blood flow to the erectile tissues. Other mechanisms include vascular disease and psychogenic impotence.

Vascular Deficiency
Although aortic bifurcation obstruction (Leriche's syndrome) is a well-recognized cause of impotence, impotence from vascular disease more frequently results from obliteration of smaller vessels such as the pudendal and profunda arteries, which leads to inadequate penile blood flow. Recent developments in phalloarteriography have uncovered such lesions in impotent men in whom there is no other evidence of peripheral vascular disease.

Neurologic Causes
Transection of autonomic neural fibers in radical prostate, bladder, or colorectal surgery may result in impotence. Chronic degenerative neurologic diseases, spinal cord destruction, and 10 to 20% of cord transections are also associated with impotence.

Endocrinopathy
Hypogonadism resulting from irregularities in any segment of the hypothalamic-pituitary-gonadal axis can cause erectile dysfunction. Other endocrine disorders such as hyper- and hypothyroidism, Addison's disease, Cushing's syndrome, acromegaly, hyperprolactinemia, and pituitary tumors can cause impotence and decreased libido as well.

Miscellaneous Causes
Peyronie's disease is a fibrosing disorder of penile structures that may cause painful erections and/or impotence. It may present with hard plaques along the shaft and glans of the penis or with lateral deviation of the penis while flaccid or erect. Anatomic defects such as hypospadias, phimosis, and hydrocele may cause erectile dysfunction. Priapism (either idiopathic or associated with sickle-cell anemia) may result in irreversible fibrosis of the corpus cavernosa, leading to impaired erectile function. Impotence also frequently coexists with severe medical illnesses, especially chronic renal failure, severe heart failure, chronic lung disease, and hepatic failure. Sometimes improvement in the underlying disease will lead to resolution of the dysfunction.

Physiologic changes that accompany aging include increasing time to reach the full erectile state, fewer and less intense genital spasms, and decreasing amounts of ejaculate. It is important to clarify for the patient that these are not premonitory signs of impending impotence.

Diagnosis

History
A thorough history of drugs taken, the specifics of previous surgery, and medical illnesses is essential. A careful sexual history should include the following: (1) A description of the dysfunction. Patients may group a number of problems under the label "impotence," including loss of libido and inability to ejaculate. (2) Whether the onset was gradual or abrupt. (3) Whether erections occur in any circumstances, that is, with masturbation, other sexual partners, during sleep, or on arising. (4) The estimated firmness of erections attained by the patient during masturbation, attempted intercourse, or on arising, on a scale of 1 to 10, with 10 being the firmest erection he has ever had. (5) Any major sources of stress in the patient's life.

Classically, organic impotence is gradual in onset with steadily progressive loss of erectile capacity. The dysfunction is present in all sexual situations, and there are diminished or absent morning or sleep erections. Functional impotence tends to be more abrupt in onset, intermittent in nature, and selective of partner and sexual situation. However, sporadic erections and successful intercourse have been reported in patients with well-documented organic impotence, including primary testicular failure, pituitary tumors, hypogonadotropic hypogonadism, hyperprolactinemia, and occlusive vascular lesions. Therefore, intermittent impotence cannot be regarded as an absolute indication of intact physiologic mechanisms.

Physical Examination
Special attention should be paid to neuroendocrine and vascular function, including evaluation of secondary sexual characteristics (beard, body hair, and testicular size), gynecomastia, and abdominal or groin bruits. Neurologic examination should include an evaluation of spinal cord integrity by deep tendon reflexes and sensory/motor examination of the lower extremities; the sacral plexus should be evaluated by means of the bulbocavernosus reflex (S2 and S4), sensation on the perineum (S2 to S5), and anal sphincter tone (S2 and S4).

Other Studies
Laboratory studies should be directed by findings on history and physical examination. A 2-hour postprandial test to detect diabetes is usually recommended, although the yield of the procedure in detecting otherwise unsuspected disease has not been reported. Serum testosterone levels are also usually recommended, although reduced levels may be secondary to reduced coital stimulation rather than disease of the hypothalamic-pituitary-gonadal system. However, knowledge of these values seems necessary before launching into the next level of investigation, particularly if testosterone therapy is considered. Other endocrine studies usually obtained in referral settings include thyroid profile, luteinizing hormone (LH), follicle-stimulating hormone (FSH), and prolactin, although it should be emphasized that none of these tests, including the serum testosterone, has proved to be a useful screening test for organic impotence.

In older patients, determination of penile blood pressure helps identify those in whom vascular disease may be important. These studies are performed in vascular laboratories, using Doppler techniques. A normal pressure supports normal blood flow, whereas a less than normal pressure suggests, but does not establish conclusively, that impotence is from vascular causes. Penile blood pressures fall after age 40; however, some aging men maintain normal erections in the face of decreased pressure measurements.

For diabetic men with erectile dysfunction, a cystometrogram may be useful in establishing the cause. A strong correlation has been noted between neurogenic bladder and impotence in diabetics; finding a neurogenic bladder makes it likely that the problem is secondary to autonomic neuropathy rather than a vascular or psychogenic cause.

Measurement of nocturnal penile tumescence (NPT) is a useful but not widely available technique for distinguishing between functional and organic impotence. Continuous measurements of penile size and sleep stage are made on three consecutive nights. Correlation of a normal erection with REM sleep is believed to represent a normal response, which is highly suggestive of a psychogenic dysfunction. However, occasional abnormal responses have been noted in patients without organic findings; whether this is true on the basis of psychogenic or undetected physiologic factors is unclear. Although NPT studies have been extremely useful, the procedure requires a specialized sleep laboratory and considerable time and expense. Therefore, they are usually limited to ambiguous situations or situations in which procedures such as penile implants are being considered.

Treatment

Management is based on the cause of the dysfunction and importance of the problem to the patient. Establishing a working relationship with both the patient and his regular sexual partner when possible helps to avoid misinformation. The treatment of functional impotence is frequently very complex, and many authorities do not believe that primary care physicians are equipped to deal with the problem. The decision of whether or not to attempt sex therapy in a primary care setting should depend on both the physician's comfort in discussing sexual matters and the circumstances of the disorder (e.g., anxiety about intercourse following a myocardial infarction versus longstanding marital discord or psychological difficulties). One frequently used technique developed by Masters and Johnson involves a prescribed series of sexual encounters without intercourse, progressing from simple caressing to genital stimulation. The purpose of these exercises is to remove performance anxiety, a major contributor to most cases of functional impotence, and to learn where in the sexual response cycle problems occur.

Treating patients with functional impotence with androgens is controversial. Although androgens have been used commonly in the past, the effectiveness of testosterone in men who do not have demonstrated hormone deficiency has not been established. Moreover, it may be detrimental in such cases, by increasing libido without improving erectile function. However, many clinicians continue to use androgens, at least as a therapeutic trial, recognizing the possibility that response represents a placebo effect, rather than some sort of "physiologic boost." Cholestatic jaundice, a potential side effect, is less likely with parenteral preparations. Androgens are contraindicated in patients with prostatic cancer.

Patients who do not respond to medical therapy, including those with long-term functional impotence, should be considered for penile prosthetic surgery. The two major types of implants are semirigid rods, which are implanted in the corpora cavernosa, leaving the patient with a permanent semierection, and inflatable prostheses consisting of rubber silicone cylinders, which may be inflated manually with fluid stored in a closed pouch behind the abdominal musculature. The inflatable prosthesis mimics normal physiology, but the devices are more complex than the semirigid rods, and failure rates are usually higher. Success rates with both types of prostheses of 85 to 90% are reported, but the expectations of patient and spouse should be sounded before surgery.

Reckless J, Geiger N. Impotence as a practical problem. *DM* 21:40, 1975.
  A comprehensive, well-written, although somewhat dated review covering normal physiology, organic and functional impotence, and therapy.
Levine SG. Marital sexual dysfunction: Erectile dysfunction. *Ann Intern Med* 85:342–350, 1976.
  The importance of the history in differentiating organic from functional impotence.
Ellenberg M. Impotence in diabetes: The neurologic factor. *Ann Intern Med* 75:213–219, 1971.
  An interesting paper that associates diabetic neuropathy with impotence by evaluating bladder function. Of 200 diabetics, 59% were impotent; therapeutic trials of testosterone were not helpful.
Karacan I. Diagnosis of erectile impotence in diabetes mellitus. *Ann Intern Med* 92:334–337, 1980.
  This brief report of 13 diabetic men, by the father of NPT measurements, is part of a supplement on diabetic autonomic neuropathy. Included are four other articles, all highly recommended, that cover normal physiology, sexual function in diabetics, psychological treatment of impotent diabetics, and the use of inflatable prostheses in diabetics.
Spark RF, White RA, Connolly PB. Impotence is not always psychogenic. *JAMA* 243:750–755, 1980.
  A somewhat controversial paper suggests that as many as 35% of impotent patients may have hypothalamic-pituitary-gonadal dysfunction, making routine screening of testosterone levels worthwhile. An excellent discussion of the methodologic shortcomings of the paper is found in JAMA 244:1558–1559, 1980, in a letter by Kavich-Sharon.
Wasserman MD, et al. The differential diagnosis of impotence. *JAMA* 243:2038–2043, 1980.
  A review of the literature on NPT measurements, giving sample case histories and suggesting that, with careful clinical examination, NPT may differentiate organic from functional impotence in 80% of patients.
Casey WC. Revascularization of corpus cavernosum for erectile failure. *Urology* 14:135–139, 1979.
  It works, but only in highly selected patients.
Masters WH, Johnson VE. *Human Sexual Inadequacy.* Boston: Little, Brown, 1970.
Kaplan HS. *The New Sex Therapy: Active Treatment of Sexual Dysfunctions.* New York: Brunner/Mazel, 1974.
Malloy TR, et al. Comparison of the inflatable penile and the Small-Carrion prostheses in the surgical treatment of erectile impotence. *Urology* 123:678–679, 1980.
  Both work reasonably well.

Scott FB, et al. Erectile impotence treated with an implantable, inflatable prosthesis. *JAMA* 241:2609–2612, 1979.

Of 245 men who has a prosthesis implanted, 234 were able to use the device to their satisfaction. There were 11 instances of mechanical failure.

Furlow WL (Ed.). Symposium on Male Sexual Dysfunction. *Urol. Clin. North Am.* 8:79–194, 1981.

A review that covers normal physiology, the clinical evaluation, NPT measurements, and psychological causes. Unfortunately, the appropriateness of the extensive workup recommended is not validated by the literature.

XII. ENDOCRINE AND METABOLIC PROBLEMS

89. DIAGNOSIS OF DIABETES MELLITUS
Jorge T. Gonzalez and John T. Gwynne

The syndrome of diabetes mellitus comprises a genetically, pathophysiologically, and clinically heterogeneous group of chronic diseases all characterized by hyperglycemia and associated with microvascular and macrovascular complications. Two major groups of syndromes are currently recognized: type I, insulin-dependent diabetes (IDDM), and type II, noninsulin-dependent diabetes (NIDDM). Other types occasionally encountered include gestational and secondary diabetes. Depending on the diagnostic criteria employed, all types of diabetes combined affect from 3 to 7% of the population. Less than 10% of diabetics develop their illness before age 20.

Diagnosis
The diagnosis of diabetes is made by demonstrating that blood glucose exceeds established limits when measured under defined conditions. Blood glucose levels are not bimodally distributed in the general population; thus, no single value infallibly distinguishes affected from unaffected individuals. Although diabetes is easily diagnosed when criterion 1 or 2 (listed subsequently) is met, criteria for diagnosis of mild diabetes remain controversial. Glucose tolerance decreases with increasing age; in the normal elderly person fasting glucose is the same as for younger people, but postprandial glucose is higher. The majority of people in their 80s have glucose intolerance as defined by the criteria listed below.

Currently the most widely accepted criteria for the diagnosis of diabetes mellitus are those formulated by the National Diabetes Data Group (NDDG), an international group of diabetologists especially convened for this purpose by the National Institutes of Health (NIH) in 1979. For nonpregnant adults at least one of the following criteria must be met to establish the diagnosis of diabetes mellitus.

1. Presence of classic symptoms of diabetes (polyuria, polydipsia, weight loss, ketonuria) together with gross and unequivocal elevations of the glycemia (random plasma glucose $\geq$ 200 mg/dl).
     or
2. Fasting plasma glucose $\geq$ 140 mg/dl
   or fasting venous whole blood $\geq$ 120 mg/dl
   or fasting capillary whole blood $\geq$ 120 mg/dl
   on more than one occasion
     or
3. Abnormal oral glucose tolerance test (OGTT)*

If criterion 1 or 2 is met, an oral glucose tolerance test should not be performed. The OGTT may be used to make the diagnosis of diabetes when fasting blood glucose is greater than 115 mg/dl but less than 140 mg/dl. The NDDG recommends the following conditions for a standard OGTT: (1) a 75-gm glucose load, regardless of weight, and (2) measurements of blood glucose every 30 minutes for 2 hours. To establish the diagnosis, both the 2-hour level and some other sample between 0 and 2 hours must exceed 200 mg/dl.

The test must be performed in the morning, after at least 3 days of a carbohydrate intake of at least 150 gm per day and an overnight fast of 10 to 16 hours. The subject must remain seated and not smoke during the test because variations from the above, as well as intercurrent illness, trauma, or use of numerous medications (including proprietary cold remedies and several antihypertensives), may affect the plasma glucose. Results from the OGTT must exceed the established criteria on at least two occasions to confirm the diagnosis.

In a survey of diabetes prevalence, 54% of patients with diabetes were detected by measurement of fasting blood sugar (FBS) alone, whereas the remainder exhibited an FBS less than 140 but had a positive OGTT. Fewer than 3% of patients whose FBS

*In interpreting glucose measurements, recall that whole blood values are about 10 to 20% lower than the corresponding plasma values because red blood cells contain less glucose per volume than plasma.

343

exceeded 140 failed to meet the criterion for a positive OGTT. Thus, an FBS greater than 140 eliminates the need for an OGTT. The NDDG has suggested that a fasting blood sugar below 115 mg/dl effectively rules out diabetes.

Impaired Glucose Tolerance

People whose OGTT is intermediate between normal and overt diabetes are said to have "impaired glucose tolerance," which is not a diagnosis of disease but is a definition of potential risk. These patients are at increased risk for developing macrovascular complications, but do not develop characteristic diabetic microangiopathy in the absence of further deterioration in glucose tolerance. Prevention of macrovascular complications depends on control of risk factors, such as hypertension, hypercholesterinemia, obesity, and smoking. Because 1 to 5% of these patients become diabetic each year, it may be prudent to follow such patients for development of diabetes by criteria 1 or 2 rather than by repeated OGTT testing.

Potential Abnormality of Glucose Tolerance

The term *potential abnormality of glucose tolerance* is applied to people who have never exhibited abnormal glucose tolerance but are at increased risk of overt diabetes on the basis of biochemical, genetic, or epidemiologic considerations. The NDDG noted the following specific risk factors for type I diabetes in decreasing order of importance: monozygotic twin of a type I diabetic (concordance approximately 50%); sibling of a type I diabetic, "especially one with identical HLA haplotype"; offspring of a diabetic; person with islet cell antibodies. For type II diabetes, risk factors include: monozygotic twin of a type II diabetic (concordance rate over 90%); all first-degree relatives of a type II diabetic; mother of neonate over 9 pounds; obesity; member of certain racial or ethnic groups (in the U.S. some American Indians, particularly the Pima).

The degree of risk associated with these factors is not well established. Based on the 1977 diabetes survey by the United States government, the sibling of any diabetic who had the onset of diabetes before the age of 19 years is 10 to 14 times more likely than the siblings of nondiabetic controls to develop some form of diabetes. The risk declines to two- to fourfold as the age of onset of the proband increases. The offspring of any diabetic who developed diabetes before the age of 19 is 20- to 40-fold more likely to develop diabetes at some time during his or her lifetime than the offspring of nondiabetic parents; the risk to the offspring declines as the age of onset of the proband increases.

Gestational Diabetes

Diabetes first diagnosed during pregnancy in a previously euglycemic woman occurs in 1 to 2% of all pregnancies. Findings associated with gestational diabetes and indications for OGTT in pregnancy include: glycosuria, family history of diabetes in a first-degree relative, history of stillbirth or spontaneous abortion, presence of fetal malformation in a previous pregnancy, a previous heavy-for-date baby, obesity in the mother, maternal age older than 30, and parity of five or more. The presence of more than one factor increases the risk further.

Diabetes is diagnosed if blood levels exceed criteria as in nonpregnant adults, or by a more restrictive modification of the OGTT. One hundred grams of glucose is administered and glucose levels are measured every hour for 3 hours. Two or more of the following values must be exceeded to establish the diagnosis:

Venous Plasma Glucose in mg/dl

Fasting	105
1 hr	190
2 hrs	165
3 hrs	145

Early recognition and treatment of even mild glucose intolerance during pregnancy prevent perinatal morbidity and mortality and decrease fetal morbidity.

Ten to fifteen percent of women with gestational diabetes remain diabetic postpartum, and diabetes develops in another 30% of those with normal postpartum glucose tolerance in the next 15 years. Women with gestational diabetes who have normal glucose tolerance after childbirth should be reclassified as having "previous abnormality of glucose tolerance" and should be re-evaluated annually to check for the development of asymptomatic overt diabetes.

Secondary Diabetes
Impaired glucose tolerance can occur as a manifestation of a large number of diseases, either directly or through unmasking latent diabetes by additionally impairing glucose tolerance. Causes of secondary diabetes include pancreatic disease, endocrinopathies such as Cushing's syndrome, pheochromocytoma and acromegaly, and a number of genetic defects. In general, patients with secondary diabetes develop microvascular complications similar to those occurring in other diabetics. It is important to consider these possibilities in every newly recognized diabetic since glucose intolerance frequently improves with treatment of the underlying illness.

Type I and Type II Diabetes
Once the diagnosis of diabetes has been established, it is important to determine the type of diabetes because therapy differs according to the clinical class. Several clinical and biochemical features distinguish type I from type II diabetes.

The most significant difference between type I and type II diabetes is dependence on insulin. Patients with type I diabetes require insulin to sustain life, and develop ketoacidosis in its absence. In contrast, patients with type II diabetes do not require insulin to sustain life and, except under extraordinarily stressful conditions, do not develop ketoacidosis in the absence of exogenous insulin. Type I generally has its onset before the age of 35 whereas type II generally presents after the age of 35. The prevalence of type II increases with increasing age and varies with race and sex, being particularly prevalent (> 10%) in black women over 50 years of age and in Pima Indians of the southern United States. At the time of diagnosis, circulating anti–islet cell antibodies are present in almost all patients with type I but are no more frequent in those with type II than in the general population (approximately 10–15%).

The type of diabetes is frequently clear from the clinical presentation.

When the type of diabetes is in doubt, measurements of glucose-stimulated serum insulin or C-peptide levels may be helpful. In type I diabetes fasting insulin levels are low and respond poorly to glucose challenge; on the other hand, in type II diabetes fasting levels are generally elevated and respond well to glucose and glucagon challenge.

Diabetes Data. 1977 DHEW Publication No. (NIH) 78-1468. US Dept. of HEW, PHS, NIH. Washington, DC: US Government Printing Office, 1978.
An authoritative collection of interesting and useful epidemiologic data regarding diabetes.
West KM. *Epidemiology of Diabetes and Its Vascular Lesions*. New York: Elsevier, 1978.
The definitive work in the rapidly evolving field of diabetes epidemiology.
National Diabetes Data Group: Classification and diagnosis of diabetes mellitus and other categories of glucose intolerance. *Diabetes* 28:1039–1057, 1979.
The consensus report of an international group of diabetologists convened by the NIH to update methods and criteria for diagnosing diabetes.
O'Sullivan JB, Mahan CM. Criteria for the oral glucose tolerance test in pregnancy. *Diabetes* 13:278, 1964.
Established criteria for interpretation of OGTT during pregnancy.
O'Sullivan JB. Long-term Follow-up of Gestational Diabetes. In RA Camorine-Davolos and HS Cole (Eds.), *Early Diabetes in Early Life*. New York: Academic, 1975. Pp. 503–519.
These studies, which determined the frequency of persistent and subsequent overt diabetes in women with gestational diabetes, indicate the need for contained re-evaluation of glucose tolerance in this population.

Hockstra JB, et al. C-peptide. *Diabetes Care* 5:439–446, 1982.
An overview of C-peptide metabolism and potential usefulness of serum and urine C-peptide measurements in the diagnosis and management of diabetes.

90. MANAGEMENT OF TYPE I DIABETES
Jorge T. Gonzalez and John T. Gwynne

The objectives of therapy for diabetes mellitus are twofold: to improve patient well-being and to prevent acute and chronic complications. The primary, but by no means sole, way of achieving these objectives is by "controlling" blood glucose.

Recent evidence, including animal models and studies at the cellular and molecular level, suggests that "tight control" of hyperglycemia may greatly retard, and may even entirely prevent, the microvascular complications of retinopathy, nephropathy, and neuropathy. The evidence that tight control can prevent macrovascular complications (e.g., athereosclerotic cardiovascular disease) is weaker. A definitive, prospective, randomized trial comparing good with even better control has not yet been completed, but one is currently under way.

The absolute level of control required to prevent microvascular complications is not known, but most evidence suggests the nearer normal the better. However, "too-tight" control is associated, in some patients, with an undue risk of hypoglycemia. Insulin-induced hypoglycemia is usually terminated by an adequate gluconeogenic response and does not cause neurologic damage. However, some patients with diabetes cannot mount an adequate gluconeogenic response to hypoglycemia and may therefore experience unusually severe and protracted hypoglycemia leading to neurologic damage.

The level of glucose control sought should be selected on an individual basis, with the participation of the patient. Maintaining glucose at almost normal levels for "tight control" requires either multiple daily insulin injections or continuous subcutaneous insulin infusion via a pump. Multiple, daily, fingerstick glucose determinations are needed to monitor therapy. In patients with nonbrittle, type I diabetes and routine lifestyles, fasting blood glucose levels of 140 ± 20 mg/dl are generally achievable, and postprandial levels rarely need rise above 200 mg/dl. During pregnancy, blood glucose levels should be maintained between 60 and 90 mg/dl at all times, even if this requires hospitalization.

The four methods that should be employed to control blood glucose levels in type I diabetes are diet, exercise, insulin, and patient education.

Diet
Dietary management of type I diabetes should be individualized to the patient's particular likes, dislikes, and life-style. The help of a trained dietitian, nutritionist, or diabetes nurse educator should be sought when available. Aids to meal planning, such as the brochure entitled "The Exchange List for Meal Planning," are available through the American Diabetes Association and the American Dietetic Association. Their use requires individualized patient instruction and planning by an experienced health professional; it is unrealistic to expect even the most sophisticated patients to adhere to such complex instructions without individual instruction and feedback. The main issues in dietary management of the type I patient are quantity of calories, composition of diet, and distribution of calories throughout the day.

Quantity
Table 90-1 summarizes the method of calculating total calories to maintain or move toward ideal body weight.

Composition
Fats should comprise not more than 30% of the daily caloric allowance; total carbohydrate, primarily fruits and starch, should comprise 50 to 65% of caloric allowance; and protein should comprise the remainder. Because cardiovascular disease is the major

Table 90-1. Calculation of caloric requirement based on ideal body weight

Estimate of ideal body weight (IBW)
Women: 100 lbs for height of 5 feet + 5 lbs per inch over 5 feet
Example: 5'6" = 100 + (5 × 6) = 130
Men: 106 lbs for height of 5 feet + 6 lbs per inch over 5 feet
Example: 5'11" = 106 + (6 × 11) = 172 lbs
For small frame, subtract 10%; for large frame, add 10%
Calculation of caloric requirement
Basal requirement = 10 cal/lb of ideal body weight
Activity allowance
Sedentary: add 20–30% of basal requirement
Moderately active: add 50% of basal requirement
Active: add 100% or more, depending on activity
Example: 5'4" women—sedentary, medium frame
IBW = 120 lbs; basal req. = 120 × 10 = 1200 cal
Activity allowance = 30% × 1200 cal = 360 cal
Final diet = 1200 cal + 360 cal = 1560 cal
Calculation of caloric requirement for weight loss
Decrease daily caloric intake by 500 cal to obtain 1–1.5 lbs of weight loss per week.
Add 500 cal per day to obtain 1–1.5 lbs weight gain per week.

cause of death in diabetes, a "prudent diet" (low in saturated fats and cholesterol) is desirable. Concentrated, refined carbohydrates should be discouraged because they induce wide "swings" in glycemia. "Dietetic sweeteners" (fructose, mannitol) have the same caloric value as glucose but induce less fluctuation of the blood sugars and are slightly sweeter per unit weight.

There is evidence that consumption of vegetable fiber blunts postprandial glycemic excursions. The precise mechanism by which fiber produces this effect is uncertain, but a diminished rate of nutrient absorption seems likely. Inclusion of 25 to 35 gm of fiber per day generally produces benefits without undue discomfort or apparent risk. Enhanced fiber consumption can be most easily achieved by substituting whole wheat for white bread and increasing the fruit and vegetables in the diet.

Distribution
The temporal distribution of caloric consumption should be related to the type of insulin regimen used as well as the patient's pattern of exercise and life-style. Peak calorie consumption and peak insulin action should occur at the same time. Unstable patients or patients with high caloric intake benefit from spreading intake over six meals or more a day.

Treatment of Hypoglycemia
Patients with type I diabetes should always have available a source of simple carbohydrates for rapid treatment of hypoglycemic symptoms. For treatment of early hypoglycemia, 10 to 15 gm of simple carbohydrate is usually sufficient. This may be consumed in the form of prepackaged, commercially available tablets or solutions of dextrose, 4 ounces of orange juice, or a nondiet soft drink. If blood glucose is still declining in 10 to 15 minutes, an additional 10 to 15 gm of glucose should be eaten. Too-vigorous treatment of hypoglycemia, such as consumption of a 12-ounce soft drink, usually leads to marked hyperglycemia and renders subsequent regulation difficult.

Exercise
Exercise increases insulin sensitivity by increasing insulin receptor activity and cellular glucose uptake. Programs should be individualized and coordinated with diet and insulin so that adequate calories are available to prevent hypoglycemia. Mild to moderate sustained exercise, such as walking or jogging, is preferable to brief strenuous exercise. Exercise should be encouraged only when hyperglycemia is well controlled; exercise in the uncontrolled, insulin-dependent diabetic may induce a disproportionate counterregulatory hormone response, worsen hyperglycemia, and induce ketosis. With-

out additional insulin, exercise should not be undertaken if the blood glucose exceeds 300 mg/dl.

Hypoglycemia associated with exercise should be prevented by the prior ingestion of extra carbohydrates. Although exact planning is difficult, mild to moderate exercise results in an extra energy expenditure of 4 to 6 calories per minute. Thus, an hour-long brisk walk might require from 240 to 360 extra calories to prevent hypoglycemia. Exercise of an extremity markedly increases the absorption of the subcutaneous insulin injected in that extremity. Abdominal injections may therefore be preferable for someone who intermittently exercises the extremities.

Insulin Therapy

Insulins available in this country differ in three major properties: source, purity, and timing of action. Most insulin is prepared from beef and pork pancreas. Recently, human insulin (produced by recombinant DNA technology) has become available. Two levels of purity of insulin, standard and improved, are now available. Under most circumstances, standard-purity insulin is suitable. Improved-purity insulin should be tried in patients with insulin resistance, high insulin antibody titers, and local or systemic insulin allergies. It is also used for patients who may receive intermittent insulin treatment, such as gestational diabetics, to diminish the anamnestic response on resumption of insulin treatment. The mean onset, peak, and duration of action of commonly employed insulin preparations are shown in Table 90-2. Considerable individual variability exists.

In general, regular crystalline and semilente can be interchanged, as can NPH and lente. If injected immediately after withdrawal into the syringe, the lente series of insulins can be combined, as can regular and NPH or regular and ultralente.

Many factors in the individual patient may alter insulin kinetics, including site of injection, exercise, and insulin antibodies. Abdominal administration generally results in slower kinetics than injection into an extremity.

Insulin Regimens

The complexity of the insulin regimen needed for adequate glucose control depends in part on residual beta cell function. Type I diabetics with some pancreatic reserve tend to be "easy" to control, whereas those with no residual beta cell function tend to be unstable ("brittle") and require more complex insulin regimens.

In a nondiabetic, 70-kg man, total daily insulin secretion is approximately 50 units. Half is secreted to maintain a constant basal serum level, and the remainder is secreted in response to meals. Currently employed insulin regimens attempt to mimic this pattern. Improved control need not always be achieved by changes in insulin therapy; in many patients changes in diet and exercise are more appropriate.

The most appropriate insulin regimen must be selected in collaboration with the patient and will depend on the patient's life-style, understanding of diabetes, and therapeutic goals. Establishing the appropriate timing and dosage can be done only through the use of an accurate monitoring technique. Alternative insulin regimens will include the following:

ONE DAILY INJECTION OF INTERMEDIATE INSULIN. In a small minority of patients with type I diabetes (< 10%), there is sufficient islet cell reserve that adequate blood glucose control can be achieved with one injection alone. However, when tight control

Table 90-2. Onset, action, and duration of commonly used insulins

Type of insulin	Onset	Action (hrs)	Duration (hrs)
Regular crystalline	Rapid	2–4	5–7
Semilente	Rapid	2–4	12–16
Lente	Intermediate	6–12	24–28
NPH	Intermediate	6–12	24–28
Ultralente	Prolonged	14–24	36+

is sought, a single daily injection of intermediate insulin is rarely adequate. Intermediate and regular insulin given once a day have insufficient duration to control blood glucose for 24 hours, whereas ultralente alone does not provide adequate postprandial peaks.

"MIXED-SPLIT" INSULIN. Both an intermediate and short-acting insulin are administered from 30 to 60 minutes before breakfast and again 30 to 60 minutes before the evening meal. Generally, the total daily insulin dosage is distributed as follows:

$\frac{2}{3}$ intermediate $\frac{2}{3}$ before breakfast
                             $\frac{1}{3}$ before evening meal
$\frac{1}{3}$ short-acting $\frac{1}{2}$ before breakfast
                             $\frac{1}{2}$ before evening meal

Twice-daily intermediate insulin sustains the basal levels, whereas regular insulin before meals provides the required increased levels for clearing meals.

Because of early-morning hyperglycemia (the "dawn" phenomenon), it may be preferable in some patients to administer the evening dose of intermediate insulin at 10:00 to 11:00 PM instead of concurrently with the regular insulin dose before the evening meal. This is perhaps the most widely used intensified insulin regimen and achieves satisfactory control in patients whose routines vary little from day to day. It requires fewer injections than treatment with regular insulin alone and does not have the risk of sustained hypoglycemia accompanying the use of ultralente. On the other hand, it does not offer quite as much flexibility for self-management as is available with the other two regimens.

ULTRALENTE PLUS REGULAR INSULIN AT MEALTIME. A single daily injection of long-acting ultralente insulin provides the basal background. Regular insulin is administered 30 to 60 minutes before each major meal. Although this regimen gives greater flexibility than mixed-split insulin, the sustained duration of action of ultralente may lead to hypoglycemia as a result of cumulative insulin effect. Moreover, since ultralente is relatively peakless hypoglycemia may be difficult to recognize, since the onset may be gradual and not heralded by the customary acute symptoms of anxiety, tremor, and diaphoresis.

REGULAR INSULIN WITH MEALS (T.I.D.) PLUS INTERMEDIATE INSULIN AT NIGHT. Because regular insulin has a duration of action from 6 to 8 hours, administration before each main meal provides both a sustained basal level and increases at each meal during the day while intermediate insulin (NPH or lente) provides basal coverage at night. The amount of insulin administered on each occasion must be determined empirically for each patient. This regimen offers considerable flexibility but demands constant attention because of the frequency of insulin administration.

CONTINUOUS SUBCUTANEOUS INSULIN INFUSION. Several different types of miniaturized pumps for continuous subcutaneous administration of regular insulin are commercially available. They provide a continuous dose of regular insulin and deliver on demand a preprogrammed dose at mealtime. The criteria for patient selection are not well defined; however, patients who have difficulty complying with an intensified conventional regimen are also likely to have difficulty with an insulin pump.

Initiation of Insulin Therapy

Intensive insulin therapy, best managed by a multidisciplinary group, can be initiated in either an inpatient or outpatient setting. If teaching and nursing resources are available, hospitalization is useful, even in nonketotic patients, because the initiation is easier to accomplish, and the hospital provides an opportunity for intensive patient education. It is hoped that intensive outpatient programs will become widely available in the future.

The simplest way to begin insulin therapy, in either outpatients or inpatients, is by administering 10 units of intermediate insulin in the morning and 5 units in the afternoon, or ultralente (0.2 to 0.5 units/kg) in the morning. The dosage should be increased gradually (2–3 units/day).

A more intensive strategy for initiating insulin treatment in hospitalized patients is sometimes used. Meals containing an equal number of calories are given three times a day. Regular insulin is given every 6 hours, before meals, and at bedtime, on the basis of blood glucose levels. For example, if blood glucose (BG) before the meal is less than 100, no insulin is given; if it is between 100 and 150, 5 units are given; if it is between 150 and 250, 10 units are given; and if it is greater than 250, 15 units are given. This regimen is repeated daily until the desired degree of control is obtained. The estimated daily insulin requirement is the sum of the regular insulin administered in a 24-hour period. This amount may then be divided between intermediate and regular insulin or ultralente and regular insulin using methods previously described.

Total basal insulin requirements for newly diagnosed patients with type I diabetes generally are 0.2 to 0.5 units/kg/day. Subsequent adjustments are made on the basis of blood glucose measurements.

Monitoring

Measurements of urine and blood glucose are both employed to monitor response to therapy and alter insulin dose.

Self-blood glucose monitoring (SBGM) has become an easy but expensive technique for monitoring control and adjusting insulin dosages. "Fingerstick" blood sugar measurements correlate well with venous blood glucose determinations. Obtaining multiple daily blood sugars allows patients to change their insulin dosages and redistribute both the amount and timing of their meals to promote optimal control.

The aims of the program, including the risks and benefits, should be explained to the patient. Several algorithms have been developed to help patients adjust insulin dosages. Although specific instructions need to be individualized, several guidelines can be offered. (1) Improvement in blood glucose control, either reduction of hyperglycemia or amelioration of hypoglycemia, can sometimes be more readily achieved through alterations of diet and exercise than through alterations of insulin. (2) In general, blood glucose levels should be measured at the times of maximum expected insulin action. Control of fasting blood glucose levels is sought first, followed by control of postprandial hyperglycemia. (3) In all cases except to prevent hypoglycemia, changes in insulin should be made gradually (1–3 units) at 2- to 5-day intervals. When initiating SBGM, patients should have ready 24-hour telephone access to a knowledgeable health professional because anxiety-provoking events may occur.

Urine glucose concentrations correlate poorly with blood glucose levels. They are usually effective in detecting marked hyperglycemia but are not useful for guiding tight control. Urinary ketones should be determined during intercurrent illness.

Hemoglobin A_{1c} values are a representation of the glycemia during the previous 6 to 8 weeks. This test is valuable for assessing the overall degree of control and the long-term effect of therapeutic maneuvers, but it provides little information regarding day-to-day blood glucose levels.

Metabolic Complications

Prevention of Diabetic Ketoacidosis (DKA)

The risk of ketoacidosis increases during periods of intercurrent illness. Perhaps the most frequent causes of DKA are lack of understanding of its causes and early manifestations and failure to take insulin. When urine sugars or blood sugars increase and ketones appear in the urine for more than 6 to 12 hours despite adequate food intake, the patient should (1) continuing administering the usual intermediate or long-acting insulin; (2) supplement with regular insulin every 6 hours according to urine or blood glucose measurements; (3) substitute a liquid diet for solids and force fluids; (4) replenish electrolytes using broth, bouillons, and crackers for sodium and orange juice, tea, and colas for potassium; (5) notify the physician if the illness lasts longer than 48 hours or if vomiting makes it impossible to retain fluids.

Nocturnal Hypoglycemia and Somogyi Effect

Elevated fasting glucoses may result from undetected nocturnal hypoglycemia (the dawn phenomenon) leading to reactive hyperglycemia (the Somogyi phenomenon). Somogyi reactions should be suspected when the patient presents with one or more of the following: an increasing fasting blood sugar accompanying increasing insulin administration; positive nocturnal urinary ketones; restless sleep or nightmares; morning headaches; or awakening with hypoglycemic symptoms.

Education
Patient education is absolutely essential to meticulous blood glucose control. The successful management of type I diabetes is a function of the patient's education as well as willingness and ability to comply. Increasingly diabetologists are delegating the responsibility of making changes in insulin and diet regimen to the well-educated and motivated patient. This goal needs the long-term commitment of the diabetes care team and the patient.

Skyler JS. Complications of diabetes mellitus: Relationship to metabolic dysfunction. *Diabetes Care* 2:499–509, 1979.
A good overview of many diverse observations suggesting that good glycemic control prevents microvascular complications.

Unger RH. Meticulous control of diabetes: Benefits, risks, and precautions. *Diabetes* 31:479–483, 1982.
Points out the potential detrimental effects of meticulous control and the need to identify patients at unusual risk of frequent, severe, or prolonged hypoglycemia.

Nuttall FQ. Diet and the diabetic patient. *Diabetes Care* 6:197–207, 1983.
An instructive discussion of the deficiencies in our data base for formulating the optimal diabetic diets. Points out the need for flexibility and individualization in dietary prescriptions.

ADA Committee on Food and Nutrition. Fructose, xylitol, and sorbitol. *Diabetes Care* 2:399–402, 1980.
Official ADA statement regarding so-called nonnutritive sweeteners.

Anderson JW, Midgley WR, Wedman B. Fiber and diabetes. *Diabetes Care* 2:369–379, 1979.
Observations on and discussion of dietary fiber in the management of diabetes by the major contributor in this field.

Lodewick PA. Think fast. *Diabetes Forecast,* May–June, p. 29, 1983.
Practical guidelines for dietary response to hypoglycemia.

Galloway JA. Insulin treatment for the early 80s: Facts and questions about old and new insulins and their usage. *Diabetes Care* 3:615–622, 1980.
A compilation and comparison of characteristics of currently available insulins.

Berger M, et al. Absorption kinetics and biological effects of subcutaneously injected insulin preparations. *Diabetes Care* 5:77–91, 1982.
A comprehensive, revealing investigation of important practical modifiers of insulin kinetics, including site of injection, exercise, and temperature.

Service FJ, Nelson RL. Characteristics of glycemia stability. *Diabetes Care* 3:59–62, 1980.
A description of normal insulin physiology and its application to understanding current principles of insulin administration.

Skyler J. Type I diabetes: Regimens, targets, and caveats. *Diabetes Care* 5:547–552, 1982.
One algorithm for altering insulin dosage in response to self–blood glucose measurements.

American Diabetes Association Policy Statement. Indication for use of continuous insulin delivery symptoms and self-measurement of blood glucose. *Diabetes Care* 5:140–142, 1982.

Schmidt MI, et al. The dawn phenomenon, an early morning glucose rise: Implications for diabetic instability. *Diabetes Care* 4:579–585, 1981.
In some patients nocturnal increases in insulin resistance may necessitate late evening administration of intermediate-acting insulin to obtain normal fasting blood glucose and prevent nocturnal hypoglycemia.

Shapiro B, et al. A comparison of accuracy and estimated cost of methods for home blood glucose monitoring. *Diabetes Care* 4:396–403, 1981.
Demonstrates potential validity and reliability of self–blood glucose measurements.

Boden G, et al. Monitoring metabolic control in diabetic outpatients with glycosylated hemoglobin. *Am Inst Med* 92:357–360, 1980.
Hemoglobin A is an accurate indicator of time-averaged blood glucose.

91. MANAGEMENT OF TYPE II (NONINSULIN-DEPENDENT) DIABETES
John T. Gwynne and Jorge T. Gonzalez

The major pathophysiologic features of type II diabetes, also known as adult-onset or noninsulin-dependent diabetes (NIDD), are deficient insulin release in response to stimuli and peripheral resistance to action insulin.

Exogenous insulin is not ordinarily required to prevent ketoacidosis but may be needed for control of hyperglycemia. With unusual stress, ketoacidosis and/or hyperosmolar nonketotic coma requiring insulin treatment may develop. Microvascular and macrovascular complications of diabetes, identical to those occurring in IDDM (type I), also occur in type II diabetes. Their relative prevalence is not well documented.

Whether euglycemia should be attempted in type II diabetics in order to prevent vascular complications cannot be definitively answered at this time. It is not known to what extent hyperglycemia contributes to complications in type II diabetes or if it has the same impact as in type I diabetes. The majority of the experimental evidence suggests that "tight" control will retard development of microvascular complications (retinopathy, nephropathy, neuropathy) but perhaps has less influence on macrovascular complications (atherosclerotic cardiovascular disease). It is doubtful that tight control will cause regression of established vascular lesions. Moreover, tight control usually requires pharmacologic treatment, which carries an increased risk of hypoglycemia, with possible cerebral injury, and is frequently associated with further weight gain, exacerbating the underlying insulin resistance in type II diabetes. It is thus difficult to advocate the intensive use of hypoglycemia agents to maintain euglycemia in type II diabetics. However, intensive insulin treatment must be used to maintain euglycemia in pregnant type II diabetics to diminish fetal and maternal complications.

The major components of treatment in type II diabetes are diet, exercise, hypoglycemic drugs (including oral sulfonylurea and parenteral insulin), and education. A reasonable goal for blood glucose control in type II diabetes is a fasting blood glucose in the range of 140 to 180 mg/dl. The acute manifestations of hyperglycemia rarely occur with fasting glucose levels in this range. Pharmacologic attempts to maintain euglycemia (blood glucose < 120 mg/dl) carry the risk of hypoglycemia, and are not justified to alleviate acute symptoms.

Diet
The objectives of dietary treatment of type II diabetes are (1) amelioration of insulin resistance by calorie restriction and attainment of ideal body weight, and (2) prevention of accelerated atherosclerosis by use of a diet low in saturated fats. Obesity causes insulin resistance, even in nondiabetics. Of the 60 to 80% of type II diabetics who are obese, clinical remission may be achieved in some patients by weight reduction, although such patients continue to exhibit clinically important abnormalities of insulin secretion and develop clinical disease if they regain weight. Most techniques for achieving weight reduction in nondiabetics can be applied equally well in type II diabetics not receiving hypoglycemic agents.

The nutrient composition and temporal distribution of calories are less important in type II than in type I diabetes. However, restriction should be placed on intake of total fat (< 35%), saturated fat (< 40%), and cholesterol (< 300 mg/day) in an attempt to retard the development of atherosclerosis, which occurs at over twice the rate in type II diabetics as in nondiabetics. It has not been shown that this type of dietary regimen prevents atherosclerosis in diabetics. However, lowering serum cholesterol in nondiabetics by drug therapy has been definitely shown to decrease subsequent coronary artery events. The hyperinsulinemia found in type II diabetes frequently leads to marked (> 500 mg/dl) fasting hypertriglyceridemia with the potential for acute manifestations such as recurrent abdominal pain or, possibly, thrombotic episodes. Because there is potential benefit and little, if any, risk, a prudent diet can be reasonably recommended.

In type II diabetics *not* taking hypoglycemic agents, caloric intake may be spread conveniently throughout the day. In type II patients taking insulin or oral hypoglycemic agents, caloric intake must be tailored to cover periods of peak pharmacologic action, as in type I patients.

Exercise
Exercise can benefit diabetics in at least three ways. It aids in weight reduction, expedites glucose clearance, and, in conjunction with diet, may lessen the risk of coronary artery disease. The timing, intensity, and duration of exercise must be tailored to the patient. Exercise should be initiated at the minimal level and increased only gradually.

Hypoglycemic Agents
In patients who fail to achieve fasting blood glucose below 200 mg/dl through diet and exercise, hypoglycemic agents may be necessary. In most large series, the majority of obese patients with type II diabetes who comply with caloric restriction require no further treatment to maintain fasting blood glucose below this level. In lean type II diabetics (10% of total), hypoglycemic agents are more often necessary. Obese type II patients who are unwilling or unable to comply with appropriate dietary and exercise therapy present a difficult decision. The use of hypoglycemic agents must be individualized, with the participation of the patient. The goals of therapy should be clearly outlined. The risk of dietary noncompliance (sustained hyperglycemia) and of hypoglycemic agents (worsening insulin resistance and potential complications of hypoglycemia) should be explained before a decision is reached.

Insulin
The use of insulin in type II diabetes is subject to the same considerations as in type I diabetes. See Chapter 90 for a discussion of insulin regimens.

Oral Hypoglycemic Agents
Oral hypoglycemic agents are often justified as in control of hyperglycemia in obese patients during weight loss and in older, type II patients unwilling or unable to use insulin. Young, mildly hyperglycemic patients should ordinarily not be prescribed oral hypoglycemics, because they are at greatest risk for possible cardiovascular complications from these drugs. This is based on the somewhat controversial University Group Diabetes Program (UGDP) study, a prospective, randomized controlled trial to determine whether treatment with insulin or oral hypoglycemics retards macrovascular complications. In 12 clinics, 823 patients were randomly assigned to treatment with one of four regimens: diet alone, diet plus insulin at a fixed dosage, diet plus insulin at a variable dosage, or diet plus tolbutamide at a fixed dosage. No treatment group manifested fewer cardiovascular complications than did the control group treated with diet alone. Patients receiving tolbutamide had greater than double the cardiovascular death rate of other groups in the study during 8 years of follow-up evaluation.

Although the UGDP study has been criticized extensively, the best available evidence agrees that tolbutamide increases the risk of cardiovascular death in mildly hyperglycemic patients. Extrapolation of the UDGP results to second-generation sulfonylureas or to diabetics with severe glucose intolerance may not be warranted.

The sulfonylureas are the only class of oral hypoglycemic agent that is currently available. These agents have at least two modes of action: they enhance acute insulin release and increase insulin sensitivity. All currently available first-generation sulfonylureas share the same basic structure, which has been modified to alter their pharmacokinetics. Table 91-1 indicates the dosage range and duration of action of first- and second-generation sulfonylureas.

The sulfonylureas largely are catabolized by the liver, with the resulting products largely excreted in the urine. Therefore, these agents should not be used in patients with impairment of liver function. Moreover, hepatic catabolism of chlorpropamide, acetohexamide, and tolazamide produces active metabolites that are excreted renally, and therefore, these agents should not be used in patients with renal failure. Many commonly used medications either antagonize or potentiate the effects of sulfonylureas. Physicians who use these agents should be thoroughly familiar with these drug interactions.

Oral sulfonylureas are not always effective; the primary failure rate is 10 to 30% and many patients (30–60%) experience secondary drug failure as well. Sulfonylureas are most effective in younger diabetic patients. However, it is this group in whom the greatest risk of accelerated atherosclerosis exists, because they are at increased risk for the greatest period of time.

Table 91-1. Oral hypoglycemic agents

	Dosage range (mg/day)	Duration of hypoglycemic action (hrs)
First generation		
Tolbutamide	500–3000	6–12
Chlorpropamide	100–500	60
Tolazamide	100–1000	12–14
Acetohexamide	250–1500	12–18
Second generation		
Glibenclamide	1.5–20	12–24
Glipizide	2.5–40	12–24
Glibornuride	12.5–100	12–24

greatest risk of accelerated atherosclerosis exists, because they are at increased risk for the greatest period of time.

During weight loss, the dosage of oral hypoglycemics or insulin should be reduced or even discontinued, depending on the degree of caloric restriction. Guidelines are not well established. For moderately hypocaloric diets (300–600 calories/day deficient), a 30% reduction in dosage seems prudent. As weight loss proceeds, and insulin resistance resolves, further reductions in dosage are necessary. For severely hypocaloric diets (total < 600 calories/day), all hypoglycemic agents should be discontinued.

Olefsky JM, et al. Insulin resistance and insulin action. *Diabetes* 30:148–162, 1981.
A review of the role of insulin resistance in the etiology of type II diabetes. Different insulin response curves can be expected, depending on the site of insulin resistance—receptor versus postreceptor.
Genuth S. Supplemented fasting in the treatment of obesity and diabetes. *Am J Clin Nutr* 32:2579–2586, 1979.
A dramatic but effective program for achieving weight loss and associated improved glycemic control or even amelioration of diabetes.
The University Group Diabetes Program. VIII. Evaluation of insulin therapy: Final report. *Diabetes* 31(Suppl. 5): 1–81, 1982.
Includes investigators' evaluation of UGDP study.
Seltzer HS. A summary of criticisms of the findings and conclusions of the University Group Diabetes Program (UGDP). *Diabetes* 21:976–979, 1972.
A succinct review that places the criticisms into several general categories.
Kilo C, Miller JP, Williamson JR. The Achilles heel of the University Group Diabetes Program. *JAMA* 243:450–457, 1980.
Raises questions of randomization in conduct of UGDP study.
Lebovitz HE, Feinglos M. Sulfonylurea drugs: Mechanism of antidiabetic action and therapeutic usefulness. *Diabetes Care* 1:189–198, 1978.
Describes pharmacology and physiology of sulfonylureas.
Rifkin, H. (Ed.). *Physician Guide to the Care and Management of Type II Diabetes.* New York: American Diabetes Association, 1984.
A concise, practical manual. It presents the current consensus of opinion in this area.

92. MANAGEMENT OF COMPLICATIONS OF DIABETES
John T. Gwynne and Jorge T. Gonzalez

Complications of diabetes include microvascular lesions, which result in retinopathy, neuropathy, and nephropathy, and macrovascular lesions, which result in cardiovascular disease. Life expectancy for diabetics is related to the duration of the disease:

during the first 10 years of illness, the life expectancy of diabetics is 80 to 90% of that found in unaffected people but falls to 60 to 70% after 20 years with the disease. The mean life span of diabetics approaches that of nondiabetics as the age of onset increases; for individuals who first develop diabetes in the sixth or seventh decade, life expectancy is virtually the same as for nondiabetics.

Cardiovascular Disease
The major cause of death for all diabetics is cardiovascular disease, with over 50% of deaths in this group attributable to heart disease. The incidence, prevalence, and mortality of coronary heart disease are two to three times as high as in nondiabetics. Because control of blood glucose does not appear to have a substantial effect in ameliorating this risk, treatment is also aimed at controlling other cardiovascular risk factors, such as hypertension, smoking, obesity, and consumption of saturated fats.

Retinopathy
Retinopathy with neovascularization leads to blindness in 10 to 30% of type I diabetics within 30 years after diagnosis of diabetes. Laser panretinal treatment can retard the development and progression of diabetic retinopathy in as many as 70% of type I patients. To be most effective treatment should be started at the earliest appropriate time. It has been shown that internists fail to detect proliferative retinopathy in as many as 50% of patients in whom it is present. Also, fluorescein retinal angiography provides a much more sensitive means of assessing retinopathy than conventional ophthalmoscopic examination. Therefore, at the first appearance of microaneurysms diabetic patients should be seen by an ophthalmologist and undergo fluorescein angiography; examinations should take place at least annually thereafter.

Neuropathy
Diabetic neuropathy can present in a variety of ways. Some of the more common presentations include:

1. Autonomic neuropathies (diabetic gastroparesis, nocturnal diarrhea, tachycardia, orthostatic hypotension)
2. Sensory neuropathies, including symptoms attributable to posterior column disease such as diminished pin prick and vibratory appreciation in a stocking-glove distribution in the lower, or occasionally upper, extremities. This neuropathy is invariably associated with diminished deep tendon reflexes, particularly the Achilles and patellar reflexes
3. Mononeuropathies, including painful segmental lesions and isolated cranial neuropathies such as ocular palsies. In general, mononeuropathies are self-limited. However, they can recur and are frequently quite disabling or painful

Little can be done to reverse diabetic neuropathy. Improved glycemic control has been shown repeatedly to improve motor and sensory nerve conduction velocity, but this is not necessarily accompanied by clinical improvement. At least two specific therapies are available. Metoclopramide (10 mg tid), given for diabetic gastroparesis, apparently results in modest improvement in symptoms in many patients. The combination of amitriptyline (25 mg at bedtime) and fluphenazine (1 mg tid) is currently given for control of pain in neuropathies; this regimen has not been tested by an adequate controlled trial.

Nephropathy
Diabetic glomerulosclerosis occurs in both type I and type II diabetes. Its occurrence in type I is much more predictable, affecting almost half of type I diabetics by 20 to 30 years after the onset of disease. The onset of disease may be heralded by proteinuria, hypertension, and/or hyperkalemic acidosis caused by hyporeninemia. Hypertension should be controlled aggressively because it accelerates the development of retinopathy and atherosclerotic complications. Beta-blocking agents should be used with care in diabetic patients receiving hypoglycemic agents since they may mask adrenergic hypoglycemic symptoms and also may inhibit residual insulin release. The treatment of orthostatic hypotension may require mineralocorticoids if severe, although slow changes in position and support stockings may be sufficient.

Hemodialysis and peritoneal dialysis in the management of diabetic patients with chronic renal failure have been associated with an increased rate of complications in comparison with nondiabetics. At this time renal transplantation is the approach of choice if possible. Because renal failure progresses rapidly when the glomerular filtration rate drops below 20 to 30 cc per minute, any diabetic patient with a serum creatinine level greater than 3.0 mg/dl should be referred for consideration of transplantation.

Foot Care

Loss of lower-extremity sensation predisposes to traumatic foot injury. This may vary from ulcer formation to Charcot deformities. In addition to sensory defects, the integrity of the feet and lower limbs may be at risk because of microvascular and macrovascular disease as well as the infectious diastasis caused by the diabetic state itself. Therefore, patients who have sensory neuropathies and/or vascular compromise should inspect the feet thoroughly every day, including between the digits; apply moisturizing lotion daily if the skin is dry; and wear well-fitted shoes that provide good support and protection.

Palmberg PF. Diabetic retinopathy. *Diabetes* 26:703–711, 1977.
  An outline of the indications and benefits of newer therapies for retinopathy, including panretinal laser treatment and vitrectomy.
Feldman M, Scheller LR. Disorders of gastrointestinal motility associated with diabetes mellitus. *Ann Intern Med* 98:378–384, 1983.
  Autonomic neuropathies can present in a wide variety of ways.
Davis JL, et al. Peripheral diabetic neuropathy treated with amitriptyline and fluphenazine. *JAMA* 238:2291–2293, 1977.
  The initial description of the effectiveness of this treatment for painful neuropathies.
Kussman MJ, Goldstein HH, Gleason RE. The clinical course of diabetic nephropathy *JAMA* 236:1861–1863, 1976.
  A description of the natural history of diabetic nephropathy in the Joslin Clinic population.
Viberti GC, et al. Monitoring glomerular function in diabetic nephropathy. *Am J Med* 74:256–264, 1983.
  Once diabetic nephropathy is established, progression is relentless.
Christlieb AR. The hypertension of diabetes. *Diabetes Care* 5:50–58, 1983.
  An outline of special considerations in the pharmacologic treatment of hypertension in patients with diabetes.
Gietz FC, Kjellstrand CM. The treatment of diabetic kidney disease. *Diabetologia* 17:267–281, 1979.
  Compares advantages, disadvantages, and outcomes of various approaches to management of renal failure in the diabetic.
Amair P, et al. Continuous ambulatory peritoneal dialysis in diabetics with end-stage renal disease. *N Engl J Med* 306:625–630, 1982.
  A promising new method of management with a surprisingly good outcome.
Sussman EJ, Tsiara WG, Soper KA. Diagnosis of diabetic eye disease. *JAMA* 247:3231–3234, 1982.
  A comparison of the ability of internists, diabetologists, senior medical residents, general ophthalmologists, and specialists in retinal disease to detect proliferative diabetic retinopathy.
Davidson MB. The continually changing "natural history" of diabetes mellitus. *Chronic Dis* 34:5–10, 1981.
  A review of the clinical course of diabetes mellitus and the death and complication rates.

93. HYPOGLYCEMIA
Rebecca A. Silliman

Almost 60 years have passed since hypoglycemia was first implicated as a cause of physical distress, yet controversy about the condition persists. There is little question that insulinomas and other tumors, alcohol intake in malnourished people, and excessive exogenous insulin in diabetics can lead to profound symptomatic hypoglycemia. On the other hand, whether or not reactive or functional hypoglycemia is a pathologic entity is more problematic. An emotion-charged literature has served to fuel the debate. Because many people have vague symptoms of malaise, fatigue, or headache that they or others believe are caused by hypoglycemia, clinicians are often called on to decide whether or not symptoms have resulted from low blood sugar.

Case Definition
Symptoms of hypoglycemia can be attributed to either adrenergic excess or insufficient central nervous system glucose. In general, symptoms caused by the former are accompanied by a rapid drop in blood glucose and those caused by the latter, by a more gradual fall. Symptoms are nonspecific but may be the major clues to the presence of an underlying process. Adrenergic symptoms include sweating, tremor, hunger, anxiety, palpitations, and tachycardia. Neuroglycopenia can cause irritability, headache, personality changes, confusion, lethargy, seizures, stupor, or coma.

The level at which a relatively low blood glucose is responsible for symptoms is controversial, particularly for functional or reactive hypoglycemia. Historically, the diagnosis of hypoglycemia was made by a 5-hour oral glucose tolerance test (OGTT). A blood glucose nadir of less than 70 mg/dl, regardless of associated symptoms, defined reactive hypoglycemia. Later, it was asserted that the diagnosis could be made from symptoms alone. However, neither of these definitions is consistent with the evidence. From 10 to 50% of normal asymptomatic people have glucose levels that are at times less than 50 mg/dl. In addition, some patients experience their symptoms with normal plasma glucose levels (ranging from 73 to 153 mg/dl in one study). These same inconsistencies have been found with oral glucose tolerance testing. Patients may have no symptoms with a glucose nadir less than 50 mg/dl but report symptoms at normal plasma glucose levels. The rate of change of plasma glucose concentration does not seem to be a relevant factor.

Because of these inconsistencies, a Mayo Clinic group has recommended that the OGTT not be used for the diagnosis of reactive hypoglycemia. Rather, they consider the diagnostic gold standard to be a plasma glucose level of less than 45 mg/dl obtained at the time of spontaneous symptoms. However, this information is often difficult to obtain.

Despite the fact that there is lack of agreement on case definition and uncertainty as to the value of the OGTT, the symptomatic patients must be approached with two goals in mind: (1) to recognize a serious cause of hypoglycemia, if it is present, and (2) to provide symptomatic relief. The causes, symptoms, and treatment of hypoglycemia are considered in three categories: fasting, iatrogenic, and postprandial.

Fasting Hypoglycemia
It is important to make the distinction between fasting and postprandial hypoglycemia, because the former has much more serious implications. Fasting hypoglycemia is a rare condition. Patients who have it usually have serious underlying disease and manifest neuroglycopenic symptoms, which can progress to permanent brain damage if untreated. A history of symptoms beginning during fasting and exacerbated by exercise points to this category of hypoglycemia. Patients report alterations in personality, behavior, or intellectual functioning, and seizures, sweating, and blurring of vision most frequently occurring in the late afternoon or in the early morning before breakfast. These disturbances also may accompany exercise. However, distress can occur at irregular intervals, confusing the picture.

Tumors of the pancreatic islet cells (insulinoma) are the most common cause of fasting hypoglycemia. Other tumors are unusual causes of hypoglycemia, including large mesenchymal tumors, hepatomas, adrenocortical neoplasms, and a wide variety of other neoplasms including bronchogenic carcinoma, carcinoid tumors, and carcinoma of the breast. Nontumor causes of fasting hypoglycemia include pituitary and adrenal insufficiency, alcohol ingestion, severe liver disease, and right heart failure. Impaired gluconeogenesis appears to be the mechanism in most instances. Both chronic alcoholics and binge drinkers experience hypoglycemia. Diagnosis may be difficult because symptoms often mimic acute intoxication or withdrawal; the presence of hypothermia may be an important clue. Severe liver disease, such as acute necrosis, or right-sided congestive heart failure may cause hypoglycemia. However, because of the considerable functional reserve of the liver, it is unusual for these conditions or cirrhosis alone to be causative.

In the approach to the symptomatic patient, the absence of complaints associated with fasting excludes the diagnosis of fasting hypoglycemia. In the few patients in whom the relation is less clear, the likelihood is increased by findings consistent with one of the underlying causes. If fasting hypoglycemia is suspected from this information, confirmation by means of laboratory investigation, with the patient in the hospital, is necessary. This includes such tests as simultaneous glucose and immunoreactive insulin determinations and a prolonged fast (up to 72 hours).

"Iatrogenic" Hypoglycemia

Excess exogenous insulin or sulfonylureas may cause iatrogenic hypoglycemia. Usually the cause is clear, but in the case of surreptitious use it is not. Patients usually are health workers with access to hypoglycemic drugs. Symptoms have no definite pattern and are not related to the fed or fasting state. The recent development of an assay for circulating C-peptide has helped to exclude other causes, such as insulinoma. This "connecting peptide" is a component of the human insulin precursor and reflects endogenous insulin production. A low blood glucose, high concentration of immunoreactive insulin, and suppressed C-peptide suggest surreptitious insulin injection. Similarly, when an inappropriately high immunoreactive insulin and high C-peptide suggest an insulinoma, sulfonylurea blood levels should be obtained to confirm the suspicion of abuse.

The sulfonylureas have a propensity to induce unanticipated hypoglycemia even at usual doses. Older patients and those with hepatic or renal impairment are particularly at risk. In addition, a wide variety of drugs can potentiate sulfonylurea action, including propranolol, phenylbutazone, salicylates, and clofibrate.

Postprandial Hypoglycemia

There is considerable controversy about the three principal types of postprandial hypoglycemia: alimentary, early diabetic, and functional hypoglycemia. This controversy has been perpetuated by problems with case definition. Nonetheless, many people are plagued by adrenergic symptoms occurring 2 to 5 hours after eating.

A history of gastrointestinal surgery suggests alimentary hypoglycemia. The physiologic explanation is that rapid carbohydrate absorption is followed by an excessive outpouring of insulin. This may be associated with any procedure that causes rapid delivery of a glucose load into the duodenum, such as subtotal gastrectomy, pyloroplasty, gastrojejunostomy, and vagotomy. Symptoms coincident with a blood glucose nadir appear 2 to 3 hours after meals. Carbohydrate restriction, smaller and more frequent feedings, and anticholinergic agents (e.g., propantheline 7.5 mg po 30 minutes before meals) seem to ameliorate symptoms in many.

Postprandial hypoglycemia can occur before the onset of overt diabetes mellitus. The defect is thought to be a delayed and increased insulin release, resulting in symptomatic hypoglycemia 3 to 5 hours after eating. Treatment includes weight reduction if obesity is present and dietary modification including carbohydrate restriction (60–100 gm/day) and increased protein (100–200 gm/day) divided among three meals and three snacks.

If other causes of postprandial hypoglycemia have been excluded, functional hypoglycemia must be considered. It is essential not to attribute disease to those with vague symptoms because labeling can lead to additional symptoms and dysfunction. The nature of the complaints and their relation to meals must be assessed carefully. Exploration of possible emotional disturbances should be included as part of a thorough medical evaluation. Depression, anxiety, or other emotional disturbances may be operant or, in fact, the underlying problem.

Although the shortcomings of the OGTT must be recognized, this test can be useful in two ways. The fact that the vast majority of symptomatic patients do not have reactive hypoglycemia can be demonstrated effectively by the OGTT. In the small percentage of patients whose symptoms coincide with the plasma glucose nadir of the OGTT and who are not symptomatic at other times, dietary changes similar to those recommended for alimentary and early diabetic hypoglycemia may be beneficial.

Exercise-Induced Hypoglycemia

In recent years there has been much interest in hypoglycemia induced by prolonged exercise. Carbohydrate loading before competition and the ingestion of glucose- and electrolyte-containing fluids have become part of the runner's armamentarium. Although hypoglycemia has been known to occur in both marathon runners and bicyclists, the relation of this to fatigue and performance is less clear. For example, in a study of healthy men exercising to exhaustion, there was no difference in endurance between those in whom hypoglycemia developed and those in whom it was prevented by the ingestion of glucose solutions. There is no sound evidence that hypoglycemia is responsible for symptoms that ordinarily occur during exercise or that ingesting sugar prevents these symptoms.

Service FJ, et al. Insulinoma: Clinical and diagnostic features of 60 consecutive cases. *Mayo Clin Proc* 51:417–429, 1976.
Experience with insulinoma at the Mayo Clinic between 1964 and 1975.

Merimee TJ. Spontaneous hypoglycemia in man. *Adv Intern Med* 22:301–317, 1977.
A discussion of glucose homeostasis, emphasizing the variability found in normal people. The causes of hypoglycemia are presented, and reactive hypoglycemia is discounted as a pathologic entity.

Kahn CR. The riddle of tumor hypoglycemia revisited. *Clin Endocrinol Metab* 9: 335–360, 1980.
An up-to-date review of the possible mechanisms and the evidence for each.

Fajans SS, Floyd JC. Fasting hypoglycemia in adults. *N Engl J Med* 294:766–772, 1976.
A thorough discussion of the mechanisms and causes of fasting hypoglycemia.

Horwitz DL, Kuzuya H, Rubenstein AH. Circulating serum C-peptide. *N Engl J Med* 295:207–209, 1976.
The indications for and interpretation of the C-peptide assay are outlined.

Johnson DD, et al. Reactive hypoglycemia. *JAMA* 243:1151–1155, 1980.
One hundred ninety-two patients underwent a 5-hour glucose tolerance test for the evaluation of hypoglycemic symptoms. The OGTT was considered unreliable as a diagnostic tool.

Felig P, et al. Hypoglycemia during prolonged exercise in normal men. *N Engl J Med* 306:895–900, 1982.
A recent study examining the role of hypoglycemia in exercise endurance. Hypoglycemic men performed as well as euglycemic men.

Lev-Ran A, Anderson RW. The diagnosis of postprandial hypoglycemia. *Diabetes* 30:996–999, 1981.
Of 118 patients carrying the diagnosis of hypoglycemia, 16 had symptoms coincident with glucose nadirs during the OGTT. However, only 5 of these had symptoms following usual meals. The authors caution against the use of the OGTT as the diagnostic criterion for reactive hypoglycemia.

94. HYPERTHYROIDISM

Robert D. Utiger

Hyperthyroidism is a rather common disorder. A recent community survey in Great Britain showed a prevalence rate of 19 per 1000 women and 1.6 per 1000 men, and an estimated incidence of 2 to 3 per 1000 women per year.

Clinical Manifestations

The manifestations of hyperthyroidism reflect increased function of various organ systems; they also may reflect the inability of an organ system to meet the demands imposed by hyperthyroidism. The diagnosis also should be considered in patients with thyroid enlargement or infiltrative ophthalmopathy. Although the clinical manifestations are similar whatever the cause, their frequency and severity are influenced by the rate of onset, age of the patient, and vulnerability of various organ systems to excess thyroid hormone. The term *apathetic* or *masked hyperthyroidism* is used to describe the condition in elderly patients who have cardiac failure, atrial fibrillation, muscle weakness, or weight loss but not the nervousness, heat intolerance, hyperphagia, and hyperactivity so common in younger patients. There is no evidence that apathetic hyperthyroidism differs pathophysiologically from "ordinary" hyperthyroidism.

Psychological Symptoms

Nervousness, physical hyperactivity, emotional lability, anxiety, and distractibility occur commonly. These changes often result in impairment of work or school performance and disturbances in home and family life.

Neuromuscular Symptoms

A fine tremor is often evident in the hands and fingers, and performance of skills requiring fine coordination becomes difficult. Deep tendon reflexes are hyperactive. Some evidence of myopathy is common. Weakness usually develops gradually, is progressive, and may be accompanied by muscle wasting.

Skin

The skin is warm and its texture smooth or velvety. Erythema and pruritus may be present. Hyperhidrosis is a common complaint. Hair may become thin and fine, and alopecia occurs.

Eyes

The noninfiltrative abnormalities are lid retraction and lid lag. Lid retracton results in "apparent" proptosis, but not in forward protrusion of the eye, and is often accompanied by symptoms of conjunctival irritation. Infiltrative ophthalmopathy, a manifestation of Graves' disease, is discussed below.

Thyroid Gland

Enlargement of the thyroid gland is very common. In Graves' disease, both thyroid lobes are usually moderately symmetrically enlarged, but thyroid enlargement may be absent. Thyroiditis results in slight or moderate diffuse thyroid enlargement; the thyroid is tender in subacute thyroiditis. Toxic multinodular goiters are large and asymmetric. A thyroid adenoma causing hyperthyroidism is usually at least 3 cm in diameter, and no other thyroid tissue is palpable.

Cardiovascular System

Dysfunction of the cardiovascular system is common, and in some instances, the only manifestation of hyperthyroidism. Heart rate and cardiac output are increased, and peripheral resistance is decreased. These changes result in palpitations, sinus tachycardia or atrial fibrillation, and heart failure. Examination reveals a prominent apical impulse, bounding arterial pulsations, accentuated heart sounds, systolic ejection murmurs, and occasionally cardiac enlargement. Other than arrhythmias, electrocardiographic changes are limited to nonspecific ST and T wave abnormalities.

Respiratory Function

Abnormalities of respiration include decreased vital capacity and decreased pulmonary compliance. They result in dyspnea and hyperventilation during exercise and sometimes at rest.

Gastrointestinal System

Increased caloric utilization is almost always present. It results in increased appetite and food intake, but compensation is usually inadequate, and modest weight loss occurs. In older patients, weight loss of 20 pounds or more is common. Increased gastroin-

estinal motility may result in increased frequency of bowel movements and even frank
iarrhea. Minor abnormalities in hepatic function are often found.

Hematopoietic System

Some patients have a modest anemia, caused by mild deficiency in one or more hema-
opoietic nutrients or increased plasma volume. Mild granulocytopenia and thrombo-
ytopenia may be present.

Energy and Intermediary Metabolism

Because of increased energy expenditure, energy production must be augmented; this
s accompanied by increased oxygen consumption and heat production. In patients with
iabetes mellitus, requirements for exogenous insulin increase because of accelerated
nsulin catabolism.

Endocrine System

In women, hypomenorrhea or amenorrhea may occur, although often no changes are
oted. In men, there may be loss of libido and impotence.

Hypercalcemia is found occasionally; it is usually neither severe nor symptomatic. It
s caused by increased bone resorption, but clinical osteopenia is rare.

Laboratory Diagnosis

Thyroid Hormones

In most patients, serum total T_4 and T_3 concentrations are increased. However, these
changes also can be caused by increased thyroxine-binding globulin (TBG) production
(e.g., as a result of estrogen therapy). Therefore, confirmation of the diagnosis of hyperthyroidism demands demonstration of increases in both total and free T_4 (or T_3)
concentrations. Free T_4 concentrations are most often measured indirectly, using the
T_3-resin uptake to calculate the free T_4 index. Rare causes of increased serum total T_4
concentrations and free T_4 index values include peripheral thyroid hormone resistance
and production of an abnormal T_4-binding albumin. The serum total T_3 concentration
should be measured only when the serum T_4 concentration and free T_4 index are normal in a patient suspected of having hyperthyroidism. A high serum T_3 concentration
establishes the diagnosis of T_3 hyperthyroidism. Some patients with hyperthyroidism
have increased serum T_4 but normal serum T_3 concentrations (T_4 hyperthyroidism).
This is a consequence of impaired extrathyroidal conversion of T_4 to T_3, caused by
concomitant nonthyroidal illness. T_3 hyperthyroidism and T_4 hyperthyroidism are
found in less than 5% of any group of hyperthyroid patients.

Thyroid-Stimulating Hormone (TSH)

Serum TSH is characteristically undetectable in hyperthyroid patients. However, the
usefulness of serum TSH measurement is limited because serum TSH is undetectable
in some normal subjects and because hyperthyroidism caused by excessive TSH secretion is very rare. Therefore, serum TSH should be measured only when there is evidence of pituitary disease. Measurement of serum TSH after administration of thyrotropin releasing hormone (TRH) is helpful in confirming a diagnosis of
hyperthyroidism when unequivocal elevations of serum T_4 and/or T_3 are not present.
A subnormal TSH response to TRH is indicative of thyroid autonomy and hyperthyroidism. The test is easily performed, requiring measurements of serum TSH before
and 10 to 15 and 20 to 30 minutes after the intravenous administration of 400 or 500
μg TRH.

Radioiodine Uptake

Most patients with hyperthyroidism have increased thyroid radioiodine uptake. Important exceptions include patients with subacute thyroiditis, painless thyroiditis, and
exogenous hyperthyroidism. The indications for measurement of thyroid radioiodine
uptake are for confirmation of a suspected diagnosis of thyroiditis or of surreptitious
thyroid hormone administration in a hyperthyroid patient, and as a prelude to ^{131}I
therapy. Thyroid scans are useful in determining regional, but not overall, thyroid
function, and therefore are not a test for hyperthyroidism. This test may be helpful in
identifying a thyroid adenoma or multinodular goiter as a cause of hyperthyroidism.

Diagnostic Strategy
A useful scheme for the evaluation of patients with suspected hyperthyroidism is as follows: First, measure the serum T_4 concentration and T_3-resin uptake or serum free T_4 concentration. If the results are elevated, the diagnosis of hyperthyroidism is confirmed. If the results are normal or equivocal, measurement of serum T_3 is indicated. When these tests do not confirm the diagnosis, a TRH stimulation test may be done. An abnormal response indicates the presence of thyroid autonomy and is compatible with, although not diagnostic of, hyperthyroidism.

Causes of Hyperthyroidism

The underlying cause of hyperthyroidism should be identified, because the causes differ in natural history and therefore require different therapy. In most patients the cause can be identified by history and physical examination alone, with particular reliance on the duration of symptoms and presence or absence of thyroid enlargement and of extrathyroidal manifestations of Graves' disease. Laboratory procedures that help to establish the cause are described below; they should be done only when specifically indicated. Graves' disease is the cause in roughly 90% of patients; the next most common causes are the various forms of thyroiditis.

Graves' Disease
Graves' disease occurs most often in young women, but it may occur in men and at any age. It consists of one or more of the following: hyperthyroidism, diffuse thyroid enlargement, infiltrative ophthalmopathy, and pretibial myxedema. Most patients with Graves' disease have both hyperthyroidism and goiter. The two usually develop concurrently and are caused by the production of thyroid-stimulating immunoglobulins (TSI). Extrathyroidal manifestations are less common, and their cause is not known. Graves' disease may remit spontaneously so that some patients remain euthyroid after antithyroid drug therapy is withdrawn. The proportion of patients who have a remission after 1 year of antithyroid therapy varies from 40 to 60% and is higher in those treated longer.

Subacute Thyroiditis
Clinical manifestations of hyperthyroidism occur in about 50% of patients with subacute thyroiditis, but this disorder is dominated by the nonspecific systemic inflammatory manifestations of the illness and by thyroid pain, tenderness, and enlargement. Hyperthyroidism lasts from a week to a month or so and then subsides, often followed by transient hypothyroidism; ultimate recovery is the rule.

Painless Thyroiditis
Hyperthyroidism caused by thyroiditis without pain or tenderness is characteristically of recent onset. Thyroid enlargement is slight or moderate. Thyroid radioiodine uptake is low. Recovery occurs in a few weeks or months and may be preceded by transient hypothyroidism.

Exogenous Hyperthyroidism
Iatrogenic or factitious hyperthyroidism is likely to occur with T_4 in dosages of 250 μg per day or more, T_3 in dosages of 100 μg per day or more, or desiccated thyroid in dosages of 180 mg per day or more. In euthyroid patients with autonomous thyroid function, smaller dosages may cause hyperthyroidism. Important clues to the presence of exogenous hyperthyroidism are the absence of thyroid enlargement, normal or low serum T_4 concentrations (with use of T_3 therapy), and low thyroid radioiodine uptake.

Toxic Nodular Goiter
Toxic nodular goiter may result in hyperthyroidism late in its natural history. The usual patient has a long history of gradually increasing thyroid enlargement and hyperthyroidism develops insidiously. There is no ophthalmopathy or pretibial myxedema.

Toxic Uninodular Goiter (Thyroid Adenoma)
Hyperthyroidism occurs in some patients with an autonomously functioning thyroid adenoma, clinically manifested as a solitary thyroid nodule. Although thyroid adeno-

mas occur in adults of all ages, most patients with hyperthyroidism are in the older age groups. The thyroid scan shows intense isotope uptake in the location of the palpable nodule and nearly complete absence of uptake elsewhere.

Other Causes
Rare causes of hyperthyroidism include iodine-induced hyperthyroidism, trophoblastic tumors, TSH-secreting pituitary tumors, and ectopic hyperthyroidism (struma ovarii).

Treatment Options
Ideal therapy for a hyperthyroid patient would be elimination of the cause so that normal pituitary-thyroid function can be restored. For most patients, however, the fundamental cause of their hyperthyroidism is not known, and no truly curative treatment is available.

Antithyroid Drugs
Propylthiouracil (PTU) and methimazole (MMI) are effective inhibitors of thyroid hormone biosynthesis. PTU also inhibits extrathyroidal conversion of T_4 to T_3. The usual initial daily dosage of PTU is 300 to 450 mg and of MMI, 10 to 30 mg, in divided doses. Some improvement usually occurs after 1 or 2 weeks of treatment, and it is usually substantial after 4 to 6 weeks. Failure of antithyroid drug therapy to control hyperthyroidism results from inadequate dosage and/or noncompliance. As improvement occurs, the dosage is reduced by 25 to 50% at 1- to 2-month intervals and the drug may be given once daily. If the patient with Graves' disease remains euthyroid with dosages of 50 mg PTU or 5 mg MMI daily for 1 to 2 months, the drug is discontinued. Decisions about dosages are made largely on clinical grounds, supported when necessary by serum T_4 determinations. Recurrences may be treated with an antithyroid drug again, although many patients choose ablative therapy.

Toxic reactions to the usual dosages of either drug are uncommon, occurring in less than 5% of patients. Most are dermatologic reactions, such as pruritus or urticaria, which subside with no treatment or with symptomatic therapy. More serious reactions include fever, arthritis, hepatitis, anemia, thrombocytopenia, and agranulocytosis; agranulocytosis occurs in approximately 0.2% of patients. Because these reactions usually develop rapidly, monitoring blood cell counts is not helpful. Patients should be carefully warned of the symptoms of such reactions and instructed to discontinue therapy and contact the physician immediately if any occur. Although a toxic reaction to one drug does not preclude use of the other, it is wiser to give ^{131}I therapy after a serious toxic reaction.

Drugs to Ameliorate Thyroid Hormone Effects
Some manifestations of hyperthyroidism are ameliorated by adrenergic antagonists. Propranolol, in dosages of 60 to 240 mg daily, results in rapid (24 to 48 hours) diminution of some common symptoms of hyperthyroidism. Propranolol alone is inadequate treatment for hyperthyroidism. Although useful for alleviating symptoms, it should not be used routinely.

[131]I Therapy
Thyroid ablation with ^{131}I is an effective treatment for hyperthyroidism due to Graves' disease. Major advantages of ^{131}I therapy are that usually only a single dose is needed, it is safe, and its cost is relatively low. Amelioration of hyperthyroidism usually requires several months. For markedly symptomatic patients, a period of antithyroid drug therapy before ^{131}I therapy is often advisable. Iodides should not be given, and care should be taken to avoid iodide-containing drugs or contrast agents if ^{131}I therapy is planned. The usual ^{131}I dosage is 8 to 15 µCi.

There are only two important untoward effects of ^{131}I therapy: persistent hyperthyroidism and hypothyroidism. Acute temporary exacerbations of hyperthyroidism, caused by radiation thyroiditis, are rare. Persistent hyperthyroidism results from inadequate therapy and is more common when lower doses of ^{131}I are given. Hypothyroidism may occur in the first few months after therapy or any time thereafter (see Chap. 95). Many physicians are reluctant to use ^{131}I therapy for treating children and young adults, because hypothyroidism is more likely to develop in patients whose life expectancy is longer, because ^{131}I might cause thyroidal or other neoplasms or gonadal damage resulting in birth defects, or because the patient might be pregnant. However,

^{131}I therapy is not a proven risk factor for thyroid or other neoplasms and the gonadal radiation dose after ^{131}I is less than the dose that results from diagnostic radiologic procedures. Because ^{131}I crosses the placenta and can destroy the fetal thyroid, pregnancy is an absolute contraindication to its use.

Surgery
Because of the simplicity, safety, and economy of antithyroid drugs and ^{131}I therapy, the only indications for subtotal thyroidectomy are hyperthyroidism during pregnancy or very large goiters.

Treatment of Specific Conditions

Graves' Disease
Antithyroid drugs or radioactive iodine (^{131}I) are both effective, safe, and relatively inexpensive forms of treatment. Neither results in cure, and both require long-term observation of the patient. The choice depends on several considerations. Antithyroid drugs are given in the hope that a remission will occur that will be sustained after withdrawal of therapy. Although this goal is not always achieved, antithyroid drugs are the initial treatment of choice for most patients. ^{131}I is simpler, although hypothyroidism nearly always develops subsequently. The most important considerations, however, are acceptability to the patient and experience of the physician in use of the therapy.

Thyroiditis
Both subacute and painless thyroiditis are transient, and the hyperthyroidism accompanying them is usually mild. If treatment of it is needed, propranolol is the agent of choice. Salicylates or prednisone effectively relieve neck pain and tenderness in patients with subacute thyroiditis.

Toxic Multinodular Goiter
Ablative treatment with ^{131}I is the treatment of choice for this permanent disorder. Large doses of ^{131}I, and sometimes multiple doses, should be used, because thyroid ^{131}I uptake is usually only slightly increased, and persistent hyperthyroidism is to be avoided in these elderly patients. Hypothyroidism rarely develops following treatment, because the thyroid gland contains suppressed tissue that can regain function.

Thyroid Adenoma
Because thyroid adenomas also cause permanent hyperthyroidism, ablative therapy with ^{131}I is the most appropriate. The dosage used should be large (20 to 25 μCi) so that the nodule is effectively destroyed. There is small risk of permanent hypothyroidism because the suppressed extranodular tissue recovers function as production of T_4 and T_3 by the nodule declines.

Extrathyroidal Manifestations of Graves' Disease

Infiltrative Ophthalmopathy
Ophthalmopathy is present in 20 to 40% of patients with hyperthyroidism from Graves' disease. It usually develops gradually, concomitantly with hyperthyroidism, but it may first appear months or years later. The symptoms include pain in the eyes, lacrimation, photophobia, diplopia, and blurring or loss of vision. The major signs are proptosis (exophthalmos), periorbital and conjunctival congestion and edema (chemosis), and limitation of ocular mobility. The diagnosis of infiltrative ophthalmopathy when hyperthyroidism is or recently was present is not difficult. The diagnosis is less certain if the patient is not or never was hyperthyroid (euthyroid Graves' disease). Orbital ultrasonography or computed tomography is the best procedure to confirm the diagnosis of ophthalmopathy due to Graves' disease and to exclude other causes of ophthalmopathy, such as orbital pseudotumor and orbital tumors.

Ophthalmopathy is at its worst in most patients before their hyperthyroidism is treated. With antithyroid treatment, noninfiltrative eye signs (lid retraction, stare), local irritative symptoms, and subjective diplopia often improve. However, in most patients there is little change in proptosis or ophthalmoplegia. When progression occurs, it is usually in the first 1 to 2 years after antithyroid treatment. There is no satisfactory treatment. For many patients, assurance that lid retraction and stare will improve with treatment of their hyperthyroidism and that progression is unlikely is adequate. Periorbital and eyelid edema may improve if patients sleep with their head elevated, and diuretics may be tried. Eye irritation and pain can be treated with 1% methylcellulose eye drops. Patients with marked inflammation or threatened vision should be treated aggressively with corticosteroids or orbital decompression. Both are reasonably effective, and there are no established criteria for the selection of either.

Spaulding SW, Utiger RD. The Thyroid: Physiology, Hyperthyroidism, Hypothyroidism, and the Painful Thyroid. In P Felig, et al. (Eds.), *Endrocrinology and Metabolism*. New York: McGraw-Hill, 1981. Pp 301–326.
  A discussion of all aspects of hyperthyroidism.
Davis PJ, Davis FB. Hyperthyroidism in patients over the age of 60 years: Clinical features in 85 patients. *Medicine* 53:161–181, 1974.
  Patients over 60 with hyperthyroidism were found to have thyroid enlargement less often, and anorexia, constipation, pulse rates less than 100, and atrial fibrillation more often than younger patients.
Kaplan MM, Utiger RD. Diagnosis of hyperthyroidism. *Clin Endocrinol Metab* 7:97–113, 1978.
  A short review of the pathophysiology of excess thyroid hormone production and the usefulness of various laboratory tests in patients with hyperthyroidism.
Kidd A, et al. Immunologic aspects of Graves' and Hashimoto's diseases. *Metabolism* 29:80–99, 1980.
  A review of the genetics and abnormalities of humoral and cell-mediated immunity found in patients with these diseases.
Woolf PD. Transient painless thyroiditis with hyperthyroidism: A variant of lymphocytic thyroiditis. *Endocrine Rev* 1:411–420, 1980.
  A review describing the diagnosis, course, and pathologic features of this illness and discussing the hypothesis that it is a form of chronic autoimmune thyroiditis.
Sugrue D, et al. Hyperthyroidism in the land of Graves: Results of treatment by surgery, radioiodine, and carbimazole in 837 cases. *Q J Med* 49:51–61, 1980.
  The outcome of therapy was studied in 837 patients. Most (91%) patients given antithyroid drug therapy for less than 2 years relapsed; the relapse rate was 49% in those treated longer. Relapse rates were much lower in patients treated with ^{131}I and surgery, but many developed hypothyroidism.
Gorman CA. Endocrine ophthalmology: Current ideas concerning etiology, pathogenesis, and treatment. *Endocrine Rev* 5:200, 1984.
  A review of the ophthalmopathy of Graves' disease, including pathogenesis, clinical manifestations, and management.

---

95. HYPOTHYROIDISM
Robert D. Utiger

The spectrum of hypothyroidism ranges from a few nonspecific symptoms, to overt hypothyroidism, to myxedema coma. The biochemical spectrum is even broader, because it includes subclinical, or compensated, hypothyroidism. Patients with subclinical hypothyroidism have thyroid disease but are asymptomatic because serum thyroid hormone concentrations are maintained within the normal range by elevated serum thyrotropin (TSH) concentrations.

The most common cause of hypothyroidism is primary thyroid disease (thyroidal hypothyroidism), but hypothyroidism may also be due to pituitary or hypothalamic disease (hypothyrotropic hypothyroidism). Hypothyroidism occurs in 3 to 6% of the adult population, but is symptomatic only in a minority of them. It occurs 8 to 10 times more often in women than in men and usually develops after the age of 30.

Clinical Features

The major symptoms and signs of hypothyroidism reflect slowing of physiologic function. Virtually every organ system can be affected. The onset of symptoms may be rapid or gradual; severity varies considerably and correlates poorly with biochemical changes. Because many manifestations of hypothyroidism are nonspecific, the diagnosis is particularly likely to be overlooked in patients with other chronic illnesses and in the elderly.

Behavioral and Neurologic Symptoms

Most hypothyroid patients complain of fatigue, loss of energy, and lethargy. Their level of physical activity decreases, and they may speak and move slowly. Mental activity declines, and there is inattentiveness, decreased intellectual function, and sometimes overt depression. Neurologic symptoms include hearing loss, paresthesias, and objective neuropathy, particularly the carpal tunnel syndrome.

Skin

Hypothyroidism results in dry, thick, and scaly skin, which is often cool and pale. Less commonly, there is nonpitting edema of the hands, feet, and periorbital regions (myxedema). Pitting edema also may be present. Hair may become coarse and brittle, hair growth slows, and hair loss may occur.

Cardiovascular System

Cardiac rate and contractility are decreased. The heart is dilated, cardiac wall thickness is increased by interstitial edema, and there may be a pericardial effusion. These findings, along with peripheral edema, may simulate congestive heart failure. However, most hypothyroid patients can increase their cardiac output normally in response to increased demand. Increased peripheral resistance may result in hypertension. The electrocardiogram may show low voltage and/or nonspecific ST and T wave changes. Hypercholesterolemia is common. Whether or not there is an increased prevalence of ischemic heart disease is controversial. Anginal symptoms, when present, characteristically occur less often after the onset of hypothyroidism, probably because of decreased activity.

Respiratory System

Dyspnea on effort is common. This complaint may be caused by enlargement of the tongue and larynx, causing upper airway obstruction, or by respiratory muscle weakness, interstitial edema of the lungs, and/or pleural effusions. Hoarseness from vocal cord enlargement often occurs.

Gastrointestinal System

Hypothyroidism does not cause obesity, but modest weight gain from fluid retention and fat deposition often occurs. Gastrointestinal motility is decreased, leading to constipation and abdominal distention. Abdominal distention may be caused by ascites as well.

Musculoskeletal System

Muscle and joint aches, pains, and stiffness are common. Objective myopathy and joint swelling or effusions are less often present. The relaxation phase of the tendon reflexes is prolonged. Serum creatine phosphokinase and alanine aminotransferase activities are often increased, probably attributable as much to slowed enzyme degradation as to increased release from muscle.

Hematopoietic System

Anemia, caused by decreased red blood cell production, occurs in about one-quarter of hypothyroid patients; it is probably from decreased need for peripheral oxygen delivery rather than hematopoietic defect. Most patients have no evidence of iron, folic acid, or cyanocobalamin deficiency.

Endocrine System

There may be menorrhagia, secondary amenorrhea, infertility, and, rarely, galactorrhea. Pituitary-adrenal function is usually normal. Pituitary enlargement from hyperplasia of the thyrotropes occurs rarely in patients with primary hypothyroidism; such enlargement also may be caused by a primary pituitary tumor, with resulting TSH deficiency. In patients with diabetes mellitus, hypothyroidism results in increased insulin sensitivity.

Laboratory Diagnosis

Serum T_4

Initial evaluation of a patient suspected of having hypothyroidism should include determination of serum total and free T_4 concentrations. The former alone is inadequate because it may be low as a result of either decreased production of serum thyroid hormone–binding proteins or decreased T_4 secretion. The serum free T_4 concentration may be measured directly or indirectly using the T_3-resin uptake test, which indicates the number of unoccupied binding sites on thyroid-binding proteins. The product of the T_3-resin uptake and the serum T_4 concentration is the free T_4 index. A low serum free T_4 index or serum free T_4 concentration is a reasonably specific and sensitive indicator of hypothyroidism. The serum free T_4 index is more widely available and less expensive. Low serum free T_4 index values may occur in seriously ill patients with nonthyroidal illness, but such patients are not likely to be encountered in ambulatory settings. Mild symptomatic hypothyroidism also may occur with serum T_4 concentrations and free T_4 index values in the low-normal range.

Serum T_3

Serum T_3 measurements are of no use in the evaluation of a patient suspected of having hypothyroidism, because levels are normal in 20 to 30% of patients with hypothyroidism and low in many patients with nonthyroidal illnesses.

Thyroid-Stimulating Hormone (TSH)

Secretion of TSH is exquisitely sensitive to small changes in serum T_4 and T_3 concentrations. Serum TSH always should be measured when hypothyroidism is suspected, for the following reasons. First, increased serum TSH concentrations are found in all patients with symptomatic primary hypothyroidism, and thus the test confirms that diagnosis. Second, modest elevations in serum TSH concentrations may identify mildly symptomatic patients with thyroid disease who have serum T_4 concentrations within the normal range. Finally, a low or normal serum TSH concentration in a hypothyroid patient makes radiologic and hormonal evaluation for pituitary or hypothalamic disease mandatory. Pituitary TSH deficiency can be distinguished from hypothalamic thyrotropin-releasing hormone (TRH) deficiency by finding an increase in serum TSH after exogenous TRH administration in patients with hypothalamic TRH deficiency; however, such testing is unnecessary.

Causes

The cause of hypothyroidism should be determined if possible because the disease may be transient and hence not require therapy. A cause is usually evident from the history and physical examination.

Primary (Thyroidal) Hypothyroidism

Primary hypothyroidism results from destruction of thyroid tissue by autoimmune mechanisms, irradiation, or surgical removal, or from genetic or biochemical inhibition of thyroid hormone biosynthesis. Chronic autoimmune thyroiditis is the most common cause of hypothyroidism. It may be goitrous (Hashimoto's disease) or nongoitrous (atrophic thyroiditis). ^{131}I therapy for hyperthyroidism results in hypothyroidism in 20 to 60% of patients within the first year after therapy and in 1 to 2% each year thereafter. Hypothyroidism also results from external neck irradiation therapy in doses of 2000 rads or more such as are used in the treatment of malignant lymphoma and laryngeal carcinoma. After total thyroidectomy for thyroid carcinoma, hypothyroidism is expected; its occurrence after subtotal thyroidectomy is extremely variable, ranging from 25 to 75% in different series. Most patients become hypothyroid within the first year after surgery, but thereafter there is a small steady increment. Rare causes of primary hypothyroidism include inborn errors of thyroid hormone biosynthesis and infiltrative disease such as cystinosis and amyloidosis. In all the above situations, hypothyroidism is permanent.

Transient Hypothyroidism

Drugs that block thyroid hormone synthesis and secretion, such as propylthiouracil, methimazole, lithium carbonate, and iodine, can cause transient hypothyroidism. Iodine can cause sustained reduction in thyroid secretion in patients with autoimmune thyroiditis or patients who have had ^{131}I therapy, but not in normal subjects. Transient hypothyroidism also occurs in the first months after ^{131}I therapy or after subtotal thyroidectomy, during recovery from subacute thyroiditis or painless thyroiditis, in the postpartum period, and from iodine deficiency.

Secondary (Hypothyrotropic) Hypothyroidism

TSH deficiency usually occurs along with other anterior pituitary hormone deficiencies and is most often caused by a pituitary tumor. Other causes include pituitary infarction, infiltrative processes, trauma, and idiopathic hypophysitis. Many of the same processes may involve the hypothalamus and thereby cause TRH deficiency.

Treatment

Patients with symptomatic hypothyroidism should be treated with 1-thyroxine (T_4) unless their hypothyroidism is expected to be transient or to subside if some medication is discontinued. Complete amelioration of all clinical and biochemical manifestations of hypothyroidism usually can be achieved with T_4 in dosages of 100 to 150 μg daily; only rarely is a larger dosage required. In young adults the initial dosage should be 100 μg daily. The dosage can be increased in 50-μg increments at 4- to 6-week intervals until clinical and biochemical euthyroidism is achieved. In older patients, lower initial dosages (25 μg) and more gradual increments are indicated. Cautious replacement is particularly warranted in patients with ischemic heart disease, because angina pectoris or cardiac arrhythmias may be precipitated by T_4 therapy. Improvement in energy and activity is usually evident within 1 to 2 weeks after initiation of therapy, but objective manifestations diminish more slowly.

The adequacy of therapy can be assessed by clinical and biochemical means. Relief of symptoms usually requires T_4 dosages that raise the serum T_4 concentration to the normal range. At that point, slight TSH hypersecretion may persist, but there is no evidence that additional increases in T_4 dosage are of any benefit. Nonetheless it seems desirable theoretically to restore the serum TSH concentration to normal as well. Once this is achieved, dosage adjustments are rarely indicated, and the patient need be seen only at 6-month or yearly intervals. The most important reason for such visits is the opportunity they provide to reinforce the need for continued therapy, because patient-initiated discontinuation of T_4 therapy is an important "complication" of treatment.

Patients with subclinical hypothyroidism probably should be treated. Some may have unrecognized symptoms and hence may benefit from therapy. Also, unrecognized symptomatic hypothyroidism may develop as time progresses. No other hazards are known to result from not treating these patients.

Thyroid preparations other than T_4, such as T_3 and natural or synthetic mixtures of T_4 and T_3, should not be used. Because they contain T_3, serum T_4 measurements underestimate the amount of hormone being given, and the risk of iatrogenic hyperthyroidism is therefore greater in patients receiving these preparations.

Spaulding SW, Utiger RD. The Thyroid: Physiology, Hypothyroidism, and the Painful Thyroid. In P Felig, et al. (Eds.), *Endocrinology and Metabolism*. New York: McGraw-Hill, 1981. Pp. 326–339.
   A discussion of all aspects of hypothyroidism.
Bigos ST, et al. Spectrum of pituitary alterations with mild and severe thyroid impairment. *J Clin Endocrinol Metab* 46:317–325, 1978.
   A demonstration of the sensitivity of thyroid-stimulating hormone secretion to small decreases in thyroid hormone secretion. Serum triiodothyronine levels were often normal in patients with mild hypothyroidism.
Tunbridge WMG, et al. Natural history of autoimmune thyroiditis. *Br Med J* 1:258–262, 1981.
   A study of the course of autoimmune thyroiditis. Clinical hypothyroidism developed

in women with positive tests for thyroid antibodies and elevated serum TSH concentrations at the rate of 5% per year.

Lamberg BA. A etiology of hypothyroidism. *Clin Endocrinol Metab* 8:3–19, 1979.
   A review of the various causes of hypothyroidism and the mechanisms by which they result in impaired thyroid secretion.

Malone JF, Cullen MJ. Two mechanisms for hypothyroidism after ^{131}I therapy. *Lancet* 1:73–75, 1976.
   Radioiodine therapy for hyperthyroidism causes hypothyroidism by acutely destroying thyroid tissue and by impairing the replicative ability of thyroid follicular cells.

Krugman LC, et al. Patterns of recovery of the hypothalamic-pituitary-thyroid axis in patients taken off chronic thyroid therapy. *J Clin Endocrinol Metab* 41:70–80, 1975.
   Thyroid therapy must be withdrawn for 3 to 4 weeks before pituitary-thyroid function returns to normal or before the characteristic findings of hypothyroidism emerge.

Stock JM, Surks MI, Oppenheimer JH. Replacement dosage of l-thyroxine in hypothyroidism. *N Engl J Med* 290:529–533, 1974.
   A study of the effects of different dosages of T_4 on serum thyroid hormone and TSH concentrations in patients with hypothyroidism. Normalization of these parameters was found to require from 100 to 200 μg of T_4 daily in almost all patients.

96. THYROID NODULES
Robert D. Utiger

A single thyroid nodule (solitary nodule) in a patient who is euthyroid and whose thyroid gland is otherwise apparently normal is most often an adenoma, cyst, or adenomatous nodule that is part of an otherwise unrecognized multinodular goiter. It also may be a thyroid carcinoma, localized thyroiditis, or, very rarely, a nonthyroid mass. Of these, only carcinoma poses any appreciable risk and hence needs to be identified; distinguishing among the other lesions is not important.

Thyroid nodules are common, occurring in about 3% of the adult population. Thyroid carcinoma is rare, with an incidence in the 1969 to 1971 national cancer survey of 3.7 per 100,000 per year, or one new case yearly per 27,000 people. The key question in dealing with a patient with a thyroid nodule is how to identify the nodule that is a carcinoma.

Clinical Findings
The vast majority of patients with a solitary nodule have only an asymptomatic neck mass. Only occasionally is there a history of pain, hoarseness, dysphagia, or rapid growth, even in those patients whose nodule is a thyroid carcinoma.

Risk factors for thyroid carcinoma include a history of head or neck irradiation in infancy (not adolescence) and family history of thyroid carcinoma. A solitary nodule is more likely to be a carcinoma in younger individuals, especially men, since benign thyroid nodules occur less frequently in them than in middle-aged or older women. Both benign and malignant thyroid nodules occur about four times more often in patients who had head and neck irradiation in infancy. The threshold radiation dose is very low and the latent period ranges from 5 to 30 years. Medullary thyroid carcinoma may be familial, occurring either alone or as one component of type II multiple endocrine neoplasia.

Physical findings that increase the chances that a thyroid nodule is a carcinoma include fixation of the nodule to underlying tissue, hard consistency, cervical lymphadenopathy, and hoarseness resulting from vocal cord paralysis.

Diagnosis
Laboratory studies should include measurement of the serum T_4 concentration and T_3-resin uptake; if hyperthyroidism is present, the nodule is an autonomously functioning thyroid adenoma, and additional workup is not necessary. Serum calcitonin should be

measured in patients who have a family history of medullary thyroid carcinoma, pheochromocytoma, or hyperparathyroidism.

Procedures for determining the function and nature of a nodule, in order to identify those likely to be a carcinoma, include thyroid scanning, echography, and fine needle aspiration. Thyroid radioisotope scanning is done with ^{99m}Tc pertechnetate or ^{123}I iodide. ^{99m}Tc pertechnetate is more convenient because the image is obtained 20 to 30 minutes after isotope administration, whereas iodide scans are done 24 hours after isotope administration. Approximately 15% of solitary nodules prove to be hyperfunctioning (autonomously functioning thyroid adenoma) and 85% are poorly or normally functioning. Thyroid carcinomas usually concentrate either isotope less efficiently than normal thyroid tissue and thus appear as hypofunctioning, or "cold," on the scan, but some are isofunctional. Most benign nodules also are hypofunctioning. Because benign nodules are much more prevalent than malignant ones, most hypofunctioning nodules are benign. Therefore, a thyroid scan does not establish a diagnosis of thyroid carcinoma. The principal values of a thyroid radioisotope scan are to discover a hyperfunctioning adenoma, which is almost always benign, and to detect nodules other than the one that was palpated, which indicates that the patient has a nontoxic multinodular goiter. When a nodule is found to be hypofunctioning, echography can be used to distinguish those that are cystic (20%), which are usually benign, from those that are solid (80%), which may be a carcinoma. With the advent of fine needle aspiration, however, echography is of little value. Fine needle aspiration biopsy is a simple and reliable way to identify thyroid carcinoma and should be done in patients whose nodules are iso- or hypofunctional. Cystic nodules are discovered readily by this procedure. Sufficient material for cytologic study is obtained by fine needle aspiration in over 95% of patients, and the procedure is complication-free. Approximately 20% of hypofunctioning solid nodules prove to be carcinomas; 80% are thyroid adenomas or other benign lesions. False-positive and false-negative cytologic diagnoses occur in approximately 5% of patients.

A patient whose isotope scan reveals a hyperfunctioning nodule and whose serum T_4 concentration is normal need only be re-examined periodically. Because most thyroid nodules are iso- or hypofunctioning, it follows that most patients are referred for fine needle aspiration biopsy. Alternative approaches are to limit needle aspiration to patients who have risk factors for thyroid carcinoma, those whose nodule increases in size during a period of observation, or those whose nodule does not decrease in size after treatment with 150 to 200 μg of L-thyroxine (T_4) daily for several months. Few thyroid carcinomas are likely to be overlooked by these more conservative approaches, but early cytologic study has intangible benefits for both patient and physician.

For patients with a history of head and neck irradiation who have no palpable thyroid abnormalities, yearly thyroid examination is all that is necessary.

Specific Types of Thyroid Nodules

Thyroid cysts probably result from necrosis and liquefaction of a thyroid adenoma, or possibly a carcinoma. A cyst is treated by aspiration, with cytologic examination of the fluid to rule out the possibility that the nodule is a cystic thyroid carcinoma. Aspiration results in substantial regression or disappearance of the cyst in most patients. Recurrence of fluid sometimes occurs; re-aspiration may be performed if the patient wishes but is not mandatory. There is no evidence that thyroid hormone therapy reduces the likelihood of recurrence.

Autonomously functioning thyroid adenomas are benign tumors that concentrate iodide and synthesize and secrete thyroid hormones. The autonomously secreted thyroid hormone inhibits TSH secretion so that function of the remaining thyroid tissue is reduced; the nodule thus appears hyperfunctioning—"hot"—on the thyroid scan. Most patients with these adenomas are euthyroid, but when the nodules are 3 cm or larger in diameter, hyperthyroidism may be present. Patients who are euthyroid do not require treatment, because later increase in either nodule size or thyroid secretion is uncommon. In a recent study of 159 patients followed for up to 15 years, 86% of patients had no change in nodule size and 93% remained euthyroid. If the patient desires treatment for cosmetic reasons or local discomfort, ^{131}I ablation is the method of choice. This therapy effectively destroys the nodule, and there is little risk of posttherapy hypothyroidism because the suppressed thyroid resumes function as nodule function declines.

Hypofunctional benign nodules are most commonly follicular adenomas, papillary adenomas, or colloid nodules. All are well encapsulated and usually compress adjacent tissue. Administration of T_4 in dosages of 100 to 200 μg daily indefinitely to patients who have such nodules diagnosed by fine needle aspiration biopsy may reduce the size of the nodule or prevent additional growth. T_4 therapy is also sometimes recommended to prevent the development of new nodules, but there is little evidence that such patients have an increased risk of developing new nodules.

Three types of *thyroid carcinoma* commonly present as a solitary nodule: papillary, follicular, and medullary carcinoma. All are treated surgically. Anaplastic carcinoma and lymphoma are rare and usually occur in patients with preexisting nontoxic multinodular goiter or Hashimoto's disease and are not discussed here.

Papillary carcinoma is the most common thyroid carcinoma, accounting for 50 to 80% of them. Nearly all carcinomas in patients who had head and neck irradiation in infancy are of this type. Papillary cancers occur at any age but most often in the third and fourth decades, and they usually present as a slow-growing asymptomatic mass. They are unencapsulated tumors that spread by invasion of surrounding thyroid tissue or lymphatics. Approximately 50% of patients have cervical node metastases at the time of initial surgery. This tumor has a very slow growth rate; although recurrences after initial therapy occur in 10 to 20% of patients, death from the cancer is very rare.

Follicular carcinoma accounts for 10 to 20% of thyroid carcinomas and occurs most often in the third and fourth decades. These tumors are characteristically well differentiated and encapsulated, and metastasize to lungs and bone by blood vessel invasion. Follicular carcinoma is also a very slow-growing tumor, although it is slightly more lethal than papillary carcinoma.

A medullary carcinoma is a tumor of thyroid parafollicular, rather than follicular, cells. It accounts for approximately 10% of thyroid carcinomas and occurs sporadically and in two familial forms. In one, affected family members have only medullary carcinoma, and in the other, affected patients and family members may have pheochromocytoma and hyperparathyroidism as well as medullary carcinoma. Because all medullary carcinomas secrete calcitonin, serum calcitonin measurements are valuable to indicate the presence of this tumor and to monitor the course of disease. Medullary carcinoma is often multicentric and is somewhat more malignant than papillary or follicular carcinoma.

Mazzaferri EL. Papillary and follicular thyroid cancer: A selective approach to diagnosis and treatment. *Annu Rev Med* 32:73–91, 1981.
This review describes the clinical features of thyroid carcinoma and how patients whose thyroid nodule is a carcinoma can be identified.

Maxon HR, et al. Clinically important radiation—associated thyroid disease: A controlled study. *JAMA* 244:1802–1805, 1980.
The authors found an excess of both benign and malignant thyroid tumors in a large group of patients who had received external head and neck radiotherapy in childhood.

Blum M, Rothschild, M. Improved nonoperative diagnosis of solitary "cold" thyroid nodule: Surgical selection based on risk factors and three months of suppression. *JAMA* 243:242–245, 1980.
Clinical risk factor assessment identified most patients likely to have carcinoma in this study of 118 patients with solitary thyroid nodules. Of 26 patients whose nodule did not shrink 50% or more during thyroid hormone therapy, 5 also had carcinoma.

Hamberger B, et al. Fine-needle aspiration of thyroid nodules: Impact on thyroid practice and cost of care. *Am J Med* 73:381–384, 1982.
Fine needle aspiration biopsy in 455 patients with thyroid nodules resulted in a marked decrease in the number of patients referred for surgery, with a correspondingly higher number found to have thyroid cancer at surgery.

Mazzaferri EL, et al. Papillary thyroid carcinoma: The impact of therapy in 576 patients. *Medicine* 56:171–196, 1977.
A comprehensive review of the clinical manifestations as well as the results of several types of treatment in patients with the most common type of thyroid carcinoma.

Hamburger JI. Evolution of toxicity in solitary nontoxic autonomously functioning thyroid nodules. *J Clin Endocrinol Metab* 50:1089–1093, 1980.
These nodules were found to change in size or function in only a small minority of a large group of patients followed for up to 15 years.

Van Herle AJ, et al. The thyroid nodule. *Ann Intern Med* 96:221–232, 1982.
  A discussion of the use of thyroid ultrasonography and fine needle aspiration biopsy in patients with a thyroid nodule. It also includes a thorough analysis of the sensitivity and specificity of tests used to identify carcinoma and of the most cost-effective ways to identify nodules that are a thyroid carcinoma.

97. GOITER

Robert D. Utiger

Visible and/or palpable thyroid enlargement occurs in 3 to 8% of adults living in areas in which iodine intake is adequate. Virtually all of these patients are clinically and biochemically euthyroid.

Thyroid enlargement may take the form of (1) a diffuse goiter, in which both thyroid lobes are more or less equally enlarged and their surfaces relatively smooth, (2) a multinodular goiter, in which both lobes are irregularly enlarged, or (3) a solitary thyroid nodule. In large groups of patients with nontoxic goiter, roughly two-thirds have diffuse or multinodular goiter and one-third have a solitary nodule. The evaluation and management of the patient with a solitary nodule are discussed in Chapter 96.

Diffuse and multinodular goiters should be distinguished because their causes, natural history, and treatment differ. Differentiation is primarily by physical examination. Laboratory tests may also be helpful. The serum thyroxine (T_4) concentration and T_3-resin uptake are used to document that the patient is euthyroid. If the serum T_4 concentration is in the low-normal range, measurement of serum TSH is indicated to detect subclinical hypothyroidism. Thyroid antibodies identify those patients with diffuse enlargement who have chronic autoimmune thyroiditis. Thyroid radioiodine uptake measurements and thyroid scans provide little information beyond that gained by palpation of the thyroid gland and should not be done routinely in patients with goiter.

Chronic Autoimmune Thyroiditis (Goitrous Autoimmune Thyroiditis, Hashimoto's Disease)

Clinical Characteristics
The goitrous form of chronic autoimmune thyroiditis is the most common cause of diffuse goiter. Most patients are women between 30 and 60 years old. The thyroid enlargement is typically moderate and symmetric, the gland surface is slightly irregular, and its texture is firm or rubbery. In clinically euthyroid patients, serum T_4 concentrations are usually low-normal, and serum TSH concentrations are normal or modestly increased. Hashimoto's disease also may result in overt hypothyroidism. The thyroid radioiodine uptake may be low, normal, or slightly increased; thyroid scans usually show either uniform or heterogeneous patterns of isotope uptake.

Pathogenesis
The pathogenesis of Hashimoto's disease is dependent on both the cellular immune system and autoantibodies, which include cytotoxic antibodies, antibodies that inhibit TSH binding to its receptor, and antibodies that stimulate thyroid epithelial growth. Variations in the nature and degree of these abnormalities in serum and cellular immunity probably explain the variations in functional impairment and response to therapy found in patients with Hashimoto's disease.

Diagnosis
The diagnosis is most readily confirmed by positive serum tests for antithyroglobulin and/or antithyroid microsomal antibodies; both are present, usually in high titer, in most patients with Hashimoto's disease. Positive tests for thyroid antibodies may also be found in patients with other thyroid diseases, especially Graves' disease, and in normal individuals, but they are not found in patients with multinodular goiter, the disorder most often confused with Hashimoto's disease.

Prognosis
The disease usually progresses slowly over a period of months or years. Thyroid enlargement may increase or diminish, and thyroid functional impairment becomes evident or worsens, particularly in patients in whom reduction in goiter size occurs.

Treatment
To reduce the size of the gland and prevent hypothyroidism, T_4 therapy, in dosages of 100 to 200 μg daily, is recommended for all patients, except perhaps those with only slight thyroid enlargement and normal serum T_4 and TSH concentrations. The patient should be re-examined after 2 to 3 months of therapy and serum T_4 measured to be sure the T_4 dosage is not excessive. Thereafter, semiannual or annual visits are appropriate. In the majority of patients, T_4 therapy gradually reduces thyroid size. Less often, the reduction occurs rapidly and is nearly complete, or there is no change. Withdrawal of therapy is almost always followed by recurrent thyroid enlargement and/or hypothyroidism; therapy therefore should be lifelong.

Sporadic Diffuse Goiter (Simple Goiter)

Clinical Characteristics
Sporadic diffuse goiter is defined as thyroid enlargement in a euthyroid patient that does not result from an inflammatory, infiltrative, or neoplastic process. Patients are usually young women, ranging in age from 10 to 30 years. The thyroid gland is usually only moderately enlarged and soft in consistency. Serum thyroid hormone concentrations are normal, although serum TSH concentrations occasionally are slightly increased.

Pathogenesis
Sporadic diffuse goiter is only a descriptive term. Such goiters undoubtedly have many causes; they are believed, at least in their early stages, to be caused by TSH hypersecretion secondary to small decreases in thyroid hormone secretion. Postulated causes of decreased thyroid secretion include mild inherited thyroid biosynthetic defects, environmental goitrogens or drugs, and iodide excess; however, firm evidence implicating any of these factors is sparse and rarely obtained in an individual patient.

Diagnosis
This diagnosis may be made when tests for antithyroid antibodies are negative in a patient with diffuse thyroid enlargement.

Treatment
Although treatment is not required, if thyroid enlargement concerns the patient, T_4 therapy may be given. Treatment results in some reduction in thyroid enlargement in the majority of patients and may limit the evolution from diffuse to nodular goiter.

Nontoxic Multinodular Goiter

Clinical Characteristics
Nontoxic multinodular goiter is a common type of thyroid enlargement, especially in women above the age of 30 to 40 years. It may be discovered incidentally or found in a patient with a long-standing history of thyroid enlargement. The patient may have local symptoms of thyroid enlargement, such as neck fullness, difficulty swallowing, or coughing, but is often asymptomatic. On palpation both thyroid lobes are irregularly enlarged, often asymmetrically; it may be possible to feel discrete nodules of varying size and consistency. Rarely a multinodular goiter reaches sufficient size to produce thoracic inlet obstruction, respiratory symptoms, or a mediastinal mass. Acute hemorrhage into a nodule may occur, resulting in sudden painful increase in its size; the pain usually subsides in a few days, and the swelling diminishes in several weeks.

Diagnosis
Thyroid hormone secretion and serum thyroid hormone concentrations in patients with nontoxic multinodular goiter are, by definition, within normal limits, as is thyroidal radioiodine uptake. Thyroid isotope scans reveal a spectrum of abnormalities, ranging from a heterogeneous uptake pattern to discrete hyperfunctioning or hypofunctioning

areas that often correlate poorly with palpable nodules. Many patients have evidence of thyroid autonomy, as indicated by subnormal serum TSH responses to thyrotropin-releasing hormone (TRH). From the practical point of view, the diagnosis is made by palpation. Euthyroidism should be confirmed by serum T_4 measurement; other tests are not usually indicated. In the absence of obvious nodules, tests for antithyroid antibodies serve to rule out Hashimoto's disease.

Pathogenesis

Nontoxic multinodular goiter is thought to evolve from diffuse goiter (see previous section) by development of local areas of autonomous hyperplasia. These areas may enlarge sufficiently to become palpable nodules and remain hyperplastic, or they may resolve in such a way that the nodules become colloid-filled thyroid follicles with decreased function. Alternatively, colloid-filled follicles may arise de novo. Some nodules lose their blood supply and become necrotic, cystic, or fibrotic. These events result in a pathologic picture that is extremely varied.

Prognosis

The natural course of nontoxic multinodular goiter is one of very gradual thyroid enlargement. Continued growth of one or more autonomous hyperplastic nodules may result in hyperthyroidism, although this is rare, even in patients with large multinodular goiters. This disorder does not result in hypothyroidism. Carcinoma in a nontoxic multinodular goiter is rare but should be suspected if a nodule is hard and enlarges during observation.

Treatment

The treatment of nontoxic multinodular goiter is controversial. If there are no pressure symptoms or cosmetic problems, treatment is unnecessary. If such symptoms are present, thyroid hormone therapy may be tried. Dosages of 100 to 200 µg of T_4 daily result in some reduction of thyroid enlargement in from 30 to 60% of patients. Therapy should be given for 6 to 12 months before being abandoned as ineffective. Complete regression is rare. T_4 therapy is not without hazard; it may cause hyperthyroidism in patients whose endogenous thyroid secretion is largely autonomous. If treated with T_4, the patient should be re-examined and the serum T_4 concentration determined after several months of therapy. The development of clinical evidence of hyperthyroidism and/or a rise in serum T_4 concentration mandates discontinuation of therapy. Very large multinodular goiters causing pressure or obstructive symptoms require surgical removal. Iodides in any form should not be administered to patients with multinodular goiter because they may induce hyperthyroidism.

Doniach D, Bottazzo GF, Russell RCG. Goitrous autoimmune thyroiditis (Hashimoto's disease). *Clin Endocrinol Metab* 8:63–80, 1979.
  A thorough discussion of the clinical and laboratory manifestations and pathogenesis of Hashimoto's disease.
Kidd A, et al. Immunologic aspects of Graves' and Hashimoto's disease. *Metabolism* 29:80–90, 1980.
  A comprehensive review of the genetics and humoral and cell-mediated immunologic abnormalities found in patients with thyroid autoimmune diseases.
Monteleone JA, et al. Differentiation of chronic lymphocytic thyroiditis and simple goiter in pediatrics. *J Pediatr* 183:3811–3815, 1973.
  Of 81 patients who had thyroid biopsies, clinical and laboratory findings were similar in both groups except for the presence of thyroid autoantibodies in patients with thyroiditis.
Beckers C. Thyroid nodules. *Clin Endocrinol Metab* 18:181–192, 1979.
  A short review of the clinical manifestations, pathogenesis, and available therapeutic strategies in patients with nodular goiter.
Shimaoka K, Sokal J. Suppressive therapy of nontoxic goiter. *Am J Med* 57:576–583, 1974.
  Therapy with T_4 or T_3 resulted in reduction in goiter size in over half of 114 patients with solitary nodules or multinodular goiter.
Vagenakis AG, et al. Iodide-induced thyrotoxicosis in Boston. *N Engl J Med* 487: 523–527, 1972.

Iodide therapy caused hyperthyroidism in half of a small group of patients with non-toxic multinodular goiter. Such therapy should be avoided in these patients.

98. HYPERCALCEMIA
Robert H. Fletcher

Hypercalcemia can cause obvious symptoms or can be a complication of a serious underlying disease, such as cancer or sarcoidosis. Usually, however, hypercalcemia is asymptomatic and discovered by accident on a serum chemistry panel performed as part of a general health examination or as an investigation of problems unrelated to hypercalcemia.

Definition
Serum calcium is ordinarily measured as the concentration of the total of ionized and bound calcium. Measurements of ionized calcium, the physiologically active compound, are not generally available. Because most calcium is bound to serum proteins, normal levels vary with concentration of serum albumin. As a rule of thumb, serum calcium levels rise or fall 0.7 mg/dl per 1 gm/dl albumin. Serum calcium levels do not vary in a clinically important way according to age and sex.

Hypercalcemia is usually defined as a serum calcium concentration above 10.5 mg/dl (2.62 mmol/L). The precise definition of the upper limit varies from one laboratory to another according to the analytic method used, the reference population, and the choice of a cutoff point between normal and abnormal.

Judgments about the presence of hypercalcemia should not be based on single determinations. Elevations are usually small (< 1.0 mg/dl), and there is broad overlap between normal levels and levels of people with diseases causing hypercalcemia. In one study, for example, 42% of patients with documented hyperparathyroidism had a mean serum calcium concentration of 10.5 mg/dl or less. Many people with a serum calcium level above 10.5 mg/dl on one determination have lower levels if the test is repeated. Therefore, serum calcium should be considered elevated only after several high levels are obtained, unless the initial levels are very high, hypercalcemia was strongly suspected before the test, or there is an associated disease that might be a cause (e.g., multiple myeloma) or a complication (e.g., renal stones) of hypercalcemia.

Symptoms
Serum calcium concentrations in the 10.5 to 11.0 mg/dl range usually are not symptomatic. In general, the faster the rise in serum calcium, the more severe the symptoms at a given serum concentration.

The classic symptoms of hypercalcemia include, in descending order of frequency, fatigue, polydipsia, mental confusion, anorexia, polyuria, nausea and vomiting, muscle weakness, and constipation. Other manifestations are related to the underlying cause or complications: bone pain, renal stones, pancreatitis, and rarely, peptic ulcer disease. Hypertension may be more prevalent in patients with hypercalcemia.

It is often difficult to detect hypercalcemia by symptoms alone. Relatively few patients have the pronounced hypercalcemia syndrome. Because the symptoms are nonspecific and common, they are easily overlooked or attributed to other diseases. Similarly, if elevated serum calcium is known to be present, it may be difficult to know, without a trial of treatment, whether it is causing symptoms.

Causes
The majority of patients with hypercalcemia—approximately 90% of those identified in a general hospital—have primary hyperparathyroidism or cancer. Other conditions causing hypercalcemia are less commonly encountered, and the elevations are usually not sufficiently severe or protracted to cause major complications.

Primary hyperparathyroidism is present in 1 to 5 adults per 1000 in the general population. It is uncommon before the age of 40 years, but the incidence increases thereafter. The disease is twice as common in women as in men. Until recently, primary hyperparathyroidism was usually discovered because of complications: renal stones, painful bone disease, peptic ulcer disease, or overt hypercalcemia syndrome. Now, because of widespread use of serum chemistry panels that include measurement of serum calcium, many patients with primary hyperparathyroidism (about half in one study of a community) are discovered because of small elevations in serum calcium. Most remain asymptomatic and without detectable complications for many years after diagnosis.

Cancer often causes hypercalcemia, with carcinomas of the breast and bronchus most common. A wide variety of other malignancies can also be responsible. Multiple myeloma usually causes hypercalcemia at some time in its course. Usually the neoplasm is overt. In one series, 75% of patients had obvious bone metastases at the time the elevated serum calcium was discovered. However, hypercalcemia can occur in malignancy without metastatic bone lesions. A variety of humoral mechanisms have been described, including peptides that activate osteoclasts or mimic the action of parathyroid hormone, prostaglandins, and rarely, exogenous parathyroid hormone production. Most malignant hypercalcemia is slight and only mildly symptomatic. Renal stones and nonmetastatic bone disease are uncommon, presumably because the duration of disease is too short for metabolic complications to occur.

Thiazide diuretics decrease renal excretion of calcium and elevate mean serum calcium slightly. In approximately 2% of patients, thiazides cause hypercalcemia. In some patients, serum calcium falls after withdrawal of thiazides, usually within a month. However, most of these patients have persistent hypercalcemia when thiazides are stopped and have parathyroid adenomas found at surgery. Chlorthalidone has the same effects but other diuretics (e.g., furosemide, ethacrynic acid, spironolactone) do not cause hypercalcemia.

Vitamin D in pharmacologic dosages (as little as 50,000 IU twice a week) causes hypercalcemia by increasing intestinal absorption. This problem is found in "food faddists" and patients treated overzealously with vitamin D.

Paget's disease occasionally causes hypercalcemia in ambulatory patients. More often hypercalcemia is precipitated by a period of immobilization, in which bone deposition is decreased and the abnormally high resorption is unmasked.

Sarcoidosis is associated with hypercalcemia at some time in its course, in as many as 10% of patients. The degree of hypercalcemia follows the activity of the disease and is rarely severe.

Lithium carbonate therapy, given for bipolar (manic-depressive) illness, apparently causes a small increase in parathyroid hormone secretion and is associated with small elevations in serum calcium concentrations, and rarely, overt hypercalcemia.

Thyrotoxicosis occasionally causes elevations in serum calcium, but rarely does it cause the symptoms and complications of hypercalcemia.

In the *milk-alkali syndrome* hypercalcemia is found in association with renal insufficiency, usually in patients with peptic ulcer disease who ingest large amounts of milk and absorbable antacids (e.g., bicarbonate of soda). The syndrome is now rarely seen, perhaps because newer approaches to ulcer therapy and other forms of antacids are widely available.

Patients with physiologic causes of low serum calcium concentrations (e.g., renal failure or malabsorption) have adaptive increases in parathyroid function, with return of serum calcium toward normal (secondary hyperparathyroidism). It has been suggested that stimulated glands occasionally become autonomous—*tertiary hyperparathyroidism*—after the hypocalcemic stimulus is removed—for example, after renal transplantation—but the evidence for this is not conclusive. Hypercalcemia rarely occurs under these circumstances, and if it does, calcium homeostasis returns to normal spontaneously.

Familial hypercalcemia is uncommon. Two types have been described. Familial hypocalciuric hypercalcemia resembles primary hyperparathyroidism in clinical presentation. It is characterized by autosomal dominant inheritance and low renal excretion of calcium. Multiple endocrine neoplasia type I (MEN I) is also inherited as an autosomal dominant and is characterized by neoplasia and autonomous endocrine activity of the pituitary and parathyroid glands and the pancreas, and, in addition, peptic ulcer disease.

Other causes of hypercalcemia include *acute adrenal insufficiency, vitamin A intoxication,* and *phosphorus depletion.*

Evaluation

Faced with newly recognized hypercalcemia, the clinician should briefly consider the evidence for each possible cause. Most of the causes—but not hyperparathyroidism—can be detected or ruled out by a simple set of observations.

Primary hyperparathyroidism, in its classic form, is manifested by repeated, distinctly high, serum calcium concentrations, depressed serum phosphate, and hyperchloremic acidosis (e.g., serum $Cl^- > 102$). There may be elevated serum alkaline phosphatase, bone changes, and subperiosteal resorption, best seen by x-ray in the finger tufts. All these are signs of late and/or severe disease. In practice, the disease is often milder and the evidence equivocal. At the present time, serum parathyroid hormone assays, even when interpreted in relation to serum calcium by means of nomogram, are not sufficiently reliable to be the sole basis of a firm diagnosis of hyperparathyroidism. Often the presumptive diagnosis of hyperparathyroidism is made by excluding other causes of hypercalcemia. The only definitive evidence for hyperparathyroidism is the finding of one or more pathologic parathyroid glands at surgery.

Does the patient take a *drug* that can cause hypercalcemia, such as a thiazide, vitamin D, lithium, or vitamin A? If the patient is a "food faddist," and the history of vitamin D ingestion is difficult to elicit, elevated serum $1,25 (OH)_2$-D_3 levels are diagnostic. If any of these drugs is responsible, serum calcium levels should fall within weeks of withdrawal.

Does the patient ingest large amounts of sodium bicarbonate or calcium carbonate (e.g., Tums, Titralac)? It is estimated that about 2 dozen doses (e.g., tablets) per day for weeks are necessary to develop milk-alkali syndrome.

Cancer is usually obvious from the history and physical examination, with particular attention to bone pain and common primary sites (breast and lung). Multiple myeloma usually has concomitant anemia or proteinuria.

Paget's disease should be considered in elderly, immobilized patients with elevated serum alkaline phosphatase. X-rays of hips, spine, or skull (according to symptoms) confirm the diagnosis.

Sarcoidosis may be associated with few chest symptoms, but there is usually chest disease that is easily seen on x-ray. Response to a therapeutic trial of corticosteroids supports sarcoidosis as a cause, although many patients with other causes of hypercalcemia also respond.

Thyrotoxicosis is usually overt, except in the elderly. When in doubt, a serum thyroid panel settles the issue.

Previous chronic severe hypocalcemia from renal failure or malabsorption is clear from the medical history. In renal failure a normal serum calcium suggests increased parathyroid activity.

Familial hypercalcemia. In practice, familial hypocalciuric hypercalcemia is recognized by family history and/or failure to respond to parathyroidectomy. MEN I is established by family history and/or evidence of autonomous activity of one of the other endocrine glands ordinarily involved (pituitary and pancreas) or the presence of peptic ulcer disease.

Management

Mild, asymptomatic hypercalcemia, of whatever cause, need not be treated. If there are no symptoms or complications, it is reasonable simply to observe patients with hyperparathyroidism, particularly if serum calcium elevations are small (e.g., < 11.5 mg/dl), the patient is at high surgical risk, or there is reason to believe the patient will not live many years. There must be reliable surveillance for changes in serum calcium concentrations or the onset of complications. Re-evaluation every 4 to 6 months is usually appropriate. It is common practice to treat hypercalcemia if serum calcium is consistently above 12.0 mg/dl; some physicians set this level as low as 11.0 mg/dl.

The following paragraphs summarize the various means of controlling chronic hypercalcemia in nonhospitalized patients. The treatment of hypercalcemia emergencies is not discussed.

Hydration and activity are the mainstays of management. Fluid intake should be at least 3 L per day, and dehydration should be avoided at all times. Inactivity reduces the rate of calcium deposition in bone and should also be avoided. For patients who might have increased calcium absorption from the gut (e.g., some patients with hyperparathyroidism or sarcoidosis), dietary calcium is often restricted. Ordinarily, this amounts to avoiding dairy products.

Drugs that aggravate hypercalcemia—thiazides and vitamin D—should be withdrawn. Several drugs have been used to lower serum calcium concentrations. Furosemide and ethacrynic acid increase renal calcium excretion but at the expense of a negative calcium balance, which, in the long term, may increase the rate at which bone disease develops. Oral phosphates (e.g., Neutra-Phos capsules, 1–8/day in divided doses) lower serum calcium concentrations, particularly in patients with hypophosphatemia. Diarrhea is a common side effect; extraskeletal calcification can occur but is not common. Corticosteroids lower serum calcium in some patients with malignant hypercalcemia and most with sarcoidosis. The onset of action is within several days. Other drugs that have been suggested, but currently have no established place in the management of chronic hypercalcemia, include estrogens, calcitonin, diphosphonates, betablockers, and histamine blockers.

Bilezikian JP. The medical management of primary hyperparathyroidism. *Ann Intern Med* 96:198–202, 1982.
   A review of the various modalities available to manage primary hyperparathyroidism when patients are asymptomatic and surgery is not done.
Christensson T, Hellström K, Wengle B. Hypercalcemia and primary hyperparathyroidism. *Arch Intern Med* 137:1138–1142, 1977.
   Of 15,903 persons undergoing health screening, 95 (0.6%) had hypercalcemia; 20 of 1034 receiving thiazides (1.9%) were hypercalcemic, and 14 of these had proven hyperparathyroidism.
Sherwood LM. The multiple causes of hypercalcemia in malignant disease. *N Engl J Med* 303:1412–1413, 1980.
   A review of the mechanisms for hypercalcemia seen with malignancy.
Heath H III, Hodgson SF, Kennedy MA. Primary hyperparathyroidism. *N Engl J Med* 302:189–193, 1980.
   A description of the incidence of hyperparathyroidism in a defined population (Rochester, Minn.), by age and sex, for 1965 to 1974.
Mazzaferri EL, O'Dorisio TM, Lo Buglio AF. Treatment of hypercalcemia associated with malignancy. *Semin Oncol* 5:141–153, 1978.
   An excellent review.
Agus ZS, Wasserstein A, Goldfarb S. Disorders of calcium and magnesium homeostasis. *Am J Med* 72:473–488, 1982.
   A thoughtful review with an extensive set of references.
Gordon DL, et al. The serum calcium level and its significance in hyperthyroidism: A prospective study. *Am J Med Sci* 268:31–36, 1974.
   Mild hypercalcemia was found in 17% of patients with hyperthyroidism.
Wong ET, Freier EF. The differential diagnosis of hypercalcemia. An algorithm for more effective use of laboratory tests. *JAMA* 247:75–80, 1982.
   An algorithm for determining the cause of hypercalcemia, based on experience with hospitalized patients.

99. ASYMPTOMATIC HYPERURICEMIA

Bernard Lo

A serum urate level greater than 8.0 mg/dl in men or 7.0 mg/dl in women is statistically abnormal, since these levels are two standard deviations greater than the population mean. This definition is plausible physiologically, since serum is saturated with monosodium urate around 8 mg/dl. All urate levels discussed here refer to the colorimetric method of measuring serum urate, which is used in most autoanalyzers. This method is nonspecific; falsely elevated results can be caused by amino acids, uremia, high doses of vitamin C, and L-dopa. The uricase method is more specific and gives levels that are 0.4 to 1.0 mg/dl lower than colorimetric measurements.

True elevations of serum urate levels occur secondary to azotemia, acidosis, and diuretic use. In one series of hospitalized patients, these factors accounted for 60% of all elevated urate measurements. Other secondary causes of increased serum urate levels are myeloproliferative diseases; psoriasis; lead intoxication from moonshine whiskey; drugs such as aspirin (in dosage under 2 gm daily), ethambutol, nicotinic acid, and L-dopa; and excessive purine intake from organ meats, anchovies, sardines, and yeast. Summer weather and life stress also can be associated with temporary increases in serum urate levels. Thus before labeling a patient hyperuricemic, the physician should correct any reversible conditions and repeat the abnormal result, preferably by the uricase method.

Risk

The risk of asymptomatic hyperuricemia is the development of gouty arthritis, renal stones, or gouty nephropathy. Our assessment of the risk of developing these conditions is based on several prospective studies that are flawed by the difficulty in determining how long patients had asymptomatic hyperuricemia before the study began. Most patients with asymptomatic hyperuricemia never develop symptoms; in others, gouty arthritis or renal stones occur after 20 or 30 years. Gouty nephropathy rarely occurs before gouty arthritis.

Gouty Arthritis

In a prospective, community-based study (the Framingham Study), the risk of gouty arthritis rose with increasing elevations of the serum urate level. Gouty arthritis developed in fewer than 2% of patients with a urate level of 7.0 mg/dl in a follow-up period of 12 years. If the urate level was between 7.0 and 7.9 mg/dl, the risk of gouty arthritis developing was 17% over the course of the follow-up period. If the urate level was between 8.0 and 8.9 mg/dl, the risk was 25%. Ten patients had a urate level above 9.9 mg/dl, and nine of them developed gouty arthritis. Only 179 women had a urate level over 6.0 mg/dl; 5% developed gouty arthritis. However, in another, shorter-term study, the incidence of gouty arthritis was lower: Of 69 men whose uric acid was greater than 9 mg/dl, only 3 developed gouty arthritis in the course of 4 years. Thus treatment to prevent gouty arthritis may be unnecessary in the short term, even at very high urate levels.

Renal Stones

The risk of renal stones is approximately 3.4 per 1000 patients with asymptomatic hyperuricemia per year, compared to a little over 1 per 1000 per year in people without hyperuricemia. It is likely that increased urinary excretion of uric acid, higher serum urate levels, acidic urine, and low urine volumes increase the risk of renal stones.

Gouty Nephropathy

A chronic interstitial nephritis, gouty nephropathy is believed to be secondary to deposits of urate crystals in renal parenchyma. It is rare in patients without gouty arthritis, and evidence linking it with asymptomatic hyperuricemia is inconclusive. In one study, fewer patients with asymptomatic hyperuricemia than controls developed an increased creatinine level. It was projected that even an elevated serum urate level of 12.0 mg/dl sustained over 40 years in an asymptomatic man would increase the serum creatinine level from 1.2 mg/dl to only 2.7 mg/dl. It is not known whether treatment of hyperuricemia can prevent this mild deterioration of renal function.

Although hyperuricemia is associated with an increased risk of coronary artery disease, this association has not been shown to be independent of other known cardiac risk factors; thus there is no reason to believe that lowering of the serum urate level prevents coronary disease.

Treatment

Considering the natural history of asymptomatic hyperuricemia, most experts recommend no treatment. Gouty arthritis and renal stones may not occur for years and can be treated readily when they are found. Little permanent or serious harm to the patient is likely if treatment to lower serum urate levels is deferred until symptoms occur.

The cost of daily drugs to lower serum urate levels (approximately $100/year), side effects, and noncompliance are substantial. See Chapter 71 for a discussion of drugs and effects. The risks and benefits of treatment should be explained to the patient, whose preferences and attitudes ultimately are decisive. The recent experience with ticrynafen, a uricosuric diuretic developed for the "problem" of thiazide-induced hyperuricemia, emphasizes the dangers of using drugs in asymptomatic patients; the drug was withdrawn because of deaths from liver disease.

Patients with persistent elevations of uric acid and coexistent renal failure are probably at greater risk for gouty nephropathy and stones than patients with normal renal function. Many patients with chronic renal failure and serum urate levels of over 13.0 mg/dl are therefore treated with allopurinol, even though no evidence exists that such treatment prevents additional loss of renal function.

There is one situation in which asymptomatic patients should always be treated. Patients with cancer starting chemotherapy should be given allopurinol and adequate hydration to prevent acute uric acid tubular blockade.

Liang MH, Fries JF. Asymptomatic hyperuricemia: The case for conservative treatment. *Ann Intern Med* 88:666–670, 1978.
   A thoughtful argument against prescribing drugs to asymptomatic patients to prevent gouty arthritis or renal disease.
Fessel WJ, Siegelaub AB, Johnson ES. Correlates and consequences of asymptomatic hyperuricemia. *Arch Intern Med* 132:44–54, 1973.
   Of 124 patients with asymptomatic hyperuricemia, gouty arthritis developed in 3, in 4 years of follow-up. Of 69 asymptomatic patients with serum urate levels over 9.0 mg/ dl, only 3 had gout.
Hall AP, et al. Epidemiology of gout and hyperuricemia. *Am J Med* 42:27–37, 1967.
   The experience of the Framingham study with asymptomatic hyperuricemia. Ascertainment bias (the clinical criteria for gout included an elevated serum urate level) may have caused the incidence of gout to be overestimated.
Paulus HE, et al. Clinical significance of hyperuricemia in routinely screened hospitalized men. *JAMA* 211:277–281, 1970.
   Although 13.2% of inpatients in a Veterans Administration Hospital had elevated serum urate levels, azotemia, acidosis, and diuretics accounted for 60% of the elevated levels.
Yu TF, Gutman AB. Uric acid nephrolithiasis in gout. *Ann Intern Med* 67:1133–1148, 1967.
   A discussion of serum urate levels, urinary uric acid excretion, and urine pH.
Fessel WJ. Renal outcomes of gout and hyperuricemia. *Am J Med* 67:74–82, 1979.
   A carefully designed, large, prospective study concluding that azotemia attributable to hyperuricemia is not clinically important until serum urate levels reach 13.0 mg/dl and that the low risk of stones justifies deferring hypouricemic drugs until after the first stone.

100. CORTICOSTEROID USE
David R. Clemmons

Corticosteroids are among the most effective and potentially dangerous drugs commonly prescribed. Their safe use requires an understanding of their physiologic effects and an awareness of the side effects that occur after prolonged administration.

Adrenal Physiology
The principal secretory product of the adrenal gland is cortisol, which is secreted at a rate of 15 to 20 mg per day under nonstressful conditions. Its secretion is pulsatile, reflecting minute-to-minute variations in pituitary ACTH release. The integrated concentration of these pulsations shows a characteristic pattern termed *diurnal variation* (e.g., the mean 8:00 AM plasma concentration is 10 μg/dl, and the 10:00 PM concentration is 2 μg/dl). The cortisol secretory rate is increased during periods of stress, pregnancy, and many illnesses. In plasma, most cortisol is bound to carrier proteins and only 1 to 2% circulates as free hormone.

Regulation of Adrenal Secretion

ACTH directly controls cortisol secretion. Pulsatile ACTH release by the pituitary gland is controlled by higher brain centers and mediated by corticotropin releasing factor (CRF), which is secreted by the hypothalamus. The diurnal variation and stress responses are also mediated through this pathway. Cortisol feeds back directly on the pituitary gland to suppress ACTH secretion and also inhibits CRF release. Stress is the most powerful stimulus to ACTH secretion; it overrides the normal basal ACTH pulsations and diurnal variation.

Therapeutic Regimens

Table 100-1 lists several corticosteroid preparations.

Pharmacology of Glucocorticoids

Synthetic analogues of cortisol have chemical properties that give them enhanced biologic potency compared to cortisol and less sodium retention at equivalent anti-inflammatory dosages. They have a longer biologic half-life (e.g., cortisol, 8–12 hrs; prednisolone, 12–36 hrs; dexamethasone, 36–54 hrs). The anti-inflammatory effect of each compound is proportional to its half-life. One milligram of dexamethasone is equivalent to 6.7 mg of prednisone and 27 mg of hydrocortisone. The most commonly administered corticosteroids—prednisone, prednisolone, methylprednisolone, and triamcinolone—have intermediate half-lives and are useful for alternate-day therapy, because hypothalamic-pituitary-adrenal (HPA) axis suppression is, in general, not apparent on the day on which no steroid is given. The salt-retaining potential of each drug varies greatly; cortisone has the greatest mineralocorticoid activity, whereas dexamethasone has the least.

HPA Suppression

Acute administration of glucocorticoids does not block the stress-mediated increase in cortisol secretion, but long-term administration is associated with considerable suppression. The exact time interval required to induce suppression is unknown, but it generally is believed to be between 2 weeks and 2 months. Higher dosages (i.e. > 30 mg prednisone/day) will result in continuous 24-hour suppression of ACTH secretion and lead to an early loss of the stress response.

During the first phase of recovery after pharmacologic steroid therapy is withdrawn, ACTH and cortisol secretion may remain subnormal for a 2- to 6-month period, depending on the degree of suppression. During the second phase ACTH secretion is increased, and adrenal mass and basal cortisol secretion return. The HPA axis stress responsiveness remains impaired, however. Recovery of the stress response may require a full year.

Replacement

Primary adrenal insufficiency and hypopituitarism require different replacement regimens; therefore, the location of the lesion and severity of the defect must be documented before treatment. In Addison's disease, both glucocorticoid and mineralocorticoid replacement are required. The usual dosage schedule is 25 to 30 mg per day of hydrocortisone or its equivalent given in two divided doses, with two-thirds of the dosage in the morning and one-third in the evening. 9α-Fludrocortisone (Florinef), 0.1 mg per day, is given to replace mineralocorticoid activity. Periods of stress require higher dosages, commonly 300 mg of hydrocortisone equivalent per day for major stress, such as a laparotomy, and 60 to 100 mg per day for minor stress, such as an upper respiratory infection. High dosages of cortisol—greater than 150 mg per day—have sufficient mineralocorticoid activity, and fludrocortisone may be omitted. Tapering of the dosage following cessation of stress is usually accomplished by a reduction of 50% of the total dosage per day, although the response to this maneuver must be monitored closely.

Secondary adrenal insufficiency (e.g., hypopituitarism) is not usually accompanied by mineralocorticoid deficiency. For chronic replacement, all that is required is glucocorticoid replacement in dosages equivalent to those given for primary adrenal insufficiency. Treatment of acute stress is identical to that listed above.

Short-Term, High-Dose Therapy

Several potentially severe conditions—for example, poison ivy and asthma—respond to acute, short-term administration of corticosteroids (e.g., 60 mg prednisone per day). The duration of therapy should be limited and the therapeutic end point determined at

Table 100-1. Corticosteroid preparations

USP name	Trade names	Approximate equivalent dosage (mg)	Anti-inflammatory potency	Mineralocorticoid potency
Hydrocortisone (cortisol)	—	20.0	1.0	1.0
Cortisone	—	25.0	0.8	0.8
Prednisone	Deltasone Meticorten	5.0	3.0–5.0	0.8
Prednisolone	Meticortelone Delta-Cortef	5.0	3.0–5.0	0.8
Triamcinolone	Aristocort Kenacort	4.0	3.0–5.0	0.5
Dexamethasone	Decadron Deronil Gammacorten	0.75	20.0–30.0	0.5
Methylprednisolone	Medrol	4.0	3.0–5.0	0.5
Betamethasone	Celestone	0.6	20.0–30.0	0.5
Paramethasone	Haldrone Stemex	2.0	8.0–12.0	0.5

the outset. Often only a 2- to 3-day course is required. If the duration of treatment is less than 2 weeks, therapy can be stopped abruptly without tapering, unless this is likely to exacerbate the underlying disease. Complications of short-term therapy include ulceration of gastric mucosa, precipitation of diabetic ketoacidosis, burning or itching of mucous membranes, acute psychosis, and masking of symptoms and signs of underlying inflammation, such as an acute appendicitis. Some patients have biochemical evidence of abnormal HPA axis function after periods of treatment as short as 5 days; however, there usually are no clinically important consequences of these abnormalities.

Prolonged Therapy
Many chronic inflammatory diseases are treated with long-term administration of corticosteroid therapy. Most patients require 75 mg per day or more of hydrocortisone equivalent. These dosages predictably cause Cushing's syndrome, with its complications of osteoporosis, hypertension, obesity, myopathy, glucose intolerance, predisposition to infection, reactivation of tuberculosis, impaired wound healing, peptic ulcer, aseptic necrosis of bone, or acute psychosis. Once this syndrome is present, tapering must be done slowly, usually over several months' time, because the HPA axis is suppressed and the stress response is impaired. Even while taking replacement dosages, patients may experience symptoms of steroid withdrawal, such as myalgias, arthralgias, weakness, and anorexia. The underlying disease also may be reactivated, which results in additional stress leading to an increased requirement for steroid. The short ACTH test may be very useful in this situation to determine the degree of adrenal impairment.

Alternate-day therapy has been advocated as a means of avoiding many of the complications of chronic steroid use. This is based on the presumption that the anti-inflammatory effects of corticosteroids last longer than the metabolic actions. Prednisolone or prednisone is generally used for this purpose because both have half-lives of intermediate length, and when administered every other day usually do not cause HPA axis suppression between 24 and 48 hours following a single dose. Most of the symptoms of Cushing's syndrome, as well as objective indices such as blood pressure, leukocyte kinetics, skin testing reactivity, urinary nitrogen excretion, and linear growth, are less abnormal with alternate-day than with daily steroids. HPA axis suppression is usually not present. In general, when suppression of the underlying disease is studied, alternate-day regimens compare favorably with daily therapy. Occasionally, diseases such as ulcerative colitis and pemphigus vulgaris do not respond. If HPA suppression is already present, changing to alternate-day therapy may be hazardous because the patient may have no effective glucocorticoid in the plasma toward the end of the alternate day or may be unable to respond to stress. Therefore, abrupt transition in a patient who has taken daily steroids for several months should be avoided. A commonly used regimen involves gradually increasing the dosage on the first day while decreasing the second-day dosage.

Withdrawal from Steroid Therapy

Problems
Sudden withdrawal from high-dose, long-term glucocorticoid therapy can result in adrenal insufficiency leading to death. Typical symptoms are arthralgias, fatigue, weakness, anorexia, orthostatic hypotension, and hypoglycemia. The duration of previous therapy and the dosage and potency of the steroid used determine the severity of HPA suppression. After prolonged therapy with a potent steroid, a period of 9 months to 1 year is necessary for complete recovery.

Evaluation of Adrenal Function During Withdrawal
Several tests are available to evaluate acute symptoms suggesting adrenal insufficiency or to assess recovery of normal basal corticosteroid secretion and response to stress in patients who are not acutely ill.

1. A 24-hour urinary cortisol excretion test can be performed on ambulatory patients, but correct interpretation requires that the patient be in an unstressed state. Creatinine excretion must be checked to ensure adequate collection. A value of less than 20 μg/24 hours indicates diminished adrenal function.

2. Eight AM plasma cortisol values of 10 μg/dl or greater are indicative of normal adrenal secretion. Pulsatile variations in cortisol secretion may make this test difficult to interpret.

3. The short ACTH test is free of many of the problems of the above-mentioned tests. It can be performed at any time of the day. Twenty-five units of synthetic ACTH are given IV or IM and a blood sample for cortisol is obtained at 30 or 60 minutes. Criteria of a normal response are baseline value greater than 5 μg/dl at the start of the test, peak response of 18 μg/dl or more, and increment of at least 7 μg/dl. The major problem in interpreting this test occurs in stressed patients, who may have high basal values and respond poorly to ACTH but in fact have normal adrenal function. In tests of patients who are withdrawing from prolonged glucocorticoid treatment a subnormal response has been shown to correlate well with loss of the stress response.

Generally patients withdrawing from prolonged steroid therapy who had normal adrenal function before suppressive therapy can be managed with these tests alone. Morning plasma cortisol values can be followed at regular intervals and used to predict recovery of basal secretion as the dosage of replacement therapy is lowered. The ACTH test is used to predict return of the stress response. If primary adrenal failure or hypopituitarism is suspected, more definitive testing is required to establish the diagnosis of adrenal failure (prolonged ACTH infusion) or to confirm the loss of the stress response (metyrapone test).

Therapeutic Regimens

Initially, the dosage of glucocorticoid should be tapered to the equivalent of 20–30 mg per day of hydrocortisone. To determine if basal cortisol secretion has returned, an 8:00 AM plasma cortisol measurement should be obtained. A value of 10 μg/dl or greater indicates return of normal adrenal function. If this is not present, maintenance of hydrocortisone therapy should be continued for at least 1 month. At this time, the daily dosage can be decreased by 2.5 mg per day until a dosage of 10 mg per day is reached. This is maintained until normal 8:00 AM cortisol values are present, at which time the maintenance dosage is stopped and supplements are used for periods of stress only. At that time, short ACTH tests can be performed at 2- to 3-month intervals until the stress response normalizes.

Axelrod L. Glucocorticoid therapy. *Medicine* 55:39–63, 1976.
   An excellent, exhaustive review that covers steroid pharmacology, withdrawal symptoms, and short- and long-term complications of steroid therapy.
Melby JC. Systemic corticosteroid therapy: Pharmacology and endocrinologic considerations. *Ann Intern Med* 81:502–512, 1974.
   A comprehensive discussion of the treatment modalities available and the pharmacology of each drug.
Byyny RL. Withdrawal from glucocorticoid therapy. *N Engl J Med* 295:30–32, 1976.
   A succinct description of the withdrawal regimens and required testing during steroid withdrawal.
Meikle AW, Tyler FH. Potency and duration of action of glucocorticoids: Effects of hydrocortisone, prednisone, and dexamethasone on human pituitary adrenal function. *Am J Med* 63:200–207, 1977.
   A detailed comparison of the pharmacologic potency, duration of action, and HPA axis–induced suppression of the major glucocorticoids.
Dixon MA, Christy NP. On the various forms of corticosteroid withdrawal syndrome. *Am J Med* 68:224–227, 1980.
   Three cases are presented to illustrate the variety of symptoms and clinical courses that may be manifested during steroid withdrawal.
Fauci AS, Dale Dc, Balow JE. Glucocorticosteroid therapy: Mechanisms of action and clinical considerations. *Ann Intern Med* 84:304–315, 1976.
   A detailed discussion of the anti-inflammatory potency of several steroid preparations and the mechanism of action of each.
MacGregor RR, et al. Alternate-day prednisone therapy. *N Engl J Med* 280:1427–1438, 1969.
   A detailed discussion of the anti-inflammatory response to alternate-day therapy and the probability of avoiding severe chronic glucocorticoid-induced complications with this treatment.

XIII. BLOOD PROBLEMS

101. ANEMIA

Peter C. Ungaro

Anemia, or low blood hemoglobin concentration, is a sign of disease rather than a disease in itself. The level of blood hemoglobin concentration below which anemia is considered to exist has been defined by the World Health Organization as 13 gm/dl in men and 12 gm/dl in adult, nonpregnant women (hematocrits of about 38 and 35, respectively); other authoritative bodies have chosen similar levels (Table 101-1). These levels are arbitrary and do not correspond to symptoms or to increased risk of serious underlying disease.

Table 101-1 summarizes the distribution of hematocrit and hemoglobin levels in the general population. Lower levels in women are explained in part by the prevalence of iron deficiency. On the average, hematocrit levels rise about 2 "hematocrit points" in postmenopausal women.

Detection

History
The symptoms attributed to anemia (fatigue, generalized weakness, dyspnea on exertion, and light-headedness) are common among people in general, in part because of the high prevalence of anxiety, depression, smoking, and overwork. Moreover, many of the diseases that cause anemia, such as cancer, are themselves responsible for these same symptoms. Although there is strong evidence that anemia does not produce an excess of symptoms above hemoglobin levels of 10 gm/dl, symptoms clearly do occur when anemia is severe. Rapidly acquired anemia, such as with blood loss or destruction (hemolysis), is more often symptomatic than comparable anemia of gradual onset caused by a production defect, such as iron deficiency or pernicious anemia. Also, anemias are better tolerated by people who do not engage in vigorous activity.

Physical Examination
If anemia is looked for by examining for pallor of the conjunctivae, mucous membranes, nail beds, and palmar creases, only severe anemia (i.e., hematocrits below 25%) will be detected. The history and physical examination are better suited for detecting clues to the cause of anemia, rather than the anemia itself.

Laboratory Tests
It is not recommended that anemia be sought routinely on periodic examination or screening (see Chap. 125). The search for anemia usually is prompted by the finding of a condition known to cause anemia, such as excessive menstrual bleeding, gastrointestinal blood loss, or a positive stool guaiac. The presence of anemia is confirmed by hematocrit or hemoglobin determinations, or by a Colter Counter complete blood count. Once anemia is found to be present, a precise cause must be sought.

Approach to Diagnosis
The diagnostic workup of anemia begins with a complete blood count, a calculated mean corpuscular volume (MCV), and a reticulocyte count. The reticulocyte count must be adjusted to the hematocrit by calculating the reticulocyte index:

$$\text{Reticulocyte count} \times \frac{\text{actual hematocrit}}{\text{normal hematocrit}} = \text{reticulocyte index (normal value is 1--3\%)}$$

The information from these readily available, inexpensive laboratory tests categorizes the anemia, thereby limiting the number of possible diagnoses and directing the subsequent evaluation.

In Table 101-2, the most common causes of anemia are characterized by reticulocyte count and MCV. The great majority of patients with anemia fall into one of the diagnostic categories in the table. Because the MCV has been shown to be the most useful RBC index, the other traditional RBC indices—mean corpuscular hemoglobin (MCH)

Table 101-1. "Normal" hematocrit and hemoglobin by sex*

Sex	Hematocrit (%)		Hemoglobin (gm/dl)	
	Mean	5th–95th Percentile	Mean	5th–95th Percentile
Men	44	38–51	14.8	11.5–16.5
Women (nonpregnant)	40	32–46	13.0	8.5–14.5

*Data from 130 men and 165 women in the general population.
Source: From WW Wood and PC Elwood. Symptoms of nondeficiency anemia: A community survey. *Br J Rev Soc Med* 20:117–121, 1966.

Table 101-2. Characterization of anemia by reticulocyte count and MCV

Anemia with reticulocytopenia (reticulocyte index < 1%)
  Microcytic—MCV < 82 cu μ
    Iron deficiency
    Thalassemia (often reticulocytosis)
    Sideroblastic anemia
    Anemia of chronic disease (sometimes)
  Macrocytic—MCV > 100 cu μ
    B_{12} deficiency
    Folate deficiency
    Chronic liver disease
    Myxedema
  Normocytic—MCV 82–100 cu μ
  (anemias that are macrocytic or microcytic are normocytic when detected early)
    Anemia of chronic disease (usually)
    Bone marrow infiltration or failure
Anemia with reticulocytosis (reticulocyte index > 3%)
(MCV is often not helpful because reticulocytosis causes macrocytosis)
  Macrocytic
    Acute blood loss (sometimes)
    Acute hemolysis (sometimes)
    Postsplenectomy
  Microcytic
    Microangiopathic
    Thalassemia
    Certain hemoglobinopathies
  Normocytic
    Acute hemorrhage (usually)
    Acute hemolysis (usually)

and mean corpuscular hemoglobin concentration (MCHC)—are not included in this table.

Microcytic Reticulocytopenic Anemia

Most adults with a microcytic reticulocytopenic anemia have iron deficiency, although early iron deficiency is often normocytic. The majority of these patients are menstruating women, many of whom have had multiple pregnancies. Their anemia is explained by iron loss in excess of intake. Menstruating women lose an average of 2 mg of iron per day, whereas the average adult diet contains only 15 to 18 gm of iron, of which only 10% is absorbed (1.5–1.8 mg/day). This imbalance is often compounded by previous, full-term pregnancies, which, even when uncomplicated, cause the loss of an additional 500 to 1000 mg of iron.

In contrast, iron loss in the adult man and postmenopausal woman occurs primarily through the shedding of epithelial cells in the gastrointestinal tract and amounts to only about 1 mg of iron per day. Therefore, iron deficiency in these patients requires an additional explanation. Usually the cause is blood loss from gastrointestinal bleeding; occasionally, it is iron malabsorption.

Dietary habits may contribute to iron deficiency. Some women do not eat adequate amounts of major sources of iron, such as liver, red meats, apricots, peaches, prunes, apples, grapes, raisins, spinach, and eggs. However, even the poorest of diets provides adequate iron for men and postmenopausal women. Laundry starch and clay, sometimes eaten in large quantities because of an insatiable craving (pica), chelate iron in the gastrointestinal tract and prevent absorption of iron.

Evaluation

Menstruating women who have microcytic anemia with reticulocytopenia and no evidence of occult gastrointestinal blood loss seldom require additional evaluation. It is safe to assume that they have iron deficiency anemia.

In other instances of suspected iron deficiency, serum iron, iron-binding capacity, and percent saturation may be obtained. Characteristic of iron deficiency are a low serum iron, elevated iron-binding capacity, and saturation of less than 16%. Unfortunately there are many false positives and negatives. The level of serum ferritin (a large iron-storage protein compound found primarily intracellulary) is more useful. A low ferritin is highly diagnostic of iron deficiency. False elevations can occur with diseases such as hepatitis that affect storage sites. Thus, a normal level does not exclude iron deficiency. The "gold standard" for diagnosing iron deficiency is the demonstration of trace or absent stainable iron on a bone marrow aspiration. However, the clinical picture and laboratory evaluation are usually sufficient, and a bone marrow aspirate is seldom necessary.

Once a diagnosis of iron deficiency is confirmed in an adult man or postmenopausal woman, a diligent search for sources of blood loss must be made. Such instances should be considered to be caused by gastrointestinal blood loss until proved otherwise. One should never assume that dietary iron has been inadequate, nor should iron therapy by given without a thorough search for the bleeding source.

Treatment

The treatment of iron deficiency is the administration of iron. Because it is inexpensive, effective, and tolerated by most patients, ferrous sulfate, 300 mg (60 mg iron) three times a day with meals, is generally considered the treatment of choice. Unfortunately, ferrous iron causes mucosal irritation. Many expensive iron preparations are advertised as better tolerated than ferrous sulfate; however, tolerance is accomplished by providing less iron or less contact with the absorptive surface and, therefore, decreased iron absorption. Ferrous gluconate tablets (300 mg, 30 mg iron) are less irritating, primarily because each of the tablets contains less iron. Enteric-release tablets are also less irritating but prevent the ferrous iron from coming in contact with the absorptive mucosa of the proximal gastrointestinal tract and, therefore, result in decreased absorption.

Taking iron with meals reduces absorption but makes the treatment more tolerable. Starting with a single ferrous sulfate tablet daily and building up to two and then three tablets per day over a period of many days seems to reduce gastrointestinal side effects in many patients. Because the hydrochloric acid in the gastric secretions promotes absorption by helping to maintain iron in solution, the patient should not take antacids and iron at the same time. It is rare that patients cannot take adequate amounts of oral iron if these precautions are taken.

Rarely, parenteral iron is necessary, usually given as iron dextran (Imferon). Administration frequently produces severe pain at the site of intramuscular injection and skin staining; anaphylaxis has been reported. Use of the Z-tract injection technique is helpful in preventing skin staining.

In the absence of continued blood loss, effective iron therapy should result by the tenth day of treatment in a reticulocytosis that seldom exceeds 10%. After 3 weeks of therapy, the hemoglobin levels should rise by more than half the difference between the initial level and the normal level for that patient. Once normal hemoglobin levels are achieved (usually in 6 to 8 weeks), iron must be continued for approximately 4 to

6 months to replenish the body stores of iron. Failure to respond to oral $FeSO_4$ is most often from not taking the medication or from inhibition of absorption caused by the innovative methods patients sometimes find to reduce gastrointestinal irritation.

Macrocytic Anemia

Anemia with reticulocytopenia and macrocytosis is often associated with liver disease in the absence of folate or vitamin B_{12} deficiency. Other causes are folate deficiency from inadequate intake and B_{12} deficiency in pernicious anemia or blind loop syndrome. The anemias of B_{12} and folate deficiency occasionally are normocytic early in the disease.

Physical Examination

Vitamin B_{12} deficiency classically produces subacute degeneration of the dorsal columns of the spinal cord with decrease in proprioception; however, a symmetric peripheral polyneuropathy and/or dementia frequently occurs. Surgical scars suggest gastrectomy, blind loop syndrome, and other surgical causes of B_{12} deficiency.

Laboratory Tests

Assessment should begin with an evaluation of the peripheral blood smear. In B_{12} or folate deficiency, oval macrocytes, hypersegmented polymorphs, and giant platelets may be found. Hypothyroidism and liver disease usually cause target cells from increased membrane lipids.

Characteristically, patients with B_{12} deficiency have a low serum B_{12} with normal serum and red cell folate, whereas patients with folic acid deficiency have low folate and normal B_{12} studies. Occasionally, folate deficiency causes low B_{12} levels, and vice versa. Moreover, the folic acid determinations are sometimes misleading for other reasons. The serum folate level is sensitive to reductions in vitamin ingestion, even in the presence of normal body stores; dietary restriction causes the serum folate to fall before anemia or megaloblastic changes occur. On the other hand, the red cell folate is less sensitive but more specific, because it may fall only after anemia and megaloblastic changes have occurred. Because of these problems, some advocate obtaining serum and RBC folate and B_{12} levels in all patients who have megaloblastic anemias. A careful examination of the peripheral smear and a bone marrow examination may be necessary to clarify the diagnosis.

After a diagnosis of B_{12} deficiency is established, testing for achlorhydria or performing a Schilling test is helpful in determining the cause of the deficiency if the clinical picture is unclear. Antibodies to intrinsic factor strongly suggest a diagnosis of pernicious anemia.

Treatment

Treatment of B_{12} deficiency anemia is with parenteral B_{12}, usually given in a dosage of 1000 μg once a month for life. This dosage is in excess of what is required, but the excess is excreted. Most experts recommend more frequent doses in the presence of neurologic disease (e.g., daily injections for 2 weeks, followed by injections every 2 weeks for 6 months, then once a month for life).

Folate deficiency, which is usually caused by inadequate dietary intake, is treated by folate, 1 mg orally every day. Vitamin B_{12} deficiency must be ruled out before administering folate, because folate alone can partially correct the anemia of B_{12} deficiency while the neurologic manifestations progress.

Normocytic Reticulocytopenic Anemia

Most normocytic anemias with reticulocytopenia are associated with chronic disease. Almost any severe chronic disease can result in anemia; the more common ones are chronic renal failure; chronic inflammatory diseases, such as rheumatoid arthritis; certain endocrine disorders, such as adrenal insufficiency; and neoplastic diseases. The diagnosis of the chronic, underlying disease is usually not difficult. The real difficulty lies in ascertaining that other important causes of anemia are not present, such as early megaloblastic or iron deficiency anemia. It is generally thought that hemoglobin must fall 2 gm% for the microcytosis of iron deficiency to be detectable. In the anemia of chronic disease, both the serum iron and iron-binding capacity are reduced, and there is either low or normal percent saturation.

In general, there is a parallel between the severity and chronicity of the chronic illness and the severity of the anemia. If the anemia is disproportionately severe, other causes must be considered.

Anemias frequently have more than one cause; in particular, the anemia of chronic disease may be complicated by folate or iron deficiency. The serum ferritin and folate levels can help sort this out; however, the laboratory evaluation of combined processes can be difficult, and bone marrow examination is often necessary. An exacerbation of a chronic anemia requires a search for a concomitant deficiency state.

Anemia with Reticulocytosis

The two common causes of anemia in which a reticulocytosis is present are acute blood loss and hemolysis. Usually the indices are not particularly helpful, especially since reticulocytes are large cells that cause the MCV to be increased.

Diagnosis

The diagnosis of hemolysis may be supported by additional laboratory tests. The serum haptoglobin is often depressed because of the formation of hemoglobin-haptoglobin complexes. However, if the hemolytic process is mild or extravascular, serum haptoglobin may be normal. Also, haptoglobin is an acute reactant that may be elevated in inflammatory states. When the binding capacity of haptoglobin is exceeded, hemoglobinuria results. Elevation of serum bilirubin and lactate dehydrogenase (LDH) provides additional evidence of hemolysis.

If there is no evidence of blood loss and the diagnosis of hemolysis is uncertain, it may be useful to observe the patient for several weeks, periodically checking for persistent reticulocytosis and anemia. When the diagnosis is uncertain, a radionuclide red cell survival study may be required to document decreased red cell survival.

Establishing a Specific Cause

A peripheral smear should be examined, particularly for spherocytes or schistocytes. Spherocytes suggest congenital spherocytosis; schistocytes suggest a microangiopathic process or heart valve hemolysis.

Certain patients, particularly blacks, may have a glucose-6-phosphate dehydrogenase deficiency. Drug-induced hemolysis in these patients affects only older, enzyme-deficient cells; the younger cells have adequate enzyme to resist the oxidant stress. Therefore, enzyme screening tests are normal immediately after hemolysis, and diagnosis may require repeat determination of the enzyme level when the older cells are once more present in the circulation. A variety of drugs can cause hemolysis by other mechanisms.

If the history, review of old records, race, or ethnic origin suggests that the process may be inherited, a sickle cell preparation, hemoglobin electrophoresis, and quantitative hemoglobin A_2 and F levels are indicated. The quantitative A_2 and F levels are helpful in detecting sickle β-thalassemia or suggesting hereditary persistence of hemoglobin F. In addition, citrate agar is needed to separate hemoglobin S from hemoglobin D, because they migrate together on routine electrophoresis.

Thalassemia occurs predominantly in Mediterraneans and blacks. The most important clue to this diagnosis is reticulocytosis with microcytosis. In β-thalassemia the quantitative hemoglobin A_2 and F levels should be obtained because elevations confirm the diagnosis. α-Thalassemia is a diagnosis of exclusion supported by the presence of microcytosis and reticulocytosis in other family members. In acquired hemolytic anemias, the direct antiglobin (Coombs') test can help identify autoimmune erythrocyte destruction. A search for splenomegaly is needed since hypersplenism may be an important factor.

Douglas SW, Adamson JW. The anemia of chronic disorders: Studies of marrow regulation and iron metabolism. *Blood* 45:55–65, 1975.
   This study of 17 patients indicates that this disorder represents a limited proliferative response primarily caused by defective availability of iron.
Eichner ER, Pierce HI, Hillman RS. Folate balance in dietary-induced megaloblastic anemia. *N Engl J Med* 284:933–938, 1971.
   Two subjects were studied to determine the interaction of poor diet, depleted body

stores of folate, and ethanol on the development of anemia and associated laboratory abnormalities.

Herbert V. The nutritional anemias. *Hosp Pract* 15:65–89, 1980.

The presentation, diagnosis, and therapy of patients with nutritional anemias are presented in a concise informative fashion.

Westerman MP. Bone marrow needle biopsy: An evaluation and critique. *Semin Hematol* 18:293–300, 1981.

A review evaluating the role of the bone marrow examination, particularly the biopsy, in multiple disease states.

Frank MM, et al. Pathophysiology of immune hemolytic anemia. *Ann Intern Med* 87:210–222, 1977.

The mechanisms of immune hemolytic anemia are reviewed, with particular emphasis on differences between warm and cold antibody-mediated disease.

Cooper RA, Shattil SJ. Mechanisms of hemolysis: The minimal red cell defect. *N Engl J Med* 285:1514–1520, 1971.

The mechanisms of hemolysis in multiple disease processes are explored and deficiencies in current understanding are pointed out.

Brewer GJ. Inherited erythrocyte metabolic and membrane disorders. *Med Clin North Am* 64:579–596, 1980.

This comprehensive review provides the practical information needed for effective patient evaluation.

Charache S. The treatment of sickle cell anemia. *Arch Intern Med* 133:698–705, 1974.

A description of the most helpful therapeutic interventions, including a useful method of partial exchange transfusion.

Cook JD. Clinical evaluation of iron deficiency. *Semin Hematol* 19:6–18, 1982.

A review article providing a detailed assessment of the testing procedures used to diagnose iron deficiency.

Fischer SL, Fischer SP. Mean corpuscular volume. *Arch Intern Med* 143:282–283, 1983.

Supports the MCV as the only RBC index that is of clinical usefulness.

102. ABNORMAL BLEEDING
Robert H. Fletcher

Abnormal bleeding from other than local causes is an uncommon event outside of hospital and referral hematology practice, but suspicion of abnormal bleeding is not. Concern about the adequacy of hemostastis arises in several situations: when patients are worried about a bleeding episode; before major surgery; and when there appears to be excessive bleeding from a known local cause, such as nose bleed or tooth extraction. This chapter discusses how bleeding from any one of the major systemic mechanisms—abnormality of platelets, coagulation, or vascular fragility—is recognized. It does not discuss the next step—assigning a specific cause to the abnormality.

Normal Bleeding
There is no precise definition of normal bleeding. As a general rule, however, bleeding from minor cuts and abrasions should subside spontaneously within several minutes; bleeding from uncomplicated tooth extractions may be brisk for up to an hour and continue as oozing for a day or two. Most people have sufficient personal experience with bleeding to judge whether or not it is abnormal.

Patients may mistake a variety of common clinical conditions for signs of abnormal bleeding. Senile purpura is a benign condition that is prevalent in the elderly. Purpuric lesions are most commonly seen on the extensor surface of the upper extremities. The lesions are usually up to 1 cm in diameter and often occur in clusters of 2 or 3. The lesions are thought to result from a loss of vascular supporting tissues and perhaps minor trauma as well. Senile purpura is a problem only because of its appearance. There is no effective prevention or treatment.

Patients with varicosities of the lower extremities but otherwise normal hemostasis may experience spontaneous bleeding, apparently from rupture of a small blood vessel. Typically, there is the sudden onset of an intense, stinging pain similar to a bee sting, occurring in an area 1 to 2 cm in diameter. Examination at the time discloses no abnormality; however, over the next 24 to 48 hours an ecchymosis develops, which resolves over 7 to 10 days.

Young people, particularly women, often report what they regard as excessive bruising after minor trauma. In the great majority of instances this is not a sign of abnormal hemostasis. Evidence against a clinically important bleeding abnormality includes location of bruises only at the sites of known trauma, or in places commonly exposed to minor trauma; absence of multiple bruises or petechiae; lack of abnormal bleeding from mucosal surfaces or with menstruation; and absence of other symptoms of poor health.

Patterns of Abnormal Bleeding

The manifestations of a bleeding disorder are related to the underlying abnormality. Platelet abnormalities tend to cause bleeding into skin and mucosal surfaces. There are petechiae or purpura, which may be spontaneous or associated with minor trauma. Bleeding follows immediately after trauma. Menstrual flow may be excessive.

Coagulation defects cause bleeding into deeper structures, such as subcutaneous tissues, muscles, and joints. Although this bleeding may begin immediately after injury, it often occurs hours or days later and frequently recurs after the initial bleeding has stopped. Menstruation can be affected by coagulation defects; however, the common ones (e.g., hemophilia) do not usually occur in women.

Tests for Abnormal Bleeding

The great majority of bleeding disorders can be detected by a screening history. The remaining disorders can be detected, with uncommon exceptions, by a battery of four laboratory tests: partial thromboplastin time (PTT), prothrombin time (PT), platelet count, and bleeding time. However, abnormal hemostasis is infrequent, and the tests are relatively expensive and time-consuming. Physicians should exercise restraint in requesting these tests and not consider them "routine."

History

Taking an appropriate history, supported by a routine physical examination, is a very sensitive—albeit nonspecific—test for abnormal hemostasis. In studies of patients admitted to a hospital or undergoing surgery, false-negative histories occurred in less than 1% of patients. A substantial proportion of the abnormal coagulation tests that were not suspected by history were normal when repeated or were not associated with clinical bleeding. False-positive histories—suggesting a bleeding disorder was present when it was not—occurred frequently—in 60 to 90% of patients. Family history alone is a relatively insensitive test for hereditary coagulation disorders; it is negative in up to 40% of patients with hemophilia A.

A screening questionnaire for abnormal bleeding has been proposed by Rapaport (see References), based on clinical experience and knowledge of the clinical manifestations of potential bleeding disorders.

Have you ever bled for a long time or developed a swollen tongue or mouth after cutting or biting your tongue, cheek, or lip?
Do you develop bruises larger than a silver dollar without being able to remember when or how you injured yourself? If so, how big was the largest of these bruises?
How many times have you had teeth pulled, and what was the longest time that you bled after an extraction? Has bleeding ever started up again the day after an extraction?
What operations have you had, including minor surgery such as skin biopsies? Was bleeding after surgery ever hard to stop? Have you ever developed unusual bruising in the skin around an area of surgery or injury?
Have you had a medical problem within the past 5 years requiring a doctor's care? If so, what was its nature?
What medications, including aspirin or other remedies for headaches, colds, menstrual cramps, or other pains, have you taken within the past 7 to 9 days?

7. Has any blood relative had a problem with unusual bruising or bleeding after surgery? Were blood transfusions required to control this bleeding?

Laboratory Tests

Platelet counts by autoanalyzer are normally approximately 200,000 to 400,000/µl; the normal range varies with the method used. If a Wright-stained blood smear is available, and a platelet count would not otherwise be ordered, the smear can be used to estimate the platelet count: several platelets per oil-immersion powered field or 1 per 10 to 20 red cells corresponds to normal levels. Bleeding from too few platelets is ruled out by counts greater than 100,000/µl; unlikely in the 30,000 to 100,000 range and plausible below 30,000/µl. In general, the risk of abnormal bleeding increases sharply below 20,000 to 30,000, and the risk of life-threatening (e.g., CNS) bleeding rises below 10,000. The risk may be modified by the underlying disease; for example thrombocytopenia seems to be better tolerated in idiopathic thrombocytopenic purpura than in aplastic anemia.

Partial thromboplastin time (PTT) is abnormal in the most frequently occurring disorders of intrinsic coagulation: hemophilia (e.g., deficiency of factor VIII, classic hemophilia, and of factor IX, Christmas disease), disseminated intravascular coagulation (DIC), and acquired anticoagulants. PTT may be normal in mild hemophilia and low grade DIC, and it does not detect deficiency of factor XIII (congenital or acquired) or dysfibrinogenemia, both extremely rare. Occasionally, high levels of one factor may mask low levels of another. PTT is also normal in the presence of liver disease, even when deficiency of vitamin K–dependent factors (II, VII, IX, X) is relatively severe.

Bleeding time (BT), ordinarily by the Ivy technique or a modification, is a test of platelet and/or vascular function. Normal values are 7 to 10 minutes. To detect subtle prolongations, one must know the normal range for the specific laboratory. However clinical bleeding is unlikely unless the bleeding time is distinctly prolonged—at least 15 to 20 minutes. If bleeding time is prolonged and the platelet count is greater than 100,000/µl, a qualitative platelet defect or vascular abnormality is suspected.

Aspirin and other nonsteroidal anti-inflammatory drugs (NSAIDs) prolong bleeding time by inactivating platelet cyclo-oxygenase. The effect lasts for the life of the platelet (several days) for aspirin and is briefer for other NSAIDs; however, clinical bleeding is uncommon if BT is less than 15 to 20 minutes. An increasing number of other drugs are reported to interfere with platelet function; thus it is wise to suspect drugs in the setting of increased BT and normal platelet count.

Abnormal vascular fragility is usually diagnosed by the presence of one of the diseases with which it is associated: scurvy, Cushing's syndrome, or one of a variety of congenital connective tissue diseases (Ehlers-Danlos or Marfan's syndrome, pseudoxanthoma elasticum, and osteogenesis imperfecta). Vascular (palpable) purpura results in petechiae, particularly of the lower extremity; it is a small-vessel vasculitis usually related to hypersensitivity and is not a systemic disorder of hemostasis.

Prothrombin time (PT) is a measure of coagulation through the extrinsic (tissue contact) pathway. It is useful for monitoring sodium warfarin (Coumadin) anticoagulation and liver disease. But it has limited value, over and above the PTT, in detecting coagulation disorders, because it is less sensitive to reduced levels than is the PTT. When PT is abnormal in the presence of liver disease, usually the condition is obvious from the history and physical examination.

Strategy for Detecting Abnormal Bleeding

Although a battery of tests will identify nearly all disorders of hemostasis, it is not recommended that the battery be performed in an all-or-none fashion. The intensity of the evaluation can be graded according to the degree of suspicion raised by the screening history. The following scheme, abreviated from a proposal by Rapaport for preoperative hemostatic evaluation, will serve for most situations in which hemostasis is in question.

Level I

If a screening history is negative and a major local challenge to hemostasis (e.g., major surgery) is not present, no additional tests are necessary, even though there have been no previous surgical tests of hemostasis.

Level II

If the history is negative, including previous surgical tests of hemostasis, and a major challenge to hemostasis (e.g., major surgery, trauma) is present, a PTT and platelet count are done.

Level III

If the screening history raises the possibility of a hemostatic defect, or if the history is negative but an unusual challenge to hemostasis is present (e.g., cardiac surgery, prostatectomy, major trauma), or if bleeding would be unusually risky (e.g., CNS surgery), then a full evaluation is recommended: platelet count, BT, PTT, and PT. Also, an assessment of clot stability is recommended.

Level IV

If the screening history leaves the physician very suspicious or certain of a hemostatic defect, a variety of tests are done in addition to those listed in level III. These include bleeding time after aspirin or in vitro tests of platelet function; specific factor VIII and factor IX coagulant activity; and thrombin time, to detect dysfibrinogenemia or weak heparin-like anticoagulants.

Consequences

If not all screening tests are performed whenever hemostasis is questioned, detectable abnormalities will occasionally be missed before bleeding occurs. What are the consequences? Nearly all disorders of hemostasis can be characterized and treated successfully after abnormal bleeding occurs. The exception is when the early manifestations of abnormal bleeding, however small, can cause irreversible damage, particularly after CNS trauma or surgery. In this situation, aggressive evaluation is prudent.

Rapaport SI. Preoperative hemostatic evaluation: Which tests, if any? *Blood* 61:229–231, 1983.
Proposes broad guidelines in which the intensity of laboratory evaluation depends on the likelihood of a bleeding disorder, based on a screening history.
Eisenberg JM, Clarke JR, Sussman SA. Prothrombin and partial thromboplastin times as preoperative screening tests. *Arch Surg* 117:48–51, 1982.
The yield of PT and PTT tests before surgery was low in the absence of evidence of a bleeding disorder from history and physical examination.
Bachmann F. Diagnostic approach to mild bleeding disorders. *Semin Hematol* 17:292–305, 1980.
The author presents his personal experience with 95 patients with mild bleeding disorders referred to a hemostasis unit in a university hospital in Switzerland.
Stuart MJ, et al. The post-aspirin bleeding time: A screening test for evaluation of hemostatic disorders. *Br J Haematol* 43:649–659, 1979.
In normal people, bleeding time was doubled 2 hours after ingestion of 600 mg aspirin. The test detected patients with mild von Willebrand's disease or qualitative platelet abnormalities, some of whom had normal bleeding times before the ingestion of aspirin.
Doan CA, Bouroncle BA, Wiseman BK. Idiopathic and secondary thrombocytopenic purpura: Clinical study and evaluation of 381 cases over a period of 28 years. *Ann Intern Med* 53:861–876, 1960.
A review of experience with a large number of patients with thrombocytopenia—271 with idiopathic thrombocytopenia and 110 with secondary thrombocytopenic purpura.
Lackner H, Karpatkin S. On the "easy bruising" syndrome with normal platelet count: A study of 75 patients. *Ann Intern Med* 83:190–196, 1975.
Approximately half of patients referred because of "easy bruising" had normal platelet function and half had a variety of abnormalities demonstrated by in vitro tests.
Harker LA, Slichter SJ. The bleeding time as a screening test for evaluation of platelet function. *N Engl J Med* 287:155–159, 1972.
A description of the relation between platelet count and bleeding time for normal and qualitatively abnormal platelets.

103. POLYCYTHEMIA
James A. Bryan II

Definition
The literal definition of polycythemia is "too many cells." The term is usually applied to any condition in which the number of red cells, as measured by a hematocrit or hemoglobin concentration, exceeds the statistical norm. By this definition, the upper limit of "normal" hematocrit values in adults at sea level is accepted as 54% for men and 52% for women. However, the judgment of "too many" red cells should be put in the context of the patient's physiology or pathophysiology. For example, acclimatized people living at 15,000 feet normally have hematocrit values of about 60% and do not have a disease. On the other hand, a hematocrit of 60% in a person at sea level usually indicates disease.

Causes
Polycythemia can occur either because too many red blood cells are produced (absolute erythrocytosis, either primary or secondary) or because of a reduction in the amount of plasma in which the red cells are suspended (relative or pseudoerythrocytosis). The causes of polycythemia are listed in Table 103-1.

The prevalence of primary polycythemia is approximately 2 per 100,000 persons; the relative frequencies of the various causes of polycythemia are not known.

Pathophysiology
Primary polycythemia (polycythemia vera) is usually associated with increased white cell and platelet counts and splenomegaly. It is considered a primary myeloproliferative disorder that can evolve into acute leukemia or myelofibrosis.

Secondary polycythemia is associated with conditions that lead to low tissue oxygen tension: lung disease, hypoventilation syndrome, and congenital heart disease with venous to arterial vascular shunting. Cigarette smoking, which increases carboxyhemoglobin levels, causes a moderate polycythemia. Abnormal hemoglobins that are associated with high oxygen affinities can also lead to low tissue oxygen tensions and polycythemia. About 60 different abnormal hemoglobins have been identified, but all are rare. When systemic oxygen tension is reduced, erythropoietin is released, possibly from the kidney, and red cell production is stimulated. If iron, vitamin B_{12}, folic acid, and protein are available, more red cells and hemoglobin are made. Other causes of secondary excess red cell production are listed in Table 103-1. The mechanisms by which they are associated with polycythemia are unknown.

Table 103-1. Causes of polycythemia

Primary polycythemia (polycythemia vera)
Secondary polycythemia
   Pulmonary disease
   Heart disease with right-to-left shunts
   Hypoventilation syndromes
   Renal disease
      Polycystic disease
      Hypernephroma
   Tumors
      Ovarian thecoma
      Large uterine leiomyoma
      Cerebellar vascular tumors
   Congenital hemoglobinopathies
   Cigarette smoking
Decreased plasma volume
   Gaisböck's syndrome
   Diuretics
   Dehydration

Decreased plasma volume causes high hemoglobin concentrations and hematocrits, with normal total body red cell mass. When there is no apparent dehydration, the condition is called "Gaisböck's syndrome." The biologic mechanism for the syndrome is not known, but the condition is usually found in men who smoke, are under stress, are overweight, and have hypertension. The hematocrit values rarely, if ever, exceed 58%. Chronic use of diuretics is responsible for small decreases in plasma volume; the resulting hematocrit rarely exceeds 54%.

Complications

It has been difficult to establish a level of hematocrit above which symptoms or complications occur. As hematocrit values rise, viscosity rises, flow diminishes, and oxygen transport is impaired. This can translate into increased work for the heart, with heart failure and/or a tendency toward vascular occlusions, particularly stroke. These complications occur more frequently in patients with primary or secondary polycythemia, particularly at hematocrits above 55%. Some physicians believe that concomitant elevation in platelet counts increases the risk from hyperviscosity in polycythemia vera compared to other causes of polycythemia. Cerebral blood flow apparently also is reduced by high hematocrits. In one study, only 2 of 19 patients with hematocrits above 50% had normal cerebral blood flow, whereas only 3 of 21 patients with hematocrits below 46% had abnormal cerebral blood flow.

Evaluation

If a high hematocrit (over 52%) is found, a sequence of simple maneuvers helps to sort out the many possible causes.

History

In polycythemia vera there may be a variety of nonspecific symptoms, including headache, weakness, pruritus, and dizziness; however, none occurs in greater than 50% of patients. In secondary polycythemia, symptoms are from the underlying disease, unless symptoms of hyperviscosity intervene. Diuretic or cigarette use may be associated with a mild polycythemia.

Physical Examination

Usually there are few physical findings except for a ruddy complexion and splenomegaly in polycythemia vera, the findings of an underlying pulmonary cardiovascular disease, or a mass associated with a tumor in secondary polycythemia.

Laboratory Evaluation

If polycythemia is mild (hematocrit 52–54%) and the patient is otherwise normal, additional workup is unnecessary, provided there is a likely explanation such as a history of smoking or diuretic use. Although measuring carboxyhemoglobin may identify patients whose polycythemia is caused by smoking, the same information can be obtained by repeating hematocrit values a few weeks after smoking has been stopped.

For patients with more pronounced polycythemia (HCT > 55%), a minimal objective laboratory evaluation should include a complete blood count with smear examination for white cell, red cell, or platelet structural abnormalities, as well as a platelet and reticulocyte count. Qualitative or quantitative abnormalities in the cellular elements of the blood imply a primary myeloproliferative process, particularly if there is a palpable spleen. Other studies include a urinalysis, looking for hematuria (i.e., kidney pathology); chest x-ray, for heart or lung disease; and arterial oxygen saturation, looking for occult deoxygenation states. Second-level studies such as CAT scans or pulmonary function tests including nocturnal blood gas evaluation are obtained in those in whom pulmonary problems seem likely or an occult malignancy is possible. Hemoglobinopathies are detected by hemoglobin electrophoresis.

Radioisotope studies of red cell mass discriminate between increased numbers of red cells and diminished plasma volume. Although many experts suggest beginning with this study, it is an expensive test and is often unnecessary because causes of polycythemia can be found by history, physical examination, or inexpensive screening tests. It is necessary only after secondary causes have been ruled out, and the discrimination is between polycythemia vera and Gaisböck's syndrome.

Treatment

Polycythemia vera, or primary polycythemia, may require chemotherapy (busulfan or melphalan), radiotherapy (usually administered as the isotope P^{32}), and/or phlebotomies. Vascular occlusive episodes can be reduced considerably by reducing hematocrit from over 55% to below 48% (and platelets to below 400,000/mm^3).

Treatment of *secondary polycythemia* is directed at the management of the underlying primary disease. If the primary condition cannot be controlled, one is forced to deal with the secondary polycythemia as well as the primary disease. In these instances, it is generally believed to be beneficial to maintain the hematocrit below 55%. This can be accomplished by regular phlebotomy, usually 500 ml of blood with normal saline replacement on a weekly basis until a lower hematocrit is obtained. In some patients, improvement in oxygenation through low-flow oxygen administration also aids in controlling the polycythemia.

Russell RP, Conley CL. Benign polycythemia: Gaisböck's syndrome. *Arch Intern Med* 1143:734–740, 1964.

A descriptive paper on the clinical findings and course.

Dinterfass L. A preliminary outline of the blood high viscosity syndromes. *Arch Intern Med* 118:427–435, 1966.

A review of the effects of blood viscosity in various diseases.

Hurtado A. Some clinical aspects of life at high altitudes. *Ann Intern Med* 53:247–258, 1960.

A fascinating description of high-altitude physiology and pathophysiology.

Thomas DJ, et al. Cerebral blood flow in polycythemia. *Lancet* 2:161–163, 1977.

Convincing data on keeping hematocrits low to improve brain functional integrity.

Pearson TC, Weatherly-Mein G. Vascular occlusive episodes and venous hematocrit in primary proliferative polycythemia. *Lancet* 2:1219–1222, 1978.

The relation between the incidence of occlusive episodes and the hematocrit and platelet count shown in a retrospective study.

Smith JR, Landow SA. Smokers' polycythemia. *N Engl J Med* 298:6–10, 1978.

Red cell volume is increased and plasma volume reduced with increased mean hematocrits in the 22 smokers of 54, and elevated carboxyhemoglobins—11.6%.

XIV. NERVOUS SYSTEM PROBLEMS

Evaluation

Almost 80% of the population suffers each year from at least one headache. Of these perhaps 50% have severe or recurrent headaches, and 10 to 20% of sufferers consult their physicians.

In most cases, headache occurs in the context of common primary headache syndromes such as tension headache, cluster headache, migraine headache, or other vascular headache. While these painful syndromes may be quite disabling, they are not progressive. However, in a minority of cases, headache is the presenting manifestation of progressive and life-threatening conditions. Subdural hematoma, subarachnoid hemorrhage, brain tumor, and meningitis are some of the conditions that often present as headache with few other symptoms or signs and are medical emergencies requiring immediate diagnostic evaluation and treatment.

History

For almost all patients with headache, the diagnosis and treatment are based on the history. Certain key points need emphasis to distinguish the more common primary headache syndromes from the less common, but more dangerous, secondary headaches. Nevertheless, it is often difficult to make the distinction with the first headache.

TIME COURSE. Headaches may be chronic, subacute, or acute. Primary headache disorders (tension, vascular, and cluster headaches) frequently are chronic; while there are exacerbations and periods of relative remission, the pattern does not change rapidly. If the headache has been present for years, it is very important to establish why the patient has presented to the doctor. A change in the pattern of the headache may be the result of new stresses in the patient's life, the superimposition of a new type of headache on the pattern of a chronic headache, or an exacerbation of the old headache.

The subacute onset of new headaches is likely to be associated with underlying organic disease. Attacks that become increasingly frequent and increasingly painful suggest intracranial mass lesions or chronic meningitis. Brain tumor causes headaches in about 50% of cases and presents with headaches in 30%; nevertheless brain tumors account for less than 1% of all headaches.

The acute onset pattern is also associated with life-threatening disease. Subarachnoid hemorrhage is suggested in a patient who presents with the worst headache of his life. However, even the severe acute headaches frequently turn out to be trigeminal neuralgia or migraine headaches.

Pain from subarachnoid hemorrhage peaks within 1 to 5 minutes, but pain from vascular headaches builds less rapidly. Many patients who initially state that their headache was of sudden onset will, on more careful questioning, indicate that pain built up over 30 minutes to 1 hour. In subarachnoid hemorrhage, about 50% of patients lose consciousness briefly at onset, an uncommon pattern in recurrent vascular headaches. History of loss of consciousness or obtundation can be a sign of grave disease.

LOCATION AND QUALITY. The location and quality of the pain may suggest a cause. Dural structures, including the tentorium and the middle and anterior fossa, refer pain to the forehead. Posterior fossa lesions, cervical vertebral disease, and high blood pressure cause occipital pain. Tension headaches are generalized and often described as squeezing or "like a band around the head." Unilateral pain is seen in migraine, tic douloureux, and cluster headache. In migraine, temporal localization contrasts to the orbital pain of cluster or the maxillary pain of tic. Lower facial pain is also seen in a variant of migraine. The pain in migraine is conventionally thought to be throbbing, corresponding to the pulse, but in one study only half the patients reported pulsatile pain.

TIME OF DAY. Tension headaches characteristically start in the afternoon, last until evening, but seldom interfere with sleep. They may also be present shortly after arising in patients who are having constant pain. Migraine headaches may occur at any time of day but frequently occur in the early morning or at night, waking the patient from sleep. They also occur following periods of stress. Because the supine posture tends to increase intracranial pressure, early morning occurrence suggests increased intracranial pressure, particularly if the pain remits shortly after rising. Headaches from common causes such as sinus congestion, glaucoma, and hypertension also have this pattern. Conversely, "low-pressure" headache following lumbar puncture is characteristically worsened by upright posture and relieved by a supine position

ASSOCIATED SYMPTOMS. Associated symptoms such as nausea and vomiting are characteristic of migraine and advanced cases of elevated intracranial pressure. Photophobia, motion sickness, and tenderness of the scalp are very characteristic of migraine. In temporal arteritis there may be tenderness of the artery or jaw claudication.

Certain foods, such as packaged meats containing nitrates, or withdrawal from alcohol or coffee can precipitate headaches. Birth control pills increase the severity and frequency of migraine, and some medications, such as nitroglycerine, characteristically cause headaches. Headaches are a frequent adverse reaction to many medicines, such as indomethacin (Indocin). Other precipitating factors such as head trauma, emotional stress, menses, fatigue, and infections should be sought. See Table 104-1 for a summary of historical features.

Physical Examination

Certain points of the general examination require particular attention. Eyes should be examined for impaired vision, glaucoma, optic atrophy, subhyaloid hemorrhage, and signs of papilledema. The head and neck should be examined for craniocervical bruits over the eyes and carotid and vertebral arteries and palpated for painful areas, masses, or evidence of trauma. The scalp, sinuses, and temporal arteries specifically should be palpated. In 35 to 77% of patients with temporal arteritis, the artery is firm and enlarged and may be tender. The neck should be examined for unusual proportions (suggesting craniocervical junction abnormalities), masses, and range of motion and nuchal rigidity.

Any abnormalities of neurologic examination are clear indicators for neurologic consultation and/or further evaluation. Full, detailed neurologic exam is essential.

Diagnosis: Common Headache Syndromes

TENSION HEADACHE. Tension is probably the most common cause of headache, accounting in one study for 40% of patients referred to a headache clinic. However, in the general, nonspecialty clinics the prevalence may be even higher. Women are affected three times as frequently as men, and in a high percentage of cases there is a family history of headache, including migraine. The clinical picture is typically that of bilateral headache with dull, constant pain in a tight band around the head. Pain precipitated by stress often occurs in the latter part of the day. Headaches may occur daily for years. The headache may be associated with abdominal bloating and mild nausea and is frequently associated with depression or anxiety and contraction of jaw, face, and neck muscles. However, atypical cases exist. The pain can be throbbing rather than constant, and in 10% of cases the pain is unilateral. In addition, tension headache and migraine can coexist. This possibility requires careful consideration in patients with premonitory symptoms of frequent unilateral headaches.

Vascular factors do seem to operate in tension headaches. Moreover, the high proportion of important psychological factors in both migraine and tension headaches and the overlapping family history have lead some authors to suggest that the two conditions are the extremes of a single disorder.

MIGRAINE. About 4 to 15% of the population suffers from migraine, with a 3:1 female predominance. Migraine headaches, although usually unilateral, are bilateral in up to 40% of patients.

Classification of migraine is based on the characteristics and timing of the aura: classic migraine headache is preceded by an aura; in interposed migraine, the transient neurologic disturbance occurs after the onset of headache; in common migraine, no aura symptoms occur; in migraine equivalent, the aura occurs without headache; and in complicated migraine, the neurologic deficit of the aura becomes permanent.

The typical migraine patient has the onset of headaches between the ages of 10 and 30 years old; only 10% begin after age 40. In 20 to 50% there is a family history, but the genetics of inheritance are unclear. About 60% of patients had motion sickness as children, and some patients may have recurrent attacks of vomiting and abdominal pain. Usually the headaches occur at intervals of 1 to 2 months, but attacks may vary from infrequent to daily. Although attacks may occur at any time, they most often happen in the early morning hours, either awakening the patient from sleep or occurring shortly after waking.

In classic migraine there is an aura, or warning, before the onset of headache. The aura is usually a visual disturbance, but virtually any neurologic deficit can occur. Frequently described disturbances include flashes of color, wavy lines, heat waves, and bright spots. About 10 to 15 minutes following the onset of the aura, the head pain begins and builds up relatively slowly over the course of 30 to 90 minutes. Occasionally the buildup is rapid. In all forms the pain is described as throbbing by only 50% of patients; in some patients, sharp, brief, ice pick–like pains may be superimposed on the more constant pain. There is pain on motion of the head and tenderness of the scalp. Photophobia and nausea with or without vomiting frequently occur, and diarrhea may occur in some patients. Some relief comes with lying in a quiet, darkened room. In 66% of patients, the pain lasts for less than 24 hours.

Common migraine accounts for the majority of cases and classic migraine for less than one-third. Other forms are relatively rare. However, for any patient the pattern of headache may not remain the same and may evolve from classic migraine in the teens to common migraine in middle age. About half of migraine patients have other headaches, usually tension headaches.

One of the most common mistakes made by physicians caring for headache patients is underdiagnosis of migraine. The majority of headaches associated with gastrointestinal disturbances and photophobia are vascular, despite the lack of aura, hemicranial pain, or pulsatile pain. Though fewer than 30% of migraine patients have classic migraine, aura symptoms can be subtle, consisting of mood changes, unsteadiness on feet, or nonspecific dizziness.

Precipitating factors important in migraine include stress and worry, menstruation, contraceptives, fatigue, lack of sleep, drop in barometric pressure, and foods, especially chocolate, alcohol, and citrus fruits. Although pregnancy frequently reduces the rate of migraine attacks, an increase in headaches may be seen during pregnancy.

The cause of neurologic symptoms and headache of migraine is not clear. In both intra- and extracranial arterial systems, vasoconstriction has been noted during the aura and vasodilatation during the headache. The most widely held belief is that the basic mechanism involves peripheral vasomotor tone. The drop in serotonin levels in the blood and the increase in its excretion during migraine headaches suggest a role for serotonin in migraine pathophysiology.

CLUSTER HEADACHE. Cluster headache, also called sphenopalatine neuralgia, ciliary neuralgia, migrainous neuralgia, and histamine cephalgia, is a relatively rare form of headache. The syndrome occurs most often in older men (men account for 85% of cases) with onset between ages 20 and 50. The headaches are excruciatingly painful and cause the patient to feel restless and agitated. The orbital pain is unilateral and associated with nasal discharge and stuffiness, lacrimation, chemosis, and Horner's syndrome. Painful episodes last 15 to 20 minutes and may occur one to several times per day. Associated symptoms include nausea and vomiting in 45%, but rarely visual symptoms. During the time of the cluster, drinking alcohol may precipitate headaches. Although clusters occur once or twice a year in most patients, headaches may occur more often. The tendency for headaches to occur in clusters, usually lasting 4 to 8 weeks, separated by several asymptomatic weeks or months, has given rise to the name "cluster headache."

Recently some variant forms of cluster headache have been described. Chronic cluster headache is a cluster-type headache occurring without pain-free intervals. Chronic paroxysmal hemicrania affects women more frequently than men and is characterized by frequent painful attacks occurring without remission.

During headache, elevated blood histamine levels may be seen, but treatment with antihistamines has rarely been successful. No clear-cut changes in scalp or intracranial blood flow have been noted. The etiology of the syndrome remains obscure.

POSTTRAUMATIC HEADACHE. Headache occurs in up to 80% of head injuries, ranging from severe injuries with brain damage to injuries with only concussion or even milder findings. Posttraumatic headache develops most commonly following accidents at the work place or in motor vehicles and develops more frequently in patients who were premorbidly considered "nervous" or "neurotic." The probability of developing

Table 104-1. Headache syndromes

Syndrome	Location of pain	Time course	Associated signs and symptoms
Primary headaches			
Migraine	Unilateral or bilateral temporal pain	Onset in early AM; last 2–12 hr, occurring infrequently or daily	Nausea, vomiting, photophobia, varied neurologic signs and symptoms in aura phase
Tension	Bifrontal and/or occipital	Daily or frequent; worse in later afternoon	Associated anxiety and stress
Cluster	Orbital area, unilateral	Onset at night, waking from sleep, or during day; bouts of pain lasting 15–45 min, occurring in clusters lasting a few weeks	Ipsilateral tearing, rhinorrhea, Horner's syndrome
Trigeminal neuralgia	Facial, in 5th nerve dermatome, unilateral	Daily pain occurring in brief 1–5 min bouts	Trigger area, lack of neurologic findings
Psychogenic	Vertex or localized	Often constant pain	Associated psychosis or neurosis
Sinusitis	Over involved sinus (referred frontal or vertex in sphenoid sinusitis)	Occurrence increased in allergy seasons	Associated URI, sinus tenderness, postnasal drip
Posttraumatic	Unilateral or bilateral, frontal or occipital	Starts immediately following trauma, may persist for 2 yr or more	Associated dizziness, occasional syncope, mild thought disorder
Post–lumbar puncture	Generalized	Following lumbar puncture	Worse in upright posture, relieved in supine position; associated nausea and vomiting
Secondary headaches			
Pseudotumor	Variable, often generalized	Weekly to daily; often worse in AM; relieved by erect posture	Visual obscurations, 6th nerve palsy, papilledema

Temporal arteritis	Unilateral pain in temporal area	Onset over age 45	Visual symptoms, polymalgia rheumatica jaw claudication, tender palpable temporal artery
Costen's syndrome (TMJ syndrome)	Temporal, behind ear	Daily	Anxiety, dental occlusion problems, "blocked" sensation in ear
Gradenigo's syndrome	Eye or frontotemporal pain	Constant	Lesion of apex of petrous bone, 6th nerve palsy
Raeder's syndrome	5th cranial nerve distribution, usually forehead	Constant	Horner's syndrome, 5th nerve and 6th nerve palsies, internal carotid artery or middle fossa lesion
Cervical spondylosis	Occipital	Constant	Neck pain, history of neck trauma
Eye disease	Ocular	Frequent	Glaucoma, refraction problems
Meningitis	Generalized	Acute or subacute onset, increasing pain over hours or days	Fever, lethargy, variable neurologic signs, stiff neck
Subdural hematoma	Variable, depending on location of hematoma	Subacute onset, constant pain	Dulling of sensorium, focal neurologic signs
Tumor	Variable	Increasing in frequency and intensity, constant in late stages	Worse in supine position, improved in vertical posture; focal signs; projectile vomiting
Hypertensive	Generalized	Often acute onset	Need to rule out hemorrhage
Subarachnoid hemorrhage	Generalized; worst headache in patient's life	Acute onset	Family history, loss of consciousness, meningeal signs, focal neurologic signs (especially 3rd nerve pain)

posttraumatic headaches is not affected by the presence or absence of brain damage, nor is it correlated with the duration of loss of consciousness. Such headaches occur concurrently with objectively defined deficits in attention span and memory, reductions in rate of information processing, increase in irritability, and occasionally abnormalities on electrophysiologic testing.

The posttraumatic headache often occurs within 24 hours of injury, but may be delayed. It may resemble either a tension or migraine headache. Vertigo and light-headedness occur in a high proportion of cases, but syncope occurs in only 10% of patients. Scalp injuries tend to result in localized pain superimposed on a background of tension headache. The headache occurs frequently and tends to worsen for a few weeks or months before improving. The problem is self-limited and resolves in less than 1 year in 70% of cases and in less than 3 years in 85%.

Because litigation is often involved and because the patients may have multiple complaints in the absence of findings, there is a tendency for physicians to dismiss posttraumatic patients as hysterics or malingerers. The cognitive deficits in this syndrome are often not assessed by the usual clinical examination, and an unsympathetic attitude on the part of the physician may contribute to the development of anxiety, depression, or other psychiatric problems. It is difficult to determine, often, whether psychiatric components are primary or secondary.

Late sequelae of head injury include hydrocephalus, seizures, and chronic subdural hematoma, each of which may present with only subtle neurologic signs but require prompt, specific treatment. Neurologic consultation may therefore be indicated for patients with persistent posttraumatic headache.

Laboratory Evaluation

If the history suggests a primary headache syndrome and general and neurologic examination are normal, extensive laboratory evaluation is not needed. A number of studies show that few CT scan abnormalities leading to a change in therapeutic approach are found in such patients. Routine screening for unsuspected medical conditions (e.g., anemia) may be helpful and an ESR in older patients to rule out temporal arteritis is mandatory. Skull, cervical, or sinus x-rays are useful in selected cases.

CT scanning is necessary when secondary headache is suspected, but many give confounding results in primary headache syndromes. As many as 30% of patients with classical migraine attitudes may have transient focal low-density parenchymal lesions maximally 3 to 4 days following attacks. There have been reports of increased incidence of cortical atrophy in severe migraine and in tension headache patients, but the significance of these changes is unclear.

EEG abnormalities are probably more frequent in primary headache patients. Migraine patients may have epileptiform changes and other nonspecific EEG abnormalities. Focal slowing has been reported during migraine attacks.

Abnormal findings on CT or EEG may lead to further unnecessary diagnostic testing. Normal studies may lead to a false sense of security. Headache from chronic meningitis, nasopharyngeal tumor, or craniocervical junction abnormalities among other secondary causes is compatible with a normal routine CT scan. There is no formula for an adequate headache workup: Testing must be individualized using clinical judgment.

Ancillary studies are clearly indicated in four circumstances: (1) when the examination is abnormal, (2) when the history suggests a specific diagnosis other than a primary headache, (3) when chronic syndrome headaches develop new features, and (4) when there are atypical features, for example, new onset of migraine in an elderly patient. When these indications for further workup do not exist, it is reasonable to follow the patient's clinical course.

Treatment

There is a common background of patient education that underlies treatment of all patients with primary headaches. Patients should be reassured that the headache does not represent a serious disease and instructed that they must participate in their treatment. Because finding the best therapy may require several trials, patients should not expect immediate cure.

The first step is to attempt to modify triggering factors and stresses that contribute to the headache. Medicines, dietary factors (e.g., citrus fruit, chocolate, caffeine with drawal) and habits (e.g., smoking, alcohol) that may worsen headache should be explored with the patient and appropriate changes or modifications made. Birth control pills, which may exacerbate migraine headaches, should be discontinued. Work and domestic stresses should be discussed and modified if possible. Sometimes psychotherapy is useful.

Relaxation training or biofeedback training has been shown to be effective in some cases. Various techniques are available, including conditioning methods, biofeedback using hand or head temperature or scalp electromyography, hypnosis, acupuncture or even transcendental meditation. One study found only transient relief in 136 of 309 patients after 8 to 10 acupuncture sessions. Much of the success of these measures may be from placebo effect. Simple relaxation techniques that require no special equipment should be attempted before more elaborate and expensive alternatives. Instructing friends or relatives in massage of the affected painful area may also be helpful.

Often psychological support, attention to precipitating factors, and some form of relaxation therapy are all that are required (especially for simple tension headache or for headaches related to acute stress). The question should not be *which* medication to start a patient on but *whether to start any* medication at all. If headaches are disrupting the patient's life or if the pain is perceived as quite severe, and if simple measures have failed, pharmacologic treatment should be considered.

Medication for headaches can be given in three different ways: (1) for symptomatic relief of an acute painful episode, (2) for prevention of headache after warning signs have appeared (abortive therapy), and (3) as prophylactic therapy to reduce the frequency of occurrence of headaches. Infrequent headaches without aura require only symptomatic therapy. In classic migraine with a clear-cut aura, abortive therapy can be tried. The decision to attempt prophylactic therapy should be made only after symptomatic therapy has failed. The patient must clearly understand the purpose of prophylaxis and not take the medicine for symptomatic relief.

Symptomatic Treatment for Tension/Migraine Headache

If aspirin and acetaminophen are not effective, codeine may be added for more severe headaches, especially if they are infrequent. More frequent headaches often respond well to Fiorinal, a proprietary combination of aspirin, and caffeine with a small amount of barbiturate. Because of their addictive potential, narcotic medications should be avoided in treating headaches. However, some physicians recommend intramuscular meperidine (Demerol) for very severe attacks of migraine. Such attacks are probably the most acutely uncomfortable headaches in the range of primary headaches. For such severe attacks no medication will completely relieve the pain; the goal should be to make the patient as comfortable as possible while the headache runs its course. In migraine, there is also the theoretic consideration that after only a few days of use, narcotics may cause a mild withdrawal syndrome with recrudescence of the headache. For severe headaches, sedatives such as choral hydrate or benzodiazepines, which allow the patient to sleep until the pain subsides, may be more effective than narcotics. Before undertaking such therapy, one must be very secure in the diagnosis.

Abortive Treatment

Tension headache can occasionally be aborted by escaping from the precipitating situation or by massage.

In classic migraine, abortive therapy should be used if an aura is clearly identifiable. Various preparations of ergotamine, including Cafergot and Bellergal for oral use, Ergomar for sublingual use, and a medihaler for inhalation, are available. Patients may have nausea and vomiting at the outset of an attack, making dosing difficult. The sublingual and medihaler forms help to circumvent this difficulty. Nausea and vomiting as well as tingling and numbness of the extremities are side effects of these drugs. They are contraindicated in patients with hypertensive cardiovascular disease, hepatitis, or renal failure and in pregnancy. Isometheptene is effective for both abortive and prophylactic treatment of migraine.

For cluster headaches, abortive therapy is more difficult because of the relatively rapid buildup of pain. However, ergotamine compounds have been found effective in aborting attacks for 80% of patients. Sublingual or inhalant medications are more

Table 104-2. Medications for prophylaxis of headache

Medication	Indication	Dosage	Effects and Advantages	Adverse Effects
Propranolol (Inderal)	Migraine	20 mg bid to start Up to 240 mg/day	Side effects relatively rare; effective β-adrenergic blocker	Bradycardia; contraindicated in chronic renal failure, congestive heart failure, asthma; rebound cardiac effects; expensive; increased depressive symptoms; bid or tid dosing
Amitriptyline (Elavil)	Migraine, tension	10–25 mg hs to start Up to 100–150 mg/day	Antidepressant action (separate from antiheadache action) may be beneficial; once daily dosing; effective; blocks serotonin uptake at nerve terminal	Sedation, dry mouth, orthostatic hypotension, rare urinary retention
Methysergide (Sansert)	Migraine, cluster	2–8 mg/day	The most effective prophylaxis for migraine and cluster; serotonin antagonist	Abdominal discomfort, peripheral vasoconstriction, angina muscle cramps; retroperitoneal, endocardial, and pleural fibrosis
Cyproheptadine	Migraine	12–24 mg/day	Physiologic effects similar to methysergide without side effects	Sedation, nausea, light-headedness, pedal edema, dry mouth, occasional diarrhea
Bellergal (contains ergotamine, belladonna, and phenobarbital)	Migraine, tension	1 tid	Few side effects; somewhat effective for tension headaches	Sedation, ergot side effects

Drug	Headache type	Dose	Comments	Side effects/contraindications
Midrin (contains isometheptene, dichloralphenazone, and acetaminophen)	Migraine, tension	For acute attack 2 po; 1 g hr up to 5 capsules in 12 hr For prophylaxis 1–2 q8h	Effective for aborting migraines, may be useful prophylactically for tension headaches	Contraindicated with glaucoma, heart and liver disease, and hypertension
Diazepam (Valium)	Tension	2–10 mg/day	Muscle relaxant	May induce dependence with withdrawal syndrome; increases depression
Aspirin	Migraine	325 mg qid	Inexpensive, simple, but relatively unconventional treatment; effective in some patients	GI side effects, antiplatelet activity
Lithium	Cluster	Start at 200 mg tid and adjust according to serum levels	Especially effective in chronic cluster	Nephrogenic diabetes insipidus, tremor, GI symptoms, confusion
Indomethacin (Indocin)	Chronic paroxysmal hemicrania, ice pick headaches	25–100 mg tid	Mechanism unknown but effective	GI side effects; may induce headache
Corticosteroids (Prednisone)	Cluster, migraine	60 mg/day for 7–10 days with rapid taper	Very effective in majority of cases of severe acute exacerbation	Cataracts, induced diabetes, osteoporosis, Cushing's syndrome, mood changes

likely to be effective because of their more rapid onset of action and their availability despite vomiting. Another form of therapy, which is effective, has no contraindications or side effects, and can be used at home, is oxygen inhalation. In one study this was as effective as ergotamine.

Prophylactic Treatment
Tension headaches, migraine headaches, and cluster headaches can all be treated by prophylactic medication when indicated. Prophylaxis should only be used after other modes of therapy have proved ineffective. In all cases, trials of prophylactic medications should be made for a period of 3 to 6 months, and if the headaches remit, the drug should be tapered off to prevent the chronic side effects of medication.

For migraine, a wide choice of medications allows individualization treatment. While both amitriptyline and propranolol are effective in a wide range of patients, treating depressed patients with amitriptyline and hypertensive patients with propranolol reduces the number of medicines needed to manage both conditions. A useful approach in refractory migraine patients is to rotate through a series of medications for a trial period of 2 to 3 months until the most effective treatment is found. The patient's cooperation will be improved if it is explained that an empirical approach will be taken.

The method of trying a series of prophylactic medications for 2- to 3-month periods is also effective for tension headache, although the range of medications is much more limited (see Table 104-2).

Cluster headaches can be effectively prevented by a variety of medications, as outlined in Table 104-2. Lithium and methylsergide are both quite effective, but both require close follow-up by a physician familiar with their use. The daily headaches of chronic paroxysmal hemicrania, a recently described form of cluster headache, can be effectively prevented by relatively low doses of indomethacin.

Conclusions
The major principle of treatment is to adopt the simplest effective approach. This means reassuring the patient of the benign nature of the condition and taking the time to explain the importance of avoiding precipitating factors. When medications are unavoidable, the simplest and safest should be tried first. When medications fail or when there is a question about the diagnosis, early referral to a neurologist or neurosurgeon is indicated. One study of the effect of such referrals found that in more than two-thirds of cases an evaluation by a specialist reduced the frequency of doctor visits for headache. The authors believed that the reason for this decrease was the reassurance that no underlying disease was present.

Caviness VS, O'Brien P. Current concepts: Headache. *N Engl J Med* 302:446–450, 1980.
  Concise overview of the primary headache syndromes.
Dalessio DJ (Ed.). *Wolff's Headache and Other Head Pain* (4th ed.) New York: Oxford University Press, 1980.
  A classic text brought up to date, this book includes data on the mechanisms of many headache syndromes.
Dickman RL, Mastern T. The management of non-traumatic headache in a university hospital emergency room. *Headache* 19:391–396, 1979.
  Stresses the benign nature of most headaches and the importance of a proper workup.
Friedman AP (Ed.). Symposium on headache and related pain syndromes. *Med Clin North Am* 62:427–621, 1978.
  Reviews each major syndrome with guidelines for treatment.
Kudrow L. *Cluster Headache.* New York: Oxford University Press, 1980.
  Most complete single text on cluster headache.
Lance JW. *Mechanism and Management of Headache* (4th ed.). Boston: Butterworth, 1982.
  Reviews a large clinical experience and provides updated discussion of the mechanisms of headache as well as detailed suggestions for treatment. One of the best sources.
Lance JW. Headache. *Ann Neurol* 10:1–10, 1981.
  Briefly reviews selected topics in headache diagnosis and management, with review of recent work on underlying mechanisms.

Matthew NT. Indomethacin responsive headache syndromes. *Headache* 21:147–150, 1981.

Reviews syndromes responsive to indocin including a new group of patients with a cluster headache variant that responds to indomethacin.

Raskin NH, Appendzeller O. Headache. *Major Problems in Internal Medicine.* 19:1–244, 1980.

This is one of the best sources for information on the diagnosis, pathogenesis, and treatment of headache.

Sargent JD, et al. Use of CT scans in an outpatient headache population: An evaluation. *Headache* 19:388–390, 1979.

The CT scan reveals abnormalities in substantial numbers of migraine and tension headache patients, but the rate of finding abnormalities that change therapy is quite low.

105. SEIZURES: EVALUATION
Robert W. Eckel

Seizures result from synchronous firing of an abnormally active group of neurons. When such activity occurs in a localized cortical area, a focal or partial seizure is produced whose manifestations depend on the normal function of the area affected. When abnormal discharges occur in deeper brain structures, a generalized seizure is produced. Because these abnormal discharges disrupt the ongoing activity of both cerebral hemispheres (and may also affect the reticular activating system), generalized seizures are always associated with a loss of consciousness. However, a partial seizure may sometimes progress to a generalized seizure with loss of consciousness.

Because they are sudden events, seizures and transient loss of consciousness are frequently seen as emergencies. In a recent study of all patients presenting to a big city emergency room, patients with transient loss of consciousness accounted for 3% of visits. Of 198 cases that could be fully evaluated, 29% were seizure disorders, 3% were other neurologic problems, 40% were of vasovagal or psychogenic origin, 7% were related to drugs or metabolic disturbances, and 8% were cardiac problems. The cause remained undetermined at 12 months in 13% of cases.

Classification
Seizures are classified as partial (focal) and generalized. The complete classification is given in Table 105-1.

Partial Seizures
Partial seizures are either simple or complex. When consciousness is not impaired, they are referred to as simple partial seizures. Those in which awareness and responsiveness are impaired (other than unresponsiveness due to paralysis, aphasia, or apraxia) are referred to as complex partial seizures. Complex seizures may be accompanied by automatisms, which can be complex motor behaviors, emotional mimicry, chewing or swallowing, or spoken words.

Partial seizures are characterized by a warning or aura that precedes the attack. When a partial seizure proceeds to secondary generalization, the aura helps to localize the earliest site of epileptic activity. The manifestations of simple partial seizures are quite varied and may consist of

1. Typical focal motor symptoms.
2. A variety of sensory symptoms such as tingling or coldness of an extremity or flashes of light and visual hallucinations. Perhaps the best known sensory seizure is the olfactory hallucination; usually this consists of an unfamiliar unpleasant smell, but pleasant smells can occur.
3. Autonomic signs and symptoms, which include blood pressure changes, epigastric sensations, unilateral or bilateral pupillary changes, and sweating or pallor.
4. Psychic symptoms, which vary from déjà to jamais vu, forced thinking, and dreaming

Table 105-1. Proposed international League Against Epilepsy Seizure classification

I. Partial (focal, local) seizures
   A. Simple partial seizures
      1. With motor signs
      2. With sensory or special sensory symptoms
      3. With autonomic symptoms
      4. With psychic symptoms
   B. Complex partial seizures (with impairment of consciousness)
      1. With impairment of consciousness only
      2. With clonic components
      3. With atonic components
   C. Partial seizures evolving to secondarily generalized seizures
      1. Simple partial evolving to generalized seizures
      2. Complex partial evolving to generalized seizures
      3. Simple partial evolving to complex partial evolving to generalized seizures
II. Generalized seizures (convulsive and nonconvulsive)
   A. Absence and atypical absence
   B. Myoclonic seizures
   C. Clonic seizures
   D. Tonic seizures
   E. Tonic-clonic seizures
   F. Atonic seizures
III. Unclassified epileptic seizures

Source: From Proposal for revised clinical and electroencephalic classification of epileptic seizures. *Epilepsia* 22:495–501, 1981.

states. Emotional symptoms (most often fear, but occasionally anger or amusement) are less common. Patients may also have complex, structured hallucinations.
5. Automatisms can be simple gustatory movements (e.g., lip smacking, sucking) or can be quite complex. In some cases, normal behavior such as walking, eating, or driving continues during the seizure. Most often the behavior consists of gestures such as scratching of the head, rubbing body parts, or clasping hands. Occasionally the automatisms are bizarre: opening cupboards and throwing dishes to the floor, undressing, or simulating the motions of sexual intercourse. When the seizure abates, the patients cannot recall what happened during the seizure.

Simultaneous video and electroencephalographic (EEG) monitoring of patients with complex partial seizures has revealed several distinct types of spells. In some (type I), an aura precedes a period of motionless staring followed by automatisms such as lip smacking or chewing, blinking, or swallowing. In other seizures (type II), there is no aura or any motionless staring; the patient develops clonic movements of the face, assumes a fencing posture, develops contraversive movement of head and eyes, or displays automatisms. Some patients develop "temporal lobe syncope," and an EEG is needed to distinguish this from other causes of syncope.

Convulsive Generalized Seizures
Convulsive generalized seizures ("grand mal" or generalized tonic-clonic seizures) begin with a sudden generalized onset of rigid tonic muscle tone without a warning and often are associated with an epileptic cry and incontinence of bowel and bladder. After the tonic phase, lasting 1 to 2 minutes, generalized jerking movements of the extremities occur (the clonic phase). The frequency of the clonic activity diminishes slightly as the attack proceeds. The clonic phase usually lasts no more than 5 minutes. After the attack, there is a postictal phase during which the patient is at first unarousable, then successively stuporous and confused. The duration of the postictal phase is quite variable and can last for 1 to 2 hours.

Primary generalized seizures are not focal at their onset, and there is no lateralization during the postictal phase. This is in contrast to generalized tonic-clonic seizures evolving from partial seizures, which clearly have a focal onset and which may show transient focal signs during the postictal phase.

Nonconvulsive Generalized ("Absence") Seizures
Nonconvulsive generalized ("absence") seizures are brief interruptions of consciousness lasting one to several seconds. Attacks may occur several hundred times a day. Often the patient is not aware that the spells are occurring. They are not accompanied by loss of muscle tone or syncope, and patients resume tasks at the point they left off. Absence seizures are sometimes accompanied by fluttering movements of the eyelids, nystagmoid eye movements, or facial movements. The syndrome occurs in children between the ages of 4 to 5 years and puberty and may progress after puberty to primary generalized tonic-clonic attacks. These seizures are accompanied by a characteristic three per second spike-and-wave EEG pattern during the attack.

Recognizing nonconvulsive partial seizures and absence seizures requires a high index of suspicion on the part of the physician. It should be normal practice in interviewing patients who have seizures to inquire about aura, incontinence, and postictal fatigue or confusion. When inquiring about aura it is helpful to inquire specifically about motor, autonomic, sensory, and psychic symptoms. Many patients may not be aware of the significance of these symptoms and, because they are often bizarre, may be too embarrassed to mention them unless specifically asked.

Differential Diagnosis of Transient Loss of Consciousness
The first step in evaluating transient loss of consciousness is to decide if the spell was a seizure. Syncope is the condition most frequently confused with seizures. Ordinarily, following a faint due to postural hypotension from any cause, normal blood pressure and brain perfusion are restored by the supine position. If the head and upper body are unwittingly propped up during a syncopal episode, blood flow to the brain may not be rapidly restored and a generalized seizure can follow. A seizure that is secondary to the postural hypotension does not require specific therapy.

Other conditions associated with spells that may be confused with seizures include hyperventilation syndrome, psychiatric disorders and hysterical seizures, drop attacks with vertebral basilar artery insufficiency, and migraine headaches. Hyperventilation syndrome can present with a wide range of neurologic complaints such as dizziness, confusion, paresthesias, or blackouts; having the patient over-breathe for 2 to 3 minutes reproduces the symptoms. Drop attacks occur without loss of consciousness. Usually such patients have other symptoms referrable to the brain stem such as diplopia, vertigo, dysarthria, or dysphagia. Migraine headaches occasionally cause syncope in association with neurologic symptoms.

Evaluation: Transient Loss of Consciousness

History
Because the history is the major basis on which seizures are differentiated from other kinds of spells, the account of an eyewitness must be sought. Certain features are particularly useful.

1. *Precipitating circumstances:* Seizures can occur any time; however, they are often associated with falling asleep or waking. Some forms of seizures, known as reflex epilepsy, can be precipitated by external stimuli; flashing lights (e.g., the flicker of the television tube) are the commonest of these precipitants. Seizures are not precipitated by postural changes, unless the patient is propped in a sitting or standing position. Psychogenic hysterical and hyperventilation spells often occur in highly charged emotional circumstances, or with anxiety, and almost always occur in the presence of other people. Personal injuries can result from seizure and from syncope, but usually not during psychogenic spells.

2. *Auras* may be quite bizarre but are usually stereotyped and repetitive and can be prolonged. If the aura is not followed by a generalized tonic-clonic convulsion, it is a partial seizure. In contrast, patients with syncope have a brief feeling of dizziness or of "darkening of vision." Hyperventilation may produce tingling in hands and feet and around the lips.

3. *Muscle tone* is rigid during the tonic phase of generalized tonic-clonic convulsions. Complete loss of tone may occur with complex partial seizures and with syncope.

4. *Incontinence* is most characteristic of seizures but occurs rarely in hysterical seizures as well.

5. *Duration* of the convulsive phase of a typical generalized tonic-clonic seizure is 1 to 5 minutes. Consciousness may not be fully regained for as long as 1 to 2 hours. Syncope is typically much briefer.

6. *The postictal phase:* Following generalized tonic-clonic seizures, consciousness may be impaired for 1 to 2 hours, and fatigue and muscle tenderness may last as long as 24 hours. Following partial seizures, there is often brief postictal confusion. By contrast, recovery of consciousness following syncope is typically immediate and complete.

7. *Skin color* usually does not change during seizures but is pallid just before a faint because of generalized vasoconstriction.

Physical Examination
The physical examination includes evaluation of postural changes in blood pressure and pulse, cardiac examination, and careful neurologic examination for focal findings that localize the central nervous system (CNS) disease. A postictal (Todd's) paralysis may persist for as long as 24 hours after a seizure. Hyperventilation for 3 minutes will often reproduce the spells in hysterics and hyperventilators.

Laboratory Tests
Immediately following a spell, laboratory evaluation is useful in identifying medical problems associated with seizures. Helpful studies include electrocardiogram, Holter monitoring electrolytes, calcium, magnesium, liver and renal function tests, VDRL, and blood glucose.

During a generalized convulsion, the EEG is always abnormal; it is usually abnormal during partial seizures and is always normal during hysterical seizures. An EEG taken postictally is of limited usefulness. It may reveal abnormalities not seen beyond the postictal period—local slowing or interictal spikes. Slowing can occur 12 to 24 hours following both seizures and syncope but not hysteria. Moreover, in patients with epilepsy, an EEG taken more than 1 week after an attack may be normal in as many as 20% of patients, while some conditions such as migraine may show focal spike activity.

Evaluation: Seizure
When it is clear that seizures are the cause of the spells, it is still necessary to answer two other questions: (1) are the seizures generalized or focal, and (2) if focal, what is the focus?

Primary generalized epilepsies are more often inherited, commonly have onset in childhood, and presumably are due to inheritable errors of brain metabolism. Acquired generalized epilepsies are more often due to alcohol or barbiturate withdrawal or are associated with hyponatremia, hypoglycemia, hypotension, fevers, or a variety of other systemic insults. Focal seizures in any age group are more likely to be related to intracranial pathology such as vascular disease, infections, tumors, trauma, and demyelinating, degenerative, and autoimmune diseases.

There are two peak ages for the onset of seizures. One is in patients up to age 20 and the other after age 50. The early-onset group has about half generalized seizures and one-third to one-quarter partial complex seizures. After age 50, there are proportionally more focal seizures and more simple partial seizures. The overall frequency of brain tumor, while quite variable in different studies, is from 8 to 10% in adults with seizures. Patients with simple partial seizures are more likely to have tumors (as many as 20–30%). Eighty-five percent of generalized seizures are idiopathic. In one large study of patients of all ages with seizures, 25% had identifiable causes. Of these cases, 22% were caused by trauma or surgery, 22% were related to vascular disease, either bleeding or thrombosis, 18% were due to tumor, 17% were due to congenital disease including the neurocutaneous syndromes, 12% were related to infections, and 4% were related to degenerative disease.

All patients with new seizures or with a significant change in the pattern of seizures should have a computed tomography (CT) scan of the head and an EEG. Patients with an exacerbation of seizures should have anticonvulsant levels drawn. If no lesion has been found, a lumbar puncture should be performed after CT scan has ruled out hydrocephalus or mass lesion. This is useful in establishing some diagnoses that cannot be established any other way, such as cerebrospinal fluid infiltration of tumor, encephalitis, meningitis, or CNS syphilis. Arteriography or nucleotide brain scans occasionally may be needed to study questionable areas or to detect intracerebral, subdural, or epidural bleeding.

When seizures are poorly controlled and an EEG diagnosis has not been established, a number of specific maneuvers may help to increase the yield of the EEG. Sleep sometimes activates epileptiform activity, and sleep-derived EEGs exploit this fact. Nasopharyngeal and sphenoidal leads, although uncomfortable for the patient, may help electrically "visualize" the medial temporal lobe. Further information can occasionally be gained by prolonged records (the usual EEG records only 20 or 30 minutes of cerebral activity) with or without video monitoring. Despite such procedures, the EEG may remain normal in a small proportion of epileptics.

The pace of evaluation for seizures can vary depending on the clinical situation. Frequent seizures, especially those accompanied by abnormalities of the general or neurologic examination, fever, or head trauma, require rapid evaluation and hospitalization for observation, usually by a neurologist or neurosurgeon. Single, isolated seizures can sometimes be evaluated in the outpatient department over the course of 1 to 2 weeks.

Lum LC. Hyperventilation and anxiety state. J R Soc Med 74:1–4, 1981.

Magarian GJ. Hyperventilation syndromes: Infrequently recognized common expression of anxiety and stress. *Medicine (Baltimore)* 61:219–236, 1982.

Lum and Magarian present guidelines for diagnosis of this often missed diagnosis.

Cleland PG, et al. Prognosis of isolated seizures in adult life. *Br Med J* 283:1364, 1981.

Hauser WA, et al. Seizure recurrence after first unprovoked seizure. *N Engl J Med* 307:522–527, 1982.

Day SC, et al. Evaluation and outcome of emergency room patients with transient loss of consciousness. *Am J Med* 73:15–23, 1982.

These three papers illustrate that it is not uncommon for a patient to have only one seizure. Caution in diagnosing epilepsy is recommended.

Victor M. The pathophysiology of alcoholic epilepsy. *Res Publ Assoc Res Nerv Ment Dis* 46:431, 1968.

Classic study of these commonly seen withdrawal seizures.

Proposal for revised clinical and electroencephalic classification of epileptic seizures. *Epilepsia* 22:489–501, 1981.

Penry JK, Porter RJ. Epilepsy: Mechanisms and therapy. *Med Clin North Am* 63:801–812, 1979.

So EL, Penry JK. Epilepsy in adults. *Ann Neurol* 9:3–16, 1981.

All three papers above present excellent reviews including prognostic factors and recommendations for surgical and medical therapy.

Daly DD. Ictal clinical manifestations of complex partial seizures. *Adv Neurol* 11:57–83, 1975.

An extensive cataloging of seizure symptomatology.

Hauser WA, Kurland LT. The epidemiology of epilepsy in Rochester, Minnesota 1935 through 1967. *Epilepsia* 16:1–66, 1975.

A detailed analysis of seizures that occured in that city over 32 years including prevalence, causes, and prognosis.

106. SEIZURES: TREATMENT
Robert W. Eckel

Once initial workup has ruled out a treatable underlying cause (e.g., encephalitis, brain tumor), therapy of seizure disorders is empirical and aimed at suppression of seizures and at helping the patient live with the condition. With modern anticonvulsants, the majority of patients can be seizure-free or have greatly reduced numbers of seizures. The two major errors in the treatment of seizures are overtreatment with pharmacologic agents and inadequate patient education. The prognosis in epilepsy is more closely related to the underlying condition than to the effects of seizures. The only true emergency in epilepsy is grand mal status epilepticus.

General Measures
All patients with epilepsy need to be instructed about the dangers of their condition. Driving, swimming, bathing, and working with machinery, fire, or electricity or on heights may be hazardous. Specific vocational rehabilitational services are available in many parts of the country for retraining epileptics.

Driving
Driving poses both legal and medical problems. The law varies from state to state, but it is usually illegal for a person with uncontrolled seizures to operate a motor vehicle. In most states, the physician's legal responsibility is to advise the patient that he must inform the authorities, but not to report the patient to the licensing agency. Driving licenses in most cases will be suspended until the patient has been seizure-free for some specified time, usually 1 or 2 years. Physicians must become familiar with the laws applicable to their region.

Factors that Tend to Precipitate Epilepsy
Factors that tend to precipitate epilepsy should be avoided. Some of these are

1. Insufficient sleep
2. Excessive alcohol, which can lower seizure threshold, particularly during the withdrawal phase
3. Drugs such as antidepressants and major tranquilizers, which lower seizure threshold
4. Stimuli such as strobe lights
5. Psychological stress and anxiety
6. Febrile illnesses

Avoiding the precipitants of seizures may be all that is necessary for therapy in some patients. Rushing into long term pharmacologic therapy is not always warranted, particularly in patients who have had a single seizure that is related to known precipitants.

Anticonvulsant Therapy
Patients with recurrent seizures should be treated with anticonvulsants. The fundamental principle is to give as little of a single drug as needed to keep the patient seizure-free. More than one drug should be given only when a patient continues to have seizures despite consistent therapeutic levels of an appropriate agent and re-evaluation confirms that the diagnosis of etiology and seizure type was correct. If more than two drugs appear to be necessary, the patient should be referred for evaluation by a neurologist. No patient should be treated with more than three anticonvulsants because effectiveness is usually not increased, but interactions and toxicity are.

Serum Levels
Serum levels are useful for establishing a baseline therapeutic level, detecting noncompliance or other causes of lowered serum levels if seizures recur (e.g., drug interaction or fast or slow acetylation), and establishing a maximum nontoxic dose when seizures continue. Drug levels represent a total of both the protein-bound and free fractions of the drug. These fractions usually exist in a fixed relationship, and the total levels correspond well with brain levels. However, if this proportion is upset, as it is in renal disease, in hypoalbuminemia, or when two drugs compete for a serum protein binding site, it may be necessary to check free serum levels. Generally, levels should be checked when a drug is in steady state for a given dose. A steady state usually occurs after a patient has been on the dose for 5 half-lives of the drug.

Choice of an Agent
The choice of an agent for initial therapy depends on the type of seizure. Dosage schedule is summarized in Table 106-1. For absence seizures, ethosuximide, clonazepam, or valproic acid is appropriate. Ethosuximide is specific for absence seizures and ineffective against other types. For primary generalized tonic-clonic (grand mal) seizures, phenytoin, phenobarbital, carbamazepine, or valproic acid is used. For initial therapy of generalized seizures, phenobarbital or phenytoin is best, but there is no clear choice

Table 106-1. Guidelines for use of anticonvulsants

Anticonvulsant	Therapeutic level	Serum half-life	Initial dosage	Maintenance dosage
Phenobarbital	20–50 μg/ml	96 ± 12 hr	1 mg/kg/day	1.5–3.0 mg/kg/day
Phenytoin	10–20 μg/ml	24 ± 12 hr	5 mg/kg/day 300 mg/day	4–8 mg/kg/day 300–600 mg/day
Carbamazepine	4–10 μg/ml	8–60 hr	200 mg/day	800–1200 mg/day
Primidone	5–15 μg/ml	12 ± 6 hr	Child: 125 mg/day Adult: 250 mg/day	Child: 500–750 mg/day Adult: 1–2 gm/day
Ethosuximide	40–100 μg/ml	30 ± 6 hr	3–6 yr: 250 mg/day > 6 yr: 500 mg/day	Up to 1.5 gm/day
Clonazepam	20–70 μg/ml	27 ± 5 hr	Child: 0.01–0.03 mg/kg/day Adult: 1.5 mg/day	Child: 0.1–0.2 mg/kg/day Adult: less than 20 mg/day
Valproic acid	40–100 μg/ml	10 ± 2 hr	15 mg/kg/day	30 mg/kg/day

between them. For partial seizures, the drugs used for primary generalized seizures are appropriate; in addition, for intractable cases surgical therapy should be considered.

Phenobarbital

Phenobarbital is the oldest and one of the least toxic of the anticonvulsants. It can be given orally, intramuscularly, or intravenously. Some patients may exhibit paradoxic hyperactivity. Withdrawal of phenobarbital after prolonged therapy can result in seizures if the withdrawal is too sudden. Idiosyncratic allergic reactions, with cross-reaction with phenytoin, occur in 10 to 25% of patients. Loading doses and overdoses can result in coma, sometimes with focal neurologic signs. Toxic levels may increase seizure frequency especially in children.

Phenytoin

Phenytoin (Dilantin) is the mainstay of antiepileptic therapy. The therapeutic dosage of phenytoin is about 5 mg/kg daily. Because of the long half-life, a single, daily dose is possible. The drug is useful in status epilepticus because traumatic levels can be achieved quickly with minimum sedation.

Phenytoin is 90% protein-bound. Large changes in free concentration, without change in total concentration, can occur from drug interactions. When this happens, toxicity can occur, even at total drug levels within the therapeutic range.

Dose-related toxicity results in nystagmus, diplopia, dizziness, and ataxia. Relatively high blood concentrations (usually > 40 μg) are required before sedation appears. Hyperglycemia is seen in some patients. Common side effects include hypertrichosis, gingival hypertrophy, and facial coarsening, particularly in children. All of these may be quite distressing to patients and may require withdrawing the drug. Uncommon idiosyncratic reactions include skin eruptions, lymphadenopathy, hepatitis, blood dyscrasias, and a lupus syndrome.

Both phenobarbital and phenytoin interfere with folate metabolism and can cause megaloblastic anemia and peripheral neuropathy. Both drugs also can reduce vitamin D levels, leading to hypocalcemia and osteomalacia.

Carbamazepine

Carbamazepine (Tegretol) is a relatively new anticonvulsant, which is useful in suppressing generalized and focal seizures. Blood and brain levels are comparable. In the blood the drug is 70% protein-bound. Because carbamazepine induces the enzymes necessary for its own metabolism, the half-life is quite variable (from 8–60 hours) and depends on the age of the patient and chronicity of treatment. Because of this great variability, it is best for adults to start with a low dosage, 100 mg two times a day. By following blood levels, dosage can be gradually increased one tablet per day each week to a total of 1 gm per day. Because of its short half-life in chronic treatment, the drug should be given two to four times a day. The therapeutic range in serum is from about 4 to 8 μg/ml.

Side effects may occur at low blood levels during the initiation of therapy. Nystagmus, diplopia, and ataxia of gait are particularly common. Dose-related side effects, seen above therapeutic levels in chronically treated patients, include dizziness, vertigo, and unsteadiness. Blood dyscrasias including aplastic anemia, which were a major concern when the drug was introduced, are rare and occur in the first 12 weeks of therapy. An initial pretreatment complete blood and platelet count should be followed by monthly determinations for 4 months. After this, only biannual determinations are needed. Hepatic toxicity, which has been reported, seems to be quite rare. Renal toxicity and an inappropriate ADH syndrome are occasionally seen.

Valproic Acid

Valproic acid (VPA), the most recently introduced anticonvulsant, appears to be effective in generalized, absence, and myoclonic seizures. The drug is a branched-chain carboxylic acid, which may act by increasing brain levels of GABA, an inhibitory central neurotransmitter. It has a short half-life of 6 to 15 hours, which requires frequent dosing, and wide fluctuations in plasma levels can occur.

Side effects include nausea and vomiting in up to 50% of patients. Manufacturers are now making available coated tablets, which may greatly reduce this side effect. It is more common in children and tends to disappear with continuation of therapy. Sedation may occur at high dosages. Other central nervous system effects include tremor similar to benign essential tremor, diplopia, and ataxia. Valproic acid causes coagulation disturbances including alterations of platelet aggregation and prolongation of prothrombin time and partial thromboplastin time in a small number of patients. The most serious toxic reaction to VPA is toxic hepatitis. Death due to liver failure has occurred in a small number of cases. More frequent is a transient elevation of hepatic enzymes, which subsides in 10 to 12 weeks. However, there is no way to predict when toxic hepatitis will occur. The drug should be withdrawn when serum liver enzyme levels rise to more than three times normal. Pancreatitis has rarely been reported. Hyperammonemia and a Reye's syndrome-like reaction have occurred. In combination with other anticonvulsants, sedative effects out of proportion to drug levels are occasionally seen.

Before beginning chronic therapy, a single dose of 250 mg should be given to test for gastrointestinal side effects. Therapy should be started at a low dosage of 7 to 10 mg per day and gradually increased. The range of therapeutic blood levels is 50 to 100 μg/ml. Deterioration of seizure control may occur with excessive levels.

Benzodiazepines

Benzodiazepine drugs used in seizure control include diazepam (Valium) and lorazepam (Ativan) for status epilepticus and clonazepam (Clonopin), which is useful for myoclonic and absence seizures. The usefulness of all benzodiazepines is limited by the rapid development of tolerance to their effects. This is so rapid in the case of Valium that the drug should never be used for chronic therapy. In addition to tolerance, chronic therapy may result in a withdrawal syndrome on discontinuation of the drug. Intravenous therapy with benzodiazepines can also result in respiratory depression and hypotension. Occasionally, benzodiazepines paradoxically increase the frequency of seizures in children.

Common Clinical Problems

Poor Seizure Control on a Single Drug

If seizures continue on a single drug, one should first check anticonvulsant levels and increase the dosage to the upper therapeutic range. Phenytoin dosage should be increased cautiously when levels are in the therapeutic range because small increases in dosage can lead to big increases in serum levels. Dosages should not be increased more than 50 mg per day, and adequate time (5 half-lives) should be allowed for the drug to reach equilibrium before re-evaluating phenytoin levels.

If the drug is at the upper limit of the therapeutic range and producing toxicity, and seizures continue, a second drug should be added. There are significant interactions between antiepileptic agents. For example, VPA and phenytoin are both highly protein-bound and compete for binding sites; adding one to the other increases the free fraction of both. Because toxicity is correlated with the free drug levels, toxicity may occur when the new drug is added unless the dosage of the original drug is reduced at the same time. Phenobarbital strongly induces liver enzymes and, when given to a patient taking phenytoin, may increase degradation and reduce blood levels of phenytoin. However, because both drugs are metabolized by the same enzymes, the addition of phenobarbital may result in competition for hepatic enzymes, with reduced metabolism of both drugs and increased levels. Carbamazepine may reduce phenytoin levels, while phenytoin may paradoxically also reduce carbamazepine levels. Valproic acid added to other antiepileptic medications may cause stupor, even without toxic drug levels.

Because it is often difficult to predict what the result of the addition of a given agent to a regimen will be, it is important to follow blood levels when making changes. When the use of more than two agents is considered, it is best to consult with a neurologist. No patient should receive more than three drugs.

If a trial of appropriate drug regimens fails to control the seizures, referral for evaluation of surgical therapy should be considered. If addition of a second drug results in seizure control, the physician should consider tapering the first drug.

Discontinuaton of Drug Therapy.

Adults who have been seizure-free for at least 2 years have a 40% recurrence rate, usually within the first year after therapy is discontinued. There is no consensus in the literature about factors, including electroencephalographic, that predict the outcome of discontinuation of drugs. However, some factors seem to predict recurrence: focal seizures are more likely to reappear than generalized seizures, and only 30 to 40% of patients who have had a single isolated spell go on to have further seizures with or without anticonvulsants. In addition, presence of generalized spike-and-wave activity on prewithdrawal EEG is associated with increased risk of recurrences.

In general, patients should be encouraged to continue anticonvulsants. If the patient strongly wishes to stop medications after 2 to 4 seizure-free years, slow tapering of medications over several months can be attempted. Rapid withdrawal may induce withdrawal seizures or even status epilepticus. The patient should be warned that seizures may recur.

Epilepsy in Pregnancy

During pregnancy, seizures usually increase in frequency, but they may also decrease or remain unchanged. One reason for the increase in seizures may be that phenytoin levels drop in pregnant women, apparently because of decreased oral absorption.

The major problem of epilepsy in pregnancy is the dangers to the fetus posed by drug therapy. Congenital anomalies are reported in 2.5% of offspring of nonepileptic mothers and in 4.2% and 6.0% of untreated and drug-treated epileptic mothers, respectively. All anticonvulsants are potential teratogens. A characteristic syndrome of anomalies including cleft palate, cleft lip, cardiac septal defects, and mental retardation has been reported with phenytoin. Another fetal problem is bleeding from vitamin K deficiency in newborns of mothers taking phenytoin, phenobarbital, or trimethadione. Vitamin K should routinely be given to all newborns of epileptic mothers.

A decline in carbamazepine and phenobarbital blood levels is also seen in pregnancy. This results in an increased risk of seizures and status epilepticus during pregnancy. Careful monitoring of blood levels in pregnant patients may reduce this risk.

Brain J, Willmore J. Epilepsy and pregnancy. *Can J Neurol Sci* 6:345–349, 1979.

Montouris GD, et al. The pregnant epileptic: A review and recommendations. *Arch Neurol* 36:601–603, 1979.

These two articles provide overviews with recommendations for this vexing group of patients.

Penry JK, Newarak ME. The use of antiepileptic drugs. *Ann Intern Med* 90:207–218, 1979.

Excellent review of the pharmacologic properties of drugs in use for epilepsy.

Browne TR. Drug therapy: Valproic acid. *N Engl J Med* 302:661–666, 1980.

Haruda F. Phenytoin hypersensitivity: 38 cases. *Neurology (NY)* 29:1480–1485, 1979.

These articles provide data on these anticonvulsants.

Spenser SS. Depth electroencephalography in the selection of refractory epilepsy for surgery. *Ann Neurol* 9:207–214, 1981.

Review of indications for surgery in intractable seizures.

Hopkins A. *Epilepsy for Patients.* New York: Oxford University Press, 1980.

An excellent guide for physicians as well as for patients, providing a simplified view of seizure pathophysiology and an excellent review of the pragmatic implications of seizures in everyday life.

107. TRANSIENT ISCHEMIC ATTACKS AND CAROTID BRUITS

John S. Kizer

Transient ischemic attacks (TIAs) are focal neurologic deficits that spontaneously resolve within 24 hours. They are sometimes the initial manifestation of arteriosclerotic cerebrovascular disease.

Prognosis

The onset of TIAs indicates an increased risk for future cerebral infarctions. Estimates of the risk of stroke during the 5 years following the onset of TIAs range from 5 to 40%. However, estimates based on prospective follow-up of patients with TIAs indicate a 5-year risk closer to 5 to 15%, with the majority of new strokes occurring within the first 6 to 12 months after the onset of TIAs. The same studies suggest that over a 5-year period about 50% of the patients presenting with TIAs become asymptomatic. No more than 25 to 30% of patients with cerebral infarctions have antecedent TIAs. Thus, if one assumes that cerebral infarctions account for two-thirds all strokes (with hemorrhagic and embolic strokes constituting the majority of the other third), over 80% of all major cerebrovascular events occur without warning.

Pathogenesis

The pathogenesis of TIAs is not understood. It is clear that transient cardiac arrhythmias and episodic hypotension are unlikely causes. It is currently postulated that TIAs result from in situ platelet microaggregates, subintimal hemorrhage into existing atheromas, and fibrin and platelet microemboli from ulcerated stenoses of intra- and extracranial vessels.

While the immediate cause of TIAs is uncertain, it is quite clear that the presence of TIAs implies diffuse cerebrovascular disease, which in turn is part of a diffuse systemic vasculopathy. Thus, the presence of TIAs is a marker not only of risk for future stroke but also of increased risk for death from other cardiovascular diseases. Death from myocardial infarction occurs even more frequently than death from stroke. Therefore, therapeutic interventions to prevent the development of stroke in patients with TIAs must take into account that the onset of TIAs represents a late stage in the development of progressive systemic vascular disease.

Evaluation

In the majority of patients, TIAs are associated with cerebrovascular disease. Other illnesses that can present as transient focal neurologic deficits include polycythemia, thrombocytosis, migraine, focal seizures, hypoglycemia, disorders of the labyrinthian systems, hyperviscosity syndromes, aneurysms, tumors, emboli, multiple sclerosis, and hemoglobinopathies.

The diagnosis of obstructive cerebrovascular disease may be supported by the presence of cranial or carotid bruits and confirmed by a variety of noninvasive studies: oculo–ear lobe plethysmography, ultrasound imaging of the extracranial vessels, dynamic brain scans, and spectral analysis of Doppler ultrasound scans of extracranial vessels. The sensitivity and specificity of these noninvasive diagnostic procedures are quite variable when compared to standard arteriography. For example, oculoplethysmography may be falsely negative in as many as 50% of patients in the presence of bilateral carotid stenoses because this procedure depends on a comparison of pulse delays between the right and left sides. Two-dimensional imaging coupled with spectral analysis of a Doppler scan, on the other hand, appears to be 90 to 96% sensitive for detecting carotid artery disease. False-positive results from both procedures occur in approximately 5 to 10% of all cases.

Arteriography remains the most accurate procedure for delineating disease of the cranial vessels. However, arteriography is associated with a significant morbidity—between 1 and 5% depending on the patients studied. Currently, therefore, arteriography should be reserved for clarification of diagnosis when other serious and treatable causes cannot be excluded or prior to surgical treatment if surgery is seriously considered. Visualizing the carotid circulation by means of computerized digital subtraction angiography is safe with little or no morbidity and few contraindications; however, this test yields less precise images than classic arteriography.

Noninvasive tests like ultrasound are inferior to arteriography in the diagnosis of ulcerative plaques of the carotids. However, there is uncertainty about the relationship between ulcerative disease, its treatment, and prevention of future strokes, so the importance of this deficiency is difficult to assess.

Treatment

Medical therapy includes modifications of risk factors such as diabetes and hypertension and attempts to alter the consequences of established cerebrovascular disease.

Modification of Risk Factors

There is reasonable evidence that treatment of hypertension will prevent the initial occurrence of strokes but will not prevent the occurrence of a second or third stroke. On the other hand, there is no evidence that improved control of diabetes by generally available means lessens the risk of future stroke.

Anticoagulant and Antiplatelet Drugs

Attempts to modify the progression and sequelae of ischemic cerebrovascular disease with either anticoagulants or platelet antiaggregants are based on the rationale that platelets and the coagulation cascade are intimately involved in atherogenesis and cerebral infarction. Implicit in this rationale, however, is the untested assumption that the pathogenesis of TIAs and cerebral infarction is similar.

Over the past 20 years, numerous controlled and uncontrolled studies have investigated the hypothesis that chronic oral anticoagulation of patients presenting with TIAs prevents the occurrence of strokes. These studies have not shown any significant protection from future development of stroke, although overall cardiovascular mortality may have been reduced.

Of the major studies investigating the potential of platelet antiaggregants in the prevention of stroke, the two largest studies indicate that the administraton of aspirin to patients with TIAs decreases overall cardiovascular mortality and reduces the frequency of TIAs but not future strokes. Reduction in TIAs was observed only in men and was not enhanced by the addition of other platelet antiaggregants such as dipyridamole or sulfinpyrazone.

Vasodilator Therapy

There is no evidence to support the use of vasodilators in cerebrovascular disease, except as they are indicated in the control of systemic hypertension.

Surgical Therapy

The surgical approach to the treatment of TIAs is based on the belief that extracranial vascular disease is a cause of TIAs and a harbinger of cerebral infarction. It is postulated that TIAs result from fibrin and platelet microemboli, embolizing from ulcerated and stenotic portions of extracranial vessels to distal branches in the cerebral circulation. Implicit in the surgical approach to cerebrovascular disease is the as yet unproved assumption that the majority of extracranial stenoses will progress to a major vascular occlusion.

The most common surgical approach to the treatment of TIAs is carotid endarterectomy. Surgery of the vertebrobasilar system is rarely undertaken because this area is relatively inaccessible and because of the disputed belief that TIAs in the distribution of vertebrobasilar arteries have a better long-term prognosis than TIAs occurring in the distribution of the internal carotid arteries.

There has been only one long-term, randomized prospective study to evaluate the role of extracranial carotid surgery in the management of TIAs. The authors of this study concluded that surgery of the carotid system may be justified for the prevention of stroke. However, these conclusions are based on analyses that exclude from consideration those patients who had either a perioperative stroke or surgical death. If the risk for the development of stroke alone is calculated for all initially randomized patients, there is no evidence that carotid endarterectomy improves survival or decreases the risk of stroke in patients presenting with TIAs.

There are also numerous uncontrolled trials of carotid endarterectomy in the management of TIAs in which selected groups of patients with TIAs have appeared to benefit from carotid surgery when compared either to historical controls or to groups of patients presenting with TIAs who were considered unfit for surgery. The improved operative mortality and morbidity in these recent studies have been cited as evidence that the controlled trial described above is now obsolete. Such studies are not persuasive because it was not established that the process of surgical evaluation did not select a group of patients with TIAs who would have done well irrespective of the treatment they received. A newer carotid bypass procedure (in which the superficial temporal artery is connected to the middle cerebral artery) is being evaluated by a national controlled study.

At present, the best available evidence does not suggest that extracranial carotid surgery results in a significant long-term reduction in mortality or the incidence of new strokes.

Asymptomatic Carotid Bruits

Asymptomatic carotid bruits are found in approximately 5 to 7% of adults; they are nearly equally distributed between men and women, and their frequency increases with age. Patients presenting with a carotid bruit have an increased risk of overall cardiovascular mortality, with the frequency of myocardial infarction exceeding that of stroke. In patients with asymptomatic carotid bruits, the 8-year incidence of stroke is between 10 and 15%, a risk two to four times greater than the risk in patients who do not have a carotid bruit.

Carotid bruits are a marker of cerebrovascular disease, rather than the direct cause of future strokes. Only two-thirds of subsequent strokes in people with carotid bruits are secondary to cerebral infarction; subarachnoid and intracerebral hemorrhage and embolic strokes account for the majority of the remaining third. Also the majority of cerebral infarctions that occur in patients with asymptomatic carotid bruits are located in vascular territories unrelated to the carotid bruit. Only about 10% of all cerebral infarctions (all distributions) have an antecedent carotid bruit.

Many clinicians have advocated carotid endarterectomy for patients presenting with asymptomatic carotid bruits, arguing that surgery reduces the long-term risk of stroke and death. There is little evidence to support this approach. In patients with asymptomatic carotid bruits, fully two-thirds of all future strokes occur in the distribution of arteries outside the stenotic carotid and cannot be prevented by isolated carotid endarterectomy. Furthermore, assuming an operative mortality for carotid endarterectomy of 1 to 3%, carotid sugery must be 100% effective in preventing death from stroke before the results of surgery approach those of nonsurgical treatment.

At the present time, care of the patient presenting with an asymptomatic carotid bruit includes modification of risk factors for stroke (hypertension and diabetes) and other risk factors for total cardiovascular mortality.

Hypertension Detection and Follow-up Program Co-operative Group. Five year findings of the hypertension detection and follow-up program: I. Reduction in mortality of persons with high blood pressure, including mild hypertension. *JAMA* 242:2562–2571, 1979.

Veterans Administration Co-operative Study Group on Antihypertensive Medications. Effect of treatment on morbidity in hypertension. *JAMA* 213:1143–1152, 1970.

Bauer RB, et al. Joint study of extracranial arterial occlusions. *JAMA* 208:501–518, 1969.
Randomized prospective study of carotid endarterectomy in the patient presenting with TIAs.

Joint Committee for Stroke Resources. XIV. Cerebral ischemia: The role of thrombosis and of antithrombotic therapy. *Stroke* 8:147–175, 1977.
Comprehensive review of studies relating to use of anticoagulants for prevention of stroke in the patient with TIAs.

Heyman A, et al. Risk of stroke in asymptomatic persons with cervical arterial bruits. *N Engl J Med* 302:838–841, 1980.

Wolf PA, et al. Asymptomatic carotid bruit and the risk of stroke—the Framingham Study. *JAMA* 245:1442–1445, 1981.

Canadian Co-operative Study. Randomized trial of aspirin and sulfinpyrazone in threatened strokes. *N Eng J Med* 299:53–59, 1978.

Fields WS, et al. Controlled trial of aspirin in cerebral ischemia (the aspirin in TIA study—AITIA). *Stroke* 8:301–315, 1977.

The Anturane Reinfarction Trial Research Group. Sulfinpyrazone in the prevention of sudden death after myocardial infarction. *N Engl J Med* 302:250–256, 1980.

Yutsu F, Hart R. Asymptomatic carotid bruit and stenosis: A "reappraisal." *Stroke* 14:301–304, 1983.

Faught E, Trader SD, Hanna GR. Cerebral complications of angiography for transient ischemia and stroke: Prediction of risk. *Neurology (NY)* 29:4, 1979.
Eighteen of 147 patients (12.2%) had cerebral complications; 8 (5.4%) were present at discharge from the hospital.

108. PARKINSONISM
Axalla J. Hoole

Parkinsonism is not a single disease but a clinical syndrome characterized by resting tremor, slowing of voluntary movements, muscle rigidity, and gait abnormalities. It may appear as the predominant problem or as an incidental finding in patients with other diseases.

Causes
Most patients with parkinsonism have idiopathic Parkinson's disease (paralysis agitans). This disease develops in patients over 50 years old and affects men and women equally and whites slightly more frequently than blacks. Von Economo's encephalitis lethargica was recognized as a cause of parkinsonism after the pandemic of 1918 to 1920. Other viruses have occasionally been associated with sequelae that have parkinsonian features, but infection has not been established as a major cause of parkinsonism.

Drugs such as phenothiazines (especially chlorpromazine), butyrophenones (especially haloperidol), and less commonly methyldopa, metoclopramide, and reserpine have been associated with a dose-dependent form of parkinsonism. Symptoms have been reported within days following high dosages, but the usual course is for symptoms to develop after weeks of therapy. Parkinsonism usually disappears within weeks of stopping the drug but may persist longer following depot injection.

Other conditions in which some manifestations of parkinsonism are often present include cerebral atherosclerosis and Alzheimer's disease as well as less common problems such as progressive supranuclear palsy and Shy-Drager syndrome. In these conditions, the parkinsonism is generally a less significant part of the overall picture. Occasionally, cerebral atherosclerotic disease may be indistinguishable from Parkinson's disease, but in atherosclerosis, parkinsonism usually appears as a part of a stepwise progression of little strokes, other local neurologic deficits are identifiable, and tremor is frequently absent. In Alzheimer's disease, dementia is the principal finding; the dementia associated with idiopathic parkinsonism is less profound and is not an early finding. However, as intellectual function is being more thoroughly evaluated, dementia is emerging as a more important finding.

Parkinsonism may also be associated with or be a sequela of severe metabolic disorders, such as hypoglycemia, hyponatremia, anoxia, and renal or hepatic failure. Normal pressure hydrocephalus, which presents as a gait disturbance as well as incontinence and deteriorating intellectual ability, may also be confused with parkinsonism. Frontal lobe neoplasms, such as meningioma, may closely mimic the features of parkinsonism and should be considered when there is a rapid onset of symptoms.

The prevalence of parkinsonism is estimated to be 1 case per 100 people over 50 years old. Before the advent of levodopa (L-dopa), parkinsonism was associated with an increase in the death rate. Since then, studies of patients taking L-dopa have shown a decrease in the deaths attributable to parkinsonism.

Manifestations
The major features of established parkinsonism are tremor, bradykinesia, and muscle rigidity. Early symptoms of parkinsonism are muscle aches and fatigue; early signs include decreased strength of speech, decreased spontaneous blinking, and unilateral gait disturbance with decreased arm swinging.

The characteristic resting "pill-rolling" tremor of the thumb and forefinger is seen in approximately two-thirds of patients. The tremor worsens with anxiety or tension, usually diminishes with movement of the limb, and disappears with sleep. Although the tremor starts in the hand, it frequently involves the arm and leg on the same side and eventually the head and opposite extremities.

Bradykinesia results from an inability to start or stop motion. This is often the most disabling aspect of the disease. Because patients have trouble adjusting positions, maintaining balance is difficult and falls are frequent.

Rigidity is bilateral and affects both extensor and flexor muscles; however, there is loss of strength. Resistance to passive motion is continuous ("plastic rigidity"), unless a superimposed tremor imparts a "cogwheel" effect to the rigidity.

The gait of patients with parkinsonism is characteristic. Early in the course of disease there is a unilateral loss of arm swinging; later both arms are involved. Starting walk becomes more difficult and the patient eventually develops a gait pattern in which the upper part of the body is thrust forward to initiate walking and then the patient goes forward with small rigid steps chasing his center of gravity (festinating gait). Finally, stopping and turning become a problem.

Characteristic changes also occur in voice, facial features, and handwriting. Hoarseness is an early sign and may be followed by loss of vocal strength. Ultimately there little face or lip movement, and speech becomes blurred and hard to understand. Facial expression is characteristic and referred to as "mask-like." Changes are bilateral, as opposed to the usual unilateral changes in patients with seventh nerve lesions. The glabellar response is positive: when the patient is asked not to blink and then tapped on the bridge of the nose, he will blink with each tap and not have the usual spontaneous suppression of response to the tap. Handwriting becomes smaller and may show the regular movements of the tremor.

Other clinical findings are blepharospasm (fluttering of the eyelids after they are shut) and sialorrhea (production of a greasy, thick sebum) accompanied by a scaly dermatitis.

Evaluation

Diagnosis is almost entirely based on clinical findings. Laboratory tests are not included unless evaluation suggests that the course is unusual, there is a focal neurologic deficit, or the parkinsonism is associated with an underlying disease that requires further testing. When the differential diagnosis includes normal pressure hydrocephalus progressive supranuclear palsy, computed tomography (CT) scanning may be helpful.

Differential Diagnosis

When only one feature of the disease is present, diagnosis may be difficult. In younger patients, in whom tremor is minimal or absent, rigidity and postural problems are the predominant complaints. In these patients, parkinsonism may be difficult to distinguish from early Huntington's disease or Wilson's disease. Rarely, patients in whom only the muscles controlling phonation are involved present with a speech disorder.

The tremor of parkinsonism should not be confused with postural tremors and cerebellar intention tremor. Postural tremor is worsened by positioning (as when the arms are outstretched), is diminished by rest, and is not accompanied by rigidity or bradykinesia. Postural tremors are found in patients with benign essential tremor, a disorder that may be sporadic or may be inherited, and in patients with metabolic problems such as thyrotoxicosis, hypomagnesemia, or alcoholism.

Benign essential tremor can frequently be identified in first- and second-degree relatives of the patient. It may diminish or disappear with alcohol consumption (a finding reliable enough to be considered a clinical test by some neurologists). These patients may respond to propranolol, 60 to 120 mg per day in divided doses, but not to L-dopa or anticholinergics.

The intention tremor of cerebellar dysfunction worsens with purposeful use of the hands. A confusing factor may be that up to 10% of patients with parkinsonism may also have an intention component to their tremor.

Parkinsonism may also be confused with problems associated with diminished facial movement and flat expression, including hypothyroidism and psychiatric disorders such as depression.

Treatment

Because the side effects of treatment are frequently uncomfortable and severe, they must be weighed against the potential benefits. Treatment is begun only after all drugs that can cause parkinsonism have been withdrawn. Patients may be followed without treatment if they have only mild symptoms or if parkinsonism is a part of an underlying disease that demands attention first.

In parkinsonism there is a decrease in midbrain levels of the neurotransmitter do-

426 XIV. Nervous System Problems

pamine in the substantia nigra, which suppresses striatal systems that are stimulated by acetylcholine. Decrease in dopamine or blockage of its effects by such drugs as phenothiazines leads to uncontrolled effects of acetylcholine. Drug treatment of parkinsonism is based on manipulating this system with either dopaminergic or anticholinergic agents, or both. The most frequently used drug is L-dopa, which crosses the blood-brain barrier and is decarboxylated to dopamine. Other drugs sometimes employed are bromocriptine, which is a dopaminergic agonist, and amantadine, whose mode of action is unclear but is believed to stimulate release of dopamine from neurons. The two most frequently used anticholinergic drugs are trihexyphenidyl (Artane) and benztropine mesylate (Cogentin).

If tremor is the cause of disability, anticholinergics alone may be sufficient treatment. Also, in mild to moderate disease anticholinergics or amantadine may be used. In more severe disability, L-dopa is used alone or in combination with a decarboxylase inhibitor. If symptoms are still bothersome, but side effects prevent further increase in L-dopa, amantadine may be added. Anticholinergics or bromocriptine may be substituted for the amantidine if symptoms persist.

Anticholinergics
Anticholinergics are used in mild cases and in relief of tremors. Frequently used agents are trihexyphenidyl (Artane), given 2 to 5 mg, two to three times a day, and benztropine mesylate (Cogentin), 1 to 2 mg two to three times a day. Neither of these agents has an established benefit over the other, and patients who do not respond to one may respond to the other. Other anticholinergics used occasionally include procyclidine (Kemadrin), biperiden (Akineton), and diphenhydramine (Benadryl).

L-Dopa
L-Dopa has its greatest effect on bradykinesia but also may be useful for treatment of all clinical features of parkinsonism except intellectual dysfunction.

The use of L-dopa is associated with many uncomfortable and potentially dangerous side effects. Because of these problems, L-dopa is now frequently given with carbidopa a decarboxylase inhibitor that prevents conversion of dopa to dopamine outside the brain. A carbidopa/L-dopa combination (Sinemet) is available in several strengths. The use of this combination allows a smaller total dose of L-dopa and results in a decrease in nausea and vomiting and postural hypotension, but not psychotogenic effects and dyskinesias.

One method of initiating therapy is to start L-dopa at 250 mg two times a day and add 250 mg every third day until there is a good clinical response, unacceptable side effects intervene, or the total daily dose is 8 gm. Best results are found if doses are taken at 2- to 3-hour intervals. If gastrointestinal or hypotensive side effects interfere carboxylase inhibitor can be added with a reduction of about 75% in the dose of L-dopa. Because the decarboxylase inhibitor will potentiate the effects of L-dopa remaining from the test dose, the L-dopa should be discontinued for at least 8 hours (i.e., overnight) before the carbidopa/L-dopa combination (Sinemet) is started.

Beginning with L-dopa rather than a carbidopa/L-dopa combination provides more variability in dosing schedules and the simplicity of one drug over two. However, many neurologists prefer to start with a combination drug. Therapy can be started with one 10/100 tablet three times a day. One tablet can be added each week until a good clinical response, a total daily dose of 1 gm of L-dopa, or unacceptable side effects occur. If nausea and vomiting occur rapidly, a 25/100 tablet can be tried. However, with this combination the total daily dose of L-dopa should not exceed 400 to 500 mg.

The most frequently encountered early side effects are nausea and vomiting. These symptoms, which are improved by stopping and restarting at a lower dosage or by adding antacids, usually disappear with chronic administration. Another common problem, postural hypotension, may be helped by support stockings.

The central nervous system side effects are not helped by including a decarboxylase inhibitor. Of these problems, the dyskinesias are the most frequently seen. Almost any movement can develop, but orofacial dyskinesia is most frequently found, followed by athetoid movements, such as those found in Huntington's disease, and dystonic posturing. These effects are dose related and usually diminish with decreasing dosage, but may appear at dosages previously tolerated.

Psychiatric disturbances associated with L-dopa range from depression to frightening hallucinations, or manic psychosis, and appear most often in patients with a history of previous psychiatric disease. Hallucinations may disappear or decrease in frequency by experimentally reducing the dosage of any drug associated with this side effect.

An "on-off phenomenon" is noted after therapy is well established, usually after 1 to 3 years. This is a fluctuation in response to drugs; during the day patients may quite suddenly become markedly bradykinetic or dyskinetic. Spells may last only minutes but tend to grow longer. Symptoms usually improve by giving smaller doses more frequently. Also noted are early-morning problems because of insufficient dose, and end-of-dose deterioration, which is a shortening of the effective duration of therapy.

Other specific but uncommon effects of L-dopa are cardiac arrhythmias and exacerbation of narrow-angle glaucoma. Other minor side effects are blackening of urine or sweat and change in taste.

Amantadine
Amantadine, 100 mg two times a day, may improve symptoms of parkinsonism for a short time (weeks or months). It has fewer side effects than L-dopa but is only useful in mild cases or as an adjunct to L-dopa.

Bromocriptine
Bromocriptine has a structure and action very similar to those of L-dopa. Its use has not been fully evaluated, and it is now primarily used as an adjunct to L-dopa.

Loss of Efficacy
In some patients, drugs may eventually lose their efficacy. These patients may benefit from a "drug holiday." During this time, the patient is hospitalized, and all drugs are stopped for about a week and then reinstituted. In some patients there may be significant improvement, and lower maintenance doses may be required.

Hill JW. Parkinson's disease. *NZ Med J* 90:300–304, 1979.
A practical review of parkinsonism.
Reynolds, NC. The tremor syndrome: Is it Parkinson's disease? *Wis Med J* 80:29–30, 1981.
A short review of the differential diagnosis of tremors.
Mental symptoms and parkinsonism (editorial). *Br Med J* 2:67(e), 1973.
A discussion of the causes of these problems.
Clinical therapeutic rounds: Individualization of drug therapy for the parkinsonian patients. *JAMA* 233(11):1198–1201, 1975.
Stresses the need for adapting therapy to individual patients.
Duvoisin RC. *Parkinson's Disease (A Guide for Patient and Family).* New York: Raven, 1978.
A good guide for both family and physicians.
Teychenne PF, et al. Bromocriptine: Low dose therapy in Parkinson's disease. *Neurology* 32(62):577–783, 1982.
Describes effectiveness of a low dosage of bromocriptine in conjunction with L-dopa.
Bauer RB, McHenry JT. Comparison of amantadine, placebo and levodopa in Parkinson's disease. *Neurology* 24(8):715–720, 1974.
Well-designed study showing the usefulness of amantadine.
Klawans HL, Glantz RH. Ten years of L-dopa in parkinsonism. *Guidelines Neurosci* 4:1, 1980.
An up-to-date review of persistent therapeutic dilemmas.

---

109. BELL'S PALSY
Robert S. Dittus

Bell's palsy (idiopathic facial paralysis) is an acute peripheral paretic or paralytic condition of the seventh cranial (facial) nerve for which a specific etiology cannot be detected. It is not an uncommon affliction, having an incidence of about 20 per 100,000 population per year.

The specific causes of Bell's palsy are unknown. A variety of pathophysiologic mechanisms, including hereditary, mechanical, vascular, and inflammatory processes, have been postulated, but none is supported by conclusive evidence. Perhaps more than one cause will be found to account for the cases now grouped under this single heading. The best-supported theory invokes a viral inflammatory and secondary immunologic injury to the facial nerve. In some cases the facial nerve is the only clinically symptomatic nerve in a more diffuse polyneuropathy.

Risk Factors
Bell's palsy occurs with a fairly uniform distribution worldwide. It can occur at any age. The median age of onset is 40 years old; it is less common below age 15. Men and women are equally affected. The incidence appears to be increased in pregnancy, especially during the third trimester. Ten percent of patients with Bell's palsy have had a previous episode. Eight percent give a positive family history for the condition, although a true familial predisposition has not been established. Hypertension and diabetes mellitus appear to be more prevalent among patients with Bell's palsy.

Clinical Manifestations
Prodromal symptoms and their relative frequencies include facial numbness (32%), facial spasm (22%), upper respiratory infection (20%), headache (10%), fatigue (3%), and fever (2%). Weakness in the distribution of the facial nerve occurs acutely and unilaterally and can range from a mild paresis to complete paralysis. There is no predilection for either side of the face.

Other presenting signs and symptoms include epiphora (tears collecting in and flowing over the lower eyelid—68%), pain (62%), ageusia (57%), hyperacusis (29%), and diminished tears (17%). The pain is usually in or behind the ear, may be moderate to severe, and does not usually persist beyond 7 to 10 days. Retroauricular tenderness or edema may occur, and the chorda tympani may be erythematous. Hypesthesia involving the distribution of cranial nerves V and IX is not uncommon.

Paralysis of the facial musculature produces a loss of all voluntary, associated, and emotional movements of the affected side of the face. Although sparing of the forehead musculature is often claimed to be an absolute discriminant in separating central from peripheral etiologies of facial nerve paresis, in one large series 5% of patients with Bell's palsy had sparing of the forehead musculature. As a result of the weakness, the affected side is expressionless, with a smoothing of the forehead wrinkles, a widening of the palpebral fissure, and a loss of the nasolabial fold. The corner of the mouth sags on the affected side, and the mouth is drawn to the unaffected side. The ipsilateral eyebrow may be lowered or elevated. The patient loses the ability to wink, and Bell's phenomenon occurs (attempted eye closure results in incomplete closure on the affected side while the eye rotates upward).

Diagnosis
Bell's palsy is by definition a diagnosis of exclusion. Five groups of disorders compose 98% of all cases of isolated facial nerve paralysis: Bell's palsy (60–70%), trauma (15–20%), otitis media (5–10%), herpes zoster oticus (4–6%), and tumors (3–5%). The remaining 2% occur in the presence of a variety of other disorders including infectious diseases (chickenpox, coxsackievirus, encephalitis, mastoiditis, infectious mononucleosis, influenza, meningitis, rubella, syphilis), metabolic abnormalities (diabetes mellitus, hyperthyroidism), and neurologic syndromes (cerebrovascular disease, Guillain-Barré syndrome, multiple sclerosis, myasthenia gravis).

When a patient presents with an acute unilateral facial weakness, the history and physical examination, including careful otologic and neurologic examination, are the most helpful guides in establishing a diagnosis. The following findings suggest a diagnosis other than Bell's palsy: simultaneous bilateral facial palsies, unilateral facial weakness that slowly progresses over 3 weeks with or without facial hyperkinesis, and failure of facial function to return within 6 months after an acute onset. Tumors are found in 30% of patients with recurrent unilateral facial palsies.

Many additional tests have been used to screen for primary causes and to attempt to locate the site of the lesion. Audiology can detect hearing loss (which is not consistent with the diagnosis of Bell's palsy). A Schirmer's test to assess the adequacy of lacrimation can be used for management; if tearing is diminished, patients should be treated with eye lubricants. Additional tests should be considered on an individual basis. Tests that are sometimes performed but have been shown not to be helpful routinely include sedimentation rate, glucose, VDRL, fluorescent treponemal antibody absorption (FTA-ABS), heterophil test, serum viral titers, cerebrospinal fluid analysis, mastoid x-rays, and temporal bone computerized axial tomography (CAT) scans.

Natural History

Approximately 50% of patients with Bell's palsy suffer a partial loss of strength in the distribution of the facial nerve. Untreated, almost all will recover with normal function: nearly 90% within 3 to 6 weeks and the remainder within 3 to 6 months. Those few whose recovery is not complete will have a result that is functionally and cosmetically quite satisfactory.

The other half of patients develop a complete paralysis, usually within a few days but occasionally within the first week following the onset of paresis. Of these patients, 50 to 60% will have a normal full recovery, 20 to 30% will have a satisfactory result, and 10 to 20% will be left with a severe palsy with disfiguring contractures and synkinesis. Resolution of symptoms occurs over several months. Rarely will patients have no detectable recovery.

Currently there is no way of making a more accurate prognosis early in the course of the disease. On the average, the younger the patient and the earlier the onset of recovery, the better the ultimate degree of recovery. Other clinical signs and symptoms have no consistent prognostic significance.

Diminished lacrimation occurs in 40% of patients whose recovery is ultimately incomplete; its presence increases the likelihood of an abnormal recovery from 25 to 50%. Diminished salivary flow also occurs in less than half of the patients whose recovery will be abnormal and again increases the likelihood of an abnormal recovery about twofold. A variety of electrical tests have been used to follow the course of nerve degeneration in hopes that this information will have early prognostic value. None has met with universal acceptance, although electroneurography, which determines the percentage of degenerated nerve fibers, has become increasingly popular.

Treatment

Therapy for Bell's palsy is controversial. There is no evidence that vasodilatation or electrotherapy alters the course of the disease. Because it is currently believed that inflammation and edema of the facial nerve play a role, both steroids and surgery have been advocated in order to decompress the nerve physically in its potentially confining pathway through the fallopian canal. Several studies exist both claiming and refuting the efficacy of both steroid therapy and surgical intervention. However, because of flaws in study design, none of the published series offers conclusive evidence for or against the use of either therapy. Both continue to be offered and investigated. In patients with no contraindications, the usual steroid therapy has consisted of 60 to 80 mg of oral prednisone daily initially and for several days with subsequent dosage reduction to a completion of therapy in 2 weeks.

Because the eyelids may not close completely, attention should be given to supportive care of the eye by providing adequate lubrication (in the form of artificial tears) and protection (by an eye patch) if necessary. If a patient has suffered permanent severe dysfunction, a variety of rehabilitative surgical procedures may be considered to improve facial appearance and function.

May M, Hardin WB. Facial palsy—interpretation of neurologic findings. *Laryngoscope* 88:1352–1362, 1978.
Detailed discussion of otoneurologic findings in 400 patients with Bell's palsy.

Adour KK, et al. The true nature of Bell's palsy: Analysis of 1,000 consecutive patients. *Laryngoscope* 88:787–801, 1978.
Review of epidemiologic, clinical, and laboratory data.
Huizing EH, et al. Treatment of Bell's palsy. *Acta Otolaryngol (Stockh)* 92:115–121, 1981.
Analysis of the literature on therapy.
May M. Facial nerve disorders. *Am J Otol* 4:77–88, 1982.
Review article with special attention to rehabilitative surgery.
Adour KK. Diagnosis and management of facial paralysis. *N Engl J Med* 307:348–351, 1982.
Review of facial paralysis including Bell's palsy.
Peitersen E. The natural history of Bell's palsy. *Am J Otol* 4:107–111, 1982.
Description of the natural history of Bell's palsy in 1011 untreated patients.

110. DEMENTIA IN THE ELDERLY

Alan K. Halperin and Paul Beck

Altered mental status is a common finding in the elderly. Approximately 5 to 10% of people older than 65 years of age and 20% of those older than 80 years have clinically important intellectual impairment. In nursing homes and mental hospitals, as many as 50% of the patients may be demented. It is estimated that 15% of all patients with dementia have a potentially reversible cause and that another 20 to 25% can improve function with medical intervention.

Causes

Irreversible Causes

Younger patients are more likely to have potentially reversible causes of dementia than older ones. The major irreversible causes of dementia in the elderly and their relative frequencies include Alzheimer's disease (54%), multi-infarct dementia (8%), and Huntington's disease (5%). Until the 1960s, the dominant view was that arteriosclerotic vascular disease caused senile dementia. However, pathologic examination of the brain of most patients with senile dementia usually reveals a degenerative process involving cortical neurons, with no evidence of significant ischemic lesions. This process, first described by Alzheimer, is characterized clinically by a gradual and progressive decline of intellectual function. In contrast, patients with dementia secondary to multiple cerebral infarctions frequently have stepwise decline in intellectual functioning.

Potentially Reversible Causes

Potentially reversible causes of dementia and their relative frequencies include normal pressure hydrocephalus (6%), alcoholism (5%), intracranial masses (5%), drugs (3%), and miscellaneous causes (9%). Depression is the cause of symptoms in approximately 4% of patients with apparent dementia.

Normal pressure hydrocephalus results in progressive dementia, gait disturbances, and urinary incontinence. In most patients, the cause is unknown, although it may be secondary to a blockage of cerebrospinal fluid reabsorption. In some patients, it is secondary to other central nervous system diseases such as previous subarachnoid hemorrhage, meningitis, or tumors.

A variety of disorders, none by itself very common, accounts for a significant number of dementias. A partial list includes metabolic problems such as hyperthyroidism, hypothyroidism, Addison's disease, Cushing's disease, steroid administration, hypoglycemia, hypercalcemia, and hypopituitarism; metabolic and electrolyte disturbances such as hepatic encephalopathy, hyponatremia, and uremia; nutritional deficiencies such as Wernicke-Korsakoff syndrome found in alcoholics, anemias associated with vitamin B_{12} or folic acid deficiency, and pellagra; cerebral infections such as tuberculosis and fungal meningitis, brain abscess, and neurosyphilis; and dehydration from diuretics, poor fluid intake, or excessive fluid losses.

Diagnostic Strategy

It should never be assumed that dementia is irreversible until a careful evaluation has been completed. However, familiarity with the reversible causes of dementia, a thorough history and physical examination, and a few laboratory and x-ray tests are frequently all that are needed.

History

The history should be directed at characterizing the nature and progression of the dementia and uncovering clues to causal or contributing factors such as drugs, underlying illnesses, or depression. If the patient is unaware of disability, close family members can be helpful in assessing the severity and progression of impairment and behavioral or intellectual changes.

The dementia associated with Alzheimer's disease begins with subtle memory loss and somatic complaints. Later, impairments in judgment, orientation, intellect, and memory become more prominent. The ability to comprehend, assimilate, and integrate new information is impaired and attention to usual social amenities is decreased. In the late phase, the patient's personality and identity can be totally lost. Mood disturbances frequently occur, ranging from apathy and listlessness to suspiciousness and anger. The factors influencing the progression of disease are unknown, and the rate of progression is variable. In cases of multi-infarct dementia, patients or their families may be able to remember a specific time when intellectual and cognitive function began to deteriorate. A family history of dementia suggests the possibility of Huntington's disease.

Dementia must be differentiated from depression presenting with loss of cognitive abilities, which is termed pseudodementia. Findings that help distinguish the two are summarized in Table 110-1.

Taking an accurate drug and alcohol history is important because many widely used common drugs can cause or exacerbate dementia. The most commonly implicated are alcohol, tranquilizers, sedatives, hypnotics, antidepressants, antihypertensives including sympatholytics and diuretics, anticonvulsants such as phenytoin and barbiturates, anticholinergics, and miscellaneous drugs such as levodopa, corticosteroids, and cimetidine.

Patients should also be asked about prior treatment for syphilis, focal neurologic symptoms, and brain trauma. Chronic subdural hematomas and subarachnoid hemorrhages can cause reversible dementia. Acute intellectual changes may be superimposed on a chronic level of dysfunction. The review of systems may rule out coexisting systemic diseases contributing to the dementia.

Physical Examination

A detailed, thorough physical examination is necessary to rule out systemic diseases that can cause reversible dementia. Neurologic examination begins with a quick screen of mental status to confirm the presence of dementia. The level of consciousness is not

Table 110-1. Findings that differentiate between dementia and pseudodementia

Dementia	Pseudodementia
Insidious onset, slow progression	Rapid onset and progression
Does not complain of cognitive and memory loss	Complains of cognitive and memory loss
Tries hard to perform tasks and is easily frustrated	Makes little effort to perform tasks
Retention of social skills	Loss of social skills common
Labile and shallow affect	Pervasive affective change

impaired in dementia, unless there is a superimposed delirium. Impairment of memory can be detected by digit or object recall (short-term memory) and questions about historical events that are compatible with the patient's educational background. Intellectual function can be tested by simple calculations or interpretation of proverbs.

Frontal lobe signs such as the grasp reflex, oral responses, palmar-mental reflex, and glabella tap reflex are signs of diffuse cerebral dysfunction and are frequently present in dementia. Cranial nerves should be checked for papilledema (an indication of increased intracranial pressure), visual field defects (lesions of optic pathway), disturbances of extraocular movements (cranial nerves III, IV, VI dysfunction), and pupillary reactivity (tertiary syphilis). Abnormal movements such as tremors (Parkinson's disease) and tardive dyskinesia should be observed. The presence of gait disturbances may also aid in diagnosis. Focal gait abnormalities may be secondary to stroke or tumor; small shuffling steps and unstable gait may result from normal pressure hydrocephalus, ataxia or cerebellar disease secondary to alcoholism, tumors, strokes, or hypothyroidism. A shuffling and rigid gait is characteristic of Parkinson's disease, and a slapping, wide-based ataxic gait suggests tabes dorsalis or subacute combined degeneration. A sensory examination should be performed to rule out the dorsal and lateral column disease of vitamin B_{12} deficiency.

Laboratory Tests
Diagnostic tests are done to discover potentially reversible causes of dementia. The recommended battery includes complete blood count; liver, renal, and thyroid function tests; serum electrolytes and calcium, B_{12}, and folate levels; serologic tests for syphilis; urinalysis; and chest x-ray.

If none of the above tests leads to a definitive diagnosis, further neurologic testing is indicated. Computed tomography (CT) scans of the head should be done in all cases where no obvious cause is found, since they can detect subdural hematomas, intracranial tumors, normal pressure hydrocephalus, multi-infarct dementia, and atrophy consistent with Alzheimer's disease. An electroencephalogram (EEG) is usually of little value in the evaluation of dementia. A lumbar puncture should not be performed routinely, but should be done when tertiary syphilis or other central nervous system infection is suspected. Because the diagnostic tests used to confirm the presence of normal pressure hydrocephalus are controversial, a neurologist and neurosurgeon should be consulted when this diagnosis is suspected. The evaluation of dementia is best done on an outpatient basis because changes in environment such as hospitalization can exacerbate symptoms.

Treatment

Specific Therapy
Specific therapy of potentially reversible dementias is directed at the underlying cause. If depression is present, tricyclic antidepressants should be used cautiously. Nortriptyline and desipramine tend to have a lower frequency of anticholinergic side effects, which makes them preferable in elderly patients. These agents should be started at very low dosages (25 mg a day), and the dosage should usually not exceed 75 mg per day.

The effectiveness of therapy for normal pressure hydrocephalus is controversial. Improvement with shunt therapy is more likely if the condition is secondary to a prior cerebral insult and in patients in whom the gait disturbance precedes dementia.

It is controversial whether drugs improve cognitive function in demented patients. Hydergine has been the most extensively studied. Numerous uncontrolled and placebo-controlled studies have yielded conflicting results. Hydergine is begun at 1 mg three times per day and continued for at least 2 months for an adequate trial. Use of papaverine, a vasodilator, is also controversial. The use of lecithin, choline, and physostigmine for patients with Alzheimer's disease, in efforts to increase deficient amounts of acetylcholine in the brain, has not been shown to produce consistent improvement in memory or cognitive function.

Supportive Therapy
Although there is no specific treatment for most cases of dementia, supportive measures may help stabilize and improve functional capacity regardless of the cause. General principles include the following:

1. Coexistent medical conditions should be aggressively treated.
2. Changes in the environment should be minimized because they frequently result in mental deterioration. Thus, hospitalization and nursing home admission should be avoided if possible.
3. Drugs should be used very carefully. Use of sedatives and psychotropic drugs should be avoided. If severe agitation is present, haloperidol (Haldol) in low doses of 0.5 to 1.0 mg daily may be helpful. If nocturnal wandering or sleep disturbance is a problem, a short-acting benzodiazepine, such as oxazepam (Serax), may be useful.
4. Sensory impairments, such as visual and hearing deficits, should be corrected.
5. Support groups for families of patients with Alzheimer's disease may help them to have more realistic expectations and fewer feelings of guilt and anger.
6. Social services such as visiting health nurses, homemaker aides, home-delivered meals, physical therapy, respite care, senior citizens centers, and day care centers for the elderly can be invaluable resources to patients and family.

Beck BC, et al. Dementia in the elderly: The silent epidemic. *Ann Intern Med* 97:231–241, 1982.
  A symposium that includes information on causes, clinical presentation, and appropriate patient workup.
Mace NL, Rabins PV. *The 36-Hour Day: A Family Guide to Caring for Persons with Alzheimer's Disease, Related Dementing Illnesses, and Memory Loss in Later Life.* Baltimore: Johns Hopkins University Press, 1981.
  A practical and detailed reference book designed for families of demented patients, but an excellent resource as well for clinicians who advise them.
Wells CE. *Dementia* (2nd ed.). Philadelphia: Davis, 1977.
  Excellent review of all aspects of dementia.
Wells CE. Pseudodementia. *Am J Psychiatry* 136:895–900, 1979.
  Review of psychiatric illness (depression) that can mimic dementia.
Task Force Sponsored by the National Institute on Aging. Senility reconsidered: Treatment possibilities for mental impairment in the elderly. *JAMA* 244:259–263, 1980.
  Review of reversible causes of dementia.
McEvoy JP. Organic brain syndromes. *Ann Intern Med* 95:212–220, 1981.
  Brief review of all organic brain syndromes.
Smith JS. The investigation of dementia: Results in 200 consecutive admissions. *Lancet* 1:824–827, 1981.
  Lists the frequency of different causes of dementia.
Hughes CP, et al. Adult idiopathic communicating hydrocephalus with and without shunting. *J Neurol Neurosurg Psychiatry* 41:961, 1978.
  Review of surgical results of normal pressure hydrocephalus.
Kennie DC, Moore JT. Management of senile dementia. *Am Fam Physician* 22:105–111, 1980.
  Practical aspects of treatment.
Barnes RF, et al. Problems of families caring for Alzheimer patients: Use of a support group. *J Am Geriatr Soc* 29:80–85, 1981.
  Experience of support group.

For information about patient care and educational programs, contact Alzheimer's Disease and Related Disorders Association, 32 Broadway, New York, NY 10004.

XV. PSYCHIATRIC PROBLEMS

Patients with a problem of "nerves" account for about 10 to 30% of encounters in a general medical practice. They may complain of being "shaky," "tense," "irritable," or "uptight," or the diagnosis may be made in the course of evaluating a somatic complaint. The major dilemmas facing the clinician are deciding which patients require special treatment and choosing between pharmacologic and nonpharmacologic treatment approaches.

Evaluation

The information required for initial treatment planning should include a full description of symptoms and the life circumstances surrounding their onset, which can be obtained in about 30 minutes of uninterrupted interviewing. The following specific questions should also be asked:

1. What has been the overall course of the symptoms? Anxiety disorder typically begins in early adult life and recurs intermittently. Anxiety arising for the first time in middle or late life often indicates another disorder such as depression or occult somatic disease.
2. Does the patient have a chaotic or stable life pattern? Frequent moves, shifting relationships, or doctor switching, for example, suggests an unstable personality disorder and diminishes the possibility that antianxiety medication can be used successfully.
3. Does the patient's drinking pattern suggest alcoholism? The most sensitive indicators are the need for a morning eye-opener and annoyance over criticism about drinking.
4. Has there been chronic sedative use? If so, the anxiety may be caused by drug withdrawal.
5. Are there vegetative symptoms of depression? These include loss of appetite, weight loss, early morning awakening, loss of energy, decreased libido, and diurnal mood variation (feeling worse in the morning).
6. Does the patient have fears of public places or sudden attacks of panic that might indicate the agoraphobic syndrome?
7. Is the patient being abused or exposed to other real life threats?

Diagnosis

Although the majority of cases do not fit into specific diagnostic categories, there are a handful of overlapping conditions that require special treatment approaches. These generally account for 10 to 30% of anxious patients.

Depression

Depressive illness is the most common psychiatric disorder in general medical practice, more often appearing in the guise of nonspecific nervousness than as the "classic" retarded depression described in psychiatric textbooks. It is important to recognize these patients, since primary depression is specifically responsive to antidepressant medication. The diagnosis can usually be made by inquiring into vegetative symptoms. Persistence of two or more of these symptoms beyond 1 to 2 weeks generally implies the presence of a medication-responsive depression. Anxiety appearing for the first time after age 40 should probably be considered evidence of depression until proved otherwise.

Alcohol and Drug Abuse

Alcoholism, which is the most frequently encountered form of drug abuse, is the underlying factor in at least 5% of cases of chronic anxiety in general clinic settings. Anxiety may be a part of either intoxication or withdrawal states. Problem drinking can usually be uncovered by straightforward questioning about drinking patterns. It is usually unproductive to attempt to treat anxiety while drinking continues. Other drugs that may be associated with anxiety syndromes when abused include amphetamines, over-the-counter sympathomimetics, hallucinogens (particularly PCP), cocaine, and sedative-hypnotics.

Unstable Personality Disorders (Borderline Syndrome)

Identifying features of unstable personality disorders include familiarity with multiple sedatives, past history of repeated suicide gestures, a demanding presentation, and angry, disparaging attitudes toward clinical providers. Sedatives offer no real benefit for the kind of anxiety experienced by these patients and should be avoided. The best approach is to offer a firm, consistent doctor-patient relationship, a task requiring no small degree of skill and tolerance.

Hidden Violence and Other "Unmentionable" Traumas

Unrecognized spouse abuse was found to be the main underlying factor in half of the female mental health referrals from a rural primary care clinic. These patients usually presented with nonspecific manifestations of anxiety. The history of traumatic beating, easily elicited on questioning, was largely overlooked by the primary providers, who simply prescribed sedatives for their patients' symptoms. Women who have been raped, and members of stigmatized minorities are additional examples of individuals who may feel inhibited about disclosing the real traumas underlying their anxiety.

Undiagnosed Physical Illness

Undiagnosed physical illness underlies anxiety in about 4% of cases. Common culprits include hyperthyroidism, cardiovascular disease, and medication (e.g., steroids, aminophylline, anticholinergics, sympathomimetics, and occasionally sedatives).

Panic Disorder/Agoraphobia

Sudden, recurrent panic attacks (choking, palpitations, dyspnea, and extreme apprehension) along with fears of being in public places characterize this dramatic subgroup of anxiety disorders. Although not common, this syndrome occurs frequently enough to justify inquiring about these symptoms. Panic anxiety disorder is frequently mistreated with sedatives but often responds quickly to a combination of antidepressant medication and behavior modification. Psychiatric referral is usually indicated.

Acute Psychotic Decompensation

Although generally self-evident, acute psychoses may occasionally be hidden under vague anxiety complaints and superficially intact thinking. Bizarre bodily concerns or fears of bodily "disintegration" are tip-offs to the presence of psychosis, which nearly always calls for a major tranquilizer (e.g., chlorpromazine, thioridazine, haloperidol) along with expeditious psychiatric referral.

More typically the anxious patient does not fit into the above groups but presents with complaints of fatigue, irritability, and autonomically-mediated symptoms. Combinations of these symptoms have usually recurred intermittently since early adulthood, although the patient's life has generally been relatively stable and free of extraordinary psychosocial perturbations. This familiar pattern describes *generalized anxiety disorder* (formerly anxiety neurosis or neurasthenia). It is not clear whether this condition represents a psychological or physiologic process or where anxiety disorder stops and "normal anxiety" begins.

Prognosis

A number of well-constructed follow-up studies have shown that most patients with untreated anxiety disorder have no more than mild disability 20 years after initial diagnosis, although symptoms usually return intermittently throughout life. Despite the proliferation of therapeutic techniques and agents, treatment has not been shown to alter the life course of this condition.

Treatment

These findings argue for a treatment approach that emphasizes long-term management over short-term cure.

At present there are four basic options to consider for the patient with generalized anxiety disorder: (1) reassurance in the context of an ongoing doctor-patient relationship, (2) medication, (3) psychotherapy, and (4) relaxation techniques. Flexibility is recommended, with the major emphasis determined by the clinician's working style and the availability of treatment resources. The psychological makeup of individual patients, cost, and possible adverse effects should all be considered.

Reassurance

Reassurance alone is indicated when daily functioning is relatively unimpaired, when the patient fears dependence on medication, or when the interview itself has an observable calming effect on the patient. The relationship with the physician is the active ingredient, and reassurance is more likely to be successful when supplemented by regular visits, adequate listening, and skillful use of suggestion.

Medication

Despite recent controversies, the bulk of evidence seems to support the utility of the benzodiazepine antianxiety agents in properly selected cases. In clinical studies, their overall effectiveness in relieving subjective anxiety is 70 to 75%, as compared to 35% for placebo. These drugs blunt hyperarousal regardless of cause and reduce symptoms in both idiopathic and reality-based anxiety states. Excluding the specific diagnostic categories mentioned earlier, other psychotropic drugs offer no significant advantages in the treatment of anxiety.

The benzodiazepines have relatively few major adverse effects. Dependence and withdrawal have now been well documented but are relatively rare. Psychological dependence is estimated at 1%. Withdrawal symptoms usually require the equivalent of at least 40 mg of diazepam (Valium) per day for more than 20 weeks. Unlike most of the other sedative-hypnotics, these drugs have amazingly little effect on respiration and other basic life-support functions; death due to deliberate or accidental overdose is extremely unusual.

Most authorities recommend intermittent use with treatment intervals limited to 1 to 4 months. A useful strategy is to inform the patient of the time-limited nature of the symptoms and then to explain that medication will prove most effective when limited to periods of undue stress. This often provides the stimulus for a previously avoided review of the patient's life circumstances and identification of mutually agreed upon "red flag" situations that will signal the need for future courses of medication.

All the benzodiazepines are roughly equivalent in terms of efficacy and side effects. Choosing between different benzodiazepines is largely a matter of choosing between drug half-lives. The long half-lives of the most commonly used drugs (50 hours for diazepam and 30 hours for chlordiazepoxide) are generally considered an advantage in young, physically healthy patients. In patients with impaired metabolism (particularly the elderly), a long half-life can lead to toxic drug accumulations; in such patients, drugs with a short half-life, such as oxazepam (Serax), are preferable.

Although a single daily dose of the longer-acting drugs is sufficient to maintain a pharmacologic steady state, a three-times-daily dosage schedule is widely utilized. The advantage lies in the placebo effect and/or subjective "boost" that occurs during the 4- to 6-hour period of rising blood levels following oral ingestion. Within these bounds the clinician has considerable flexibility and should choose a regimen based on the needs of the patient. Typical starting dosages are 10 to 20 mg per day of diazepam, 25 to 50 mg per day of chlordiazepoxide, or 30 to 60 mg per day of oxazepam.

Propranolol is given to some patients whose symptoms are predominantly sympathetic (e.g., palpitations from sinus tachycardia, tremulousness), particularly if dread of these symptoms contributes to anxiety.

Psychotherapy

Psychotherapy requires a relatively large investment of effort by both patient and therapist, making it the most costly alternative in the treatment of anxiety. The indication for psychotherapy lies less in the anxiety symptoms themselves, which are time-limited anyway, than in the potential benefit of resolving persistent underlying problems affecting human relatedness, achievement, or self-concept. Controlled studies give no edge to any particular school of psychotherapy but do indicate that patients in therapy improve at a greater rate than do controls: up to twice as many patients improve depending on outcome criteria. Patients who preferentially respond to psychotherapy generally (1) can identify (or be helped to identify) a specific source of emotional turmoil, usually interpersonal, (2) are willing to accept partial responsibility for difficulties, as well as motivation to changes, and (3) are able to tolerate expression of anxiety-producing emotions.

Relaxation Techniques
Relaxation techniques are thought to work by breaking an anxiety feedback loop maintained by overly responsive voluntary muscle contraction. Modalities include meditation, systematic desensitization, and biofeedback. Teaching the patient to achieve deep muscle relaxation is the basic component of all three. Programs can be found in many university medical centers, Veterans Administration hospitals, or freestanding stress treatment units. Reported success rates as high as 90% may reflect self-selection and may not necessarily generalize to clinic or practice populations. Attempts have been made to make some of this technology available to physicians in the form of commercially marketed relaxation tapes that can be given to patients for self-instruction. Although these may prove useful in relatively mild cases, experience indicates that relaxation is insufficient in itself and must be combined with individualized behavioral interventions in the hands of an experienced trainer to exert full benefit. Treatment can often be completed in a matter of months. Overall, these techniques work best for people who are somewhat compulsive and task oriented or have identifiable anxiety cues and a predominance of symptoms related to motor tension.

Marks IM, Lader M. Anxiety states: A review. *J Nerv Ment Dis* 156:3, 1973.
  A comprehensive review of the clinical literature on anxiety states, covering studies of prevalence, outcome, and phenomenology.
Sheehan DV. Panic attacks and phobias. *N Engl J Med* 307(3):156–158, 1982.
  Describes the appearance and treatment of panic/agoraphobic syndromes.
Wheeler EO, et al. Neurocirculatory asthenia (anxiety, neurosis, effort syndrome, neurasthenia). *JAMA* 142:878–889, 1950.
  A cohort of 167 cardiology patients with anxiety neurosis were followed up 20 years after initial diagnosis. Twelve percent were fully recovered, 15% disabled, and the rest intermittently symptomatic with minimal disability.
Noyes, R, et al. The prognosis of anxiety neurosis. *Arch Gen Psychiatry* 37:173–178, 1980.
  A 6-year follow-up of 112 anxiety neurotics. Sixty-eight percent were improved but not cured. Poorer outcomes were associated with symptom duration exceeding 1 year.
Greenblatt DJ, Shader RI. *Benzodiazepines in Clinical Practice.* New York: Raven, 1974.
  The single most comprehensive review of available data on the benzodiazepines. Covers efficacy, toxicity, and patterns of use, among other topics.
Hollister LE, et al. Benzodiazepines 1980: Current update. *Psychosomatics* 21(90), 1980.
  The entire issue is devoted to the benzodiazepines. A concise update on the social and pharmacologic issues surrounding these drugs.
Kutash IL, et al. *Handbook on Stress and Anxiety.* San Francisco: Jossey-Bass, 1980.
  An in-depth presentation of theory and practice. Chapters on behavior therapy and biofeedback training provide useful descriptions of relaxation-based procedures.
Hall RCW. Anxiety. In RCW Hall (Ed.), *Psychiatric Presentations of Medical Illness.* New York: Spectrum, 1980.
  An exhaustive, well-referenced compilation of medical conditions known to cause anxiety states.

112. DEPRESSION
John J. Haggerty

Depressed feelings affect an estimated 12 to 40% of patients encountered in primary care practices. The main task of evaluation is to identify out of these the 5% of patients who have the specific psychobiologic disorder that is known to respond to medication.

Diagnosis

Major Depression
The clinical differentiation between the medication-responsive disorder and the nonspecific symptom is not always simple. Superficial attributes of the presenting complaint, such as the intensity of emotional distress, or the presence or absence of exogenous stressors are no longer thought to be helpful in making this distinction.

At present, the most frequently used approach is to determine the extent to which depressive mood is accompanied by signs and symptoms that have been shown to be markers of the medication-responsive disorder. These are thought to reflect underlying hypothalamic dysfunction and include the following:

1. Decreased appetite or, less typically, increased appetite, along with weight change
2. Insomnia, particularly with early-morning awakening
3. Observable change in psychomotor activity, either agitation or retardation
4. Persistent inability to enjoy usually pleasurable activities, including sex
5. Fatigue, which is often worse in the morning
6. Feelings of worthlessness or guilt
7. Slowed thinking or decreased concentration
8. Recurrent thoughts of death or suicide

The daily presence of four or more of these, along with sadness or apathy, for at least 2 weeks is generally taken as unequivocal evidence for a depressive disorder. If the patient is experiencing a depressive syndrome for the first time, it is usually possible only to make the general diagnosis of major depressive episode. Subsequent clinical course may lead to a more specific diagnosis of a unipolar or bipolar disorder (see Unipolar Versus Bipolar Disorder).

In primary care settings, most patients do not have an unequivocal major depressive episode. The issue of whether or not to give antidepressant medications to patients with only two or three criteria was addressed in a 3-year follow-up of 100 patients who felt depressed but did not fully meet diagnostic criteria for a major depressive episode. Forty percent eventually developed the full-blown syndrome and so might have been helped by medications. Family history of depression and abrupt onset of dysfunction helped in identifying potentially treatment-responsive patients.

There are reports that patients with depressive disorder fail to suppress cortisol secretion normally with a dexamethasone suppression test (DST). However, it is not clear that the test provides information over and above what is available through clinical judgment. Also, the test distinguishes least well among patients with equivocal depression, the situation where it is needed the most. The DST may be useful, on the margin, when additional diagnostic certainty is needed, such as when concurrent illness increases the risk of medications.

Depression is particularly likely to escape attention in elderly patients, where it frequently presents as dementia. Cultural expectations that the elderly are naturally either sad or confused add to the oversight. Since it is not uncommon for first episodes of depression to occur in old age, clinicians should be certain to inquire about telltale changes in mood, sleeping, eating, and activity whenever evaluating generalized decline in elderly patients.

Contributing Causes
Undiagnosed medical illness often presents as depression. It should be considered in the evaluation of any depressed patient, particularly those with endocrine dysfunction, infectious disease, and neoplasm, notably pancreatic cancer. Depression may be mimicked by these conditions or be an independent condition requiring treatment in its own right. Commonly used medications that can cause the depressive syndrome include propranolol, methyldopa, reserpine, antianxiety drugs, and corticosteroids.

Unipolar Versus Bipolar Disorder
It is usually helpful to determine whether the underlying pattern of illness fits best with a diagnosis of unipolar or bipolar (manic-depressive) disorder. These are now thought to represent distinct illnesses with different modes of inheritance and response to treatment. Since these depressive disorders produce indistinguishable symptoms, it is usually necessary to rely on past history to decide in which category a depressed

patient belongs. In unipolar disorder, there are one or more episodes of depression alone, whereas in bipolar disorder manic episodes are also observed at some point in the patient's lifetime. Have there been any extended periods in the past of elevated mood, ability to get by with minimal sleep, or buying sprees? Have any family members been diagnosed as manic-depressive? If the answer to any of these questions is yes, the patient may have bipolar disorder, and psychiatric consultation is advisable. Unipolar disorder occurs at least 20 times more frequently than bipolar disorder. Therefore, it is usually safe to assume a unipolar disorder for nearly all first episodes of depression. Nevertheless, it is useful to make the distinction whenever possible because of the exquisite responsiveness of bipolar disorder to lithium.

Course and Prognosis
Regardless of the type of depressive disorder, dysfunction is usually episodic and circumscribed, rather than chronic and progressive. In fact, the latter course is often reason to rethink the diagnosis. Recurrence is the rule, and 75% of patients can expect to have more than one episode during their lifetime. When untreated, symptomatic intervals average 4 to 8 months. Intervening asymptomatic periods vary in length from months to decades but as a rule are longer than symptomatic intervals. The first episode of unipolar depression generally occurs after age 30. However, onset can occur as early as infancy.

Patients with depressive disorder typically function well when not depressed. Prognosis for return to premorbid function is usually quite good, particularly if treatment is prompt and complete. However, up to 15% of patients with depressive disorder attempt suicide. This is about 30 times the population average. Also, patients' actions during symptomatic intervals may have lasting consequences.

Drug Therapy

Non-Monoamine Oxidase Inhibitor Antidepressants
Non-monoamine oxidase inhibitor antidepressants are the treatment of choice for most patients suffering a major depressive episode. This category of drugs includes the tricyclics and tetracyclics, as well as several newer, chemically distinct agents (trazodone, buproprion, and others).

All drugs in this class demonstrate similar overall effectiveness in placebo-controlled studies, that is, improved mood and vegetative functioning in around 60 to 70% of patients with clear-cut depressive syndrome. A given patient, on the other hand, may respond to one drug but not another. Although the biochemical reasons for this are partially understood, this has not led to clinically useful predictions of which drug to start. Since individual patients' response patterns to drugs do not change and are often familial, it is useful to ask which drugs have proved effective in the past, either for the patient or for family members.

If this information is unavailable, the next best approach is to select an antidepressant on the basis of its side effects. Sedative, anticholinergic, and hypotensive effects appear in different proportions in each drug. Amitriptyline and doxepin have relatively high sedative and anticholinergic properties. Trazodone is a strong sedative but a very weak anticholinergic. Imipramine is lower on both but has powerful hypotensive effects. Sometimes, these differences can be used to the patient's advantage. For example, amitriptyline will fit a patient with insomnia, imipramine someone who fears oversedation, and trazodone a man with benign prostatic hypertrophy.

Drug dosage is quite variable, mainly due to large individual differences in drug metabolism. Primary care physicians often prescribe insufficient amounts. Usually, a healthy middle-aged adult will require 150 to 250 mg per day of antidepressant (higher for trazodone). The long half-life of all drugs of this class allows lumping as much of the daily total as possible in a single bedtime dose.

Typical practice is to start with an initial 50-mg nighttime dose and then increase to 150 mg in stepwise fashion over the next 5 to 10 days. The patient should be advised to expect dry mouth, constipation, dizziness on standing, and sedation. Some will also experience tremulousness and increased anxiety, particularly with imipramine. If any of these symptoms become excessive, the dosage should be held at tolerable levels for 1 to 2 weeks. Since patients tend to develop tolerance to side effects, it is often possible to resume increasing the dosage toward therapeutic levels after such a wait. If adverse effects are still excessive, a different antidepressant should be tried. Dosage changes should be approached more cautiously in the elderly, who are more likely to develop side effects of all types. A pretreatment electrocardiogram is generally advisable in patients over the age of 45, as well as a brief review of medicines, both prescription and over-the-counter, that might potentiate anticholinergic effects.

Symptoms respond to medication at different rates. Sleeping usually responds quickly. Mood, appetite, and energy, however, may take 4 to 6 weeks to improve. If a patient has not responded to a presumably adequate dosage (up to 250 mg per day of most antidepressants) by this time, drugs should be changed or the diagnosis reconsidered. Accurate blood levels are now available for most of the standard antidepressants and are useful in determining whether nonresponse represents wrong dosage, noncompliance, or wrong treatment. Patients who fail to respond to trials of at least two different drugs probably warrant psychiatric referral.

Once response occurs, medication should be continued for the 6 to 8 months that the depressive syndrome would normally run. When the drug is discontinued, it should be weaned over several weeks to minimize the cholinergic rebound that accompanies rapid withdrawal. Individuals with frequently recurring depressive episodes may benefit from long-term maintenance on antidepressants.

All the antidepressants are potentially toxic. Single doses exceeding 2 gm are frequently fatal. In normal doses, the main areas of concern are central nervous system toxicity in the elderly (who often respond to one-third to one-half the usual amount) and potential cardiotoxicity in patients with preexisting heart disease. Most cardiac problems result from the quinidine-like effect. Complications include worsening heart block and hypotension. Although caution is warranted, it should also be noted that the risk of medication-related death is lower than the risk of suicide associated with untreated depression.

The main advantages of the newer, second-generation antidepressants are decreased toxicity and side effects, particularly anticholinergic effects. Claims of more rapid onset of action are controversial, and none of the newer agents available at the time of this writing have greater overall effectiveness than the older antidepressants.

Lithium
Lithium clearly blunts acute manic attacks and, when taken chronically, will prevent both manic and depressive episodes in bipolar disorder. It may also help some patients with unipolar depression, but this is still controversial, and lithium is not yet a treatment of first choice in this situation.

Monoamine Oxidase Inhibitors
Monoamine oxidase inhibitors are receiving increased attention in the treatment of depressive episodes that do not respond to the tricyclic antidepressants. They seem particularly useful for patients with a marked degree of anxiety. They are not, however, drugs of first choice for primary care physicians.

Thyroid Hormone (T_3)
Thyroid hormone (T_3) has been reported to potentiate antidepressant drug response and decrease side effects in some treatment-resistant depressions. This has important research implications but is not yet an approved indication.

Neuroleptic/Antidepressant Combinations
Neuroleptic/antidepressant combinations are rational treatments only for patients with psychotic depressions or during the first days of an agitated depression. The neuroleptic adds unwarranted risk for tardive dyskinesia that is otherwise best avoided.

Non-Drug Therapy

Electroconvulsive Therapy
Recent public sentiment has obscured the fact that electroconvulsive therapy has a higher overall efficacy than any drug presently available for the treatment of depression and is no more dangerous. Present indications include psychotic depression and drug failure. Complications are rare with modern techniques. Transient and circumscribed memory loss may occur; however, controlled studies have not documented other significant alterations in mental functioning.

Psychotherapy
Depression is one of the few illnesses for which it has been clearly demonstrated that medication and talking have an additive effect. Antidepressants, for example, are less effective than psychotherapy for self-esteem, social functioning, and suicidal feelings. It is generally recommended, therefore, that depressive patients receive both treatments concurrently.

The literature favors an active, encouraging approach that focuses on current interpersonal functioning and downplays the exploration of deep-seated psychodynamics. Fortunately, the recommended technique for accomplishing these aims is generally within the abilities of most nonpsychiatrists.

A typical course of psychotherapy might involve weekly 30- to 45-minute sessions over 2 to 3 months. The initial aim is to help the patient diminish feelings of guilt and to relax excessive self-demands. This is accomplished by explaining that diminished functioning is the result of a treatable and nonvolitional illness, by legitimizing slowing down as necessary to recovery from any illness, and by being willing to tolerate the patient's temporarily increased dependency. Deep exploration of feelings in the early stages of treatment is likely to increase guilt and is best avoided at this point.

As the patient starts to improve (3–4 weeks), the focus should move to exploration of the patient's current interpersonal milieu. The goals now are to allow catharsis, to identify current precipitants, and to facilitate repair of relationships that have been damaged by the depressive syndrome. In the final stages of therapy, the clinician and patient work together on a cognitive level to identify distorted self-views involved in the depression and to characterize situations that might lead to future depressions. Not all patients are capable of reaching this last stage, and in many cases, the provider will have to be content with simple symptom reduction and catharsis. Individuals who unearth difficulties with emotional adjustment that persist beyond resolution of the depressive syndrome, and who are sufficiently verbal, should be considered for referral to more intensive psychotherapy.

Berger PA. Management of Depression and Anxiety in Primary Care Medicine. In AM Freeman, RL Sack, and P Berger (Eds.), *Psychiatry for the Primary Care Physician.* Baltimore: Williams & Wilkins, 1979.
  A practical and lucid expansion of the topics in this chapter geared for primary medical providers. Covers when to hospitalize, assessment of suicidal risk, indications for medication, drug toxicity, and psychotherapy.

Nielsen AC, Williams TA. Depression in ambulatory medical patients. *Arch Gen Psychiatry* 37:99–1004, 1980.
  Five hundred medical group practice patients were evaluated for depression. Twelve percent were at least mildly depressed, and 4 to 5% had moderate depression of the type that would probably respond to medication. Physicians identified only one-fourth of the latter group. The merits of routine screening for depression are discussed.

Akiskal HS, et al. Differentiation of primary affective illness from situational, symptomatic and secondary depression. *Arch Gen Psychiatry* 36:635–643, 1979.
  One hundred cases of "neurotic" depression were followed for 3 years. Forty percent developed clear-cut evidence for bipolar or unipolar disorder. The remaining 60% were a heterogeneous mix of personality disorder, adjustment reaction, and other miscellaneous problems. Strong family history was the best predictor of "true" depressive disorder.

Carroll BJ, et al. A specific laboratory test for the diagnosis of melancholia. *Arch Gen Psychiatry* 38:15–22, 1981.
  Describes dexamethasone suppression test. Includes data on sensitivity and specificity, standard procedure, and conditions that give false-positive results.

Dimascio A, et al. Differential symptom reduction by drugs and psychotherapy in acute depression. *Arch Gen Psychiatry* 36:1450–1456, 1979.
  In a randomized treatment study, ambulatory patients receiving a combination of antidepressants and short-term weekly psychotherapy did better than those receiving either treatment alone. Treatments affected different symptom clusters and had an additive effect when used together.

Veith RC, et al. Cardiovascular effects of tricyclic antidepressants in depressed patients with chronic heart disease. *N Engl J Med* 3067:954–959, 1982.
  Case reports may overemphasize the cardiotoxicity of antidepressants. In this con-

trolled study, 24 patients with depression and chronic heart disease developed no changes in ejection fraction or exercise tolerance on usual doses of imipramine or doxepin. Premature ventricular contractions decreased with imipramine.

Jefferson JW, Greist JH. *Primer of Lithium Therapy.* Baltimore: Williams & Wilkins, 1977.
   An excellent source of basic information on this increasingly useful drug. Available in paperback.

Beck AT, et al. *Cognitive Therapy of Depression.* New York: Guiford, 1979.
   Specifically deals with the psychotherapy of depression. Describes an active, time-limited approach that can be used with some modification in primary medical practices. Contains case vignettes and a useful chapter on how to combine psychotherapy with medication.

---

113. INSOMNIA
Jeffery J. Fahs

Sleep requirements vary considerably from one individual to another. Insomnia can be defined as the subjective perception of inadequate sleep, accompanied by disturbed daytime functioning, with complaints such as irritability, difficulty concentrating, or fatigue. Approximately one-third of the adult population has insomnia in a given year, and 15 to 20% of these people consult a clinician with the problem. In order to initiate appropriate treatment, it is helpful to establish the cause of the sleep disorder.

Transient Insomnia
Transient insomnia affects most people at some time in their lives and is often brought on by environmental events. It generally lasts less than 3 to 4 weeks and remits with resolution of the precipitating circumstances. Phase-shift insomnias, such as are caused by "jet lag" or changing work shifts, result from a dyssynchrony between the individual's sleep-wake pattern and external demands. This insomnia resolves when the sleep schedule becomes resynchronized with the prevailing clock time or work demands. Transient insomnia can be treated with the short-term use of a hypnotic agent.

Persistent Insomnia
This heterogeneous group of disorders is generally defined as more than 4 weeks of difficulty sleeping.

Psychophysiological Insomnia
Psychophysiological insomnia usually results from a combination of factors leading to a conditioned arousal at bedtime. Negative associations often develop with the usual nightly routine and setting, resulting in a vicious cycle of anxiety and apprehension about not being able to fall asleep. Often there is improvement in sleep when this cycle is disrupted, such as by a vacation. This type of insomnia may be difficult to treat and is often confounded by the long-term use of sleeping medications. The basic treatment is instruction in sleep hygiene, as described under Sleep Hygiene Measures. The chronic use of hypnotic agents should be avoided, though intermittent, short-term use may be warranted. Some success has been reported with behavioral therapy and psychotherapy.

Psychiatric Disorders
Patients with an underlying affective disorder may present with a primary complaint of insomnia. They often have disturbances of other vegetative functions (e.g., appetite, weight change, sexual activity), feelings of sadness or elation, suicidal ideation, and previous psychiatric treatment. If depression is believed to be the cause of the insomnia, and if pharmacologic therapy is indicated, a bedtime dose of one of the sedating tricyclic antidepressants (e.g., amitriptyline or doxepin) is a logical choice. Insomnia associated with a psychotic condition is suggested by presence of a thought disorder, hallucinations, or delusions; for these, referral to a psychiatrist is usually appropriate.

Drugs

Hypnotics often paradoxically exacerbate insomnia. As tolerance develops to a previously effective agent, patients may increase the dose, only to find that sleep continues to worsen. In these cases, it must be assumed that the agent is no longer beneficial, and a gradual hypnotic withdrawal is necessary. Symptoms may be temporarily worsened while the drug is being discontinued. Alcohol may be an effective short-term hypnotic, but it is also a cause of insomnia; chronic alcoholism is associated with sleep disturbance.

Nocturnal Myoclonus and "Restless Legs" Syndrome

Nocturnal myoclonus and "restless legs" syndrome are especially common among the elderly. Nocturnal myoclonus is a sleep-related movement disorder marked by rhythmic, periodic contractions of the leg muscles that lead to partial or full arousals, often without knowledge of the leg movements and sometimes without memory of the repeated arousals. Restless legs syndrome involves uncomfortable, but not painful, dysesthesias, usually in the calves. It is relieved only by moving the legs and thus interferes with sleep onset (see Chap. 72).

Delayed Sleep Phase Syndrome

Delayed sleep phase syndrome is an entity in which sleep onset and wake time are both later than desired. Affected patients are unable to fall asleep until several hours past the conventional bedtime but are required to wake at conventional times because of occupational or social demands. The result is a sleep deficit, disturbed daytime functioning, and a complaint of insomnia. However, if patients are allowed to sleep as desired, the quality and quantity of sleep are normal.

Other Conditions

Many medical problems, especially those accompanied by pain or other discomfort, may be associated with insomnia. *Sleep apnea syndrome* can cause either insomnia or excessive daytime sleepiness. Sleep is punctuated by repetitive apneic episodes with arousals marked by gasping for air, choking, or even cacophonous snoring, of which the patient may be unaware.

Diagnostic Strategy

The "sleep history" is the most important source of information for determining the etiology of a sleeping difficulty. Transient insomnias are differentiated from persistent insomnias by the duration of the problem. Other data should include the following.

Nature of the Complaint

Is the problem in falling asleep, staying asleep, or waking too early? Difficulty initiating sleep may point to a psychophysiological insomnia with anxiety or a phase-shift disorder, while early awakening is classic for depression. If there are multiple awakenings, the cause of arousals should be determined (e.g., nocturia or pain). Excessive daytime sleepiness may indicate the sleep apnea syndrome, in which case the presence of auxiliary symptoms must be clarified.

What are the initiating, aggravating, and alleviating factors? The presence of a clear environmental stressor may indicate a psychophysiological or psychiatric insomnia. Drugs may be implicated. A work schedule change may point to a phase-shift disorder. The position of the bed or number of pillows may alter the insomnia associated with gastroesophageal reflux or pulmonary disease, while a change in setting may alleviate the persistent psychophysiological insomnia. The clinician should also attempt to quantitate the patient's perception of the problem (e.g., how long it takes to fall asleep) in order to have a relative measure by which to gauge treatment response.

Sleep Patterns

What are the activities and rituals before bedtime? Physically or mentally stimulating activities in the evening contribute to insomnia, while relaxing activities and a regular ritual may pave the way for sleep. When does the patient sleep, and are there daytime naps? Answers to these questions may point to a phase-shift disorder or fragmented sleep. A 24-hour sleep-wake diary may be helpful for diagnosis as well as in quantitating the problem. What is the sleep environment? For example, is the bed comfortable, is it too hot or cold, are there noises, lights, and so on?

Sleep-Related Phenomena
Are there repeated leg movements, suggesting nocturnal myoclonus, or loud snoring and choking, which may indicate periods of apnea? Questioning the bed partner may be invaluable in detecting these problems.

Drug History
A drug history must include all current and recently discontinued prescription medications, as well as illicit drugs, over-the-counter preparations, alcohol, caffeine, and nicotine. The insomnia due to administration of stimulants and withdrawal from sedatives is well recognized, but other commonly prescribed medications, such as propranolol, can also cause insomnia. In addition, the tricyclic antidepressants may worsen nocturnal myoclonus and its associated insomnia.

General Health
Any medical condition, such as rheumatoid arthritis, in which pain is a problem may cause insomnia. In other medical conditions, such as hyperthyroidism, insomnia may be a prominent symptom.

Emotional Status
Is a primary psychiatric disorder present? History should particularly note signs and symptoms of depression.

Further Evaluation
In most cases, an accurate diagnosis of a sleep disorder can be made in the clinician's office on the basis of the history, physical and mental status examination, and additional laboratory studies and consultations as indicated. Some patients may require referral to a sleep center for further evaluation and treatment planning. These include patients in whom sleep apnea is suspected and those in whom insomnia is persistent and refractory to appropriate and adequate treatment.

Treatment Strategies
Treatment should be directed toward the underlying cause of the sleep disorder whenever this is possible. However, there are certain general treatment strategies that are helpful.

Reassurance, Education, and Counseling
Explaining the general nature of sleep, the varying individual needs for sleep, and the lack of long-term detrimental effects from short-term sleep loss may reassure the patient, elicit cooperation, and help to avoid the inappropriate and excessive use of sleeping medications.

Sleep Hygiene Measures
Sleep hygiene measures are largely common sense, with some laboratory and clinical validation. They are the backbone of treatment in a variety of sleep disorders and include the following measures:

1. Establish regular retiring and arising times.
2. Avoid daytime naps.
3. Make the environment comfortable for sleep.
4. Use the bed only for sleep (or sexual activity), not for eating, watching television, or lying awake.
5. Avoid evening stimulation. Physical exercise during the day may contribute to improvement of sleep, but late in the day will lead to physiological arousal. Mental stimulation before sleep will likewise contribute to arousal.
6. Engage in relaxing presleep activities, possibly including structured relaxation training.
7. Avoid late afternoon and evening use of stimulants (e.g., caffeine).

Hypnotic Drugs
The clearest role for sleeping medications is in the short-term treatment of transient insomnia; they may be taken prophylactically when the patient knows that he will suffer from insomnia. In addition, there is some justification for the intermittent and

short-term use of hypnotics in some cases of persistent insomnia, including nocturnal myoclonus, persistent psychophysiological insomnia, and selected psychiatric disorders. However, chronic use should generally be avoided, and hypnotics are contraindicated in sleep apnea, pregnancy, alcoholism, and situations requiring nighttime alertness. Hypnotics play a relatively minor role in the rational treatment of persistent insomnia.

The benzodiazepines are presently the drugs of choice. Any of them may be used, although only three, flurazepam (Dalmane), temazepam (Restoril), and triazolam (Halcion), are currently approved in the United States specifically for use as hypnotics. If a patient is already taking a benzodiazepine during the day, that same benzodiazepine should be used at bedtime for sleep to avoid polypharmacy. If a patient is not taking a sedative-hypnotic drug, treatment can be initiated with one of the hypnotic benzodiazepines taken about 30 minutes before retiring. The usual adult dosage of flurazepam, a long-acting benzodiazepine, is 30 mg; however, this dosage has only slightly greater clinical efficacy than 15 mg, and treatment should usually be initiated at the lower dosage. Patients should be told that they can expect greater hypnotic efficacy on the second and subsequent nights of administration as the drug accumulates. The shorter-acting benzodiazepines, temazepam and triazolam, should also be prescribed initially in their lower available dosages, although because of their lessened accumulation the maximum hypnotic response may be seen on the first night of administration. A transient worsening of sleep may occur following discontinuation of hypnotics, even after short-term administration. Patients on benzodiazepines may have daytime "hangovers," with impairment of cognitive and psychomotor function, of which they are sometimes unaware. Long-term, continuous effectiveness has yet to be clearly established for any of the hypnotic benzodiazepines, and dependence and withdrawal may develop with chronic use. Therefore, these drugs must be prescribed judiciously, for only short periods (usually no more than 2 weeks), and monitored carefully lest the patient's difficulty be exacerbated.

L-Tryptophan has been reported to be an effective hypnotic when taken in doses of about 1 gm. While its use in the treatment of insomnia has yet to be clarified and widely accepted, a trial may be worthwhile in some patients.

A number of other "pharmacologic" treatments of insomnia are entrenched in the cultural wisdom and deserve mention. Judicious use of alcohol may be an effective short-term hypnotic. However, withdrawal effects and fragmented sleep may result even during the first night, and chronic use definitely leads to disrupted sleep. Late-night snacks (e.g., warm milk) have helped many an insomniac get to sleep and may be worth trying.

Association of Sleep Disorders Centers. Diagnostic classification of sleep and arousal disorders, 1st ed., prepared by the Sleep Disorders Classification Committee, Roffwarg HP, Chairman. *Sleep* 2:1–137, 1979.
The complete differential diagnosis and classification system of all sleep disorders; complete description and bibliography for each disorder.
Coleman RN, et al. Sleep-wake disorders based on a polysomnographic diagnosis: A national cooperative study. *J Am Med Assoc* 247:997–1003, 1982.
The first large survey of sleep-wake disorders using the ASDC diagnostic classification system. The most common causes of sleep disorders evaluated at sleep centers were sleep apnea and narcolepsy, both presenting as excessive daytime sleepiness, and insomnia associated with psychiatric disorders. Evaluation, treatment, and referral suggestions.
Hauri P. *The Sleep Disorders* (2nd ed.). Kalamazoo: Upjohn, 1982.
This clinically-oriented monograph reviews basic aspects of sleep and sleep disorders, including an especially good chapter on sleep hygiene.
Hauri P. Evaluating disorders of initiating and maintaining sleep (DIMS). In Guilleminault C (Ed.), *Sleeping and Waking Disorders: Indications and Techniques.* Menlo Park, California: Addison-Wesley, 1982. Pp. 225–244.
An excellent and concise chapter that reviews the office evaluation of the insomniac patient, treatment, guidelines for referral to a sleep center, and the use of polysomnography in the evaluation of insomnia.
Institute of Medicine. *Sleeping Pills, Insomnia, and Medical Practice.* Washington, DC: National Academy of Sciences, 1979.
This monograph provides a very thorough and well-balanced picture of insomnia and

the difficulties associated with hypnotic drug treatment. Well worth obtaining from the National Academy of Sciences (publication IOM-79-04).

Solomon F, et al. Sleeping pills, insomnia, and medical practice. N Engl J Med 300:803–808, 1979.
A brief summary of the complete Institute of Medicine report that concentrates on the adverse effects and public health problems of hypnotic drugs.

Weitzman ED, et al.: Delayed sleep phase syndrome: A chronobiological disorder with sleep-onset insomnia. Arch Gen Psychiatry 38:737–746, 1981.
Clinical and laboratory description of this recently described cause of insomnia with treatment recommendations.

Zorick FJ, et al. Evaluation and diagnosis of persistent insomnia. Am J Psychiatry 138:769–773, 1981.
Insomniacs do not constitute a homogeneous group; clinical and polysomnographic evaluation lead to a diagnosis in all cases, with treatment implications.

114. PROBLEM PATIENTS
Douglas A. Drossman

Within every clinical practice, physicians can identify patients they designate as "problem" patients. These patients comprise a heterogeneous group who may have no specific medical or psychiatric diagnosis but are characterized by the behavior they exhibit within the health care system and the reactions they elicit in the physicians caring for them. Consider a typical case history:

> A patient presents with long-standing physical complaints that are difficult to characterize. Review of past workups is unrevealing. With each new doctor visited, more invasive procedures were done to exclude "organic disease." Treatment has been empirical, unsuccessful, and sometimes harmful. The patient states that others have concluded "nothing is wrong," or "it is in my head," but he knows it is real. He hopes you will find the answer and help where others have failed. By the end of the visit, additional studies seem unnecessary, yet with no specific diagnosis, you wonder if something has been overlooked. The patient strongly states that there are no emotional problems. He demands that something be done *now* for these unbearable symptoms.

Although psychosocial factors play a part in the illnesses of many medical patients, problem patients are typically unwilling or unable to acknowledge an association between stress or emotional factors and their illness. As a result, the physician finds it difficult to obtain relevant data for diagnosis or treatment. Such patients may see each new problem within a long history of chronic or recurrent symptoms as another acute episode that requires immediate relief. Their demands for the doctor to "do something" tend to heighten the physician's sense of uncertainty and may also produce feelings of ineffectiveness. This may result in any of several inappropriate physician behaviors: pursuit of unneeded diagnostic studies in an attempt to ameliorate the sense of uncertainty ("furor medicus"), anger toward the patient in whom "nothing is wrong," or dismissal with a statement that the problems are emotional, sometimes accompanied by an undesired referral to a psychiatrist. Since the "problem" with "problem patients" exists to a great degree within the physician-patient interaction, the physician who recognizes these maladaptive behavior patterns early may forestall unneeded studies and treatment and make more effective plans of patient care.

Recognition
Although problem patients do not fall into any specific diagnostic categories, they commonly exhibit a number of identifiable behavior patterns. These include the following:

1. Personalized or bizarre description of the symptoms (e.g., pain "as if seared by hot coals")

2. Persistent complaints with demands for the physician to "do something"
3. Symptoms determined in whole or part from a meaningful fantasy or experience (e.g., chest pain developing after the death of a parent from cardiac disease)
4. Temporal association of the symptoms to stress events
5. Long history of nonspecific complaints and poorly documented illnesses
6. Reluctance to accept the role of psychosocial factors in the illness
7. Resistance to improvement due to the presence of benefits derived from illness (e.g., family attention, disability, expiation of guilt feelings through suffering)

Evaluation

Evaluation should include an initial history and physical examination, which should be repeated as needed when new or different symptoms develop. The story of the illness should be obtained in as unbiased a fashion as possible and in relation to the events that may have contributed to its onset and presentation. The approach should communicate the physician's willingness to hear all aspects of the illness, whether biologic or psychologic. The interview should encourage the spontaneous reporting of information through the patient's own associations. Leading questions or those that elicit "yes" or "no" answers should be avoided at first. More direct and specific questions can be asked later to characterize the illness better and to help confirm the diagnostic possibilities.

Specific Disorders

Patients with certain psychiatric disorders or personality patterns also commonly present with physical complaints and may interact with their physician in ways that result in their being labeled as problem patients. However, early recognition of these specific disorders can lead to more directed and appropriate plans of patient care. These entities include the following.

Psychophysiologic Reaction

Psychophysiologic reaction is an exaggerated physiologic response to anxiety-producing situations, with symptoms such as palpitations, diarrhea, or the hyperventilation syndrome. Many individuals may develop these reactions at one time or another. However, some patients may present with frequent episodes as part of an underlying chronic anxiety disorder. The physician should try to determine possible stressors and, if not possible to remove them, encourage patient adaptation through support, counseling, or appropriate referral.

Conversion Reaction

Conversion reaction is an unconscious adaptive process whereby mental distress is ameliorated through its symbolic representation as a physical symptom. Conversion reactions can occur in any individual as a response to stress (e.g., development of chest pains in the grieving spouse of a heart attack victim). More frequently they develop in patients with the propensity to focus on somatic concerns. Disorders may be manifest as loss of bodily function, such as paralysis, or symptoms of pain. Treatment will vary depending on the nature of the stress, the patient's personality and coping style, and the degree of impairment in daily function. When the condition is disabling, psychiatric consultation is usually needed.

Hypochondriasis

Hypochondriasis is a personality variant in which patients maintain a chronic preoccupation with bodily function. They display an unrealistic interpretation of physical sensations as being abnormal, maintain a persistent fear of harboring serious disease, and are preoccupied with a variety of vague and shifting complaints. Many of these patients have limited social relationships outside of the health care system, and their complaints serve to maintain self-esteem and to provide a means of social communication. Treatment often includes accepting them without challenging the illness and maintaining a commitment to regular brief office visits without a need to respond to every complaint.

Pain-Prone Personality

Individuals with this disorder report a long-standing history of numerous dramatic events, operations, and pain episodes. They also seem to display an intolerance of success manifested by difficulty holding jobs, a proclivity to submit to demeaning experiences, and the development of symptoms during relatively good periods of life. Patients with this personality pattern often come from an early environment of violence, deprivation, and physical abuse, with parents who displayed inconsistent behavior or rigid discipline. Alcoholism and broken marriages in the family are common. It is believed that the pain and suffering serve as a means of atonement for early established feelings of self-devaluation and guilt. The physician should recognize that these patients often succumb to a variety of iatrogenic procedures and have a high potential for drug abuse.

"Depressive Equivalent"
The "depressive equivalent" disorder has been called a "masked depression," for the patient attributes sadness, sleep disturbance, and loss of weight and appetite to bodily complaints rather than to an emotional disorder. This misinterpretation can also be made by the physician who fails to explore the circumstances preceding the onset of illness. These patients may respond to supportive psychotherapy or antidepressant medications.

Somatic Delusion
Patients with somatic delusions describe bizarre beliefs about their symptoms (e.g., a headache is caused by the brain being split into pieces). The symptoms are not described metaphorically; the patients truly believes it is happening. These patients have significant psychic disorganization (e.g., schizophrenia) and require psychiatric referral.

Treatment
The therapeutic approach to problem patients must be individualized. The following guidelines are useful.

Establish a Therapeutic Relationship
Establish a therapeutic relationship with a mutual sense of trust and understanding of both physician and patient needs and expectations. The physician's goals should be the following: (1) Accept the adaptive value of the illness, and do not attempt to achieve premature resolution. Often the illness has existed for many years and has resulted in secondary benefits (e.g., increased attention from family, privilege of the "sick role"). (2) Make no promises that cannot be met (e.g., for quick symptom relief). (3) Involve the patient in the treatment plans. This frees the doctor from the implied obligation to be the one responsible for the patient's well-being and fosters a greater sense of patient independence and emotional maturity. (4) Accept a commitment for possibly long-term treatment. Initially one to three appointments per month for 15 to 30 minutes are recommended. During these sessions, continued efforts should be made to elicit the patient's own associations and affective state. When symptoms are reported, the physician should not always feel compelled to treat them. When the patient recounts the misfortunes of continued pain and suffering, the physician should communicate understanding of how difficult it must be to go on with such distress. When the patient focuses on significant thoughts and feelings, the physician should gently encourage them without forcing their disclosure. As symptoms improve, the visits can be decreased in frequency. It is probable that a commitment to continued care through regular though infrequent visits (twice per year when the patient is well) will reinforce the doctor's interest and minimize late-night calls and "emergency" visits.

Do Not State That the Problem Is "Emotional"
Problem patients are unable to accept the significance of emotional factors in their illnesses. For this reason, it is best to reassure those with unwarranted fears and volunteer nothing more than they are prepared to accept. To state that the problem is "emotional" may set some patients up as adversaries. If asked by a patient whether or not the problem is "all in my head," the physician should state that it is important to consider the role of all factors in the illness, be they psychological or otherwise. The doctor needs to communicate a desire to work with the patient, not to diagnose an illness to treat.

The patient's awareness of an association between emotional factors and illness is not necessary for improvement and should not be a goal of treatment.

Resist the Impulse to Order Unnecessary Diagnostic Studies
The decision for diagnostic studies should be based on careful evaluation of the objective clinical data, not solely on the patient's demands. When a reasonable assessment of the problem has developed from the history and physical examination, the physician must have the confidence *not* to order unnecessary diagnostic studies just to "rule out organic disease." If the complaints are not readily understood, it is wiser to temporize than to commit oneself to a treatment plan with uncertain effectiveness. In time, as the issues become clarified, better diagnostic and treatment choices can be made.

Accept Illness as the Interaction of Biological and Psychological Determinants
The identification of psychological factors does not exclude a concurrent somatic illness. The physician must also be alert to the development of new disease in patients who "cry wolf."

Reset Goals for Clinical Improvement
To derive satisfaction from the care of these patients requires that the physician set realistic treatment goals. Often improvement should be gauged by the patient's level of daily function (e.g., work, church, social activities) *despite* the illness rather than by resolution of the symptoms.

Be Aware of Personal Attitudes
The patient's maintenance of the sick role is not necessarily countertherapeutic, but it can be frustrating to the physician whose goal is to make the patient symptom-free. Labels such as "crock" or "turkey" applied to such patients signal the physician's frustration and sense of helplessness. Medicine is not an exact science, and physicians must tolerate uncertainty; however, recognition of the psychosocial dimensions of these patients' illnesses can often lead to greater physician security as their patients' problems are put into clear perspective.

Drossman DA. The problem patient: Evaluation and care of medical patients with psychosocial disturbances. *Arch Intern Med* 88:366–372, 1978.
Presents in more detail the characteristics of problem patients and offers a treatment approach.
DeVaul RA, Faillace LA. Persistent pain and illness insistence: A medical profile to proneness to surgery. *Am J Surg* 135:828–833, 1978.
This paper identifies the "polysurgery" patient and reports behavioral patterns that lead to physician errors in clinical judgment.
Somatoform Disorders. *Diagnostic and Statistical Manual of Mental Disorders* (3rd ed.). Washington, DC: American Psychiatric Association, 1980. Pp. 241–252.
This is the current standardized psychiatric nomenclature for patients who somatize.
Altman N. Hypochondriasis. In JJ Strain and S Grossman (Eds.), *Psychological Care of the Medically Ill: A Primer in Liaison Psychiatry.* New York: Appleton-Century-Crofts, 1975. Pp. 76–92.
A discussion of hypochondriasis from a psychodynamic perspective.
Engel GL. Psychogenic pain and the pain-prone patient. *Am J Med* 26:899–918, 1959.
A classic presentation of the adaptive value of pain and suffering for a subgroup of patients with chronic pain.

115. GRIEF

Eric W. Jensen

Grief, the reaction to loss, is a defined syndrome with predictable psychological and somatic symptoms, which occurs in response to various types of losses, such as the loss of a loved one, a body part, or self-esteem. It involves a process of realization that helps an individual accept inwardly the reality of an event that has already occurred in the external world. The term *bereavement,* often used interchangeably with *grief,* usually refers to the normal reactions and behaviors following the death of an important person in one's life.

Accumulating clinical research indicates that loss contributes to the development of a wide range of somatic and psychological disorders. While the relationship between bereavement and ill health is not necessarily a causal one, the altered emotional state seems to contribute to the development of disease. Recent work has demonstrated that the bereaved state is associated with a measurable abnormality in immune function and higher mortality and morbidity during the first year of bereavement.

Although most people regard the feelings of grief as "normal" and do not seek professional help, others may turn to physicians for relief of grief-related symptoms, such as anxiety, insomnia, anorexia, or depression. An increase has been noted in the frequency with which individuals consult general physicians for physical and emotional symptoms in the 12 to 18 months after a loss. An inquiry about recent losses during the initial evaluation of patients presenting with perplexing physical and psychological problems may help identify unresolved grief reactions, thereby circumventing the need for extensive laboratory studies and procedures.

Timely recognition and treatment of abnormal grief reactions can help prevent the physical and psychological complications that can result from failure to grieve completely and prevent the prolongation of a grief reaction.

Uncomplicated Grief Reactions
Much of our understanding of grief reaction is based on case descriptions and theoretic/conceptual formulations. Recently, a few studies that examine the epidemiologic, endocrine, and immunologic aspects of grief have appeared. Although death of a loved one is used here as an example of a grief reaction, similar reactions may occur in response to other losses.

Phases and Duration
Most uncomplicated grief reactions proceed in a predictable fashion through three stages lasting approximately 2 to 3 months. First, there is an initial phase of shock and disbelief in which denial is prominent; this phase lasts a few days. Next, a developing awareness of the loss is marked by sadness, guilt, and helplessness; crying and a sense of emptiness; anorexia, sleep disturbance, and other somatic symptoms; and loss of interest in usual activities and impairment of work performance. This stage ordinarily lasts a few weeks. Finally, a prolonged third stage occurs during which the patient is able to overcome the loss and a state of health and well-being is reestablished. The uncomplicated reaction to loss may not be immediate but usually occurs within the first 2 to 3 months.

Modifying Factors
The duration and intensity of a grief reaction can vary markedly. People differ in their inherent ability to adjust to loss and change. Those individuals who are more dependent or have significant unresolved conflicts with the deceased experience more difficulty in grieving. The loss of a close relation, such as a parent, spouse, or child, is usually felt more intensely than that of a more distant relation. Social supports and institutionalized rituals tend to facilitate the grief process, while societal or cultural values that discount the impact of loss and minimize the expression of grief can inhibit the timely completion of grieving. And finally, a major loss in childhood appears to make subsequent grieving more difficult.

Incomplete or Pathologic Grief

Failure to Grieve
Failure to grieve may occur when the grief process is excessive, prolonged, delayed, or inhibited.

Social factors that contribute to the failure to grieve include population mobility, which may separate the bereaved person from family and other traditional supports; societal expectations to be "strong," which may make it difficult for individuals, especially men, to express their sorrow; and a loss that is unrecognized or even denied, such as after an abortion or when a loved one dies while committing a crime.

Psychological factors may lead to denial or muting of the painful character of the loss, even though it is recognized intellectually. This may occur when there was marked ambivalence toward or excessive dependence on the lost person, or when the present loss awakens an old loss that was extremely painful and not fully resolved. The grieving process may also be overwhelmed by the impact of multiple losses, as when several family members die in an accident.

Pathologic Grief States
Pathologic grief states are distortions of the normal or uncomplicated grief process. They can present to the physician in a number of different forms including depression, hypochondriasis, conversion disorder, development of medical illness or exacerbation of a preexisting somatic condition, and exacerbation of underlying organic brain syndromes or psychotic states. Other manifestations include perpetual mourning with persistent loss of patterns of social interaction; altered relationships with friends, relatives, and others characterized by reclusive behavior or furious hostility; and behavior detrimental to one's social and economic existence, such as excessive generosity, foolish economic dealings, drugs, or promiscuity.

Diagnosis
Because of the multiplicity of presentations and the ubiquitous nature of loss in everyday life, it seems prudent that every medical history should include some exploration of recent and past object loss in the patient's life.

Uncomplicated Grief Reactions
Uncomplicated grief reactions proceed through the stages previously described. In addition, the clinician should be able to recognize certain acute symptoms, which have been characterized (Lindemann, 1944):

1. Somatic distress: Feelings of tightness in the throat, choking with shortness of breath, an empty feeling in the stomach, loss of muscular strength, and intense subjective distress described as tension or mental pain may occur in waves lasting 20 minutes to 1 hour at a time.
2. Preoccupation with the image of the deceased may include vivid visual and auditory components in which the bereaved speaks with or sees the deceased. The intensity of these images may frighten the bereaved who fears they indicate loss of contact with reality.
3. Feelings of guilt: Grief-stricken individuals may blame themselves for negligence or failure to do right by the deceased.
4. Hostile reactions: Friends, relatives, and physicians who seek to comfort may be the objects of seemingly inexplicable anger, irritability, and withdrawal.
5. Loss of patterns of conduct: The bereaved may experience great difficulty initiating or attending to daily tasks, is often restless, and searches aimlessly for something to do.

Pathologic Grief
Pathologic grief should be strongly considered when a patient has failed to grieve following a significant loss. The individual may have refrained from crying, avoided participating in the funeral, memorial services, or visiting the grave, and sought to put thoughts of the deceased out of mind. Symptoms that occur on or around the anniversary of a loss may indicate unresolved grief and may be accompanied by an inability to discuss someone who has died some time ago without becoming extremely emotionally distraught. Interviews characterized by themes of loss suggest pathologic grief, particularly when the patient, well beyond the normal period of grief, appear to have bodily symptoms similar to those of the dead person. Chronicity of normal grief symptoms with persistent guilt, lowered self-esteem, and impaired relationships with friends and relatives is also indicative of an abnormal grief state.

Treatment
Although the clinician should be alert for evidence of abnormal grieving, it is not necessary to intervene if the response to loss is proceeding as expected. If the grief process is impaired for any reason, timely intervention and treatment may facilitate grieving and thereby prevent prolonged and serious alterations in the patient's social adjust-

ment and physical and mental health. For pathologic grief reactions, the physician seeks to correct the distortion by recognizing the importance of the loss and encouraging the individual to experience the feelings and thoughts that have been avoided. This serves to transform the pathologic grief state into a normal grief reaction, which can then be dealt with directly.

Many uncomplicated and pathologic grief reactions can be treated effectively by the primary care physician. Since our current technologic society discourages grieving and puts a premium on a quick return to the former level of functioning, physical symptoms are often more acceptable and hence frequently substituted for painful feelings of loss. Non-psychiatric physicians are often consulted for these symptoms and are well suited to provide the necessary treatment for the underlying grief reaction. One can generally expect to help resolve most grief reactions in 6 to 10 weeks. During this time, the patient might be seen weekly or every other week. Complicated or severely pathologic reactions may take longer. Difficult and prolonged cases should be referred for more extensive psychiatric treatment.

To understand and treat the bereaved person a physician must learn the specific ways in which the deceased was important to the individual. For example, it should not be assumed that the loss of a parent or spouse means the same thing to all people. The clinician must also learn the typical coping patterns of the grieving individual, the specific family resources for dealing with loss, and the attitude toward death and loss within the individual's social and cultural setting. Understanding these dimensions permits the physician to use the following general principles of treatment to make individual patient plans:

1. Listen carefully, and allow the expression of thoughts and feelings about the deceased. Encourage a discussion of the loss, and offer support during the grief process. The physician's presence and support can itself be therapeutic.
2. Reassure and inform the person that he or she is undergoing a normal experience and is not medically ill or losing mind. Patients must recognize that grieving is necessary for putting the past in the proper perspective.
3. Facilitate the reconstruction of memories to elicit feelings. Specific questions might assist those who have difficulty grieving (i.e., What did she look like? What happened when you spoke with him last?).
4. When ambivalence inhibits grieving, it is important for the individual to express the negative feelings. Encourage but do not confront. Recognize the strength of the individual's positive feelings as well. In describing the negative feelings, words such as "disappointment," "irritation," and "aggravation" usually are better than "anger."
5. Deal with multiple losses one at a time.
6. Sedative-hypnotics may be useful during the acute stages of bereavement, but their use should be limited in order not to alter the grief process.
7. Express personal feelings when appropriate and helpful, but seek to remain objective. The physician should guide and facilitate, not interfere with the necessary grieving.

Lindemann E. Symptomatology and management of acute grief. *Am J Psychiatry* 101:141–148, 1944.
   The classic article in the field. Observations of 101 patients who experience loss provide the basis for a description of the symptomatology and course of normal grief reactions. Distortions of normal grief, issues in the management of grief reactions, and anticipatory grief are also discussed.
Epstein G, et al. Research on bereavement: A selective and critical review. *Compr Psychiatry* 16:537–546, 1975.
   This review examines the literature dealing with parental loss during childhood, conjugal loss, adult mortality following loss, and predictors of unfavorable bereavement outcome. The 54 references cover work in these areas through 1972.
Helsing KJ, Szklo M. Mortality after bereavement. *Am J Epidemiol* 114:41–52, 1981.
   This prospective study found that widowed men experienced higher mortality than married men of the same age, even after adjusting for possible confounding factors. Interestingly, mortality rates for widowed and married women did not differ significantly.

Burgess AW, Lazare A. The Bereaved. In *Community Mental Health: Target Populations.* Englewood Cliffs, NJ.: Prentice-Hall, 1976. Chap. 6.
   This chapter provides a useful overview of grief, why some people fail to grieve, and the diagnosis and treatment of pathologic grief.

Bartrop RW, et al. Depressed lymphocyte function after bereavement. *Lancet* 1:834–836, April 1977.
   A prospective study of immunologic function in healthy people undergoing the stress of bereavement. A measurable depression in T-cell function was demonstrated. Further work in this area may provide important clues to the immunologic basis of diseases thought to be stress related.

Speak PW. *Loss and Grief in Medicine.* London: Bailliere, Tindall & Cox, 1978.
   A short book that examines the experience of loss and grief and looks at the occurrence of these in the medical setting. Particular attention is paid to these experiences of loss that do not involve the death of a loved one. A third section looks at the influence of culture and religious belief on an individual's experience of loss.

Parkes CM. *Bereavement: Studies of Grief in Adult Life.* New York: International Universities Press, 1972.
   A more detailed treatise on the reactions of bereavement and the determinants of the grief process. Atypical grief presentation, approaches to helping the bereaved, and reactions to other types of loss are also discussed.

116. ALCOHOLISM

Richard M. Aderhold and Phillip A. Mooring

Alcoholism is the continuation of drinking despite physical, social, or occupational problems related to alcohol use. The prevalence of problem drinking is estimated to be 10% in the general population and 8 to 42% for adult outpatients.

Physicians detect and/or treat alcoholism in less than half of the cases. Uncertainty about what level of drinking warrants intervention, forgetting to assess patients for the problem, pessimism regarding the value of intervention, fear of alienating patients by confrontation, and little training in detecting and managing alcoholism are factors related to lack of detection and/or treatment.

Natural History

There is great variation among individuals in the pattern and course of problem drinking and often variation within individuals over time. The disorder often exhibits remissions and relapses. Periods of abstinence have been shown to be associated with finding substitute dependencies and/or new relationships. Clinic treatment and good premorbid adjustment are not predictive of abstinence. A few persons with mild symptoms seem able to develop a light to moderate pattern of alcohol use after a period of excessive use, but presently there is little information on identifying who can do this and not progress to more severe states.

The frequency and amount of drinking that can cause a problem vary greatly. Two or three drinks daily or frequent mild intoxication can result in problems for some people. Considerable evidence now indicates genetic, metabolic differences between those who develop problem drinking and those who do not.

Detection

All patients, including teenagers, the elderly, and women, should be assessed for alcohol misuse. Determining alcohol use in women of childbearing age is very important, since even small amounts of alcohol can cause fetal malformation. Consistent use of one of several very brief (less than 1 minute) questionnaires may be helpful; they can be administered by a secretary or nurse. The CAGE Questionnaire is particularly brief and easy to administer. It consists of four questions:

1. Have you felt the need to *CUT* down your drinking?
2. Have you ever felt *ANNOYED* by criticism of your drinking?

. Have you had *GUILTY* feelings about drinking?
. Do you ever take a morning *EYE-OPENER?*

A positive answer to any of the questions warrants investigation, and two positive
nswers strongly suggest an alcohol problem. For two positive answers, sensitivity is
0% and specificity 75%. The second question is especially useful when incorporated in
review of systems or past medical history. When using a questionnaire or asking
lcohol-related questions, asking first about less emotionally charged substance use
e.g., coffee, tea, soft drinks, tobacco, sweets) will reduce defensiveness as well as pro-
ide other valuable information.

A history of more than one to two drinks or beers a day suggests a problem, as does
ny drinking to intoxication. Problem drinking is also suggested by defensiveness or
tatements such as "I can take it or leave it," "I only drink beer," "I don't drink every
lay," or "I sometimes go several weeks without drinking." Many common disorders
nd signs can be caused or aggravated by unsuspected alcohol misuse, including liver
isease, gastritis, increased mean cell volume (MCV), tremor, moderate serum liver
nzyme elevations, palpitations, work absences, depression, and family problems. Any
atient having an odor of alcohol when seen in a medical office or hospital probably
as a problem with alcohol.

Management

.ppropriate treatment can be effective. For example, in one study of alcoholism treat-
nent in several Health Maintenance Organizations there was a 75% overall reduction
a alcohol consumption, 55% reduction in absenteeism, 90% reduction in reprimands
t work, and decreased use of emergency services in treated patients. A review of 271
tudies of treatment found that approximately two-thirds of patients were reported
nproved. However, it is difficult to compare various treatment methods because most
ublished studies fall short of basic standards for therapeutic research. It is likely that
he effectiveness of different treatment methods varies from patient to patient, in ways
hat we do not fully understand. Therefore, the following recommendations are based
artly on the medical literature and partly on the experience of experts.

General Approach

Changing the social environment, especially developing involvement with religion or
Alcoholics Anonymous (AA), as well as developing a close interpersonal relationship
r a substitute dependency, is generally more related to improvement or abstinence
han clinical treatment.

Denial and defensiveness can be reduced by focusing on the effects on family, job,
ealth, and on the pattern of drinking rather than the amount. Discussing alcohol use
n a calm, nonjudgmental manner like use of sugar by someone with diabetes (i.e.,
netabolic difficulty with the substance) also may be effective.

People with drinking problems may say "I don't drink every day" or "I can stop when
want to stop" or may describe what they consider problem drinking as someone in
he late stages of alcoholism. This type of denial might be reduced by asking the person
vhat he thinks the drinking pattern would be like a few years before the late stage
evelops. Speaking to the healthy side of the person helps: "I know deep down you
ealize drinking is a problem, but it is hard to admit." Giving hope is very important
nd can be generated by asserting that alcohol misuse can be effectively treated with
he patient's cooperation.

It is very important to ask frequently about any drinking while driving because this
an be lethal to the patient and others.

Repeated discussions about alcohol use may eventually motivate resistant patients
o ask for help. Remembering that alcohol misuse usually is a disorder of remissions
nd exacerbations similar to many chronic disorders (e.g., asthma, bronchitis) may
educe the clinician's frustration and discouragement.

Depression and anxiety commonly accompany alcohol misuse, either as a cause or a
esult. Determining which situation is present can be difficult and may warrant psy-
hiatric consultation or a therapeutic trial. Alcohol misusers are one of the highest
isk groups for depression and suicide. They should be asked repeatedly about suicidal
houghts and plans.

Responsibility for Care
It is usually best if the primary physician takes an active role as treatment coordinator rather than shunting total care to a psychiatrist, AA, or a mental health center. Frequency and duration of contact with a clinician or treatment program have been shown to have greater correlation with improvement than any specific type of treatment. Persons who misuse alcohol usually have very low self-esteem, and referral to a mental health professional may accentuate this, resulting in withdrawal from help. Problem drinkers often have poor verbal skills and poor response to traditional psychotherapy yet may respond to concrete actions demonstrating interest and concern, such as help arranging a better job situation or phone calls to check on progress, especially since they often feel no one is interested in them (a factor probably related to frequent missed appointments and poor compliance). If the patient is referred, the primary physician should maintain scheduled contact with the patient to demonstrate interest and concern and to monitor progress.

Treatment Options
Treatment options, in addition to the primary physician, include community agencies, Alcoholics Anonymous, mental health centers, religious groups, psychiatrists, psychologists, and Al-Anon and Alateen for family members. Allowing the patient to choose from a variety of approaches enlists cooperation, boosts self-esteem, and engenders a personal stake in making the choices successful. Often there are several AA groups in a community, with each group composed of people with similar backgrounds or interests. It is important that the group match the patient. For example, a blue-collar worker may not respond to a primarily white-collar AA group and vice versa.

Goals
At present, the safest goal seems to be abstinence, but even sporadic, partial improvement reduces morbidity and mortality. Short-term goals are preferable—for example, no alcohol for the next 2 weeks or even for 1 day in some cases. Making goals too long-term can overwhelm a patient.

Strategies
Additional relatively simple pointers that can be used when appropriate include the following:

1. Joint meetings may be held with the patient and family/friends to enlist their participation in the treatment. Al-Anon attendance by spouse and Alateen by children can be very helpful, as can enlisting the help of employers, if the patient consents.
2. When a "slipup" occurs and a drink is taken, guilt often occurs. Patients should be warned not to attempt to "drown the guilt" with further drinking in such circumstances.
3. Methods of coping with stress and anger, other than using alcohol, should be suggested. Participation in church activities seems especially helpful. Other supportive groups, hobbies, and more involvement with family and friends also can help greatly.
4. A diary of drinking times, amounts, temptations, and so on, can increase self-awareness and understanding of problem patterns.

Medication During Alcohol Withdrawal
It is prudent not to use psychoactive medication unless withdrawal symptoms are severe or there is a history of seizures. Benzodiazepines seem to be the safest and most effective agents for reducing severe withdrawal symptoms. Titration is desirable, with the goal being to maintain the patient alert and not tremulous. It is advisable to wait 6 to 8 hours after the last drink of alcohol to start any medications that might cause central nervous system (CNS) depression. Depending on severity, usual dosages are 25 to 50 mg of chlordiazepoxide or 10 to 20 mg of diazepam every 2 to 6 hours (or equivalent of another benzodiazepine) for the first day or two and then tapering over 3 to 5 days by reducing by approximately 25 mg per day of chlordiazepoxide or 10 mg per day of diazepam. Paraldehyde has been associated with deaths, and phenothiazines can increase the risk of seizures, so neither is recommended. Thiamine and other vitamins are advisable and crucial to prevent CNS damage if intravenous fluid containing glu-

cose is given. Thiamine, 100 mg intramuscularly, should be given before any intravenous fluids are started, and fluids should contain thiamine and multivitamins as well. Thiamine, 100 mg intramuscularly two times a day for 3 days, followed by 50 mg orally two times a day for 2 weeks is reasonable; further treatment is given if there is a neurologic deficit.

If benzodiazepines are used, there should be only a short 3- to 7-day tapering course (sometimes with phenytoin if there is a seizure history) with no further use of psychoactive medication unless there is an important reason other than alcoholism for the medication. Physicians are often pressured by patients for continuation of antianxiety medication, but such medication, when used after the first few days of severe withdrawal, fosters continued reliance on chemicals and drinking is likely to occur whenever medication is not readily available.

Disulfiram (Antabuse)

A disulfiram (Antabuse) prescription can be helpful in selected cases, for example, the impulsive, reasonably intelligent drinker. When alcohol is consumed by patients taking Antabuse, nausea and vomiting result, which can be severe and death is possible. Antabuse can be presented as an insurance measure, not a crutch, that helps eliminate the need to decide several times a day whether or not to stop at the liquor store or bar. Antabuse is contraindicated for persons with schizophrenia or impaired comprehension. The primary effect of Antabuse is probably psychological, so the exact dosage is not crucial; it is usually sufficient to give 125 mg daily or in some cases as infrequently as two to three times per week. It is often helpful to have Antabuse taken in the presence of someone else (e.g., spouse or therapist).

Bernadt MW, et al. Comparison of questionnaire and laboratory tests in the detection of excessive drinking and alcoholism. *Lancet* 1:325–328, 1982.
   Comparison of eight laboratory tests and three rapid interviews employing three different brief screening questionnaires. The three interviews, each of which takes less than a minute, were found most effective, with CAGE and Reich interviews identifying over 90% of excessive drinkers.
Clark WD. Alcoholism: Blocks to diagnosis and treatment. *Am J Med* 71:275–286, 1981.
   A comprehensive review of many aspects of diagnosis and treatment, including diagnostic approaches, management of denial, counseling principles and usefulness, and various treatment modalities.
Ewing J. Recognizing, confronting and helping the alcoholic. *Am Fam Physician* 18:107–114, 1978.
   Presents a discussion on recognizing alcohol abuse through use of CAGE questions. Affirmative response to these questions should elevate the physician's suspicion that the patient is at risk. Also discusses confrontation, use of disulfiram (Antabuse), and presents an Antabuse contract.
Lisansky ET. Why physicians avoid early diagnosis of alcoholism. *NY State J Med* Sept. 1975, pp. 1788–1792.
   Discusses often unrecognized factors related to lack of alcoholism detection and diagnosis.
Thompson WL, et al. Diazepam and paraldehyde for treatment of severe delirium tremens. *Ann Intern Med* 82:175–180, 1975.
   Thirty-four patients with advanced delirium tremens were allocated randomly to treatment with diazepam or paraldehyde. Adverse reactions occurred in 9 patients, all of whom were treated with paraldehyde, and there were 2 deaths in the paraldehyde group. No adverse reactions occurred in the diazepam-treated group.
Emrick CD. A review of psychologically oriented treatment of alcoholism. *Q J Stud Alcohol* 35:523–549, 1974.
   Review of 271 studies in which at least part of treatment was psychologically oriented. Approximately two-thirds of patients were judged improved with treatment.
Boyjay TG. *Alcoholism Within Prepaid Group HMOs.* Washington, DC: Group Health Association of America, 1978.
   Assessment of alcoholism treatment effects in several health maintenance organizations.

XVI. INFECTIOUS DISEASES

In recent years, the prevalence of sexually transmitted diseases (STDs) has been increasing at an alarming rate. A relatively minor part of this increase is accounted for by the traditional venereal diseases: gonorrhea, syphilis, chancroid, lymphogranuloma venereum, and granuloma inguinale. The major part is from new syndromes caused by pathogens that were not previously considered venereal: *Chlamydia trachomatis, Ureaplasma urealyticum,* herpes simplex virus, cytomegalovirus, hepatitis B virus, and *Giardia lamblia.*

Physicians are required to report STDs to state heath agencies. Although requirements vary from state to state, reporting of the five traditional venereal diseases is mandatory. Nevertheless, statistics on the frequency of STDs are notoriously unreliable. In large part, this reflects the failure of physicians and other heath care providers to report cases. Current estimates indicate that *C. trachomatis* infections are the most frequent (4 to 5 million cases per year), gonorrhea is second (2 to 2.5 million cases per year), and herpes is third (400,000 to 600,000 cases per year). These figures are probably underestimates.

Urethritis

Urethritis is one of the most common clinical syndromes associated with STDs in men. The urethral mucosa is an initial site of infection in both sexes, and the resulting symptom is dysuria. In men there is usually an associated mucoid, mucopurulent, or grossly purulent urethral discharge, which represents a combination of white blood cells and desquamated urethral epithelium. Women may complain of dysuria and a vaginal discharge, symptoms that are easily confused with several other problems that affect the female genitourinary tract. (Dysuria in women is discussed in Chaps. 60 and 79 and will not be discussed further here.)

Diagnosis

Gonococcal urethritis typically presents acutely after a relatively recent exposure. It is more prevalent among patients who have multiple sexual contacts. The characteristic urethral discharge is profuse and grossly purulent. In contrast, nongonococcal urethritis (NGU) more commonly presents after a longer history of symptoms (2–3 weeks in some cases) in patients of high socioeconomic status who have a relatively limited number of sexual contacts. The associated discharge is relatively scant and mucoid. History of symptoms in the consort(s) suggests sexually transmitted urethritis; however, many men and women with gonococcal and chlamydial infection remain asymptomatic for an indefinite period of time (about 20–50% of men and 70–90% of women).

A Gram's stain of the urethral discharge is obtained by inserting a calcium alginate–tipped urethrogenital swab 1 to 2 cm into the patient's urethra. (Cotton contains fatty acids, which may impede bacterial growth. Unless cotton swabs are marked nontoxic, calcium alginate or other synthetic fibers are preferred.) If gram-negative intracellular diplococci are observed, the diagnosis of gonorrhea is virtually assured, and there is generally no need to send a gonococcal culture unless penicillinase-producing *Neisseria gonorrhoeae* (PPNG) is suspected because of travel to endemic areas (the Far East, Africa), active military duty, or previous treatment failure on standard regimens. A gonococcal culture is also necessary in those instances in which the Gram's stain is nondefinitive—for example, when gram-negative diplococci are present but are not clearly intracellular. When the Gram's stain is definitely negative for gonococci, some authorities are now recommending routine urethral culture for *C. trachomatis,* because of the high prevalence of this organism as a cause of NGU. However, the utility of chlamydial culture is unclear, given the cost (approximately $30), the delay in obtaining results (2–3 days or longer), the existence of other causative organisms besides *C. trachomatis* and *U. urealyticum,* and the effectiveness of empiric therapy in suspected NGU cases. Evaluation for herpetic infection is unwarranted unless the patient has dysuria associated with vesicular or ulcerative lesions.

Because the prevalence of associated asymptomatic pharyngeal and rectal gonococcal infection is high in homosexual men and in people who have orogenital contact, routine pharyngeal and rectal cultures should be done on patients at risk. The recent "epidemic" of syphilis in homosexuals (about 10% prevalence) suggests that a screening VDRL is also necessary in this population. Other screening measures may be necessary depending on the individual patient's symptoms. If there are gastrointestinal symptoms in homosexuals, stool evaluation for enteric pathogens such as *Campylobacter fetus ssp jejuni* and *G. lamblia* (recently documented to be prevalent in homosexuals) and proctoscopy are indicated. Similarly, baseline serum serology for hepatitis B surface antigen (HB_sAg) and antibody provides useful information for future reference; homosexuals are at high risk to develop acute hepatitis or to become chronic carriers of hepatitis B virus (about 5% are HB_sAg positive and about 40% are HB_sAb positive).

As is the case for all STDs, the sexual contacts of patients with urethritis should be notified and evaluated. This step offers the only hope of controlling the current epidemic. Unfortunately, the best intentioned efforts to identify, evaluate, and treat contacts are often fruitless. Those who do seek medical attention should have appropriate cultures, regardless of symptoms. Cervical gonococcal cultures are advised in female contacts. For partners of either sex, pharyngeal cultures are necessary if orogenital intercourse is practiced, and rectal cultures are warranted in those who engage in anal intercourse. When positive, these cultures alert the provider to a higher risk of treatment failure when certain regimens (ampicillin, amoxicillin—see Table 117-1) are used. (Given the complexities of this evaluation scheme, a legitimate argument can be made to treat contacts with the aqueous penicillin regimen without obtaining baseline cultures. However, the Centers for Disease Control guidelines do recommend obtaining cultural data.)

Complications
Complicated infections involve spread to another mucosal surface. In men, complications include acute prostatitis and acute epididymitis, and in women, pelvic inflammatory disease and perihepatitis (see Chap. 84). Disseminated gonococcal infection occurs in 1 to 3% of patients harboring the organism and may be associated with symptomatic infection of any mucosal site and with asymptomatic urethral, rectal, or pharyngeal infection.

The typical presentations of prostatitis and epididymitis are the same as those unrelated to venereal pathogens. In the case of prostatitis, patients complain of dysuria, frequency, and urgency associated with suprapubic and perineal pain. Epididymitis typically causes a tender, swollen testicle, which is less painful when elevated. Recent studies have demonstrated that in young, sexually active men the most common causes of both of these syndromes are STDs; 75% are due to *C. trachomatis,* and 10% are due to *N. gonorrhoeae.* In men over 35 years of age who have one sexual partner, the common urinary bacterial pathogens are the more likely causes. The evaluation of both of these complications is identical to that of uncomplicated urethritis.

Treatment
Effective treatment regimens for both complicated and uncomplicated urethritis are listed in Tables 117-1 and 117-2. Several critical points should be kept in mind when these treatments are being prescribed:

1. If the Gram's stain of urethral discharge confirms gonococcal urethritis, any of the regimens recommended for gonococcal infection may be used.
2. If the Gram's stain of discharge is questionable, tetracycline is preferred because of the probability of NGU.
3. The procaine penicillin–probenecid regimen is the only one that will *reliably* treat incubating syphilis, a major consideration in homosexual patients.
4. The ampicillin, amoxicillin, and spectinomycin regimens have a high (approximately 50%) failure rate in pharyngeal infections.
5. There is also a significant failure rate of the ampicillin and amoxicillin regimens in rectal infection. The procaine penicillin–probenecid regimen is preferred; however, this too may fail in male homosexuals, who have a relatively high proportion of infections secondary to penicillinase-producing *N. gonorrhoeae* (PPNG). Two grams of spectinomycin in a single intramuscular dose may be effective but has a high failure rate in some studies.
6. The tetracycline and doxycycline regimens are the only ones that will cure both

Table 117-1. Antibiotic therapy for gonorrhea*

Indication	Therapy
Uncomplicated gonorrhea—Single mucosal site including rectal and pharyngeal infections (see exclusions in text)	Procaine penicillin G 4.8 million units IM, injected at 2 sites, with probenecid 1 gm po *or* Ampicillin 3.5 gm po with probenecid 1 gm po *or* Amoxicillin 3.0 gm po with probenecid 1 gm po *or* Tetracycline 0.5 gm po qid for 5 days (not for use during pregnancy)
Patients with penicillin allergy	Tetracycline 0.5 gm po qid for 5 days (not for use during pregnancy) *or* Spectinomycin 2 gm IM (preferred during pregnancy)
Patients with treatment failure or penicillinase-producing *N. gonorrhoeae*	Spectinomycin 2 gm IM *or* Cefoxitin 2 gm IM with probenecid 1 gm po
Acute epididymitis	Procaine penicillin G 4.8 million units, ampicillin 3.5 gm po, *or* amoxicillin 3 gm po, each with probenecid 1 gm po; *then* ampicillin 0.5 gm po qid, *or* amoxicillin 0.5 gm po qid for 10 days, *or* tetracycline 0.5 gm po qid for 10 days (in penicillin allergy)
Disseminated gonococcal infection	Ampicillin 3.5 gm *or* amoxicillin 3.0 gm po, each with probenecid 1 gm po; *then* ampicillin 0.5 gm *or* amoxicillin 0.5 gm po qid for 7 days *or* Tetracycline 0.5 gm po qid for 7 days (not for use during pregnancy) *or* Spectinomycin 2 gm IM bid for 3 days (use for PPNG infections) *or* Erythromycin 0.5 gm po qid for 7 days *or* Aqueous crystalline penicillin G 10 million units IV per day until improvement occurs, *then* ampicillin 0.5 gm or amoxicillin 0.5 gm po qid for a total of 7 days of therapy

*Recommendations of the Centers for Disease Control.

    gonorrhea and chlamydial infections. Because the four-times-daily tetracycline regimen carries the greater risk of noncompliance, the twice-daily doxycycline regimen is usually preferable.
7. The procaine penicillin–probenecid regimen carries the highest risk of drug-related toxicity; anaphylaxis occurs in 1 in 10,000 patients, and acute psychosis secondary to procaine toxicity in 1 in 1000.
8. The recurrence of urethritis after appropriate treatment for documented gonococcal

Table 117-2. Treatment of chlamydial infections*

Indication	Therapy
Regimens of choice	Tetracycline 0.5 gm po qid for a minimum of 7 days *or* Doxycycline 0.1 gm po qid for a minimum of 7 days
Alternate regimens	Erythromycin 0.5 gm po qid for a minimum of 7 days
Treatment failure or relapse	Switch to erythromycin if tetracycline was used initially and vice versa
Recurrent treatment failure or relapse	Doxycycline or erythromycin as above for 3–4 weeks Metronidazole 2 gm po as a single dose can be tried to cover the possibility of the rare case of symptomatic trichomoniasis in men
Lymphogranuloma venereum	Above regimens continued for a minimum of 3 weeks

*Nongonococcal urethritis (chlamydial and nonchlamydial), mucopurulent cervicitis, and related syndromes.

infection may be secondary to reinfection, to the presence of PPNG, or to postgonococcal urethritis (PGU). Postgonococcal urethritis is currently attributed to *C. trachomatis, U. urealyticum,* and other presently undocumented pathogens. Treatment of gonorrhea "unmasks" the nongonococcal organisms that were probably present as concomitant pathogens on initial presentation. The treatment of PGU is outlined in Table 117-2.

9. Finally, documentation of the success of treatment is required in urethritis as in all other STD syndromes. Re-examination and reculture of the urethra and all other sites of positive cultures should be done about 7 days after the initial evaluation. As in the evaluation of contacts, there is an unfortunately high "no show" rate for return appointments.

Genital Ulcers

Sexually transmitted diseases that present as genital ulcers are difficult problems for clinicians. Determination of a specific cause based on clinical data alone is fraught with pitfalls. Unfortunately, available laboratory tests lack both sensitivity and specificity, and their results are usually not generated in time to be clinically useful. The dilemma can be lessened by an accurate epidemiologic history.

In the United States, the most common STDs producing genital ulceration in order of frequency are herpes, syphilis, and chancroid. The incidence of chancroid in the United States (less than 1000 cases per year) is very low when compared to that of the other two. In contrast, chancroid is more common in the developing countries in Africa, Asia, and South America. Acquisition of the infection from a prostitute or homosexual contact increases the likelihood of chancroid and other uncommon genital ulcer syndromes: lymphogranuloma venereum (LGV) and granuloma inguinale.

Evaluation

Table 117-3 presents an approach to the evaluation of ulcerative genital lesions. There are three broad categories of ulcerations: those associated with painful vesicles, those that are painful but not associated with vesicles, and those that are painless.

Herpes is the only STD that classically presents with painful vesicular lesions. In this case, diagnosis is made on a clinical basis. The only potentially useful laboratory test is a screening serologic test for syphilis (VDRL, RPR). If the patient's history makes exposure to syphilis unlikely, screening may be unnecessary.

The presentation of painful ulcerative lesions not associated with vesicles requires a more detailed evaluation. Although herpes is the most likely diagnosis in the United States, both chancroid and syphilis must be considered. Some authorities recommend three consecutive negative dark-field examinations to exclude syphilis, even though the luetic chancre does not classically present as a tender, painful genital lesion. This approach is supported by the fact that syphilis is statistically more likely than chancroid in the United States.

Table 117-3. Management of ulcerative genital lesions

Painful vesicular lesions	Painful ulcerative lesions	Painless ulcerative lesions
Genital herpes by clinical diagnosis alone Obtain serologic test for syphilis if patient's history warrants	1. Herpes culture and Tzanck preparation 2. Culture for *Hemophilus ducreyi* 3. Obtain serologic test for syphilis; repeat in 1 week 4. Begin sulfisoxazole 4 gm daily for 2 weeks if chancroid is highly suspect 5. Dark-field exam × 3 negatives over 3 days if clinical history is compatible with syphilis; if positive, treat as in column 3	1. Dark-field exam × 3 negatives over 3 days 2. Obain serologic test for syphilis Either test positive Both tests negative Treat patient and contacts for primary syphilis as in Table 117-4 Repeat serologic tests at 1, 6, and 12 weeks

Herpes

Herpes infections present as painful genital ulcers, with or without associated vesicles. The current epidemic of herpes and the detailed attention the infection has received in the lay press behoove the clinician to have a clear understanding of this STD.

Two herpesviruses, herpes simplex type 1 (HSV-1) and herpes simplex type 2 (HSV-2), have been implicated in genital infections. Both viruses are neurotropic and share the biologic property of latency. After a primary genital infection following genital-genital or oral-genital contact, the virus ascends the peripheral nerves to the sacral ganglia and becomes latent. When periodically reactivated, the virus descends the involved nerve and causes recurrent infection. Because of unpredictable, sometimes frequent recurrences, herpetic infections can be a devastating problem for those affected.

The average incubation period following primary exposure is 6 days. The initial symptoms of primary herpes are nonspecific and include fever, myalgia, arthralgia, and malaise. Aching, paresthesia, and pruritus usually occur in the affected genital areas. These symptoms are soon followed by the appearance of crops of vesicles containing cloudy fluid. In both sexes, multiple sites may be involved, including the penis, buttocks, and thighs in men and the labia, uterus, fourchette, cervix, buttocks, and thighs in women. Dysuria and dyspareunia may occur. Typically, the herpetic vesicles gradually rupture, leaving ulcerations that are extremely painful. Bilateral, tender inguinal adenopathy may develop during the vesicular and ulcerative stages. The final stage is that of crust formation in the ulcerated areas. Complete healing takes an average of 20 days.

Recurrent infection develops in two-thirds of all patients during the year following the primary episode. Fortunately, recurrences tend to be less severe than the primary infection. Although the specific factors that cause recurrences are poorly understood, a number of triggering stimuli have been suggested: fever, menses, trauma, sexual intercourse, fatigue, and emotional stress. Prodromal symptoms are common in both sexes and present as localized pruritus, burning, or hypersensitivity at the site of the subsequent lesion. Recurrent lesions are fewer in number and may be inconspicuous and difficult to identify. The average duration of a recurrence is 10 days. With time, recurrent episodes tend to decrease in frequency.

Complications of acute primary or recurrent infection include urinary retention (particularly in women), aseptic meningitis, proctitis, endometritis, and dissemination (during pregnancy). The urinary retention is secondary to severe pain and/or bladder hypotonia. Although the underlying pathogenesis is unclear, this complication is probably caused by herpetic involvement of the sacral nerve roots. Perhaps the most devastating complication is related to perinatal infection from direct contact with the virus during delivery or from ascending infection following rupture of the fetal membranes. Neonatal herpes has a high mortality, even with current treatment and supportive measures. This is the basis for recommending cesarean section in any woman with known infection at or near the time of delivery. Unfortunately, the maternal infection may be subclinical, and documentation requires serial herpes cervicovaginal cultures during the last 6 weeks of pregnancy in any woman with a history of previous infection or exposure.

The diagnosis of herpetic infection is often possible on clinical grounds alone, particularly during the vesicular stage. However, patients may not seek medical care until the more painful, ulcerative stage. A definitive diagnosis is preferred in order to predict the patient's future clinical course and to differentiate herpes from other infections. Cytologic examination of vesicular fluid is positive in as many as 50% of cases; the yield is much lower during the ulcerative stage. The examination is done by obtaining material from a vesicle or the base of an ulcer, staining with Giemsa or Wright's stain, and looking for Tzanck cells, which are multinucleated giant cells. If Giemsa stain is negative, a herpes culture of vesicular fluid or fluid from the base of an ulcer is necessary. Culture is positive in 90 to 95% of cases and is the definitive diagnostic test available. Serology is not helpful, since many adults already have antibodies, and titers fluctuate without relation to genital herpetic infection.

The effectiveness of preventive measures is limited because recurrences are unpredictable and sometimes asymptomatic. Asymptomatic recurrences are more common in women and are usually cervical infections. In men, asymptomatic urethral infections are known to occur. As a result, there is really no "safe" period when protection from transmission to the uninfected partner is assured, and prophylactic measures, to be effective, must always be used when there is a history of herpes in either partner. Currently, there are two commonly available barriers to genital transmission: spermicidal foams and condoms. Washing of the external genitalia with soap and water after intercourse may add some protection. All of these measures should be viewed as approaches to decreasing the risk, not as ways to eliminate the risk. The following recommendations seem most reasonable for preventing transmission of genital herpes:

1. Sexual abstinence when lesions are active.
2. Use of a condom by men with a history of genital herpes or spermicidal foam by the woman or both.
3. Use of both condom and foam in the case of the woman with recurrent herpes. Use of both measures in this case seems reasonable given the increased risk of asymptomatic infection in women.

Symptomatic therapy is usually most required during the exceedingly painful primary attack. Both systemic analgesics and topical anesthetics may palliate the symptoms. Topical antiseptics such as povidone-iodine and antibiotic ointments may slightly decrease the risk of secondary infection but probably have minimal effects on the course of the primary infection.

A large number of therapeutic regimens have been proposed. Most have not been demonstrated to be effective in rigorous clinical trials. Among these are topical idoxuridine, adenine arabinoside, proflavine and neutral red photodynamic dyes, ether, zinc sulfate, corticosteroids, herpes vaccines, and nonspecific immune stimulation with smallpox vaccination or bacillus Calmette-Guérin (BCG). On the other hand, topical Acyclovir, a nucleoside analog that inhibits viral DNA polymerase, is efficacious. For patients with primary herpes genital infection, double-blind controlled trials have shown that Acyclovir applied to all lesions 6 times per day decreases the mean duration of local pain and itching, the mean duration of viral shedding, and the mean time to healing by a few days. For patients with recurrent herpes, similar studies have demonstrated a significant decrease in the mean duration of viral shedding, but no decrease in healing time and the duration of symptoms. Acyclovir has not been shown to decrease the frequency of clinical recurrences.

Syphilis

When there is a painless ulcerative lesion, primary syphilis is the most likely diagnosis. The chancre presents as a painless papule that rapidly becomes eroded, forming a painless ulcer with indurated margins. In heterosexual men, it is located on the penis. Locations in homosexual men include the anal canal, the mouth, and the external genitalia. In women, the primary sites include the cervix and labia. There is usually firm, painless, nonsuppurative bilateral inguinal adenopathy.

Optimal evaluation should include dark-field examination and should be considered negative only after three consecutive negatives on 3 separate days. A VDRL should also be done (see Table 118-3). If primary syphilis is confirmed, treatment is as described in Table 117-4.

Chancroid

Chancroid is uncommon but should be considered more seriously in patients whose sexual contacts are prostitutes. The infection occurs more often in men than women (5:1). Infected women often do not have clinically obvious ulceration. The classic clinical presentation is that of a small inflammatory papule 3 to 5 days after sexual exposure. This lesion becomes vesiculopustular and then ulcerative within 2 to 3 days. The chancroid is a superficial, shallow ulcer of a few millimeters to 2 cm in diameter. An inflammatory, erythematous halo surrounds the lesion, and the edges of the ulcer are most often ragged or scalloped.

Chancroid can be confused with luetic chancre and with the lesions of lymphogranuloma venereum (LGV). Unlike the chancre, the chancroidal ulcer is very painful and is not indurated. The most common locations include the prepuce and the frenulum in men and the labia, fourchette, and perineum in women. In over 50% of cases, the chancroidal ulcer is associated with acute, painful, and tender unilateral inguinal lymphadenopathy, which in untreated cases progresses to a unilocular suppurative bubo. When the bubo drains, it does so through a single site. The nodes of LGV usually

Table 117-4. Treatment for syphilis*

Indication	Penicillin therapy	Therapy for patients with penicillin allergy	Comments
Early syphilis: primary, secondary, latent of less than 1 year	Benzathine penicillin G 2.4 million units total IM at a single session	Tetracycline HCl 500 mg po qid for 15 days	Before using the tetracycline regimen, cerebrospinal fluid examination should be performed to rule out asymptomatic neurosyphilis. Some authorities advise doing this before penicillin therapy also.
Syphilis of more than 1 year's duration: latent, cardiovascular, late benign	Benzathine penicillin G 2.4 million units IM once a week for 3 successive weeks (7.2 million units total)	Tetracycline HCl 500 mg po qid for 30 days	
Neurosyphilis	Aqueous penicillin G 12–24 million units per day IV, divided into q4h doses, for 10 days; follow with benzathine penicillin G 2.4 million units IM weekly for 3 doses	Confirm allergy and obtain expert consultation to determine optimal therapy	Less optimal regimens include 1. Aqueous procaine penicillin G 2.4 million units IM daily plus probenecid 500 mg po qid, both for 10 days. Follow with benzathine penicillin G 2.4 million units IM weekly for 3 doses. 2. Benzathine penicillin G 2.4 million units IM weekly for 3 doses.

*Based on Centers for Disease Control recommendations.

drain through multiple sinuses and fistulae and are bilateral and nontender. Unlike chancroid, the primary LGV genital lesion is not present concomitantly. Primary genital herpes infection also causes tender inguinal adenopathy but is associated with multiple ulcerations and/or vesicular lesions. Herpes also causes systemic symptoms of fever, myalgia, and arthralgia; chancroid does not present with constitutional symptoms.

Definitive diagnosis is dependent on culturing *Hemophilus ducreyi* from the lesion. Unfortunately, the organism is isolated in less than 10% of the cases in which the infection is strongly suspected on clinical grounds. Therefore, the decision to treat should be based on clinical suspicion and not on culture. No better test is available.

Chancroidal lesions may spontaneously heal in 2 to 4 weeks without antibiotic therapy. Nevertheless, sulfisoxazole, 4 gm daily, is the preferred therapy and should be continued until the genital lesions and adenopathy have healed. Resolution usually takes about 2 weeks. Tetracycline, 2 gm daily, is also effective. One advantage of sulfonamide therapy is that it will not interfere with dark-field examinations for syphilis in those cases where consecutive examinations are deemed necessary following the institution of empiric therapy.

Proctitis and Proctocolitis

Proctitis and proctocolitis have become progressively more important STDs because of the increasing prevalence of sexual practices that involve fecal-oral transmission of pathogens. The most common pathogens, in order of frequency, include herpes simplex, *N. gonorrhoeae*, *Treponema pallidum*, *G. lamblia*, *Entamoeba histolytica*, *C. trachomatis*, and *C. fetus ssp jejuni*.

Diagnosis

Although proctitis and proctocolitis may be asymptomatic, there is usually a change in bowel habit. The most common symptom is anal discharge, followed by rectal pain, diarrhea, constipation, bloody stools, tenesmus, abdominal pain, fever, and pruritus ani. Positive findings in most patients include obvious proctitis and leukocytes in anorectal secretions. Herpetic proctitis is usually associated with multiple rectal ulcers and systemic symptoms of malaise and fever.

The evaluation of a homosexual patient with symptoms of proctitis requires proctoscopy. Specimens should be sent for laboratory evaluation of those pathogens, listed above, considered most likely based on the clinical history. This includes bacterial cultures, herpes culture, dark-field examination for syphilis, and microscopic examination for parasites. The increased frequency of syphilis in this population warrants a screening VDRL.

Treatment of anorectal infections caused by *N. gonorrhoeae* and *C. trachomatis* is outlined in Tables 117-1 and 117-2. If *N. gonorrhoeae* is the pathogen, the preferred regimen is procaine penicillin G–probenecid because the ampicillin-amoxicillin regimen has a high failure rate in men with proctitis. Treatment for primary syphilis presenting as a rectal chancre(s) is specified in Table 117-4, along with regimens for the secondary and tertiary stages of the disease. In the case of the other "nontraditional" pathogens, the appropriate treatments are the same as when the presentation does not involve sexual transmission.

New "Nontraditional" STDs

Recent investigations have documented the existence of a new groups of "nontraditional" infections, including cytomegalovirus (CMV), hepatitis B virus (HBV), and *G. lamblia*, as well as the other enteric organisms described above. The fact that many are enteric infections suggests several factors that may be related to their rise: (1) a change in sexual habits and increasing anogenital and orogenital sex among all groups and (2) possibly the improvement of sanitation over the past 20 years. Because sanitary improvements have decreased the exposure of children to such pathogens as CMV, susceptibility as adults may have increased.

Both CMV and HBV are present in the stool, semen, and cervical secretions of infected patients. These pathogens have been related to CMV mononucleosis syndrome and hepatitis B, respectively.

Homosexual men have an increased incidence of two rare conditions: Kaposi's sarcoma and the acquired immune deficiency syndrome (AIDS), which presents with infections secondary to *Pneumocystis carinii* and other opportunistic pathogens. Immunosuppression produced by chronic CMV infection and/or other sexually transmitted suppressors of normal immunity may account for these new syndromes.

Wiesner PJ, Thompson SE. Gonococcal diseases. *DM* 26:1–44, 1980.
   A detailed review of the epidemiology, pathogenesis, clinical syndromes, and treatment of gonococcal infection.
Lebedeff DA, Hochman EB. Rectal gonorrhea in men: Diagnosis and treatment. *Ann Intern Med* 92:463–466, 1980.
   A discussion of a prospective investigation of rectal gonorrhea in men, which reviews the clinical presentation and treatment options.
Wiesner PJ. Gonococcal pharyngeal infection. *Clin Obstet Gynecol* 18:121–129, 1975.
   A review of the epidemiology, clinical presentation and course, diagnosis, and treatment of pharyngeal gonorrhea.
U.S. Department of Health, Education, and Welfare, Public Health Service, Center for Disease Control. Gonorrhea: Center for Disease Control recommended treatment schedule, 1979. *Ann Intern Med* 90:809–811, 1979.
   Lists the recommendations for treatment of all gonococcal syndromes, including special considerations such as penicillin allergy, pregnancy, resistant gonococcal infection, and the treatment of sexual partners.
Holmes KK, et al. Etiology of nongonococcal urethritis. *N Engl J Med* 292:1199–1205, 1975.
   Reviews the epidemiology and etiologies of nongonococcal urethritis in men, and provides supportive data for the importance of Chlamydia trachomatis.
Jacobs NF, Kraus SJ. Gonococcal and nongonococcal urethritis in men: Clinical and laboratory differentiation. *Ann Intern Med* 82:7–12, 1975.
   Presents a very useful clinical approach that facilitates the differential diagnosis of urethritis in men and permits immediate, definitive treatment.
Sparling PF. Current problems in sexually transmitted diseases. *Adv Intern Med* 24:203–228, 1979.
   Presents an overview of current dilemmas in the etiology, diagnosis, treatment, and control STDs.
Handsfield HH. Sexually transmitted diseases. *Hosp Pract* 17:99–116, 1982.
   A succinct review of specific clinical aspects of STDs and those caused by organisms outside the traditional sphere of venereology.
Sparling PF. Diagnosis and treatment of syphilis. *N Engl J Med* 284:642–653, 1971.
   A succinct review of the serologic diagnosis and treatment of syphilis with a focus on the pitfalls of serologic testing.
Sparling PF. Syphilis. *Cecil's Textbook on Medicine* (15th ed.). Philadelphia: Saunders, 1979. Pp. 505–518.
   A concise summary of all aspects of syphilis, including etiology, pathogenesis, host response, clinical course and manifestations, diagnosis, and treatment.
Quinn TC, et al. The etiology of anorectal infections in homosexual men. *Am J Med* 71:395–406, 1981.
   Reports the results of a prospective study of homosexual men with anorectal symptoms, and reviews the prominent features of different etiologic forms of anorectal infections.
Raab R, Lorinez AL. Genital herpes simplex—concepts and treatments. *J Am Acad Dermatol* 5:249–263, 1981.
   Presents a detailed review of the epidemiology, virology, clinical manifestations, complications, and management of genital herpetic infection.
Tummon IS, et al. Genital herpes simplex. *Can Med Assoc J* 125:23–29, 1981.
   Presents a general review of herpetic infection, which emphasizes practical clinical aspects.
Proceedings of a symposium on Acyclovir. *Am J Med Acyclovir Symposium*, July 20, 1981. Pp. 1–392.
   A highly detailed review of studies that document the chemical, pharmacokinetic, and clinical characteristics of Acyclovir. Pages 326–350 are most relevant to the use of Acyclovir in genital herpes simplex infections.

118. INFLUENZA
Timothy W. Lane

Influenza viruses are an important cause of acute respiratory illness throughout the world. Because of the constant process of antigenic change in the influenza A virus, epidemics and pandemics occur when there has been sufficient change in viral strains to diminish the effectiveness of immunity to previous strains. Infections occur with a broad spectrum of complaints. Milder or typical cases produce symptoms similar to other respiratory viruses such as parainfluenza and respiratory syncytial virus. Since treatment is usually nonspecific, a precise viral diagnosis is not essential for management. However, it is sometimes useful to make a presumptive diagnosis because the prognosis of influenza is, on the average, worse than for other respiratory infections and because specific treatment with amantadine is sometimes indicated.

The three distinct influenza viruses that infect man are designated A, B, and C on the basis of differences in nucleocapsid proteins. Influenza A and, to a lesser extent, B are responsible for outbreaks. Influenza C most likely accounts for one of many childhood viral infections and appears not to cause epidemics.

The shorthand nomenclature for influenza viruses, commonly used to identify various strains, is written as follows: virus type/location of first isolation/year isolated (hemagglutinin and neuraminidase type). For example, two recent strains are designated A/Philippines/1982 (H_3N_2) and B/USSR/1983.

Epidemiology
Influenza infection is probably transmitted by both large- and small-particle aerosols generated by coughing and sneezing. Both outbreaks persisting for 6 to 8 weeks and sporadic cases occur during the winter months in temperate regions, and, rarely, cases may be identified at other times.

During outbreaks of influenza, attack rates are highest in children, but the elderly and those with chronic diseases suffer the most morbidity. The activity of influenza in the population can be determined by regular observation of deaths attributed to "pneumonia and influenza" in selected U.S. cities as well as from the isolation of influenza viruses by sentinel laboratories. A rise above the expected numbers of deaths ascribed to pneumonia and influenza defines an epidemic. Local and state health departments and the weekly epidemiologic reports of the Centers for Disease Control (CDC) have information about influenza activity that is within 2 to 4 weeks of current.

Clinical Presentation
Classic symptoms of influenza A include the abrupt onset of chills, myalgias, malaise, nonproductive to minimally productive cough, sore throat, prominent headache, and nasal stuffiness. Dizziness, photophobia, nausea, and vomiting occur less commonly. Patients chiefly complain of the systemic effects. There may be as many subclinical and mild cases as there are symptomatic ones. In symptomatic infection, clinical findings are high fever (102–104°F), a nonexudative pharyngitis, muscle tenderness, and occasionally cervical adenopathy. Influenza B has traditionally been considered a milder disease, but local and national surveillance data suggest that it can be similar in severity.

In healthy hosts, influenza is a self-limited illness. Defervescence is usually seen by day three and resolution of remaining symptoms in 4 to 5 days. However, patients will frequently experience malaise, easy fatigability, and cough for 2 to 3 weeks after onset. Persistent cough is common, presumably because influenza virus infects nasal and bronchial ciliated epithelial cells, causing inflammation and cellular necrosis. Viremia and extrarespiratory tract infection have been documented infrequently. Interferon production is temporally related to clinical resolution and is probably important for recovery.

The incubation period of influenza is normally 2 to 3 days with a range of 1 to 7 days. Viral shedding begins within 24 hours of symptomatic onset, peaks with severity, and abates over 4 to 5 days. Adults hospitalized for influenza should be isolated during this period of viral shedding to prevent possible nosocomial transmission.

Diagnosis

The likelihood that the patient with typical symptoms actually has influenza depends on the current prevalence of influenza. During a period of epidemic influenza activity, a clinical diagnosis of a typical case has a sensitivity of 85% and is usually sufficient for patient management. In a nonepidemic situation, most cases of respiratory disease ordinarily called "flu" are not influenza.

Findings on routine laboratory testing are nonspecific, and the only accurate way to confirm the diagnosis is by isolation of the virus from nasal and throat swabs or by antibody titers. Positive tissue cultures for influenza virus can be detected within 2 to 5 days of incubation. Serologic specimens collected 3 to 4 weeks apart can be examined for a fourfold rise in either complement fixing or hemagglutination-inhibition antibodies, but the time lag diminishes clinical relevance. These techniques are expensive and slow and of little use in most situations. Experimental techniques of direct viral antigen detection in respiratory secretions are being developed and offer the possibility of definitive diagnosis within several hours.

Treatment of Uncomplicated Influenza

Supportive Therapy

Supportive therapy of uncomplicated influenza has become medical folklore: adequate fluids, bed rest, and aspirin. There is no evidence that "prophylactic" antibiotics are beneficial. Nasal congestion may be ameliorated by 0.25% phenylephrine drops or spray, used for no more than 5 days, lest a rebound phenomenon develop. Judicious use of codeine may help the patient with persistent cough. Use of aspirin has recently been questioned. Several studies linking Reye's syndrome to the use of aspirin for influenza among children have prompted the Food and Drug Administration to issue formal caution in children. Because Reye's syndrome has also been reported in young adults (in their 20s), it is probably prudent to avoid aspirin in this age group as well.

Amantadine

Amantadine has in vitro antiviral activity against influenza A. In a large majority of the clinical trials with prospective, randomized, placebo-controlled design, amantadine has been shown to reduce days of fever by about 50%. Only about half of the trials have shown a significant decrease in other symptoms. The drug is effective only when administered within 48 hours of the onset of symptoms. Usual oral dosages have been 200 mg per day for 4 to 7 days. Amantadine therapy has been recommended for those at high risk of complications, that is, the elderly and those with chronic illnesses, but clinical trials have been primarily limited to young, healthy subjects. Its use in severe influenza infections has not been adequately examined.

Five to ten percent of patients given amantadine experience dizziness, nausea, and difficulty with mental concentration; these effects are quickly reversible with cessation of the drug. Amantadine is teratogenic in animals and so is contraindicated in pregnancy. Because of these problems and the difficulty of making an early diagnosis, amantadine is of limited therapeutic value in the management of respiratory infections.

Complications

The most frequent complications of influenza involve the respiratory tract. Tracheobronchitis and sinusitis are not uncommon. Primary influenzal and secondary bacterial pneumonias are the most feared complications because of their contribution to morbidity and mortality. These sequelae may result from viral destruction of mucociliary cells, adherence of bacterial pathogens to virally infected epithelial cells, and altered cellular defenses. Radiographic pneumonia has an overall frequency of about 5%. Primary influenzal pneumonia is seen in about 1% of clinical infections. Both types of pneumonia have their onset 4 to 6 days after the appearance of typical influenza. The patient experiences recrudescence of fever and respiratory symptoms. The production of purulent sputum is a helpful clue to bacterial pneumonia. The three most common bacterial causes are pneumococcus, *Staphylococcus aureus,* and *Hemophilus influenzae;* enteric gram-negative bacilli and meningococcal infectons have also been described. Susceptibility to secondary pulmonary infection is increased in those who are elderly

(> 65 years of age) or have chronic underlying renal, metabolic (including diabetes), hematologic, immunodeficiency, or cardiopulmonary disorders.

Occasionally, influenza affects organ systems other than the respiratory tract. Neurologic complications include encephalitis, Guillain-Barré syndrome, transverse myelitis, and Reye's syndrome. Myositis and, rarely, myoglobinuric renal failure have been described in the convalescent stage of influenza. Other rare complications include perimyocarditis, parotitis, and glomerulonephritis.

Prevention

Chemoprophylaxis
Amantadine is approved for prophylaxis against influenza. Many well designed studies show a 50 to 70% efficacy in preventing influenza A infections. When there is epidemiologic evidence of influenza A activity, its use should be considered for (1) susceptible individuals with chronic diseases, (2) susceptible elderly groups in institutions such as nursing homes, and (3) persons whose activities are vital to the public welfare, such as policemen, firemen, and health care personnel. The strength of these recommendations is tempered by the lack of controlled studies of the elderly and chronically ill.

The dosage of amantadine recommended for prophylaxis is 200 mg daily, the same as that for therapy. The dosage should be reduced in patients with impaired renal function (creatinine clearance $\leq$ 50 cc/min) to lessen adverse effects. Amantadine must be administered over the usual 6- to 8-week period of an outbreak to be effective. A reasonable option is to administer amantadine and influenza vaccine simultaneously. Amantadine does not interfere with vaccine immunogenicity and can be discontinued after 10 days, when about 80% of vaccines will have developed adequate antibodies.

Vaccination
Field trials have demonstrated a 50 to 80% reduction in influenza infection after vaccination. Several retrospective reports show a 30 to 70% reduction in infection in elderly and other high-risk populations. The U.S. Public Health Service recommends annual influenza vaccination for those at risk of complications and suggests vaccination in widespread epidemics for personnel of essential public services. The rationale of immunizing those at risk is twofold: (1) the majority of excess morbidity and mortality occurs in these groups, and (2) complicated logistics and limited vaccine production make it impractical to vaccinate all susceptible people. However, even with targeted vaccination, only 20 to 25% of high-risk subjects actually receive vaccine in any year. Yearly immunization is recommended because of the short-lived immunity of killed vaccines and the frequent necessity of updating vaccine antigens. Each summer the CDC publishes its yearly recommendations for vaccination. Manufacturers make vaccine available by the early fall for administration before the beginning of the influenza season.

For those over 13 years of age, a single injection of inactivated whole virus vaccine containing antigen of the A and B strains of the preceding year is currently recommended and will induce adequate antibodies in 80 to 90%. The rare individual with a history of serious egg allergy should not receive vaccine because it contains residual egg protein. Vaccination of pregnant women should be considered on the basis of individual risk of complications. Although not known to be teratogenic, vaccine should be withheld until after the first trimester if possible. Those with chronic renal and collagen vascular disorders can be safely vaccinated, but immunogenicity may be somewhat reduced. In patients receiving immunosuppressive agents, vaccine should be given during drug-free intervals to enhance response.

Adverse reactions to vaccination are generally mild; about one-third of those vaccinated note a local discomfort at the injection site and 1 to 2% experience a 24- to 48-hour syndrome of malaise and low-grade fever. During the mass swine influenze vaccination program in 1976, an increased risk of developing Guillain-Barré syndrome in vaccinees was recognized. Fortunately, nationwide surveillance has shown no such association with subsequent vaccine formulations.

Douglas RG Jr, Betts RF. Influenza Virus. In GL Mandell, RG Douglas Jr, and JE Bennett (Eds.), *Principles and Practice of Infectious Diseases*. New York: Wiley, 1985.

A thorough and authoritative review with an extensive bibliography by two recognized experts.

Waldman RJ, et al. Aspirin as a risk factor in Reye's syndrome. *JAMA* 247:3089, 1982.
One of several reported case control studies, all of which demonstrate increased risk for Reye's syndrome in children treated with aspirin for influenza and other viral infections. Indirectly suggests caution in the use of aspirin for influenza in young adults in their 20s as well.

Hirsch MS, Swartz MN. Antiviral agents (first of two parts). *N Engl J Med* 302: 903, 1980.
A succinct, well-referenced, and critical review of amantadine's pharmacology and the evidence supporting its prophylactic and therapeutic roles.

Amantadine: Does it have a role in the prevention and treatment of influenza? A National Institutes of Health Consensus Development Conference. *Ann Intern Med* 92(Part I):256, 1980.
Generally supports a wider use of amantadine based on a review of its efficacy by experts, but appropriately points out problems very much in need of further investigation.

Horadan VW, et al. Pharmacokinetics of amantadine hydrochloride in subjects with normal and impaired renal function. *Ann Intern Med* 94(Part I):454, 1981.
Establishes much needed dosing guidelines, especially since amantadine is recommended for those with chronic renal dysfunction. Refer to the guidelines when your patient's creatinine clearance is less than or equal to 50 cc per minute.

Yolken RH, et al. Flourometric assay for measurement of viral neuraminidase: Application to the rapid detection of influenza virus in nasal wash specimens. *J Infect Dis* 142:516, 1980.
A rapid (2–4 hours) method of influenza virus detection that preliminarily appears to be sensitive. Elicits hope for broader and more specific use of amantadine but not yet fulfilled in clinical practice.

Recommendations of the Immunization Practices Advisory Committee: Prevention and control of influenza 1984–1985. *Morbidity and Mortality Weekly Report* 33:253, 1984.
The most recent yearly update from the CDC, which strongly advocates vaccine for high risk groups as well as essential health care personnel.

Hurwitz ES, et al. Guillain-Barré syndrome and the 1978–1979 influenza vaccine. *N Engl J Med* 304:1557, 1981.
Unlike the distressing experience with the swine influenza vaccine in 1976, no vaccine-associated risk for Guillain-Barré syndrome was documented for subsequent vaccine formulations by this report of a national surveillance program.

Haskins TW, et al. Assessment of inactivated influenza A vaccine after three outbreaks of influenza A at Christ's Hospital. *Lancet* 1:33, 1979.
Prospective but nonrandomized study of the efficacy of repeated influenza vaccinations, which shows failure of protection in those receiving two or more immunizations with antigenically drifted influenza A (H_3N_2) strains. A preliminary report, but casts some doubt on the presumed benefit of yearly vaccination with H_3N_2 antigens.

Baker WH, Mulloly JP. Influenza vaccination of elderly persons: Reduction in pneumonia and influenza hospitalizations and deaths. *JAMA* 244:2547, 1980.
Results: 72% estimated reduction in hospitalization and 87% reduction in deaths. Albeit retrospective and nonrandomized in design, one of few available studies demonstrating vaccine efficacy in those considered a high priority for immunization.

119. INFECTIOUS MONONUCLEOSIS
Jack D. McCue

Infectious mononucleosis (IM) results from infection with Epstein-Barr virus (EBV). Most EBV infections are asymptomatic, and the rest are usually self-limited, relatively benign diseases. Symptomatic illness rarely occurs in children under 5 years old, and even adolescents have a less than 50% chance of developing typical IM as a result of

EBV infection. Clinically apparent infections seem to occur most frequently in populations in whom primary exposure to EBV is delayed until the second decade of life, and perhaps because of this, IM is most often diagnosed in adolescents from higher socioeconomic groups. Symptomatic IM appears to be caused primarily by the host response to antigenic changes in B-lymphocytes, the primary host cells for EBV. A vigorous T-lymphocyte proliferative response to EBV-infected B-lymphocytes is largely responsible for the adenopathy and atypical lymphocytosis. The inflammatory response and killing of EBV-infected lymphocytes may also be the cause of fever, pharyngitis, and hepatitis characteristic of IM.

Clinical Manifestations
Patients with typical IM are nearly always in their teens or twenties and present to a physician with severe pharyngitis and fever. Atypical presentations in adolescents and adults under 50 years old are known to be uncommon from extensive seroepidemiologic studies. For example, the chance that a healthy adolescent who complains primarily of fatigue and has a normal physical examination has IM is small indeed.

Typical IM
After a postulated 30- to 50-day incubation period, there may be a brief nonspecific prodrome. Nearly all adolescents and adults then develop the triad of pharyngitis, fever, and adenopathy. Malaise and fatigue may be disproportionately severe.

Pharyngitis is present in over 80% of patients, and about 50% have exudate. In some (so-called anginose pharyngitis) the signs and symptoms are much more severe than in streptococcal pharyngitis. Palatal petechiae, occurring at the junction of the hard and soft palate, are commonly seen; while not diagnostic of IM, they suggest the diagnosis. The degree of fever correlates with the overall severity of the illness. Temperatures commonly reach 39°C and many exceed 40°C in acutely ill young adults. Significant adenopathy is nearly universally noted, and its absence should make one doubt the diagnosis of IM. In acute disease, the nodes may be massively enlarged and tender. Infectious mononucleosis is one of the few diseases of healthy persons causing significant posterior cervical adenopathy. About half of patients have mild to moderate splenomegaly, which may be slightly tender. Enlargement is usually greatest in the second week of illness.

Palpable hepatomegaly occurs in about one-fourth of patients, although jaundice is unusual. Mild right upper quadrant percussion tenderness is very common. In a few instances, IM may present as hepatitis.

Rashes
Rashes are not helpful in diagnosis because they are infrequent and of variable appearance. Up to 100% of patients receiving ampicillin develop an extensive maculopapular rash, presumably due to immune complexes from cross-reacting antibodies; a similar reaction occurs less often with other drugs and antibiotics.

Although uncommon in IM, facial and particularly eyelid edema is rarely encountered in other illnesses of young adults and may, therefore, suggest IM.

Atypical IM
Up to 25% of patients present with atypical illness, especially those under 10 or over 50 years old. The common atypical presentations include fever of unknown origin, leukemia or lymphoma, arthralgia-myalgia syndromes, aseptic meningitis and encephalitis, pneumonia, fever and rash of unknown cause, nonspecific gastrointestinal complaints, and mild jaundice.

Clinical Course
In the typical case of IM, sore throat and fever last about a week. Fatigue resolves more slowly; usual daily tasks can be resumed after 2 to 4 weeks. Rapid onset of symptoms and severity of sore throat and fever seem to be associated with a prolonged recovery. Most cases of prolonged fatigue probably represent post-IM depression or psychological problems unrelated to EBV infection. Mild encephalitis, manifested only by headache and a temporary fall in IQ, may be relatively common. Inability to study and perform at pre-illness levels may cause students to become further depressed when they fall behind in studies.

Cases of relapsing or chronic IM due to EBV have not been well documented and, if they do occur, are exceedingly uncommon.

Complications and Sequelae

Although very few patients experience complications from IM, awareness of the possibility can prevent the occurrence. This is particularly true for splenic rupture, which is usually due to trauma during the third and fourth week of illness, but which may also occur spontaneously and after apparent recovery. All patients with IM should be instructed to seek medical attention promptly for abdominal pain. The duration of risk for splenic rupture after IM infection is not known, but it is recommended that strenuous activity be avoided for 2 to 3 months and that participation in intercollegiate or contact sports not be resumed for 6 months.

Airway obstruction from pharyngeal edema and massive tonsillar enlargement is also rare but potentially life-threatening; patients in whom impending obstruction is suspected should be hospitalized because tracheostomy or intubation may become necessary. Interstitial pneumonitis has been noted in 3 to 5% of patients, and it usually resolves without complication. Pleural effusions have also been reported.

Hematologic complications include hemolytic anemia, which is usually mild and asymptomatic and is estimated to occur in up to 3% of patients. Mild thrombocytopenia is not uncommon, but severe thrombocytopenia and other hemorrhagic phenomena may also occur. Neutropenia, sometimes severe, has been reported.

Neurologic complications probably occur in less than 1% of cases and include meningoencephalitis, aseptic meningitis, Guillain-Barré syndrome, transverse myelitis, facial nerve palsy, seizures, optic neuritis, peripheral neuropathies, and psychoses.

Cardiac complications include myocarditis, which is usually asymptomatic and recognized by nonspecific electrocardiographic changes, and pericarditis, which is very rare.

Renal involvement may be reflected by transient minor abnormalities on urinalysis (microscopic hematuria, pyuria, and proteinuria) in up to 15% of patients. These findings are usually self-limited, and there is controversy as to whether nephritis due to IM actually occurs.

Diagnosis

Clinical Presentation

The triad of fever, adenopathy, and pharyngitis is usually due to a common viral or streptococcal pharyngitis, not IM. Nonetheless, a typical case of acute IM in a young adult is readily diagnosed clinically and confirmed by a positive heterophil test. Streptococcal pharyngitis may coexist with IM but is probably not any more prevalent in IM patients than in healthy persons. Posterior cervical adenopathy and the presence of splenomegaly help distinguish an IM pharyngitis from a streptococcal one.

Of the possible causes of atypical lymphocytosis, only infection with cytomegalovirus (CMV) is commonly confused clinically with atypical IM. Diagnosis of cases of CMV mononucleosis and the less common toxoplasmosis mononucleosis is made serologically. The syndrome of Monospot-negative persistent fatigue and pharyngitis without atypical lymphocytosis usually has another viral or psychiatric cause.

Heterophil Antibodies

The "spot" tests for heterophil antibodies are about 95% specific and about 90% sensitive. False-positive results are nearly always trace or 1+ and may occur in patients recovering from asymptomatic IM, since the spot test can remain positive for several months. False-negative results are usually encountered in atypical IM in young children and older adults. The degree of positivity of antibody test does not reliably correlate with the severity of clinical illness. A false-negative spot test will usualy turn positive in 1 to 2 weeks after the onset of symptoms. Rarely is a third spot test after two negative tests, done a week apart, justified. It is rarely necessary to confirm a spot test result with a classic Paul-Bunnell heterophil titer.

The white blood count is usually elevated in acute IM. Nearly all patients have an absolute lymphocytosis with greater than 4500 mononuclear cells per cubic millimeter and a relative lymphocytosis of greater than 50%. While atypical lymphocytosis occurs in many illnesses, it ordinarily exceeds 10% of white blood cells only in IM. Atypical lymphocytes are usually T-cells that are larger than normal lymphocytes with irregular "folded" cytoplasmic borders, an increased amount of cytoplasm with vacuoles, and an irregular nucleus.

Specific Anti-EBV Antibodies
The commonly available anti–viral capsid antigen (VCA) IgG assay has limited diagnostic value when positive because a fourfold IgG titer rise is seen in only about 10% of patients and the anti-VCA IgG remains elevated at about 1:40 for life after EBV infection. A negative test, however, virtually rules out IM, since titers peak near the time of onset of symptoms. The presence of IgM anti-VCA antibody, on the other hand, is highly diagnostic, since it rises to greater than or equal to 1:5 acutely and returns to zero within a few months. Assays for IgM anti-VCA are more difficult to perform than IgG assays but are now more commonly available. Confirmatory EBV serology should ordinarily be ordered only for atypical, usually hospitalized, cases.

Other Laboratory Abnormalities
Hemolytic anemia is rare. Mild thrombocytopenia is common.

Liver enzymes are nearly always mildly elevated. Low-grade hyperbilirubinemia is common, but elevations above 5 mg/dl or enzyme elevations over 10 times normal should suggest some other diagnosis. Nonspecific electrocardiographic changes, false-positive serologic tests for syphilis, and positive rheumatoid factor assays occur rarely.

Treatment
Most patients with IM require nothing more than symptomatic therapy, such as aspirin or acetaminophen for fever and anesthetic throat lozenges or gargles for pharyngitis. Aspirin and other nonsteroidal anti-inflammatory agents like indomethacin in high doses (150 mg per day for adults) are said to relieve some symptoms of IM, but this assertion has not been tested by controlled trials.

Isolation of patients with IM is unnecessary. Although the presumed mode of transmission is contact with EBV-containing oropharyngeal secretions, and the illness is sometimes popularly called the "kissing disease," there is little epidemiologic evidence of space-time clustering of IM or of prior exposure of IM patients to other cases of IM. Therefore, patients need not be restricted from close contact with others.

The use of corticosteroids in IM is controversial. In controlled studies, they have been proved superior to placebo in ameliorating fever and pharyngitis; they may also result in an improved sense of well-being and shortened duration of illness. The use of corticosteroids is universally recommended in cases of potential airway obstruction and favored for patients with neurologic, hematologic, or cardiac complications. The usual dosage is 1 mg/kg of prednisone daily for 3 days, then tapered over 7 to 10 days. Some proponents recommend that corticosteroids also be used in most cases of severely symptomatic but uncomplicated IM to help patients return to normal functioning more quickly and possibly to prevent post-IM depression or loss of significant time from schoolwork. Other authorities are reluctant to administer potent anti-inflammatory agents during an infection and advise against their use in routine cases.

Antibiotics are indicated only for the treatment of group A beta-hemolytic streptococcal pharyngitis and possibly for anginose pharyngitis. Foul (anaerobic) breath and massively swollen and painful oropharyngeal tissues may indicate the presence of a polymicrobial bacterial pharyngitis that may respond to treatment with penicillin or metronidazole. Antibiotics in general and ampicillin in particular should be avoided because of the very high incidence of rash.

Chang RS. *Infectious Mononucleosis.* Boston: Hall, 1980.
  Extensively referenced book covering nearly all aspects of EBV infection and IM.
Hoagland RS. *Infectious Mononucleosis.* New York: Grune & Stratton, 1976.
  Classic account of clinical IM.
Schooley RT, Dolin R. EBV. In CT Mandell, RG Douglas, and JE Bennett (Eds.), *Principles and Practice of Infectious Diseases.* New York: Wiley, 1979. Pp. 1324–1341.
Karzon DT. Infectious mononucleosis. *Pediatrics* 22:231–265, 1979.
  Comprehensive reviews of clinical and laboratory aspects of IM.
Bender CE. The value of corticosteroids in the treatment of infectious mononucleosis. *JAMA* 199:97–99, 1967.

Pront C, Dalrymple W. A double-blind study of 82 cases of infectious mononucleosis. *J Coll Health Assoc* 15:62–66, 1966.
  Two of several studies showing the beneficial effects of corticosteroids in controlled trials.

Horwitz CA. Practical approach to diagnosis of infectious mononucleosis. *Postgrad Med* 65:179–184, 1979.
  Simplified approach based on spot test for heterophil antibodies and analysis of blood smear for atypical lymphocytes.

Rutkow IM. Rupture of the spleen in infectious mononucleosis: A critical review. *Arch Surg* 113:718–720, 1978.
  An excellent review of this serious complication.

120. INTESTINAL PARASITES

Richard A. Davidson

Parasitic disease is not rare in the United States. Over 20% of people in some geographic locations are infected with intestinal nematodes. The seven most common pathogenic enteric parasitic infections of adults include the protozoal infections, giardiasis and amebiasis; and helminth infections, ascariasis, trichuriasis, enterobiasis, strongyloidiasis, and hookworm.

Parasitic infections cause a variety of symptoms and signs, most of which are nonspecific. Infection may be suspected in the presence of the clinical presentations summarized in Table 120-1.

Laboratory Diagnosis

Ordinarily an enteric parasitic infection is confirmed when the diagnostic stage of the parasite is demonstrated in stool or duodenal contents. Diarrheal stools, which are likely to contain trophozoites as well as cyst forms, should be examined by a well-trained laboratory technician within 30 minutes of passage; if a delay is necessary, the stools should be refrigerated to promote the survival of trophozoites. Formed stools most frequently contain cyst, egg, or larval forms, and prompt examination is not as crucial. A concentration technique is often used to improve the chances of detecting eggs and cysts when they are present in small numbers. At least 50% of infections with intestinal parasites can be demonstrated on one stool specimen; three specimens detect 80 to 90% of all recognized infections.

Infections with giardiasis and strongyloidiasis are occasionally not detected on stool examination alone; examination of duodenal contents by endoscopy or string test (Enterotest) is done if they are suspected and stool examinations are negative. The string test involves ingestion of an encapsulated string. The proximal end is taped to the cheek and the distal end is carried into the duodenum. After 3 to 4 hours, the string is removed and the bile-stained segment examined for the presence of parasites.

Enterobiasis, in contrast to the other intestinal parasites, is less frequently diagnosed by stool examination; the "Scotch-tape test" is performed by touching clear Scotch tape to the perineum, preferably before bathing or morning bowel movement and examining the tape under a microscope for the presence of eggs.

Eosinophilia is seen in infections with most parasites that have an extraluminal stage in their life cycle, including *Ascaris, Strongyloides,* and hookworm. Ordinarily, eosinophilia is not seen in amebic dysentery, giardiasis, and enterobiasis. Approximately 90% of patients diagnosed as having strongyloidiasis have eosinophilia, making it a good screening test for this infection. However, eosinophilia may be absent in patients taking corticosteroids and possibly patients with chronic infections. There does not appear to be an association between the degree of eosinophilia and the burden of infection.

Giardiasis

Giardia lamblia is a waterborne protozoan with widespread distribution. Infection occurs when the cyst stage, which is resistant to water chlorination, is ingested. Excys-

Table 120-1. Clinical settings in which parasitic infections should be considered

Clinical setting	Potential cause
Eosinophilia	Hookworm, strongyloidiasis, ascariasis
Unexplained anemia	Hookworm
Malabsorption	Giardiasis, strongyloidiasis
Gastrointestinal bleeding	Amebiasis, trichuriasis, hookworm
Wheezing	Ascariasis, trichuriasis, hookworm, strongyloidaisis
Pruritic urticarial and maculopapular skin rashes	Hookworm, strongyloidiasis, ascariasis
Dysentery	Amebiasis, giardiasis, trichuriasis
Rectal itching	Enterobiasis
Unexplained gastrointestinal symptoms	All
Recent immigration from endemic area (e.g., Far East, Africa, Haiti, South America)	All

tation occurs in the upper gastrointestinal tract, and motile trophozoites reproduce and live in the duodenum. Infection is usually acquired from a contaminated water supply and can occur as part of a large outbreak or sporadically depending on the source of exposure. The organism is endemic in some areas (e.g., in parts of Colorado). There is an increased incidence of *Giardia* infection in homosexuals, apparently because of person-to-person spread; outbreaks have also occurred in day-care centers.

Symptoms of *Giardia* infection vary widely from none to bouts of explosive, watery, foul-smelling diarrhea. Occasionally, a subacute or chronic form occurs, with intermittent, low-grade diarrhea. In extreme cases, alterations in small bowel mucosa lead to malnutrition, which is reversible with treatment of the infection. Eosinophilia is rarely seen. When stools are examined, the cyst stage is more frequently found than trophozoites. A single Enterotest examination may be more sensitive than three stool examinations.

Metronidazole is the drug of choice (although not approved for this use by the Food and Drug Administration) and is usually effective in a dosage of 250 mg three times a day for 7 days. Quinacrine and furazolidone are alternative therapies, with higher rates of side effects. Careful follow-up 10 to 14 days after treatment is recommended to demonstrate eradication of the organism. If there is a strong clinical suspicion of giardiasis, a therapeutic trial of medication may be worthwhile because the organism can occasionally be difficult to isolate from stool or duodenal contents.

Amebiasis

Amebiasis follows the ingestion of cysts of *Entamoeba histolytica*. Transmission is hand-to-mouth or, in homosexuals, by sexual contact. Infection manifests itself in three ways. It may be asymptomatic, with passage of cysts. Infection can result in dysentery, which may be acute, with explosive, bloody diarrhea and fever, or chronic, with intermittent milder diarrhea. Extraintestinal infection occurs without a history of dysentery in about half of cases. The most common site of extraintestinal infection is in the right lobe of the liver, as a solitary abscess with fever, malaise, and hepatomegaly. Infection can also be seen in the pleural and pericardial spaces.

Diagnosis is based on the demonstration of either cysts or trophozoites of *E. histolytica*. As many as seven forms of nonpathogenic amebae, which can be confused with *E. histolytica*, live in the gastrointestinal tract; therefore, final identification is best left to a well-trained laboratory technician. Ordinarily, trophozoites are seen only in loose stools, which are examined soon after passage; cysts are found in formed or loose stools and remain recognizable for a longer period of time.

Eosinophilia is typically absent in all forms of amebiasis. The most frequently used serologic test is the amebic indirect hemagglutination titer (AIH); it is most useful in extraintestinal disease (about 95% positive), less useful in active intestinal infection (85%), and useless for identifying asymptomatic cyst passers.

All forms of amebiasis usually respond to metronidazole, 750 mg three times a day for 5 to 10 days. When a treatment failure occurs, the choice of drug depends on the location of infection. In an asymptomatic cyst passer, diloxanide furoate is used, 500 mg three times a day for 10 days. For dysenteric disease, dehydroemetine is used, 1.0 to 1.5 mg/kg daily intramuscularly for 10 days. Extraintestinal disease is treated with chloroquine, 500 mg daily for 10 weeks, plus diiodohydroxyquin, 650 mg three times a day for 3 weeks.

Ascariasis

Ascaris lumbricoides is a common nematodal infection in the United States and is present throughout North America. The infection is contracted by ingesting the egg stage, which is usually found in fecally-contaminated soil; thus, the infection is most prevalent in children but may persist into adulthood. The worm is large (up to 35 cm in length), and the usual infection consists of 8 to 10 worms.

Eosinophilia is present during larval migration but may be absent, especially in chronic adult infections. Symptoms are usually minimal, with the main complaint being intermittent mild abdominal pain. The major serious consequences of the infection are host sensitization, which may cause an allergic reaction indistinguishable from bronchial asthma; migration of adult worms, which can cause bile duct obstruction, acute hemorrhagic pancreatitis, peritonitis, and intestinal obstruction, particularly with heavy infections and in children.

The eggs are readily demonstrable in the stool. No serologic tests are available. When a patient or mother reports passage of a worm and it is over 1 cm in length, for practical purposes it should be considered *Ascaris*.

Therapy is with piperazine citrate, 75 mg/kg by mouth daily for 2 days, although mebendazole 100 mg twice a day for three days is as effective. These drugs paralyze the worm, allowing its passage in the stool. In mixed infections, *Ascaris* should be treated first because other anthelminthics will cause it to migrate.

Trichuriasis

Trichuris, also known as whipworm, is extremely common; for example, 46% of the populaton surveyed at Hilton Head Island, South Carolina, in 1974 were infected. Eggs are ingested most frequently by children and mature in the jejunum. At maturity, the worm embeds into the colonic mucosa. Adults usually have light infections, which are asymptomatic. Heavier infections give rise to anemia, blood-streaked diarrhea, nausea, vomiting, and rectal prolapse. The eggs, which are quite distinctive, can be found in the stool. Acute infections also cause eosinophilia. Therapy is with mebendazole, 100 mg twice a day for 3 days.

Enterobiasis

As many as 200 million people worldwide may be infected with pinworm, including 18 million in the United States and Canada. The infection is spread by hand-to-mouth transmission of eggs, from scratching the perianal area. Other members of the household are often infected, presumably because eggs are in house dust and are inhaled. In one study of houses with several infected children, 222 of 241 dust samples from throughout the houses contained pinworm eggs.

The worm matures in the upper gastrointestinal tract and lives in the cecum; the gravid female migrates to the perineum to lay her eggs, causing perianal and vaginal irritation and pruritus. Eosinophilia is distinctly unusual, and the diagnosis is most effectively made by using the Scotch-tape test (see under Laboratory Diagnosis above). However, three daily tests detect only 90% of infections.

The treatment of choice is pyrvinium pamoate, 5 mg/kg in a single dose. A second dose 2 weeks later is strongly recommended. This medication stains the stool bright red and may cause nausea and vomiting. Alternative therapies include mebendazole, one 100-mg tablet, then repeat in 2 weeks; piperazine, 65 mg/kg daily for 7 days; or pyrantel pamoate, 11 mg/kg as a single dose, repeated in 2 weeks. Handwashing is the most effective way of reducing infection of household contacts; efforts to minimize house dust are often recommended as well.

Hookworm

Necator americanus, the New World hookworm, is found throughout the United States. The life cycle includes skin penetration and a molting stage in the lung, which leads to a pronounced eosinophilia. Acute infection causes few symptoms; most frequently, lassitude, dyspnea on exertion, weakness, and dizziness develop insidiously, paralleling the development of a hypochromic, microcytic anemia. The adult worm attaches and reattaches itself to the intestinal mucosa many times daily and secretes an anticoagulant that causes continuous oozing from prior attachment points. Each worm may cause from 0.03 to 0.15 ml of blood loss per day.

The usual diagnostic stage of hookworm is the egg, which is readily found in the stool in heavy infections; however, in milder cases concentration techniques may be necessary. The eggs may be confused with those of *Trichostrongylus,* a prevalent nonpathogen. Presently, the drug of choice is mebendazole, one 100-mg tablet twice a day for 3 days; pyrantel pamoate is an alternative.

Strongyloidiasis

Strongyloidiasis, while somewhat rarer than the other infections, more frequently causes fatalities. The worm is related to hookworm but does not cause a profound anemia. Like hookworm, the larvae penetrate the skin, and the adults live in the upper gastrointestinal tract. The most frequent symptoms are crampy abdominal pain, intermittent diarrhea, and nausea.

Most infections occur with an eosinophilia and can be diagnosed by finding one of the larval stages, a 2-mm worm, in the stool. (Unlike hookworm, eggs are usually not passed.) Under certain conditions, particularly those with deficient cell-mediated immunity such as corticosteroid use and transplantation, the worm undergoes a metamorphosis to a different larval stage. It then penetrates the gut wall and enters the bloodstream in large numbers, causing prostration, sepsis, and death in about half of patients ("hyperinfection").

Therapy for strongyloidiasis is thiabendazole, 25 mg/kg twice a day for 2 days; a repeat course in 1 week is recommended, particularly if the patient is immunologically deficient. The two courses are 96% effective.

Brown HW, Neva FA. *Basic Clinical Parasitology* (5th ed.). New York: Appleton-Century-Crofts, 1982.

Smith JW, Wolfe MS. Giardiasis. *Annu Rev Med* 31:373–383, 1980.
Excellent, thorough review of this common infection.

Davidson RA. Issues in clinical parasitology: I. The treatment of giardiasis. *Am J Gastroenterol* April, 1984.
A review of the major controlled trials of medications used in the treatment of this common infection. A discussion about possible risks of carcinogenesis with the use of metronidazole is included.

Krogsted DJ, Spencer HC, Healy GR. Amebiasis. *N Engl J Med* 298:262–265, 1978.
Short but complete review of clinical amebiasis with current drug recommendations.

Scowden EB, Schaffner W, Stone WJ. Overwhelming strongyloidiasis. *Medicine* 57:537–544, 1978.
Clearly defines how hazardous this infection may be when it occurs in patients with altered immune status.

Davidson RA, Fletcher RH, Chapman LE. Risk factors for strongyloidiasis. A case-control study. *Arch Intern Med* 144:321–324, 1984.
The risk of strongyloidiasis was increased in whites, males, patients taking corticosteroids, and patients with gastric surgery or a hematologic malignancy.

Beal C, et al. A new technique for sampling duodenal contents. *Am J Trop Med Hyg* 19:349–351, 1970.
A description of the currently available Enterotest, which may be used easily with little discomfort in the ambulatory setting to sample duodenal contents for Giardia, Strongyloides, and other parasites.

484 XVI. Infectious Diseases

121. RABIES PROPHYLAXIS
Jack D. McCue

Human rabies is a rare illness in the United States, accounting for fewer than two deaths per year. Possible rabies exposure, on the other hand, is common: 20,000 to 30,000 persons are vaccinated yearly, and 100 to 200 persons are bitten by animals subsequently proved to be rabid. Thus while physicians rarely if ever care for human rabies, nearly all primary care physicians prescribe rabies postexposure prophylaxis once every few years. There is no second chance for rabies prophylaxis: the decision to vaccinate must be correct and treatment must be given promptly and properly to ensure that the risk of developing rabies is minimized.

Evaluating Exposure
The risk of developing rabies varies with the type of animal responsible for the bite. High-risk animals include bats, skunks, bobcats, badgers, wolves, coyotes, weasels, raccoons, and foxes. Moderate-risk animals include stray dogs and cats; abnormally behaving dogs, cats, and farm animals; and pet skunks and mongooses. Normal dogs, cats, and farm animals present a low risk, and the risk is negligible for rodents (rats, mice, squirrels, gerbils, chipmunks, guinea pigs, hamsters) and rabbits.

Wild Animal Bites
The primary, and in many industrialized nations the only, reservoir of rabies virus is carnivorous wild animals. Since normally behaving wild animals avoid humans, most wild animal bites should be considered unprovoked and abnormal behavior even when the animal seems to be defending itself. If possible, the biting animal should be captured or killed and its brain examined for rabies. Since bats ordinarily avoid daylight and humans, a bite or daytime contact with a bat should always be considered a serious potential rabies exposure unless a laboratory examination of the animal's brain is conclusively negative.

Domestic Animal Bites
Dog and cat rabies occur mostly in areas where pets and farm animals come in contact with wild animals. Dogs and cats are equally capable of transmitting rabies and become symptomatic during or shortly after the virus appears in their saliva or urine. Those who remain asymptomatic during 10 days of observation are never subsequently found to have been infective at the time of the bite. The chance that a bite from a normally behaving rabies-immunized pet could cause rabies is nearly zero. In fact, some states have found no rabies in animals other than bats for several years. On the other hand, an unprovoked bite from a stray animal, especially in states reporting rabies in ground animals, must be seriously considered as a potential rabies exposure. The stray should either be observed for 10 days or killed and the refrigerated (not frozen) head sent to the state laboratory for examination.

State health departments with good surveillance programs can give a more precise estimate of risk and should be called before immunization. For example, a provoked bite from a stray dog in a state with no reports of rabies in ground animals would be considered a lower risk than a similar bite in an area with reports of rabies in ground animals. The Centers for Disease Control (CDC) should be consulted for advice in a presumed case of human rabies.

Non-Bite Exposures
Infected saliva deposited on fresh minor abrasions and cuts can cause rabies in experimental animals, but cuts more than 24 hours old are not easily infected. The virus can also pass through the intact conjunctivae and mucous membranes of experimental animals and probably humans. Although these non-bite means of contracting rabies are theoretically possible, documented cases of human rabies after non-bite exposure to a rabid animal are extremely rare. Reported cases of rabies in humans have occurred through corneal transplants, laboratory accidents, and inhalation of aerosolized bat urine in caves.

Treatment
Clinical trials have shown that the risk of developing rabies is negligible if guidelines from the CDC are followed. These include (1) local wound care, to reduce the infiltration of virus into tissues, and both (2) passive and (3) active immunotherapy. Tetanus may also develop from bite wounds, and tetanus toxoid should be administered to bite victims who are not adequately protected.

Local Wound Care
All wounds should be thoroughly washed with soap and water, and nonvital tissue should be debrided. This procedure decreases the risk of developing rabies, probably by reducing local tissue viral titers and thereby improving the chances that antibody and nonspecific defenses like interferon will halt infection of the peripheral nerves. Flushing with antiseptic solutions such as ethyl alcohol, green soap, and benzalkonium chloride is no longer recommended.

Head and neck bites are cause for added concern because they are often severe and difficult to debride and treat locally, thus leaving more virus to multiply in the wound. Additionally, some researchers believe the close proximity of head and neck bites to the brain and the presence of larger numbers of sensory nerve pathways may facilitate movement of virus to the central nervous system.

Active Immunotherapy
Human diploid cell rabies vaccine (HDCRV) should be given intramuscularly in five doses, on days 0, 3, 7, 14, and 28. With this regimen, good antibody levels are attained in 100% of patients; results have been so uniformly good that recommendations for follow-up antibody testing to ensure that protective levels are attained were recently withdrawn. Mild systemic or local adverse reactions are seen in about 25% of recipients.

Passive Immunotherapy
Rabies immune globulin (RIG) is made from serum harvested from human volunteers hyperimmunized against rabies. It provides immediate passive antibody protection while the patient is responding to simultaneous active immunization. Animal studies and retrospective analysis of humans treated by various regimens after known rabies exposure have consistently demonstrated a better outcome when simultaneous active and passive immunization is used. Therefore, all patients with possible rabies exposure should promptly be given RIG along with HDCRV vaccination. Rabies immune globulin should be administered in a dosage of 20 IU/kg. If possible, half should be injected into the wound site, on the assumption that passive antibody will coat the virus particles, with subsequent immobilization and killing of the virus. The remainder of the RIG is given by deep intramuscular injection. Adverse reactions are uncommon, other than pain at the injection site and low-grade fever. The cost for combined RIG and HDCRV treatment alone, exclusive of emergency room or office charge, is about $500.

Treatment should, of course, be discontinued if the biting animal is proved nonrabid, either by confinement and observation or by pathologic examination of brain tissue by fluorescent antibody techniques. The older duck embryo vaccine and horse antirabies serum are less effective and more toxic than HDCRV and RIG; they should be used only when HDCRV and RIG are unavailable within a few hours, and the new preparations should be substituted as soon as possible.

Prevention
Individuals with unusual risk of exposure to rabies—for example, veterinarians and zoo keepers—may be immunized prior to exposure. A series of three doses of HDCRV (0, 7, 28 days) produces excellent antibody levels and is presumed to be protective. Antibody levels do not ordinarily need to be measured after preventive immunization to verify protective antibody levels ($\geq 1:16$).

Rabies prevention United States. *Morbidity and Mortality Weekly Report* 33:393–402, 407, 1984.
   The latest recommendatons for pre- and postexposure prophylaxis are summarized in this report.

Hattwick MAW. Human rabies. *Public Health Rev* 3:229–273, 1974.
  An extensive historical and clinical review of human rabies.
Bahmanyar M, et al. Successful protection of humans exposed to rabies infection. *JAMA* 236:2751–2754, 1976.
  Iranian experience showing 100% successful treatment of 46 severely bitten patients.
Helmick, CG. The epidemiology of human rabies postexposure prophylaxis 1980–1981. *JAMA* 250:1990–1996, 1983.
  Postexposure prophylaxis is overprescribed; state or local health departments should be first consulted before immunotherapy is used.
Anderson LJ, et al. Clinical experience with a human diploid cell rabies vaccine. *JAMA* 244:781–784, 1980.
  Experiences with pre-exposure and postexposure use of HDCRV in 294 persons that show efficacy and low toxicity.

VII. ALLERGIC CONDITIONS

Rebecca A. Silliman

Urticaria (hives) is an eruption of transient erythematous papules or wheals resulting from dilatation of small capillaries within the dermis and extravasation of fluid into the interstitium. The lesions are pruritic and worsened by scratching. Angioedema is a related condition in which the lesions are nonpruritic and involve deeper tissues, sometimes resulting in asymmetric swelling of a body region.

About 20% of the population experiences urticaria and/or angioedema at some time during life. Severity ranges from a single fleeting episode to a chronic recurring problem. There is overlap between the syndromes of acute and chronic urticaria, and the duration of the acute illness is variably defined between 6 weeks and 6 months depending upon the source quoted. Urticaria and angioedema can occur together or separately, but since they are similar in treatment and prognosis, they are usually considered to be part of the same process.

Two syndromes can be confused with urticaria/angioedema but they have different mechanisms and clinical course. Hereditary angioneurotic edema is a rare entity characterized by recurrent episodes of angioedema, laryngeal edema, and colicky abdominal pain, frequently accompanied by a family history of sudden respiratory death. Urticarial vasculitis is an uncommon and incompletely understood syndrome with features of both urticaria and vasculitis, which should be considered in patients with atypical or chronic urticaria. It differs from urticaria in being nonpruritic, although it may cause a burning sensation. It usually persists for over 24 hours and may be associated with blisters, purpura, and pigmentary changes. Other features of immune complex disease may be present to a variable extent, including arthritis or arthralgias, hypocomplementemia, and glomerulonephritis.

Causes

Many different factors can cause urticaria or angioedema (Table 122-1). Hives are often due to an allergic reaction, but a variety of nonimmunologic factors can also induce them, including chemicals and drugs, bacteria, animal substances, physical agents, and stress. Cholinergic urticaria and dermatographism are common types of nonimmunologic urticaria. Cholinergic urticaria is triggered by emotion, heat, exercise, or temperature change and induced by acetylcholine. Dermatographism is an exaggerated response to cutaneous stimuli, in which hives result from relatively mild skin trauma such as scratching or pressure from tight clothing. With both immunologic and non-

Table 122-1. Causes of urticaria and angioedema

Cause	Examples
Drugs	Penicillin, morphine, aspirin
Foods	Nuts, berries, shellfish, chocolate, tomatoes, cheese
Infections	Streptococcus, coxsackievirus, *Candida*
Inhalants	Pollens, dust
Penetrants	Cosmetics, animal dander and saliva
Insect bites and stings	Fleas, mites
Internal disease	Rheumatic fever, lymphoma, hypothyroidism
Genetic abnormalities	Vibratory angioedema, familial cold urticaria, hereditary angioneurotic edema
Complement activation	Henoch-Schönlein purpura, systemic lupus erythematosus
Psychological factors	Stress
Physical agents	Cholinergic urticaria, cold urticaria, pressure urticaria

immunologic mechanisms, mast cells and basophils are stimulated, resulting in the release of a variety of mediators. Regardless of mechanism, reexposure may cause recurrence.

Urticaria usually appears within minutes of exposure to the offending agent, but its appearance may be delayed for more than 24 hours. Lesions should disappear within 24 hours of initial appearance; longer duration suggests another pathogenetic mechanism.

Urticaria is enhanced by heat, fever, exercise, emotional stress, alcohol, hyperthyroidism, and menstrual/menopausal status. It may be worsened by aspirin as well as by drugs that cause degranulation of mast cells (e.g., morphine, codeine, guanidine, reserpine).

Diagnostic Approach

Evaluation of the patient with urticaria is guided by the following principles: (1) a successful search for etiology is most likely in the acute syndrome, (2) a history and physical examination will provide the most valuable information in this search, (3) symptomatic treatment will be virtually the same in all cases, and (4) the identification of an etiologic agent or an underlying disease can aid therapy.

Although in more than 90% of cases the cause for urticaria is never found, the causative agents most likely to be identified are new drug and food exposures. Penicillin is the major drug offender, but almost any drug can be implicated. Aspirin can both cause and exacerbate urticaria, particularly the chronic type, and is included in many combination drugs. A careful drug history should include over-the-counter medications. Remember also that penicillin may be present in trace amounts in a wide variety of dairy products. Nuts, fish, berries, eggs, shellfish, chocolate, tomatoes, and cheese are frequent food product offenders, as are additives such as dyes or benzoic acid and naturally occuring salicylates.

Several features of the urticarial lesions themselves can suggest the etiology. One to three millimeter wheals, occasionally with satellite wheals and surrounding erythematous flares, are characteristics of cholinergic urticaria. Papular urticaria on the lower extremities of children frequently results from insect bites. Pruritic linear wheals suggest dermatographism. When the lesions are limited to exposed areas, light or cold may be to blame.

Often the etiology is not obvious from either historical data or the characteristics of the lesions. In an otherwise healthy patient, symptomatic therapy may be prescribed and the search need not be pursued. When urticaria persists or recurs, the less frequent causes should be considered. These causes may not be obvious; for instance, inapparent infections such as tinea pedis or asymptomatic vaginal trichomoniasis have been implicated. In addition, the drug and food history should be reviewed again, since these are still the most likely etiologic agents.

With chronic symptoms, a more aggressive evaluation of diet is justified. Patients should be instructed to write down all foods eaten during the 24 hours prior to each attack. While ingestion often results in the development of lesions within minutes, attacks can occur as late as 24 hours after ingestion of the offending agents; exposure more remote than 24 hours is unlikely to be related. When symptoms are frequent or continuous, a short-term trial of a rigid eliminaton diet is warranted.

Laboratory evaluation should be based on clues elicited from the history and physical findings. When no such clues are found, tests may be employed to screen for common asymptomatic disease and as an aid in reassuring the patient. These tests might include a complete blood count to identify anemia, eosinophilia, or white count abnormalities and a urinalysis to look for cells or proteins. Other tests should be ordered to follow up clues elicited from the history, physical examination, or screening laboratory tests (e.g., stool examination for ova and parasites or cryofibrinogen levels). However, without evidence of a particular agent, further testing, including skin testing, is not useful. If urticarial vasculitis is suspected, suspicious lesions should be biopsied.

In some patients, urticaria will recur for more than 6 months and persist for as long as 10 years. Because of the annoying symptoms and the frequency of inadequate response to therapy, the physician may be tempted to undertake further laboratory investigation. However, the search for cause in chronic urticaria is usually unsuccessful. A review of 236 patients at the Mayo Clinic found that the primary etiologic factor was either psychogenic (22%) or undetermined (70%) in 92% of patients.

Treatment
In those situations in which a specific etiologic agent is identified, avoidance is the most important intervention. Antihistamines and sympathomimetic drugs are the mainstay of therapy in both acute and chronic urticaria. Recurrences may be decreased by minimizing triggering or modifying factors such as psychological stress. Elimination of aspirin or aspirin-containing drugs may also help. Modulators of cutaneous vasodilation, such as alcohol, heat, or exertion, should be decreased when possible.

Sympathomimetic Drugs
Sympathomimetic drugs such as epinephrine and ephedrine are most useful in the treatment of acute or severe urticaria, particularly if it is associated with anaphylaxis. A recommended approach in acute urticaria is to administer 0.3 mg of epinephrine subcutaneously and an antihistamine orally. This initial treatment should be followed by a long-acting subcutaneous epinephrine preparation (Sus-Phrine) or oral preparation (ephedrine) and an antihistamine for the ensuing 24 to 48 hours.

Antihistamines
Antihistamines are believed to benefit about 80% of patients. A wide variety of agents is available, but the choice of drug must be made based on duration of action, side effects, and costs, since controlled trials comparing efficacy are few. Hydroxyzine (Atarax or Vistaril) in dosages of 10 to 25 mg four times a day may have a more powerful antipruritic effect and more prolonged inhibition of the wheal flare response than other antihistamines. It has been reported to be superior in the treatment of dermatographism and, like cyproheptadine (Periactin), is especially effective in cholinergic urticaria. Other antihistamines commonly used include chlorpheniramine, 4 mg four times a day, and diphenhydramine (Benadryl), 25 to 50 mg four times a day. When faced with side effects or no response, it is advisable to switch from one class of antihistamines to another.

Corticosteroids
Corticosteroids are rarely indicated but may be helpful to control severe attacks and in the therapy of serum sickness, pressure urticaria, and complement-mediated urticaria with vasculitis. There are no controlled trials to support the use of steroids, and it is generally believed that they have no place in the treatment of other types of acute and chronic urticaria.

Kelly JE. Urticaria and Angioedema. In R Patterson (Ed.), *Diseases: Diagnosis and Management*. Philadelphia: Lippincott, 1980. Pp. 395–408.
A recent review emphasizing the approach to the patient.
Monroe EW, Jones HE. Urticaria: An updated review. *Arch Dermatol* 113:80–90, 1977.
A more extensive discussion of mechanisms, diagnosis, and treatment.
Garmon WR. Urticarial vasculitis: Report of a case and review of the literature. *Arch Dermatol* 115:76–80, 1979.
Case report and an extensive literature review, which place this entity in the continuum of immune complex disease.
Green GR, Koelsche GA, Kierland RR. Etiology and pathogenesis of chronic urticaria. *Ann Allergy* 23:30–36, 1965.
A retrospective review from the Mayo Clinic, which found that in 92% of patients with chronic urticaria the primary etiologic factor was undetermined or psychologic.
Champion RH, et al. Urticaria and angioedema—a review of 544 patients. *Br J Dermatol* 81:588–597, 1969.
A retrospective review from England confirming the findings of the Mayo Clinic study. It found no association with atopy but incriminated aspirin in 21%.
Champion RH. Drug therapy of urticaria. *Br Med J* 4:730–732, 1973.
A succinct approach to drug therapy.
Guin JD. Treatment of urticaria. *Med Clin North Am* 66:831–849, 1982.
Reviews pathogenesis and patient evaluation as well as treatment.
Rhoades RB, et al. Suppression of histamine-induced pruritus by three antihistaminic drugs. *J Allergy Clin Immunol* 55:180–185, 1975.
A double-blind crossover study of diphenhydramine, cyproheptadine, and hydroxyzine. Hydroxyzine was superior in suppressing pruritus.

123. "BEE" STINGS
Rebecca A. Silliman

Stings by members of the *Hymenoptera* order (honeybees, yellow jackets, wasps, hornets, and fire ants, to be referred to as "bees" throughout this chapter) are common, but fatal reactions to these stings are not. Forty to fifty such deaths are reported annually, although experts believe that the actual number is greater. These deaths, which follow systemic reactions to stings, are characterized by urticaria and/or angioedema, respiratory distress from laryngeal edema or bronchospasm, or anaphylaxis with shock. Abdominal pain and/or nausea may also be experienced. While the majority of systemic reactions occur in children, most deaths are in adults and often have been attributed to underlying cardiovascular disease.

Bee venoms contain a wide variety of pharmacologically active peptides and amines. Although the various venoms are similar in composition, there is no antigenic cross-reactivity between honeybee and vespid (yellow jacket, hornet, wasp) venoms. Individuals sensitive to honeybees are often not sensitive to the vespids, and vice versa. Within the vespid group there does appear to be some antigenic cross-reactivity, but the role of this in clinical sensitivity is not well documented.

Local Reactions
Nonallergic local reactions are characterized by pain, itching, and swelling at the sting site. The typical appearance is a central red sting site surrounded by a clear wheal, which extends into a red flare. Edema formation is variable.

Therapy is symptomatic. If the stinger is still in the skin, it should be carefully flicked away with a fingernail or removed with tweezers. Local application of cold compresses and calamine lotion may be soothing. An aspirin tablet rubbed on a moistened sting site will also provide pain relief, which will persist with repeated moistening. Meat tenderizer, if placed on the sting site early, may also lessen pain and itching through enzymatic degradation of the venom. A mild topical corticosteroid cream (e.g., 1% hydrocortisone) and/or oral antihistamines (e.g., diphenhydramine, 25–50 mg qid) help relieve itching. Patients should be reassured that they are not at increased risk for developing the more serious systemic reactions.

Predicting Systemic Reactions
The natural history of systemic reactions is variable and unpredictable. Patients with a history of a systemic reaction, therefore, pose diagnostic and therapeutic problems. The history of a previous systemic reaction does not predict future reactions, nor does the absence of such a history mean that one is less likely to have anaphylaxis in the future. Laboratory testing can also be misleading. In one study of patients with a history of systemic reaction to sting, only 40% of those with positive tests to venom had a systemic reaction when subsequently stung. Likewise, immunoglobulin E (IgE) antibody determinations (RAST testing) are associated with both 20% false-positive and 20% false-negative rates. Experience with the combination of these two tests (skin testing and IgE measurements) has been limited, although anaphylaxis has been observed in skin test–positive and IgE-negative patients. In vitro determination of human leukocyte histamine release is even less helpful. The test requires sophisticated equipment, and cells from 15% of insect-allergic patients will fail to release histamine when challenged with anti-IgE.

Thus the clinician cannot predict accurately who is at risk for future systemic reactions, either by history or by laboratory tests. In general, however, children who have had a systemic reaction tend to experience progressively less severe reactions and lose their sensitivity altogether, while adults are more likely to retain their sensitivity.

Preventing Systemic Reactions
Since systemic reactions of any degree can be quite terrifying, patients need education about the probability of future episodes, preventive strategies, and treatment.

Avoiding Stings
Avoiding stings is an important preventive measure and can be accomplished without significant restricton of activities. Yellow jackets cause most accidental stings because

of their wide geographic distribution and because they build their nests in the ground. Wearing shoes helps protect against stings on the feet. Close-fitting clothing should be worn so that the insects cannot get to the skin. Dark-colored clothing attracts insects, but gray, white, or red materials do not. Also, shiny jewelry and scented perfume, soaps, and lotions should be avoided. Keeping garbage in containers with tight-fitting lids will deter bees. If a nest or hive is built in the vicinity of a patient's home, it should be removed, preferably by a professional exterminator. Lastly, an insect-sensitive person should drive with the car windows closed. If a bee becomes trapped in the car, the driver should stop and help the insect out using a cloth or handkerchief.

Treatment of Reactions
In addition to receiving these instructions, a sensitive person should be taught what to do if stung. The honeybee is the only member of the *Hymenoptera* order that leaves its stinger behind in the victim. A person stung by a honeybee should remove the stinger carefully because there still may be venom remaining in the venom sac. Squeezing the sac or leaving the stinger in place will force any residual venom into the skin.

Sting-sensitive patients (those who have experienced a systemic reaction) should receive a prescription for an emergency treatment kit (e.g., Ana-Kit, Hollister-Stier Laboratories). These kits contain a preloaded syringe of epinephrine and a chewable antihistamine. The kit insert should be carefully reviewed with patients to make sure that they understand how to administer the epinephrine. They also must recognize when the solution has become inactivated (it turns pink-brown) and needs replacement. Patients not on immunotherapy should be instructed to administer the epinephrine and seek immediate medical attention. Those on immunotherapy need not be seen by medical personnel unless the epinephrine fails to relive bronchospasm, laryngeal edema, or hypotension. This will allow for more intensive therapy, including fluid replacement, additional epinephrine, and bronchodilators as necessary.

Immunotherapy
While the prevention of stings and the treatment of reactions is straightforward, the prevention of systemic reactions in a sting-sensitive person is not. The first decision is whom to treat. A general, though perhaps controversial, recommendation is that any patient who has had generalized urticaria, angioedema, bronchospasm, or anaphylactic shock should be skin-tested and treated with the appropriate immunotherapy. Initial testing and immunotherapy should be performed by an allergist, although continued therapy can easily be supervised by a generalist in collaboration with an allergist.

Skin-testing should be performed at least 4 to 6 weeks after a sting to avoid false-negative results. The aim is to determine specifically which hymenoptera caused a reaction. Whole-body extracts became widely used in the 1950s, and their efficacy was reported to be 90 to 95%. However, these studies were neither well designed nor well controlled. The occurrence of treatment failures plus in vitro evidence of an immunologic response to venom but not to whole-body extract led investigators at Johns Hopkins to conduct a small controlled trial comparing venom to whole-body extract and placebo. Venom therapy was found to be superior to both placebo and whole-body extract. The study has been criticized and results questioned because of methodologic weaknesses. However, it provides the best evidence to date. The Food and Drug Administration approved the use of venom immunotherapy in 1979, and it is now considered the treatment of choice. The Johns Hopkins group reports a 98% protection rate for sting-sensitive adults. Patients should be treated with the venom of the insects to which they are sensitive. As noted previously, patients sensitive to honeybees are usually not sensitive to the vespids. Within the vespid group, there may be some cross-reactivity resulting in multiple positive skin tests. Only those patients with both positive skin tests and a history of systemic reactions to different vespids (e.g., hornet and yellow jacket) should receive more than a single venom. For example, sensitivity to both hornets (yellow and white-faced) and yellow jackets is known to occur, and a mixed venom preparation that contains these three is commercially available.

Different dosing regimens have been advocated, with varying incidences of both local and systemic reactions. These rates are comparable to those experienced in other forms of immunotherapy (e.g., ragweed hay fever). Because an average sting contains about 50 μg of proteinaceous material, 100 μg has been empirically chosen as a maintenance dose. This should fully protect patients against at least two stings. Whether a smaller maintenance dose is as effective is not known. A recent study compared three different dosing frequencies and found no difference in rates of either local or systemic reactions. However, since the immunologic response was greater and the number of injections fewer with the more rapid regimen, the authors recommend a program of seven bimonthly injections beginning with 15 μg divided into two doses separated by 30 minutes. Every 2 weeks the dose is doubled until maintenance (100 μg) has been reached. A more conservative approach begins with 0.01 μg and increases to 100 μg over 6 to 8 weeks with two to three injections per weekly visit. In either case, dose increases are adjusted in response to reactions. After the maintenance level has been attained, hyposensitivity is maintained by injections every 1 to 2 months.

The optimal duration of therapy is unknown. However, the risks of chronic therapy appear to be minimal, based on findings in a study of beekeepers and their families who have long-term and repeated exposure to honeybee venom. Therapy has been discontinued in patients whose IgE levels have become undetectable, with untoward effects observed from future stings. Further investigations, however, are clearly necessary.

Solar-Mills A. Allergy to Stinging Insects. In R Patterson (Ed.), *Allergic Diseases: Diagnosis and Management*. Philadelphia: Lippincott, 1980. Pp. 368–373.
An easily read general review of the subject with practical suggestions. The section on immunotherapy is outdated.

Lichtenstein LM, Valentine MD, Sobotka AK. Insect allergy: The state of the art. *J Allergy Clin Immunol* 164:5–12, 1979.
The best treatment of the subject to date.

Reisman RE. Stinging insect allergy. *J Allergy Clin Immunol* 64:3–4, 1979.
A companion article to Lichtenstein (above), which stresses areas where important information is still lacking.

Hunt KJ, et al. *N Engl J Med* 299:157–161, 1978.
The best controlled trial comparing whole-body extract with placebo and venom therapy. The authors conclude that venom therapy is superior.

Rubenstein HS. Bee-sting diseases: Who is at risk? What is the treatment? *Lancet* 1:496–499, 1982.
A critical appraisal of systemic reaction risk and the evidence of immunotherapy efficacy. Many questions are raised but no solutions offered. Rubenstein does not feel that immunotherapy is justified.

Yunginger JW, et al. Immunological and biochemical studies in beekeepers and their families. *J Allergy Clin Immunol* 61:93–101, 1978.
A report of two cross-sectional studies of beekeepers and their families. Compared to controls, both beekeepers and family members had higher IgE antibody levels. However, no clinically significant hematologic, renal function, or blood chemistry abnormalities were found.

XVIII. HEALTH MAINTENANCE

Suzanne W. Fletcher

The periodic health examination is a set of clinical tasks: taking a history, doing a physical examination, ordering laboratory tests, and performing simple preventive maneuvers such as counseling or immunizations. These tasks are undertaken to promote health and prevent disease or to find disease early so that it can be treated before adverse health effects occur.

Recommendations

Over the past several years, the periodic health examination has evolved from "the yearly physical," a general and untargeted checkup of presumably healthy patients, to very specific examinations designed to look for certain diseases, according to age and sex of patients. Three criteria are used for deciding whether a medical condition should be sought during a periodic health examination. In order of importance, they are (1) the treatability of the condition if it is found early, (2) the severity of the medical condition, and (3) the quality of the screening procedure (sensitivity, specificity, simplicity, cost, safety, and acceptability).

Figure 124-1 lists recommendations for the minimal set of maneuvers that should be included in periodic health examinations. There is not uniform agreement, even among "experts"; however, some of the lack of agreement is more apparent than real. The various groups used different approaches and different schedules of examinations. For instance, the American Cancer Society did not consider any examination for noncancerous conditions. Moreover, the groups sometimes differed not in whether but in how frequently some procedures should be performed (e.g., blood pressure determinations, breast examinations, Pap smears, and stool examination for occult blood). Differences also arose because the groups reported their recommendations over a period of several years. For some examinations, such as mammography, new information became available during the interval or was evaluated more carefully. Thus, mammography was not uniformly recommended in early reports, but the three groups making recommendations later all recommended mammography for some age groups.

The list of examinations outlined in Figure 124-1 is short; expert groups currently recommend fewer items than previously. For example, no group presently recommends routine chest x-rays. In the future, recommendations for the periodic health examination will change as new information is gathered and new treatments and procedures become available.

Implementation

Physicians who wish to incorporate periodic health examinations into their practices should keep in mind four problems.

First, it has been shown that practicing physicians frequently do not perform some examinations that experts recommend with a high degree of consensus, especially efforts to detect breast and colorectal cancers. Physicians performing periodic health examinations should therefore start with the items listed in Figure 124-1.

A second problem is that it is difficult to incorporate the performance of indicated examinations into care for established diseases. For example, physicians may not remember that a given patient being seen for congestive heart failure is also due for a breast examination, mammography, and stool guaiac test. Prompting systems can help. Many practices include in each patient's medical record a flow sheet similar to that in Figure 124-1; when the patient is checked in by the nurse, the flow sheet is consulted for any indicated procedures. As more practices incorporate computers into their settings, these may be used for prompting as well.

Third, physicians who screen their patients for unrecognized disease must understand that they will rarely find the disease. Even "common" diseases, such as breast cancer, are uncommon. A great many patients will be examined for each cancer found. Also, most of the abnormalities uncovered will not be due to the disease in question. For example, most stools found to be positive for occult blood are not signs of occult colorectal cancers.

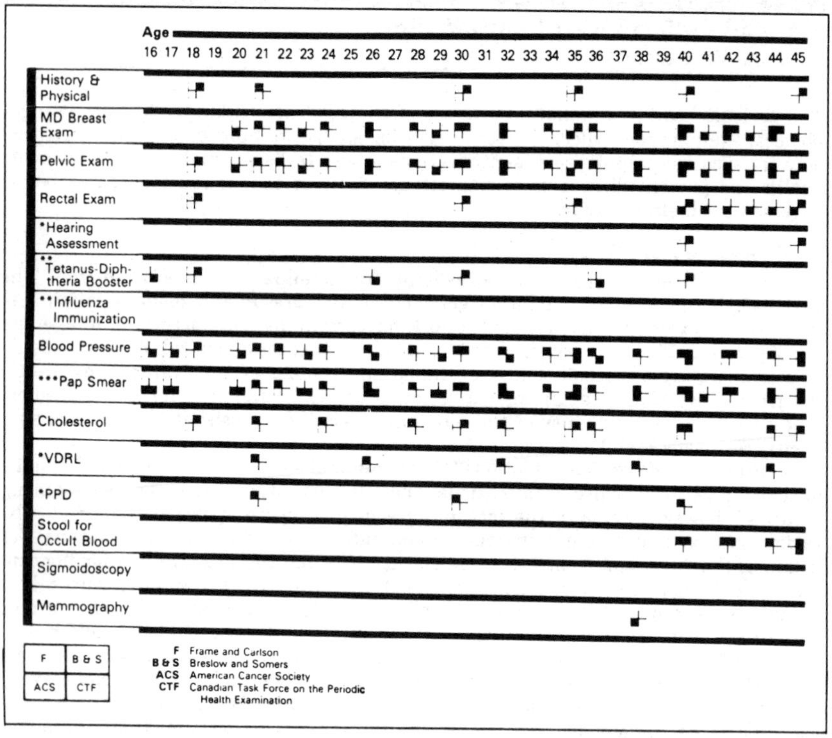

Fig. 124-1. Summary of periodic health examination recommendations by four major groups: Frame and Carlson, Breslow and Somers, the American Cancer Society, and the Canadian Task Force on the Periodic Health Examination. * = Canadian Task Force recommends that this be done on the basis of clinical judgement. ** = At first visit physician should check past immunization history per Centers for Disease Control recommendations for rubella, mumps, poliomyelitis, diphtheria/tetanus toxoids, pertussis. *** = If sexually active. A blackened square indicates that a group has considered the maneuver and recommended it. Squares left empty do not necessarily indicate that the group considered but did not recommend the maneuver. (From Periodic health examination: A guide for designing individualized preventive health care in the asymptomatic patient. Medical Practice Committee, American College of Physicians. *Ann Intern Med* 95:729–732, 1981.) Note: Since publication of this guide, the American Cancer Society has modified its recommendations for asymptomatic women age 40 to 49 years and suggests that mammography be performed on women in this age group every 1 to 2 years.

Finally, physicians should keep in mind that if enough tests are performed, on statistical grounds alone, an "abnormality" will be found in most patients. These "abnormalities" will be false-positive test results. The potential burden of financial, medical, and psychological costs among patients with false-positive tests results may be large. Physicians can guard against this potential problem by keeping the number of tests they perform to a minimum and by making sure that they search only for medical conditions meeting the three criteria outlined at the beginning of the chapter.

Frame PS, Carlson SJ. A critical review of periodic health screening using specific screening criteria. *J Fam Pract* 2:29–36, 123–129, 189–194, 283–289, 1975.
Breslow L, Somers AR. The lifetime health-monitoring program: A practical approach to preventive medicine. *N Engl J Med* 296:601–608, 1977.
Spitzer WO (chairman). Report of the Task Force on the Periodic Health Examination. *Can Med Assoc J* 121:1193–1254, 1979.

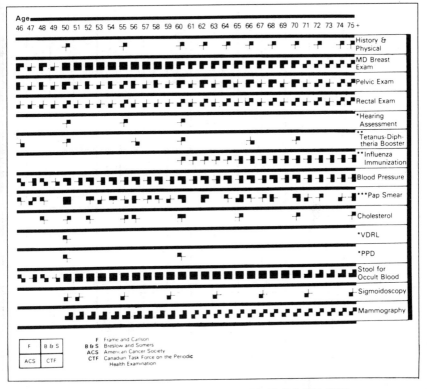

Age
46 47 48 49 50 51 52 53 54 55 56 57 58 59 60 61 62 63 64 65 66 67 68 69 70 71 72 73 74 75+

History & Physical
MD Breast Exam
Pelvic Exam
Rectal Exam
*Hearing Assessment
**Tetanus-Diphtheria Booster
**Influenza Immunization
Blood Pressure
***Pap Smear
Cholesterol
*VDRL
*PPD
Stool for Occult Blood
Sigmoidoscopy
Mammography

F	B & S		F	Frame and Carlson
			B & S	Breslow and Somers
			ACS	American Cancer Society
ACS	CTF		CTF	Canadian Task Force on the Periodic Health Examination

ACS report on the cancer-related health checkup. *CA* 30:194–240, 1980.

Preventive Services for the Well Population, Report of the Institute of Medicine, National Academy of Sciences, Healthy People (Appendices). Washington: U.S. Department of Health, Education, and Welfare, 1978. Pp. 1–22.

Mammography guidelines 1983: Background statement and update of cancer-related checkup guidelines for breast cancer detection in asymptomatic women age 40 to 49. American Cancer Society. *CA* 33:255, 1983.

Spitzer WO (chairman). The periodic health examination: 1984 update. Canadian Task Force on the Periodic Health Examination. *Can Med Assoc J* 130:1278–1285, 1984.
Recommendations of five expert groups on the content of periodic health examinations.

Romm FJ, Fletcher SW, Hulka BS. The periodic health examination: Comparison of recommendations and internists' performance. *South Med J* 74:265–271, 1981.

Wechsler H, et al. The physician's role in health promotion—a survey of primary care practitioners. *N Engl J Med* 308:97–100, 1983.
Two studies comparing recommendations for periodic health examinations to actual practices and beliefs of physicians.

125. PREMARITAL EXAMINATION

Mary L. Field

Requirements

Every state in the United States requires some form of medical examination and/or testing before granting a marriage license. Most states require specific information about venereal disease, such as certification that both partners are free from venereal

Table 125-1. 1982 Medical inquiry requirements for marriage license application

State	Certificate of freedom from VD	Exam for VD	Culture or serology for VD	Rubella immunity test	RH test	Sickle cell test	Mental competence
Alabama	+						
Alaska		+	+ (Serology)				
Arizona			+ (Serology)				
Arkansas		+ (Syphilis)	+ (Serology)				
California		+ (Syphilis)		+			
Colorado		+		+	+		
Connecticut	+	+ (Serology)					
Delaware	+		+ (Serology)				
D.C.	+		+ (Serology)				
Florida		+	+ (Serology)				
Georgia		+					
Hawaii	+						
Idaho				+			
Illinois	+					+|	

State							
Indiana	+					±	
Iowa	+						
Kansas	−	−		−	−	−	−
Kentucky	+	+	+				
Louisiana	+	+					
Maine	−	−		−	−	−	−
Maryland	−	−		−	−	−	−
Massachusetts	+	±					
Michigan	+	+ (Serology)					
Minnesota	−	−		−	−	−	−
Mississippi		+ (Serology)					
Maryland	−	−					
Montana	−	+ (Serology)		−			
Nebraska	+	+ (Serology)	+				
Nevada	−	−		−	−	−	−
New Hampshire	−	−		−	−	−	−
New Jersey		+ (Serology)					

Table 125-1. (continued)

State	Certificate of freedom from VD	Exam for VD	Culture or serology for VD	Rubella immunity test	RH test	Sickle cell test	Mental competence
New Mexico		+ (Serology)					
New York		+ (Serology & GC)				±	+
North Carolina[a]			+				+
North Dakota	+	+ (Serology)					
Ohio			+ (Serology)				
Oklahoma		+	+ (Serology)				
Oregon		−	−	−	−	−	−
Pennsylvania		+					
Rhode Island		+ (GC also)	+ (Serology)	+			
South Carolina		−	−	−	−	−	
South Dakota		+ (Syphilis)					
Tennessee		+					
Texas		+					

Utah[b]	+			
Vermont	+	+		
Virginia		+		
Washington		+ (No medical exam required)		
West Virginia	+			
Wisconsin	+	+		
Wyoming	+	+		

Source: Compiled from *Martindale, Hubble Law Directory,* Vol. VIII. Summit, N.J.: Martindale-Hubble, 1982.
±Test or advise at discretion of physician.
[a]Certificate states free of TB also.
[b]Counseling if divorced.

disease on the basis of examination and/or culture and serology. Fewer states require rubella immunity, Rh antibodies, sickle cell test, mental competence testing, and tuberculosis screening (Table 125-1).

Specific Tests

Syphilis

When serologic testing is not required by law, the examining physician must make a judgment about its value. Arguments in favor of serologic testing are that syphilis (early and late) can be detected, prevented, or treated; that congenital syphilis can be prevented; and that requiring the test motivates patients to seek treatment before the examination to avoid embarrassment.

Much of the criticism of requiring serology has centered on the cost-effectiveness of the practice. It has been shown that only 0.6% of cases of primary and secondary syphilis reported in 1978 were identified by premarital syphilis serologies and only 4% of serologic tests require further investigation. Also, in 1976, 46.3% of cases of infective syphilis occurred in homosexuals; by and large, these cases will not be detected by premarital examinations. Thus, serologic testing before issuing a marriage license would seem to do little to prevent congenital syphilis or the spread of disease.

Rubella

Testing for rubella immunity is required in six states. In one state, 14.4% of blood tests showed a titer of less than 10%. Of the women with low titers who were followed up (the minority) 41% had been immunized, 21% were pregnant, and 25% were sterile or using some method of contraception. In another study, when immunization was rec-

Table 125-2. Actions to be considered during a premarital examination

History
  Medical: emphasis on diseases that might preclude childbearing; cardiovascular, renal and chronic disease history; menstrual and reproductive history
  Family: emphasis on genetic diseases
  Psychosocial: history of relationship with future spouse; support systems, family of origin's composition and characteristics of client's relationship with family members; job/career experiences, goals, frustrations; coping mechanisms; leisure interests; major anxieties with particular regard to impending marriage, religion
Physical examination
  Dental assessment
  Blood pressure check
  Breast examination and patient instruction about self–breast examination
  Pelvic examination and Pap smear if not done within a year or on request, with assessment of need for hymenal dilatation; diaphragm or IUD fitting or referral for fitting if requested
Laboratory studies
  Gonorrhea culture if required or indicated by history or physical examination
  Observation for signs of primary or secondary syphilis
  Rubella immunity testing in females if required, desired, or indicated
  Urine dipstick for protein and sugar
Therapeutics
  Tetanus immunization if patient not immunized within the past 10 years
  Counseling and education
    1. Open, direct offer of information about sexual functioning and adjustment, lifestyle adjustment concerns and contraceptive measures
    2. Recommendations regarding early prenatal care
    3. Smoking, alcohol, and drug use counseling as indicated
    4. Diet and exercise recommendations
    5. Information about recommended periodic examination for cancer detection, hypertension, diabetes, and at risk conditions specific to the client
    6. Community resources for further information and assistance in all above areas

ommended, only 20 to 50% of women complied. Therefore, the decision to perform rubella immunity testing during the premarital examination should be individualized unless the test is required by law.

Recommendations
The premarital examination is an opportunity for health promotion and disease prevention, over and above that required by law. The examination usually occurs at the stage in life, between childhood and middle age, when many people do not use health services, yet are at risk for a variety of preventable diseases. Therefore, elements of the periodic health examination, as indicated for age and sex, should be performed (see Chap. 124). In addition, counseling can be done, based on individual patients' needs. Table 125-2 summarizes a variety of aspects of the examination that should be considered.

It is best not to assume that patients who do not ask questions lack interest. It has been shown that patients ask more questions about sex and contraception if physicians introduce the topic rather than leave it up to the patient to initiate the discussion. There is also evidence that people want more from a premarital examination than they ordinarily receive. In a study conducted in Michigan, 89% of women favored having a vaginal examination performed; only 35% actually received a physical and pelvic examination. A survey of North Carolina college students showed that only 25% understood the purposes of the premarital examination, but 93% wanted an extended examination—that is, pelvic examination, as well as sex and contraceptive counseling.

Farber ME, Finkelstein SN. A cost-benefit analysis of a mandatory premarital rubella-antibody screening program. *N Engl J Med* 300:856–859, 1979.
Studies the effect of mandatory rubella screening in Massachusetts.
Felman YM. Should premarital syphilis serologies continue to be mandated by law? *JAMA* 240:459–460, 1978.
Discusses the cost and effect of premarital syphilis screening and proposes that the mandatory serologies are of questionable value.
Judson FN, et al. Mandatory premarital rubella serologic testing in Colorado: A preliminary report. *JAMA* 229:1200–1202, 1974.
Presents the methods used and results of the enactment of a Colorado law requiring that each female marriage license applicant have a serologic test for rubella.
Kingon RJ, Wiesner PJ. Premarital syphilis screening: Weighing the benefits. *Am J Public Health* 71:160–162, 1981.
Martindale, Hubble Law Directory, vol. VIII. Summit, N.J.: Martindale-Hubble, 1982.
A directory of the laws of the states in concise summary form.
Nash EM, Louden LM. The premarital medical examination and the Carolina Population Center. *JAMA* 210:2365–2369, 1969.
Report of a study of NC college students' perceptions of and needs during the premarital exam.
Polonoff DB, Garland MJ. Oregon's premarital blood test: An unsuccessful attempt at repeal. *Hastings Cent Rep* 9:56, 1979.
Account of issues raised in the Oregon legislature regarding the repeal of the requirement of a syphilis serology and addition of a requirement for rubella testing.
Stahaman RF, Hiebert WJ. *Counseling in Marital and Sexual Problems.* Baltimore: Williams & Wilkins, 1977.
Trainer JB. Premarital counseling and examination. *J Marital Fam Ther* 5:61–78, 1979.
Comprehensive approach to premarital counseling and examination described with assessment tool included.
Trythall SW. The premarital law: History and survey of its effectiveness in Michigan. *JAMA* 187:900–903, 1964.
Reveals the inadequacy of premarital medical examination and actual fraud regarding serologies found in a study in Michigan. Makes case for the importance of the examination and laboratory studies.

126. ATHLETIC PHYSICALS
Desmond K. Runyan

Although much has been written about preparticipation athletic physicals, there is little agreement about the objectives, frequency, and content of the ideal examination. Current recommendations are not based on formal evaluation of the recommended diagnostic maneuvers but rather on clinical experience, surveys, or "expert opinion." This chapter will summarize those recommendations that have the strongest support and present a rational outline for the athletic physical.

Objectives
Most experts in sports medicine would limit the preparticipation examination to a search for problems of special concern to the athlete. Others point out that the athletic examination is frequently the only regular contact with the health care system for young adults and so advocate a more extensive evaluation of general health status and physical fitness. However, there is no evidence favoring the extensive examination. The limited, focused athletic physical offers protection while decreasing expenditure of time and money.

Format
The personal physician has the advantage of access to records, rapport with the patient, and often a more comfortable setting. Group examinations involving serial organ system examinations by different examiners have the advantages of special equipment and expertise, at relatively low cost. The relative advantages of these two approaches have not been studied. The personal physician's advantages may ultimately prove most important; athletic injuries are frequently re-injuries, and the history has proved most useful in identification of the injury-prone.

Single-file "lineup" examinations by a solo examiner provide inadequate conditions for physical diagnosis and patient privacy and have been soundly condemned by both the American Academy of Pediatrics and experts in sports medicine.

The frequency of examination is controversial. Traditionally, examinations are done yearly or even for every sports season, but this practice is inefficient and inappropriate. In healthy young athletes, the yield of disqualifying conditions on initial examination is low (0.3%–1.3%) and will be even lower on repeat examination. Since most unsuitable candidates are disqualified on the initial examination, a comprehensive first physical with subsequent evaluation limited to review of medical history will be adequate for the vast majority of athletes. Other examinations will be needed only to evaluate the rehabilitation status of acquired conditions.

History
The majority of disqualifications of athletes will be based on history alone. With a limited goal of identifying those conditions that proscribe athletic participation, a brief and focused history should include (1) general health status, (2) past injuries or hospitalizations, (3) drug and alcohol use, (4) limitations of function, and (5) cardiac, pulmonary, and musculoskeletal review of systems. There is little need for review of other systems or for family or social histories.

It has been suggested that athletes with the potential for sudden death may be identified in advance by asking about syncope during exercise and about a family history of sudden death, because sudden death in young athletes has been associated with hypertrophic cardiomyopathy, for which syncope is a well-described symptom. However, in a recent review of 29 athletes dying suddenly, most did not have evidence of risk on prior histories or physical examinations. Since the prevalence of syncope in the general population is unknown, the risk of sudden death for an individual with a history of syncope is not established but is likely to be very small.

Physical Examination
The yield from physical examination is small, reflecting the low prevalence of disqualifying conditions among young athletes. The majority of physical findings noted and referred for consultation in two recent reports were false positives. Since no patients

were disqualified because of physical findings alone, the researchers concluded that a routine physical examination was unnecessary for preparticipation screening assessment of athletes.

Cardiopulmonary Examination
Despite a paucity of data, it is reasonable to see that each athlete receives a cardiopulmonary examination early in his or her career. This should include blood pressure measurement, palpation of peripheral pulses, and auscultation of the heart. Several authorities recommend that each athlete be required to run and/or walk for 12 minutes and then be examined immediately afterward for evidence of hemodynamic abnormality or exercise-induced asthma.

Experience with large numbers of preparticipation physicals suggests that otoscopy, ophthalmoscopy, and the traditional hernia examination are neither important nor useful in the absence of a relevant history. These maneuvers may be safely deferred in the majority of athletic examinations.

Orthopedic Examination
The orthopedic examination is perhaps the most useful part of the physical. The objectives of the orthopedic athletic examination are (1) examination of the site of old injuries to determine whether there are residual deficits and (2) examinations of the knees and ankles for ligamentous laxity. Examination should be detailed for the knee and ankle, the joints at most risk, but it can also be tailored to include other joints involved in specific sports.

Evaluation of knee strength should be part of a routine examination. A study of West Point cadets in athletic competition suggested that the majority of leg and knee injuries are actually re-injuries. Cadets found to have a difference of as little as 10 pounds in strength between legs on extensive knee-strength testing were referred to a program to rehabilitate the weaker leg, and the subsequent rate of knee injuries fell precipitiously. Similar reductions of knee injuries among high school athletes have been described after general voluntary preconditioning programs.

Knee strength is most accurately determined using a weight-lifting apparatus. Measurement and comparison of the midthigh muscle bulk of each leg, along with clinical muscle strength testing, may prove a reasonable proxy for more elaborate measurement, but the diagnostic accuracy of this approach has not been established.

The relationship between flexibility or ligamentous laxity and sports injuries remains unclear. One study of professional football players showed an eight times higher risk of subsequent ruptured knee ligaments for players with flexible knees and ankles compared to "tight" players. However, a recent review of the evidence of high school players found no difference in injury rates between "loose" and "tight" players. Although there is no basis for disqualifying an athlete from competition because of joint flexibility, referral of exceptionally flexible athletes to physical therapy may prove a useful maneuver for prevention of injuries. Five simple flexibility tests have been described by Nicholas [1970]. They are the ability to

1. Place the palms flat on the floor while bent at the waist with the knees locked.
2. Supinate the hands so that the hypothenar eminence is higher than the thenar eminence with the arms held out in front of the body and elbows hyperextended.
3. Demonstrate more than 15 degrees of recurvatum or hyperextension of the knees when standing or bending over at the waist.
4. Externally rotate the legs so that the feet can be directed 180 degrees from each other with the heels still touching. (A practical measure of the "cutting" ability of the athlete.)
5. Sit in a classic "Lotus" position with the plantar surfaces of the feet opposed and the ankles and knees parallel to the floor.

Ability to perform one or more is normal; to perform all five is rare.

Genitalia
Examination of the genitalia of the peripubertal athlete has been reported to be useful in the reduction of injuries in school competition. Athletes who have not reached Tanner stage III (marked development of secondary sex characteristics) in pubertal development should be encouraged to participate in contact sports only with developmental peers or limit participation to noncontact sports.

Table 126-1. Summary of disqualifying conditions for sports participation

Condition	Absolutely	Temporarily[a]	Until risks acknowledged[b]
Acute infections (i.e., hepatitis, herpes)		S,C	
Absence of body part (eye, kidney, testicle)			C
Enlarged liver or spleen		C	
Acute cardiovascular disease			
Arrhythmias	S[c]		
Pulmonary hypertension	S		
Angina	S		
Myocarditis	S[d]		
Cyanosis	S		
Hypertension			S[e]
Syncope of exercise	S		
Diagnosis of IHSS	S		
Uncontrolled diabetes		S	
Uncontrolled epilepsy		C	
Physiologic immaturity			C
History of multiple concussions			C
Spinal abnormality	C		

[a]Until resolution of acute problem.
[b]The athlete and/or his parents may elect to participate after being informed of the risks.
[c]Goldberg B, et al. Pre-participation in sports assessment. *Pediatrics* 66:736–744, 1980.
[d]Strong W, Sted D. Cardiovascular function of the young athlete. *Pediatric Clin North Am* 29:1325–1329, 1982.
[e]Smilkstein G. Health evaluation of high school athletes *Physician Sports Med* 9(8):73–80, 1981.

C = contact sports; S = strenuous sports.

Source: D. Runyan. The preparticipation examination of the young athlete: Defining the essentials. *Clin Ped* 22:674–679, 1983.

Laboratory Testing

There is no evidence that routine testing of the blood or urine is of any benefit in the evaluation of athletes. In neither of the previously cited studies of athletic physicals (Linder et al, 1981, and Goldberg et al., 1980) were any potential athletes excluded because of an abnormal laboratory test. In the absence of a positive history, hemoglobin analysis is unlikely to reveal an anemia that will have an adverse impact on performance. Urinalysis is also unproductive. One study noted that 40 of 701 children had abnormal urine protein on screening, but none was found to have any urinary tract abnormality upon more extensive evaluation. Other screening tests are only indicated in populations where the prevalence of some disqualifying condition (e.g., tuberculosis) is sufficiently high to warrant screening in the absence of symptoms.

Disqualifying Conditions

Conditions calling for disqualification from sports participation are summarized in Table 126-1. Disqualification from nonstrenuous noncontact sports is rarely necessary, but disqualification from strenuous or contact sports may be necessary either during an acute illness or because of chronic disease.

Linder CW, et al. Pre-participation health screening of young athletes. *Am J Sports Med* 9:187–193, 1981.

A review of the findings of preparticipation screenings of 1268 children in public school.

Goldberg B, et al. Pre-participation sports assessment—an objective evaluation. *Pediatrics* 66:736–744, 1980.

The most analytic report of the athletic physical to date. A review of the findings among 701 children screened prior to athletic participation. It does not relate the positive findings to subsequent problems during participation.

Strong W. The uniqueness of the young athlete. *Am J Sports Med* 8:372–376, 1980.

A discussion of acute and chronic diseases that may influence athletic performance. The cardiovascular examination is elaborated in detail.

Maron BJ, et al. Sudden death in young athletes. *Circulation* 62:218–229, 1980.

A case-series of the history and pathologic examinations of 29 athletes (ages 13–30) who died in training or actual athletic competition. Twenty-eight of the 29 had structural cardiac abnormalities, although only 7 had heart disease suspected in life. Idiopathic hypertrophic subaortic stenosis was the most common abnormality.

Nicholas J. Injuries to knee ligaments. *JAMA* 212:2236–2239, 1970.

A prospective study of the relationship between "loose" and "tight" knee ligaments and the subsequent development of ruptured ligaments.

Abbott H, Kress J. Preconditioning in the prevention of knee injuries. *Arch Phys Med Rehabil,* July 1968, pp. 326–533.

A report of a conditioning program instituted at West Point Military Academy to reduce the frequency of knee injury.

Davies G, Larson R. Examining the knee. *Physician Sports Med* 6:51–67, 1978.

An encyclopedic summary of techniques for the knee examination.

Godshall R. The predictability of athletic injuries: An eight year study. *Sports Med,* Jan. 1975, pp. 50–54.

This report is anecdotal in style and analysis. The author's opinions are based on 2800 preparticipation physicals. He shares some data suggesting that gradual reduction in joint laxity is a normal developmental phenomenon.

Runyan D. The preparticipation examination of the young athlete: Defining the essentials. *Clin Ped* 22:674–679, 1983.

A summary article on the athletic physical and contraindications to participation in sports.

127. IMMUNIZATIONS
Philip D. Sloane

There are two forms of immunization, passive and active. Passive immunization consists of the use of antibody-containing serum or concentrates of serum. It is useful in postexposure prophylaxis of hepatitis and tetanus and in both postexposure prophylaxis and short-term prevention of hepatitis A. Active immunization, in contrast, consists of the induction of an individuals's own immunity by injecting all or part of the offending organism or of a similar, cross-reactive organism. Active immunization results in prolonged and often permanent immunity, whereas passive immunization provides only transient protection. Therefore, active immunization is preferable and is the principle behind all routine vaccinations.

A number of different substances can be used for active immunization. These include whole organisms killed by heat or chemicals, extracted cellular fractions, toxoids (toxins that have been inactivated), benign organisms offering cross-immunity, or live, attenuated organisms. The live organism vaccines induce a subclinical infection and thus are usually contraindicated in immunocompromised individuals.

Routine Immunizations
It is recommended that all children receive routine immunizations according to the schedule outlined in Table 127-1. Primary immunization for children not immunized in infancy is similar but can be shortened by giving three doses of diphtheria toxoid,

Table 127-1. Recommended immunization schedule for normal infants and children

Ages	Vaccines
2 months	DTP and TOPV
4 months	DTP and TOPV
6 months	DTP and TOPV
15 months	MMR
18 months	DTP and TOPV
5 years	DTP and TOPV
14–16 years (and every 10 years thereafter)	dT

DTP = diphtheria toxoid, tetanus toxoid, and pertussis vaccine; TOPV = trivalent oral poliomyelitis vaccine; MMR = measles, mumps, and rubella vaccine; dT = adult form of diphtheria and tetanus toxoid vaccine.

tetanus toxoid, and pertussis vaccine (DTP) or DT with trivalent oral poliomyelitis vaccine (TOPV) at 2-month intervals and then again 6 to 12 months later and giving measles, mumps, and rubella vaccine (MMR) 1 month after the first visit.

For adults who have not received any childhood immunizations, only one immunization is routine, the adult diphtheria-tetanus toxoid (dT), given as a primary series of four injections followed by boosters every 10 years. Measles and mumps immunization is recommended for many young adults and rubella for nonimmune women of childbearing age. Pertussis and poliomyelitis immunizations are not recommended in adults because both diseases are so rare in adults that vaccination is considered to be riskier than remaining unimmunized.

Details of the individual routine immunizations are discussed below.

Tetanus

Tetanus toxoid is probably the safest and most effective (nearly 100%) of the routine immunizations. Local reactions to tetanus are not uncommon, but generalized anaphylactic reactions are extremely rare. One recent study of 740 patients with a history of adverse reaction to tetanus did not uncover a single case of immediate hypersensitivity. Because more than half the cases of tetanus occur in adults over age 50, tetanus immunization status is particularly important in the elderly. Adults with no history of tetanus immunization should receive a dT and be instructed to return 2, 4, and 10 to 16 months later for boosters. If they have a wound that places them at risk for tetanus, they should begin active immunization and receive tetanus immune globulin as well.

Diphtheria

Diphtheria toxoid is over 90% effective in producing immunity. The injection comes in two forms, the childhood (D) and adult (d) preparations; the adult preparation contains approximately one-tenth that of a childhood dose to minimize febrile reactions. Primary immunization consists of four doses at the appropriate intervals (see Table 127-1). For adults who have not had a primary immunization, four injections of the adult immunization are done on the same schedule. Local and mild self-limited febrile reactions are common, but generalized reactions are rare.

Pertussis

Pertussis (whooping cough) vaccine is combined with diphtheria and tetanus vaccines in childhood formulations. It is not recommended for children over 6 years old because adverse reactions are more common in older children and adults and because pertussis is a milder disease in older people. The efficacy and safety of the vaccine are controversial. Full immunization does not guarantee permanent protection. The vaccine consists of a suspension of killed bacteria, a formulation that is notoriously less dependable than other vaccine types. Adverse reactions are unusual but more common than with diphtheria and tetanus immunizations. Rare but severe reactions include convulsions and a screaming phenomenon in infants. A convulsion after a DTP is a contraindication to further pertussis immunization.

Measles
Measles is the most severe of the "childhood" viral diseases; the case fatality rate is 1 per 1000 cases. Encephalitis, pneumonia, and otitis media are the most common complications. The vaccine is an attenuated, live-virus vaccine that produces a benign infection and provokes long-standing antibody protection. Because the virus is inactivated by maternal antibodies, the immunization should be deferred until 15 months of age unless there is a measles epidemic in the community. Measles vaccine is commonly combined with mumps and rubella vaccines. Its effectiveness is excellent. Vaccination failures usually result from inactivation of the vaccine by exposure to sunlight (for as briefly as 2 minutes) or from administration prior to 15 months of age. Adverse effects are rare. Encephalitis occurs approximately once per 1 million doses.

Measles is more severe in adults than children, with a higher rate of encephalitis. Therefore, susceptible adults should be considered for immunization. The problem is that there is no good method for identifying and vaccinating susceptible adults, and the revaccination of young adults has a relatively high incidence of fever, eye pain, and flu-like symptoms. Before the early 1950s epidemic, measles provided natural immunity, but adults born between approximately 1954 and 1963 who did not have the vaccine and have no history of measles, plus those who were vaccinated with the killed virus vaccine used from 1963 to 1967, are candidates.

Rubella
Rubella is a benign disease of children and adults. The main threat is teratogenesis in infants of women infected during pregnancy, particularly the first trimester. Therefore, the target population for immunization is women of childbearing age. A single dose of the attenuated, live-virus vaccine generally provides lifelong immunity. About 30% of adolescents are seronegative; therefore, serum antibody titers against rubella should be obtained on all adolescent and young adult women, and those who are seronegative should be vaccinated. An alternative approach, which is used in Great Britain, is to vaccinate all girls in early adolescence.

Because the vaccine contains a live virus, it is theoretically dangerous during the first trimester of pregnancy. Vaccination should therefore be avoided in pregnant women, and women who receive the vaccine should avoid pregnancy for 3 months. The subclinical vaccine-induced infection is not contagious, so the vaccine can be administered safely to infants of unimmunized pregnant women. Adverse effects, particularly of arthralgia and arthritis beginning 2 to 4 weeks after immunization, are rare in children but relatively common in adults.

Mumps
Childhood mumps is a benign disease that rarely causes complications. In adults, mortality is rare. However, orchitis occurs in 20% of postpubertal males; it rarely causes sterility but it is associated with considerable discomfort.

The main attraction of the vaccine, an attenuated, live virus, is that it can be combined with the measles and rubella vaccines at a single immunization. When individuals are vaccinated as children, data are incomplete on whether protection is lasting, but it appears that the current vaccination is effective into adulthood. Adverse reactions are uncommon and usually consist of mild fever and, rarely, parotitis.

The vaccine was licensed in 1967. Therefore, young adults have the lowest rate of immunity to mumps because many were not vaccinated as children yet failed to get the disease because epidemic mumps was limited by the vaccination of others. Serologic testing for immunity is unreliable, as is the mumps skin test; therefore, the Centers for Disease Control recommend vaccination of all adults born after 1957 who do not have a history of symptomatic mumps or of immunization.

Poliomyelitis
The trivalent oral polio vaccine (TOPV) is a live, attenuated poliovirus preparation containing all three polioviruses, types 1, 2, and 3. Vaccination results in serologic conversion in over 90% of recipients. It is advocated that a full series consist of four or five doses to increase the chance that immunity to all three strains will result. The vaccine causes a subclinical infection and has been known to cause paralytic poliomyelitis. In fact, currently more cases of polio in this country are caused by the oral polio vaccine than the wild virus strain, although the numbers are quite small (five cases in 1978). Vaccine-induced immunity fades with time, but polio is so rare in this country

that booster doses of the vaccine are not recommended for adults unless they travel to an area where polio is endemic.

Immunizations for Select Patient Groups

A wide variety of immunizations of varying quality are available for selected patients. The following discussion outlines some of the most commonly used vaccines.

Hepatitis
See Chapter 59 for discussion of gamma globulin and hepatitis B immune globulin.

Influenza
See Chapter 118.

Pneumococcal Vaccine
The pneumococcal vaccine consists of purified polysaccharide agents from 14 types of pneumococci representing the causative agents of 80% of bacteremic pneumococcal pneumonias. Adverse reactions consist of frequent local discomfort, with approximately 5% of vaccine recipients having mild fever for 1 or 2 days. Severe systemic reactions are rare (1 in 100,000) and self-limited. The vaccine is recommended for patients who are at increased risk of developing or dying from pneumococcal bacteremia and who possess the ability to respond immunologically to the vaccine. These include patients with asplenia (including those with sickle cell anemia), chronic lung disease, congestive heart failure, cirrhosis, diabetes, renal failure, and certain other chronic illnesses. Studies with broader population groups and with the elderly have thus far failed to show that the vaccine decreases morbidity and mortality from pneumococcal pneumonia. Therefore, wider use of the vaccine remains controversial, but many recommend its use in all elderly patients.

Meningococcal Vaccine
There are three vaccines licensed against meningococci. These contain purified bacterial capsular polysaccharide antigens from serogroup A, serogroup C, and a bivalent A-C. The vaccines should be used to control outbreaks of meningococcal disease.

BCG (Bacillus Calmette-Guérin) Vaccine
The BCG vaccine, an attenuated tuberculosis bacillus, is used to protect against tuberculosis, but its protective efficacy is low. Persons who receive BCG become permanently tuberculin skin test–positive even when not effectively protected against tuberculosis. Therefore, disease control in this country is better done by epidemiologic and chemotherapeutic methods. The vaccine should be considered, however, for tuberculin-negative persons who have repeated exposure to patients with sputum-positive pulmonary tuberculosis. In addition, it should be considered for certain communities with high rates and ineffective surveillance, such as some groups of migrant workers and vagrants.

Prophylaxis for International Travelers

International travel is common in today's society, and physicians are often consulted for information on immunization. Specific requirements and recommendations vary depending on the countries visited and even on which sections of certain countries. In addition, advice on immunoprophylaxis depends on the duration of stay and the activities while traveling. For example, a businessman on a short trip to a large city has a low risk of acquiring exotic illnesses and should receive only the required immunizations. In contrast, a botanist spending months in the bush in the same country will probably need much more extensive prophylaxis.

The Centers for Disease Control publishes annually an update of the requirements country by country and the United States' Public Health Service recommendations for international travelers. This publication is entitled *Health Information for International Travel* and is published as a supplement to the *Morbidity and Mortality Weekly Report*. The supplement is available in county health departments and can also be obtained from the Centers for Disease Control in Atlanta. The World Health Organization provides a standard yellow vaccination card that should be used for listing all immunizations that international travelers receive.

The following presents some recommendations for international travelers. In some cases, measures other than immunizations are more effective for prophylaxis and are included.

Traveler's Diarrhea

Traveler's diarrhea is usually a self-limited illness caused by enterotoxigenic *Escherichia coli* and occasionally by shigellae; doxycycline, 200 mg initially and then 100 mg daily for 3 weeks, appears most effective for prevention. Treatment is started when entering the endemic area.

Malaria

Malaria chemoprophylaxis may be the most important advice for travelers to third-world countries. Because the risk of malaria changes rapidly, local health departments should be consulted for current information on malaria risks. The type of prophylactic medication travelers should take depends on whether chloroquine-resistant *Plasmodium falciparum* has been reported in the areas to which they are traveling.

Travelers to areas without resistant *P. falciparum* should take 500 mg of cholorquine phosphate once weekly beginning 1 week before traveling and continuing 6 weeks after leaving the endemic area. To prevent an attack from *P. vivax* or *P. ovale* after leaving an endemic area, many experts additionally prescribe primaquine phosphate, one tablet containing 15 mg of base daily, during the last 2 weeks of chloroquine prophylaxis. (Primaquine can cause hemolysis in patients with glucose-6-phosphate dehydrogenase deficiency.) Patients visiting areas with resistant *P. falciparum* should take 25 mg of pyrimethamine plus 500 mg of sulfadoxine once a week in addition to chloroquine.

Hepatitis

A single injection of 2 ml of gamma globulin (immune serum globulin) is suggested for preexposure prophylaxis of travelers to high-risk areas for hepatitis A. Protection lasts up to 3 months.

Typhoid

Typhoid vaccine consists of killed bacteria and is not fully protective. It is recommended for travelers to high-risk areas (i.e., those with poor sanitation). Immunization consists of two doses of vaccine at least 4 weeks apart and then a booster every 3 years. Reactions commonly consist of 1 to 2 days of pain at the injection site, occasionally accompanied by fever, headache, and malaise.

Yellow Fever

Yellow fever vaccine, consisting of an attenuated, live virus, is required by certain countries and recommended for travelers to infected areas. The existence of yellow fever outbreaks is variable, and current information should be sought from the health department. The vaccine is given as a single 0.5-ml dose and is effective for 10 years. It is contraindicated in patients with egg allergy.

Smallpox

Smallpox vaccine is still required by a few countries. However, since the risk of vaccination outweighs the risk of disease in all individuals at this time, this vaccine should be no longer be given. World Health Organization international health regulations stipulate that a traveler need not be immunized if a physician verifies that vaccinating that individual is contraindicated on medical grounds. It is therefore recommended that physicians provide patients with a signed statement on letterhead stationery saying that the smallpox vaccination is contraindicated for health reasons, without being specific about those reasons.

Cholera

Cholera vaccination is generally not recommended for tourists because the risk of illness is low even for persons traveling to endemic areas and the vaccine itself is of limited effectiveness. Some countries require a single dose within 6 months of entry, so the vaccine is given primarily to protect travelers from border harassment when entering and leaving countries requiring cholera vaccination. A full immunization series consists of two doses given at least 1 week apart. Side effects are common (25%), usually consisting of a sore arm and a moderate febrile reaction.

Typhus
Typhus contact is unlikely in most travelers, and the vaccine is not generally recommended. The vaccine is no longer manufactured in the United States.

Health Information for International Travel, published periodically as a supplement of
  Morbidity and Mortality Weekly Report and available from the Superintendent of
  Documents, US Government Printing Office, Washington, DC 20402.
  The most authoritative information on international travel.
Mortimer EA. Immunization against infectious disease. *Science* 200:902–907, 1978.
  Reviews the types of immunizations commonly used in medical practice.
Shaw ED. Commentary on immunization. *Am J Dis Child* 134:130–132, 1980.
  Discusses controversial issues in immunization of children.
Centers for Disease Control. Mumps vaccine. *Ann Intern Med* 92:803–804, 1980.
  A review.

128. CARDIAC RISK FACTOR MODIFICATION
Mark A. Hlatky and Stephen B. Hulley

Coronary heart disease (CHD) is the leading cause of death in the United States today, as well as a major cause of suffering, disability, and expense. Some individuals are more likely to develop CHD than others; characteristics associated with an increased likelihood of subsequent CHD are known as risk factors. This chapter will focus on four aspects of risk for CHD: (1) What are the independent risk factors? (2) How strong is the relationship between the risk factor and disease? (3) Is an efficacious and feasible intervention available? (4) Does reduction in the risk factor reduce risk?

Risk factors for CHD most consistently observed in prospective studies include high blood pressure, cigarette smoking, serum total and high-density lipoprotein (HDL) cholesterol, obesity, glucose intolerance, type A behavior, and sedentary life-style. Each of these factors independently increases an individual's risk of CHD by two- to three-fold. Moreover, risk factors interact so that CHD risk may be over 10 times higher in individuals who have several risk factors than in those who have only one. In general, there is an increasing risk of CHD with increasing "dose" of risk factor, with no clearly apparent breakpoint or threshold.

Age, sex, and a family history of premature CHD are also important factors that predict CHD, but since the risk attributable to them cannot be modified, they will not be discussed further.

Effect of Risk Factor Reduction on CHD

Hypertension
A diastolic pressure of 90 mm Hg is conventionally used to diagnose mild hypertension. Patients with high levels on several visits should reduce salt intake and, if obese, lose weight. Drug treatment should be considered in those patients whose diastolic pressure remains above 95 after a few months of nonpharmacologic treatment, particularly in older patients and those with other risk factors. Randomized, controlled trials of treating patients with hypertension have demonstrated a substantial reduction in total mortality, due primarily to a lower incidence of stroke and other complications of hypertension. An effect on CHD has not been established (see Chap. 31).

The need to treat isolated systolic hypertension in the elderly remains uncertain. While there is no doubt that such individuals are at an increased risk of stroke and heart disease, they may also be at higher risk of drug-induced complications. Because it is not certain that the benefits of drug treatment exceed the risks in these individuals, a conservative approach limited to salt restriction and weight reduction seems prudent.

Smoking
The CHD risk associated with cigarette smoking rises steadily with increasing cigarette consumption and is not appreciably diminished by the use of filtered, as opposed to unfiltered, cigarettes. Pipe and cigar smokers who do not inhale do not appear to be at increased risk of CHD, although they are at higher risk for cancer of the oropharynx.

Several observations strongly suggest that cessation of cigarette smoking reduces the risk of CHD. In the Framingham Study, the CHD incidence, after adjusting for other risk factors, was more than 50% lower in persons who quit smoking as compared with those who continued to smoke. Similarly, another cohort study, which controlled for potential confounding by other CHD risk factors, found that the risk of CHD among those who had quit smoking for at least 1 year was similar to the risk of lifelong nonsmokers. The evidence regarding smoking and CHD, combined with the studies linking cigarette smoking with cancer and chronic lung disease, supports vigorous efforts at smoking cessation (see Chap. 130).

Total Cholesterol and HDL Cholesterol
The potential efficacy of interventions aimed at changing the levels of these lipids is discussed in Chapter 133.

Glucose Intolerance
Diabetes is a strong, independent risk factor for the development of CHD, but the efficacy of therapy on risk reduction is not known. Insulin injections and oral hypoglycemic agents reduce hyperglycemia, but neither eliminates the underlying metabolic disorder. While treatment of diabetes can control symptoms due to hyperglycemia and may forestall microvascular diabetic complications, its value for the prevention of CHD is not established.

Type A Behavior
The popular view that aggressive, competitive, chronically rushed individuals are more likely to die of heart disease has been confirmed by some epidemiologic studies but not by others. The efficacy of interventions to alter type A behavior remains to be established, and it is not known whether changes in behavior change CHD risk. While it seems reasonable to advise patients to reduce the stress in their lives, in order to be more comfortable if nothing else, more extensive interventions on "coronary-prone behavior" are of uncertain benefit.

Sedentary Life-Style
Many nonexperimental studies have demonstrated that vigorous, active people develop heart disease less often than sedentary individuals. There has been controversy about whether exercise is actually protective or whether people who choose to exercise are at lower risk for other reasons. The balance of current evidence favors protection (see Chapter 129). Experimental studies of exercise in CHD prevention have been inconclusive, chiefly due to the small numbers of individuals studied and the unwillingness of many sedentary people to increase their habitual level of physical activity. Although the direct effect of exercise on CHD risk remains uncertain, its beneficial effects on other risk factors, such as serum HDL cholesterol, psychosocial stress, and obesity, are established. Thus, an exercise program is an important adjunct to CHD prevention.

Obesity
Obese individuals have a high incidence of CHD, even when other risk factors are taken into account. It also affects CHD risk by increasing other risk factors. Weight loss reduces blood pressure, improves glucose tolerance, increases HDL cholesterol, and lowers total (or low-density lipoprotein) cholesterol. Thus, interventions aimed at obesity are a valuable component of any CHD risk reduction program.

Practical Implications
With the exception of hypertension and hypercholesterolemia treatment, the interventions discussed have not been unequivocally shown by randomized clinical trials to be effective in preventing CHD. However, the evidence for quitting smoking, becoming physically fit, and avoiding obesity is persuasive. Moreover, the recent decline in heart

Table 128-1. Modifiable risk factors and their potential for CHD prevention

Risk factor	Treatment goal	Appropriate target for intervention	Comment
Cigarette smoking	Nonsmoker	Yes	Top priority
Hypertension	Diastolic BP < 90 mm Hg	Yes	Use of drugs for mild hypertension is controversial
Total cholesterol > 240 mg/dl	> 10% decrease	Yes	Diet probably also effective in reducing risk
Obesity	Ideal weight	Probably	Both direct and indirect effects
Sedentary life-style	Physical fitness	Probably	Direct, indirect effects likely
HDL-cholesterol	?	Rarely	Increased by exercise
Type A behavior	?		Risk factor status uncertain
Glucose intolerance	Good control	No	Evidence for CHD discouraging reduction

disease mortality, which may be related to improved control of risk factors, provides additional encouragement for preventive efforts. On this basis, the objectives in Table 128-1 are offered as guidelines for physicians and patients interested in taking steps to prevent CHD. On the other hand, it is undeniable that CHD does develop in individuals without risk factors, and that some individuals with multiple risk factors remain free of CHD. These facts should caution us from being judgmental or overly dogmatic in dealing with healthy asymptomatic individuals, for there is still much to learn about coronary disease and its prevention.

The first step in any intervention program is an assessment of modifiable risk factors, including the patient's smoking and exercise history, and measurements of weight, blood pressure, and serum cholesterol. After this assessment, the physician can discuss the overall risk of the patient's developing CHD, explore patient attitudes, and formulate specific, individualized recommendations. Since no single factor causes CHD, preventive measures should be based on an integrated approach to multiple risk factors. Intervention seems particularly likely to benefit younger individuals and those who have several risk factors, because the risk associated with any one factor is greater in the presence of other risk factors.

Many measures directed at CHD prevention can be initiated in the doctor's office; the treatment of hypertension and hypercholesterolemia are examples. Other measures, such as smoking cessation and dietary modification, may be aided by referral to special intervention programs.

Compliance with a preventive program is often difficult for asymptomatic patients, since the disease may not strike until many years in the future. The physician should transmit conviction of the value of the recommendations wholeheartedly and consider the life-style and family setting of the patient in developing advice. For some measures, such as smoking cessation, weight loss, and exercise, the immediate benefits in well-being, improved body image, and social interactions may prove more of a motivation than the potential long-term benefits in CHD prevention. Educational pamphlets, posters, and other materials (available from the American Heart Association and other organizations) can reemphasize the consequences of risk factors and outline specific skills helpful in achieving life-style changes.

Kannel WB. Some lessons in cardiovascular epidemiology from Framingham. *Am J Cardiol* 37:269–82, 1976.

A concise review of epidemiologic methods and results from the classic Framingham Study.

Stern MP. The recent decline in ischemic heart disease mortality. *Ann Intern Med* 91:630–640, 1979.

An overview of data concerning the decrease in CHD mortality, with a discussion of possible mechanisms.

Feigal D, Hulley SB. The treatment of hypertension. *West J Med* 141:515–517, 1984.

A review of the evidence.

Guidelines for the treatment of mild hypertension: Memorandum from a World Health Organization/International Society of Hypertension meeting. *Lancet* 1:457–458, 1983.

A concise, authoritative guide to mild hypertension.

O'Malley K, O'Brien E. Management of hypertension in the elderly. *N Engl J Med* 302:1397–1401, 1980.

A succinct review of the special considerations in the diagnosis and treatment of hypertension in persons age 65 and older.

Kannel WB. Update on the role of cigarette smoking in coronary artery disease. *Am Heart J* 101:319–328, 1981.

A recent review, including data from the Framingham Study on the effect of smoking cessation.

Friedman GD, et al. Mortality in cigarette smokers and quitters: Effect of baseline differences. *N Engl J Med* 302:1407–1410, 1981.

A cohort study that examines the effect of smoking cessation while controlling for many potential confounding factors.

University Group Diabetes Program. Effects of hypoglycemic agents on vascular complications in patients with adult-onset diabetes: VII. Mortality and selected nonfatal events with insulin treatment. *JAMA* 240:37–42, 1978.

A late report from this well-known study, which failed to demonstrate a beneficial effect of treatment on vascular complications. Earlier reports from this study on the adverse consequences of oral hypoglycemic drugs are cited.

Brand RJ, et al. Multivariate prediction of coronary heart disease in the Western Collaborative Group Study compared to the findings of the Framingham Study. *Circulation* 53:348–355, 1976.

A prospective study demonstrating the independent risk of type A behavior, which also provides confirmation of the quantitative risk estimates for CHD from the Framingham Study.

Froelicher V. Exercise and health. *Am J Med* 70:987–988, 1981.

A concise editorial review of the effects of exercise, particularly on the heart.

Simopoulos AP, Van Italie TB. Body weight, health, and longevity. *Ann Intern Med* 100:285–295, 1984.

An overview of the effect of obesity on health and the definition of desirable body weight.

129. EXERCISE
David S. Siscovick

Clinicians are frequently asked how exercise affects health. Unfortunately, answers are difficult to come by because studies of the potential benefits and risks of exercise appear contradictory.

Benefits
Potential benefits that have been attributed to exercise include (1) reduced risk of coronary heart disease (CHD) morbidity and mortality; (2) reduced levels of cardiovascular risk factors; (3) increased functional capacity, effort tolerance, or work capacity; and (4) improved sense of well-being including less anxiety and depression, better sleep, and better "quality of life."

Coronary Risk

Several studies have suggested that asymptomatic persons who do not engage in vigorous exercise have two to three times the risk of clinical CHD, (i.e., angina pectoris, myocardial infarction, sudden cardiac death) compared to vigorous persons. This relationship appears to be independent of other risk factors for CHD. Thus, lack of vigorous exercise is associated with an increase in CHD risk comparable to that for hypertension and cigarette smoking.

It has been suggested that persons with other risk factors, particularly people who are older, obese, or have a history of hypertension, might benefit the most from vigorous activity. Continued participation in vigorous exercise appears to be necessary to maintain the beneficial effect. However, it is not known whether persons who begin vigorous exercise late in life achieve the same benefit as those who have engaged in exercise throughout life. Because these observations have been based on nonexperimental studies, some consider the available evidence that supports the role of exercise in the prevention of clinical CHD to be inconclusive.

Cardiovascular Risk Factors

Exercise has been shown to increase high-density lipoprotein cholesterol, fibrinolysis, and insulin sensitivity and to decrease very-low-density and low-density lipoprotein cholesterol and premature ventricular contractions. Furthermore, associations apparently exist between vigorous exercise and control of hypertension, obesity, glucose intolerance (in maturity-onset diabetes mellitus), and hyperlipidemia. The efficacy of vigorous exercise in either the prevention or long-term treatment of these latter conditions is not established. However, it is generally acknowledged that exercise is favorably associated with factors related to cardiovascular risk.

Functional Capacity

Physiologic studies have repeatedly demonstrated that vigorous exercise increases functional capacity. However, there is disagreement about the time needed for an exercise program to change functional capacity, the magnitude of the increase in functional capacity achievable, and whether older persons differ in their responsiveness to such exercise. Exercise adequate to achieve fitness clearly increases physical work capacity or effort tolerance—a benefit that both patients and doctors consider clinically significant.

General Well-Being

Based on uncontrolled studies of volunteer participants in organized exercise programs, it has been suggested that exercise improves sleep and enhances a person's "sense of well-being." Additionally, exercise has been reported to increase brain endorphine levels. It is a common clinical impression that exercise decreases anxiety and depression; however, proper studies supporting the efficacy of exercise in either the prevention or treatment of anxiety or depression have not been reported. Despite the absence of controlled evidence, exercise appears to affect the mood of many patients favorably and has been commonly recommended for this purpose.

Risks

Because exercise has been shown to precipitate myocardial ischemia and potentially fatal arrhythmias in certain individuals, it is generally believed that there is an increased risk for coronary events (myocardial infarction, arrhythmias, and sudden death) during exercise. Studies that compare the incidence of acute events observed during or immediately after exercise with the incidence of these events during nonexercise periods support this assertion. Fortunately, acute coronary events occurring during or immediately after exercise are rare in clinically healthy people. In a recent study, the annual incidence of sudden death during jogging among asymptomatic men was estimated to be as high as 1 death per 4000 to 26,000 middle-aged joggers. The rate of death during jogging was seven times the estimated sudden death rate during more sedentary activities.

Pre-Exercise Evaluation

Medical evaluations before beginning vigorous exercise have been suggested to identify persons for whom exercise might be harmful. Several groups have arbitrarily recommended that all persons over 35 years of age and persons less than 35 years of age with either a history of cardiovascular disease or CHD risk factors should "see their physician" before increasing their physical activity. In part, this recommendation is based on the conventional wisdom that persons who are at increased risk for CHD are those for whom execise might be harmful and that unusual activity is particularly likely to be dangerous. Pre-exercise evaluations have also been recommended to identify persons with other cardiac (e.g., aortic stenosis, congestive heart failure, hypertrophic cardiomyopathy) and noncardiac (e.g., acute infections) contraindications to exercise.

A variety of diagnostic maneuvers have been recommended as part of a pre-exercise evaluation: history, physical examination, chest x-ray, electrocardiogram, exercise tolerance test, complete blood count, urinalysis, fasting blood sugar, creatinine, cholesterol, arterial blood gas, pulmonary function tests, echocardiogram, and Holter monitoring. Unfortunately, it is not known whether any of these maneuvers helps identify those otherwise healthy persons for whom exercise increases risk.

Routine exercise testing of all asymptomatic adults before exercise training does not appear to be justified given the low absolute risk of exercise-related death. The likelihood of CHD in an asymptomatic population is low (approximately 5%). As a result, most positive exercise tests in an asymptomatic population would be falsely positive, and a negative test would merely confirm the low likelihood of CHD. Also, it is not known if recommendations for exercise in the prevention of clinical CHD should differ for asymptomatic persons with positive exercise tests.

For asymptomatic patients presenting for a pre-exercise evaluation, maneuvers other than a careful history and physical examination should not be obtained initially. Those patients with possible cardiac symptoms or a history of heart disease should be more fully evaluated (including an exercise tolerance test) before initiating an exercise program. Many patients and physicians have come to expect that extensive pre-exercise testing be done. The yield from doing so is certainly small, and this practice is not justified by evidence of benefit, over and above reassurance.

Exercise Prescription

Guidelines for the quantity and quality of exercise required to develop and maintain "fitness" have been suggested by the American College of Sports Medicine. These recommendations were derived from studies of endurance training programs. Improvement in fitness, measured as maximum oxygen intake, was directly related to the frequency, intensity, and duration of activity. For healthy persons, the usual recommendation is for rhythmic aerobic activity involving large muscle groups—that is, activities like jogging, swimming, tennis, and cross-country skiing that require an intensity of 60 to 90% of maximum heart rate reserve. This amounts to a heart rate of approximately 130 to 135 beats per minute in a young person (50–80% of maximum oxygen intake), of 15 to 60 minutes' duration per occasion, 3 to 5 days per week.

In prescribing exercise, the initial level of fitness is an important consideration. Persons with low levels of fitness (e.g., older persons) can achieve a significant training effect with a sustained heart rate as low as 110 to 120 beats per minute. It is commonly recommended that persons check their pulse during exercise to ensure the proper exercise intensity. However, a rough guide to attaining the necessary intensity is the "perspiration test"; exercise that results in perspiration is usually associated with a pulse above 70% of maximum. Additionally, persons should feel pleasantly fatigued rather than exhausted at the end of a workout. For joggers, a useful guide is the "talk test"; jogging should be at a pace that allows the runner to carry on a conversation with a fellow runner.

When exercise above the minimum threshold of intensity is performed, fitness development is a function of the total kilocalorie energy expenditure in such activities. This training effect appears to be independent of the mode of dynamic exercise. While the minimum level of physical activity necessary to maintain fitness is unknown, there is physiologic evidence to suggest that exercise must be maintained on a "regular" basis to maintain the "training effect." If vigorous exercise is discontinued for several months, fitness levels appear to return to pretraining levels.

When initiating an exercise program, asymptomatic persons should be advised to gradually increase the intensity and duration of their activity over a 1- to 4-week period. If symptoms consistent with cardiovascular disease occur, patients should discontinue exercise and contact their physician. Non–weight-bearing activities, such as swimming as opposed to jogging, appear to be associated with fewer debilitating injuries (e.g., foot, leg, or knee injuries) in beginning exercisers. "Overuse" injuries are common and usually result from engaging in an excessive training load for too long without adequate rest. Performance of exercises of increasing intensity to "warm up" before engaging in endurance activity and of decreasing intensity to "cool down" after intense exercise is commonly recommended.

Morris JN, et al. Vigorous exercise in leisure-time: Protection against coronary heart disease. *Lancet* 2:1207–1210, 1980.
   First clinical episodes of coronary heart disease in 17,944 middle-aged male British civil servants prospectively followed for 8½ years are reported in relation to leisure-time physical activity status.
Paffenbarger RS, Wing AL, Hydge RT. Physical activity as an index of heart attack risk in college alumni. *Am J Epidemiol* 108:161–175, 1978.
   Follow-up study of 16,936 Harvard male alumni, aged 35 to 74 years, where risk of first attack was related inversely to energy expenditure in physical activity.
Paffenbarger RS, Hale WE. Work activity and coronary heart mortality. *N Engl J Med* 292:545–550, 1975.
   Follow-up study of 6351 San Francisco longshoremen where the intensity of physical activity, classified according to individual work experience, was related to coronary mortality.
Siscovick DS, et al. Physical activity and primary cardiac arrest. *JAMA* 248:3113–3117, 1982.
   This population-based, case-control study supports the hypothesis that vigorous leisure-time physical activity reduces the risk of primary cardiac arrest.
Cooper KH, et al. Physical fitness levels vs. selected coronary risk factors: A cross-sectional study. *JAMA* 236:116, 1976.
   Prevalence study of nearly 3000 men showing an inverse relationship between the level of physical fitness and selected risk factors.
Thompson PD, et al. Incidence of death during jogging in Rhode Island from 1975 through 1980. *JAMA* 247:2535–2538, 1982.
   This study estimates the incidence of death during jogging among men 30 to 64 years as one death per 396,000 man-hours of jogging.
American College of Sports Medicine. Position statement on recommended quality and quantity of exercise for developing and maintaining fitness in healthy adults. *Med Sci Sports* 10:vii–xi, 1978.
   Presents guidelines, rationale, and research background for current recommendations for exercise prescription in healthy adults.
Pedo DST (Ed.). Exercise—a prescription for health? *Br J Sports Med* 12:211–237, 1979.
   Proceedings of a conference held at the Royal Society of Medicine in 1978, which focused on the medical evidence for benefits and risks of exercise.

130. SMOKING CESSATION
Suzanne W. Fletcher

With 30 to 40% of adults smoking cigarettes, there is abundant evidence that cigarette smoking is associated with excessive mortality, morbidity, and disability, particularly from lung cancer and cardiopulmonary diseases. It is reasonable to inquire what part physicians can play to help patients stop smoking.

Although most physicians are aware that smoking is decreasing in the United States, they are probably not aware of the number of ex-smokers. Approximately one-third of men and women who habitually smoked at some time in their lives are no longer smoking. Cigarette smoking is clearly a habit that can be broken; less clear

ecause less work has been done on the question) is how to break the habit and how
ysicians can help.

Theoretically, physicians can help patients become ex-smokers in at least three
ays: (1) by counseling, (2) by prescribing medication, and (3) by referral to specific
rograms to help people stop smoking. This chapter will review what is known about
ch of these.

hysician Counseling Against Smoking

any doctors think that it is a waste of time to advise smokers to stop. However,
veral studies on the effect of such efforts suggest that physician intervention does
lp. In general, gains are proportional to the amount of effort made.

In one study in England, smoking patients were counseled by their general practi-
oner for 1 to 2 minutes during the course of a visit for other problems and given a
amphlet published by the government on how to stop smoking. They were also told
ey would be followed up. One month later, 7.5% of these patients reported they had
opped smoking, and 1 year later, 5.1% were still abstinent. This compared to 0.3% of
ntrol patients.

In another study of male civil servants at high risk for coronary artery disease, much
eater efforts were made, and correspondingly larger results were achieved. A physi-
an spent 15 minutes with each patient during a specially arranged appointment,
scussing the risks of smoking and emphasizing the benefits of giving up smoking.
ollow-up appointments, letters, and smoking record cards were also used. One year
ter, 51% of the men stated they were smoking no cigarettes at all, and 3 years later,
6% were still abstinent. In the control group of men who had received no counseling,
0% had given up cigarettes after a year, and 14% after 3 years.

Other studies, with pregnant patients in England and with patients of family prac-
tioners in Canada, also showed that physician efforts to get smoking patients to stop
ere effective.

All of these studies were randomized, controlled trials, but none of them included
ochemical measurements to confirm claimed abstinence from smoking. Overall, how-
ver, the evidence suggests that organized efforts by physicians in their own practices
sult in some of their patients giving up smoking.

edications

he only pharmacologic substance that has been shown to be effective in helping pa-
ents to stop smoking is nicotine chewing gum. It was recently released for use in the
nited States. Use of the gum appears to help people to stop smoking by decreasing
ithdrawal symptoms. In one randomized, controlled trial conducted in a smoking ces-
ation clinic, 47% of subjects given 2-mg nicotine gum were not smoking 1 year later,
mpared to 21% of subjects given placebo gum.

Nicotine gum comes in two strengths, 2 mg and 4 mg. Absorption of the nicotine
nds to be slow—30 minutes as opposed to 5 to 10 minutes for a cigarette. Suggested
structions include starting patients on the 2-mg gum and advising them to chew a
ece of gum whenever craving for a cigarette occurs (average 8 per day). For those
eeding more than 15 per day, the 4-mg gum should be used. Patients who are still
moking after a month should not continue using the gum. Abstainers should be en-
uraged to use the gum for 4 months, to prevent relapse, and then the dosage should
e slowly tapered.

The gum may reduce the tendency to gain weight when giving up smoking. It is less
ddictive than cigarette smoking, has lower levels of blood nicotine, and gives no pleas-
nt sensation on chewing it. On the negative side, it has an unpleasant, often irritating
ste and can cause nausea, stomachache, and dizziness.

Other pharmaceuticals, including tranquilizers and tobacco substitutes (e.g., lobeline
r Indian tobacco), have not been shown to be effective in helping patients stop smok-
g.

moking Cessation Manuals and Group Programs

ost ex-smokers have stopped smoking by themselves, without any formal instruction.
or patients who need help, Table 130-1 lists some of the kits, books, and group pro-
rams that are available.

Table 130-1. Nationally available smoking cessation aids

A. *Self-Help Manuals and Kits*
   1. The American Cancer Society's "I Quit Kit." (Includes hints, calendar, buttons, and phonograph record. Available free of charge from local chapters of ACS.)
   2. The American Lung Association's "Freedom from Smoking" manuals. (Two manuals that lead the smoker through behavior modification techniques to complete cessation by the sixteenth day. Maintenance is stressed. Achieved a 1-year success rate of 20%. A nominal contribution of approximately $5.00 is requested.)
   3. Pomerleau CS. *Break the Smoking Habit.* Champaign, Ill.: Research Press Company, 1977. (Eight-week program with gradual cigarette reduction and behavior modification techniques.)
   4. Danaker BC, Lichtenstein E. *Become an Ex-Smoker.* Englewood Cliffs, NJ: Prentice-Hall, 1978. (Stresses maintenance and behavior modification.)
   5. Ross WS. *You Quit Smoking in 14 Days.* New York: Berkley Medallion, 1976. (Gives 50 self-help methods.)
B. *National Nonprofit Clinics*
   1. The American Cancer Society's "Quit Smoking Clinic." (Weekly meetings of 20–25 people over 4–6 weeks. Approximately 25% 1-year success rate. The charge is nominal, $5–35.)
   2. The American Lung Association. (Weekly meetings of 20–50 people for 4–6 weeks. Smoker must quit "cold turkey" by third meeting. The charge is $25–35.)
   3. The Seventh-Day Adventist Five-Day Plan. (More than 14 million smokers have attended these programs. Consists of five daily lectures on fitness, diet, smoking, and health life-styles. One year abstinence rates reported at 14–38%. Nominal $10 charge is sometimes made for educational materials.)
   4. The American Health Foundation. (Four consecutive evenings of groups of 20–30 people. Uses relaxation techniques and aversion methods. An in-house study showed a 1-year success rate of 40%. In New York, the charge is $125.)
C. *Commercial Organizations*
   1. The Smokenders Program. (Eight-week program using positive reinforcement. So far attended by more than 300,000 people. One year abstinence rates of 20–40% reported by independent researchers. Charge ranges from $345–445.)
   2. Schick Centers for the Control of Smoking. (Uses aversion therapy—rapid puffing, shock treatment, smoke satiation. Sessions are on five consecutive days followed by five weekly instructions on how to remain a nonsmoker. One-year success rate among persons finishing the program and followed up was 77% in an in-house study. Charge is $675; the program is available only in the western United States.)

Self-help books and kits are reasonably inexpensive or, in some cases, free of charge. Reported 12-month success rates are 15 to 20% (most relapses occur within the first 12 months). Self-help programs usually use behavior modification techniques, exploring the smoker's motivation for smoking and discussing techniques for stopping, handling withdrawal symptoms, and maintaining abstinence.

Group programs are run by both nonprofit and commercial organizations. The programs of nonprofit groups are much cheaper, use group meetings, and tend to stress behavior modifications. One commercial program stresses aversion techniques and employs electric shock, rapid puffing, and smoke satiation.

In general, commercial programs claim higher success rates than those of nonprofit organizations. However, often the follow-up studies by these various groups are not performed comparably, so that results are difficult to interpret. Also, the types of smokers attending these groups differ in their motivation to give up smoking in the first place.

In addition to these nationally run programs, there are hundreds of locally available programs, many using similar techniques and others concentrating on methods such as hypnosis and acupuncture. Most have not been evaluated rigorously.

Laboratory Confirmation

Many patients (20–40%) who claim they have stopped smoking have not. Laboratory confirmation tests that can be ordered to confirm abstinence include thiocyanate and carbon monoxide blood levels. Physicians do not routinely employ these tests, but if the need arises, they are available.

Low Tar and Nicotine Cigarettes, Cigars, and Pipes

Many cigarette smokers try to avoid the health consequences of smoking by turning to low tar and nicotine cigarettes, cigars, or pipes.

A recent publication report of the Surgeon General reported the risk for lung cancer (thought to be related primarily to tar ingredients) among smokers of low tar and nicotine cigarettes to be approximately half the risk of those smoking regular cigarettes, but still much higher than that of nonsmokers. Evidence regarding the risk for coronary heart disease (thought to be related primarily to nicotine and carbon monoxide) is less clear. Some studies have shown a slight reduction in risk with cigarettes low in tar and nicotine, while others have shown no effect or even a worsening effect on the risk of coronary heart disease.

Cigarette smokers who switch to pipes or cigars benefit only if they inhale less smoke than formerly; studies have shown that ex-cigarette smokers tend to inhale much more smoke from cigars and pipes than people who never smoked cigarettes. There is also an increased risk of mouth and tongue cancer among cigar and pipe smokers. This risk, however, is minor compared to the risk of lung cancer from cigarette smoking.

Russell MAH, et al. Effect of general practitioners' advice against smoking. *Br Med J* 2:231–235, 1979.

Rose G, Hamilton PJS. A randomized controlled trial of the effect on middle-aged men of advice to stop smoking. *J Epidemiol Community Health* 32:275–281, 1978.

Donovan JW. Randomized controlled trial of anti-smoking advice in pregnancy. *Br J Prev Soc Med* 31:6–12, 1977.
Studies of the effect of physicians' advice to healthy persons to stop smoking. Although the patient populations in these three studies were different and the intervention programs varied, all of these randomized, controlled trials showed a positive effect of physicians' efforts.

Jarvis MJ, et al. Randomized controlled trial of nicotine chewing-gum. *Br Med J* 285:537–540, 1982.

Russell MAN et al. Effect of nicotine chewing-gum as an adjunct to general practitioners' advice against smoking. *Br Med J* 287:1782–1785, 1983.
Randomized, controlled trials to evaluate the effectiveness of the use of nicotine gum in helping patients to stop smoking. Biochemical validation of reported abstinence was used.

US Public Health Service. *The Health Consequences of Smoking: The Changing Cigarette.* DHHS Publ No (PHS) 81-50156. Washington, DC: US Dept Health and Human Services, Public Health Service, 1981.
A report of the Surgeon General.

Bass F. Invalidating Tobacco. In RB Taylor, JR Ureda, and JW Denham, *Health Promotion: Principles and Clinical Applications.* Norwalk, Conn.: Appleton-Century-Crofts, 1982.

Cummings SR. Kicking the habit: Benefits and methods of quitting cigarette smoking (Topics in Primary Care Medicine). *West J Med* 137:443–447, 1982.

Schwartz JL. Review and evaluation of methods of smoking cessation, 1969–77. *Public Health Rep* 94:558–564, 1979.

Pederson LL. Compliance with physician advice to quit smoking: A review of the literature. *Prev Med* 11:71–84, 1982.
The above four articles are general reviews of methods to stop smoking.

131. BREAST CANCER SCREENING
Suzanne W. Fletcher

Breast cancer occurs more commonly and kills more often than other nonskin cancer in women. One in eleven North American women will get this disease, almost always after the age of 40; approximately 20% of cases occur between ages 40 and 50, 30% between 50 and 60, and 40% over age 60. Once a woman gets the disease, her chances of survival are about the same as they were several decades ago; one-third of women with breast cancer will die within 5 years. Part of the reason for this high mortality is that presently less than 50% of breast cancers are found before they have metastasized to axillary lymph nodes.

Effectiveness of Screening
There is good evidence that breast cancer can be found and treated early enough to prevent one-third of the breast cancer deaths in women ages 50 to 59. Breast cancer is one disease where most physicians should increase their efforts in screening, especially in this age group of women. The strongest evidence for this position comes from a single study, done by the Health Insurance Plan of Greater New York (HIP). Beginning in 1964, approximately 62,000 women, ages 45 to 60, were randomly allocated either to a screening group, in which each woman was offered an annual physical examination and annual mammography for 4 years, or to a control group, in which women were not offered either but were simply followed. After 9 years, 91 women in the screening group had died of breast cancer, compared to 128 women in the control group, a 29% reduction in mortality. Most of the lives saved were among women who were in the 50- to 59-year age group when they got cancer (40 versus 67 deaths). There was no difference in mortality between the two groups in women under age 50 (17 deaths in both groups). There were too few women over age 60 to give a clear answer regarding the effectiveness of screening in this age group; after 9 years, there were 23% fewer deaths among women in the screening group (34 deaths compared to 44 deaths among women in the control group), but this difference did not reach statistical significance.

Case fatality rates differed markedly in the screening group according to how the breast cancers were found. Women whose breast cancers were detected only on mammography had a very low 7-year case fatality rate of 9%, while those in whom the cancers were detected only by physical examination had a rate of 20%. If the cancers were detected by both mammography and physical examination, the case fatality rate jumped to 41%. The very low case fatality rate for women whose breast cancers were found by mammography alone may mean that this screening technique was particularly good at picking up early cancers.

A more recent report, summarizing the 5-year results of the Breast Cancer Detection Demonstration Project (BCDDP), suggests that with modern technologic improvements mammography has become even more sensitive as a screening technique. The BCDDP began in 1973 and conducted over 1 million annual examinations, during which time 3557 breast cancers were detected at screening sessions. Forty-two percent (1481 of 3557) of the cancers were found only by mammography (with negative physical examinations), and these particular cancers accounted for over half of the tumors with the best prognosis—that is, cancers that were less than 1 cm in size and noninfiltrating.

Physical Examination and Mammography

Physical Examination
Physical examination can pick up over half the cancers found on screening, some of which will be missed by mammography. The most important components of the examination are adequate time and thoroughness, because to be of real help to the patient, the lesion should be found when it is less than 1 cm in size.

After careful inspection for visible lumps, contraction or discharge from the nipple, or orange-skin dimpling of the skin (all rather late signs of cancer), each breast should be palpated carefully. The palms of the middle three fingers should press the breast tissue flat against the chest wall with a gentle but firm circular motion. The entire area of the breast should be covered; this is usually done in enlarging concentric circles around the breast. The procedure should be done with the patient lying down. Often the breast can be made flatter by a pillow or blanket folded under the shoulder blade and with the patient's forearm positioned behind her head. The patient's axilla should then be examined for nodes. Finally, many authorities suggest repeating the breast examination with the patient sitting. However, if time is a problem (and it usually is in office practices), one careful examination is probably more valuable than two quick ones.

The classical picture of breast cancer on physical examination is a hard, not freely movable, irregular mass. Often, however, early breast cancers cannot be distinguished clinically from benign breast disease. In fact, when physicians in the HIP study categorized breast masses before biopsy according to their size, consistency, regularity, and mobility, many of the masses that proved to be cancer on biopsy had characteristics that suggested benign disease.

Mammography

Mammography picks up both single breast masses that physicians miss (usually < 1 cm in size) and areas of microcalcifications associated with cancer, sometimes without any clearly discernible mass. The major problems with mammography are the cost and the unknown risk of future breast cancer caused by radiation.

Although the actual cost of mammography has been reported to be as low as $25, most women receiving mammography will be charged $50 to $125, making mammography the most expensive routine screening test recommended. Many women will have to bear this expense themselves because third-party payers usually do not cover charges for screening tests.

Concern regarding risk of radiation-induced breast cancers has lessened now that newer mammographic techniques have decreased radiation exposure markedly. Currently, an examination can be made using approximately 100 millirads (one-tenth of earlier doses). The original concerns arose from studies showing increased risk of breast cancer among women treated with x-radiation for postpartum mastititis, women receiving multiple chest x-rays for follow-up of pulmonary tuberculosis, and Japanese women surviving atomic bomb irradiation. Although all these groups received more radiation than women receiving mammography, extrapolating from these cases, it has been estimated that for each rad of exposure to both breasts, radiation will cause between 3.5 and 7.5 breast cancers per million women after a latent period of 10 years. The risk appears to decrease with age.

Current Recommendations (Table 131-1)

Women Ages 40 to 49

Most of the controversy surrounding breast cancer screening concerns the routine use of mammography in women ages 40 to 49. Although these women are at risk for breast cancer, the HIP study did not show benefit of screening. This fact, plus the possible increased sensitivity to radiation exposure among younger women, led the organizers of the large BCDDP to abandon routine periodic mammography in this age group. Nevertheless, the American Cancer Society recently modified its recommendations regarding mammography and now suggests mammography every 1 to 2 years for women age 40 to 49.

One problem with screening for breast cancer in young women is the high false-positive rate when breast lumps are found because most lumps in this age group are due to benign breast disease. In the BCDDP, among women ages 40 to 44, over nine women underwent breast biopsy for every cancer found. The ratio dropped to less than 4:1 in women ages 55 to 59.

Most expert groups suggest routine physical examinations ages 40 to 49. It should be understood that the effectiveness of this procedure alone among such women has not been established.

Women Ages 50 to 59

Presently all major groups making recommendations for periodic health examinations suggest annual physical examinations and annual mammography for women in this age group (Table 131-1). While a great deal of controversy remains about screening for

Table 131-1. Recommendations for breast cancer screening

| Group | Type of test | | |
	Physical examination (by age)	Teach self-examination	Mammography (by age)
Breslow & Somers	q 5 yrs until 40 q 2½ yrs 40–50 q 1 yr over 50	Yes	Yearly over 50
Institute of Medicine	q 5 yrs until 40 q 2½ yrs over 40	Yes	Yearly over 50
Canadian Task Force	Yearly 50–59	No	Yearly 50–59
American Cancer Society	q 3 yrs for women 20–40 Yearly for women over 40	Yes	Once between 35–40; every 1 to 2 years for women 40–49; yearly over 50

breast cancer, it is important for clinicians not to lose sight of the consensus and solid evidence for screening in this age group.

Women Ages 60 and Older
These women are at greatest risk for breast cancer, and several groups recommend yearly physical examinations and mammography for them, despite the fact that no controlled study has shown clear benefit to screening women in this age group. Possible risk of radiation decreases in older women, both because of decreased susceptibility and because of the latency period.

High-Risk Women
Women under 50 years of age are at high risk for breast cancer if they have a personal history of breast cancer or a mother or sister with a history of breast cancer. Women with first-degree relatives who had bilateral breast cancer before menopause appear to be at extraordinarily high risk for breast cancer (30–50% lifetime incidence), especially if the cancer occurred in both the mother and a sister. Some groups suggest that high-risk women receive both periodic physical examinations and mammography.

Many other possible risk factors for breast cancer have been studied, including history of fibrocystic disease, high socioeconomic status, late age at first birth, and late age of menopause—all having a positive (but small) correlation with increased incidence of breast cancer. It has not been established that women with any of these risk factors would benefit from aggressive searches for breast cancers before age 50.

A new approach to picking out women who are at high risk for breast cancer is to classify their mammographic parenchymal pattern. There is some evidence that women whose breasts are composed mainly of fat and with few fibrous tissue strands (Wolfe's classification N1) are at low risk of developing breast cancer. Those with increasingly prominent duct patterns (Wolfe's classifications P1 and P2) are at higher risk of breast cancer, while women with exceedingly dense parenchyma on mammography (DY) are at highest risk. Whether this approach will prove useful in defining a subgroup of women under age 50 who should receive a more aggressive screening program is not yet known.

Other Methods of Early Detection

Thermography
Because thermography measures breast surface temperatures and involves no radiation, it was hoped that this particular screening method would prove useful in breast cancer screening. However, both the sensitivity and specificity of this method are too poor for clinical use. In one study, when experienced readers read thermograms of patients known to have cancer, only 24% of the cases were identified, and among patients without cancer, 44% were falsely identified as having a positive result. After reviewing the evidence regarding thermography, the organizers of the BCDDP discontinued using it as a routine screening procedure.

Breast Ultrasound Scanning
Another nonradiation examination technique is ultrasonic scanning of the breasts. Preliminary reports comparing the sensitivity and specificity of this technique with mammography in symptomatic patients are encouraging. The technique's usefulness in screening asymptomatic women for breast cancer has not yet been determined.

Breast Self-Examination
Teaching women to examine their own breasts has been recommended by many groups (see Table 131-1). Most recommendations are for monthly self-examinations. If the woman is still menstruating, self-examination is recommended each month following the menstrual period. Pamphlets instructing women in the procedure are available from many organizations, including the American Cancer Society and the National Cancer Institute.

Breast self-examination as a method of screening for breast cancer is appealing because it is noninvasive and entails no expense. Physicians who adopt this strategy, however, should be aware of several limitations. Even physicians often miss small masses. It has not yet been established how well women can be taught to find early breast cancer. Also, important psychological effects may occur when a woman is asked to search for cancer on herself every month.

Shapiro S. Periodic breast cancer screening in reducing mortality from breast cancer. *JAMA* 215:1777–1785, 1971.
Venet L, et al. Adequacies and inadequacies of breast examinations by physicians in mass screening. *Cancer* 28:1546–1551, 1971.
Shapiro S. Evidence on screening for breast cancer from a randomized trial. *Cancer* 39(Suppl):2772–2782, 1977.
Shapiro S. et al. Ten to fourteen-year effect of screening on breast cancer mortality. *J Natl Cancer Inst* 69:349–355, 1982.
Reports of the HIP study are presented in these four references.
Baker LH. Breast cancer detection demonstration project: Five-year summary report. *CA* 32:194–225, 1982.
Initial findings of the BCDDP are presented.
Summary report of the Working Groups to Review the National Cancer Institute–American Cancer Society Breast Cancer Detection Projects. *J Natl Cancer Inst* 62:647–709, 1972.
The group was formed to review the ongoing BCDDP. It suggested several mid-course changes, including more restrictive use of mammography and abandoning thermography.
Final reports of the National Cancer Institue Ad Hoc Working Groups on Mammography in Screening for Breast Cancer and a summary report of their joint findings and recommendations. *J Natl Cancer Inst* 59:468–531, 1977.
These groups were formed to evaluate the benefits and risks of mammography. Excellent summaries of the evidence on mammography.
Wolfe JN. Risk of breast cancer development determined by mammographic parenchymal patterns. *Cancer* 35:2486–2492, 1976.
Retrospective study suggesting correlation between breast parenchymal patterns and risk of breast cancer.

Moskowitz M, et al. Lack of efficacy of thermography as a screening tool for minimal and stage I breast cancer. *N Engl J Med* 295:249–252, 1976.
Demonstrates poor sensitivity and specificity of thermography.

Cole-Beuglet C, et al. Ultrasound mammography: A comparison with radiographic mammography. *Radiology* 139:693–698, 1981.
Among 709 symptomatic women, sensitivity for ultrasound in detecting breast cancer was 69% compared to 74% for mammography.

Cole P, Austin H. Breast self-examination: An adjuvant to early cancer detection. *Am J Public Health* 71:572–574, 1981.
Good review of breast self-examination.

Breslow L, Somers AR. The lifetime health-monitoring progam: A practical approach to preventive medicine. *N Engl J Med* 296:601–608, 1977.

Preventive Services for the Well Population, Report of the Institute of Medicine, National Academy of Sciences. *Healthy People* (appendices). Washington, DC: US Department of Health, Education and Welfare, 1978. Pp. 1–22.

Spitzer WO (chairman). Report of the Task Force on the Periodic Health Examination. *Can Med Assoc J* 121:193–254, 1979.

American Cancer Society. ACS report on the cancer-related health checkups. *CA* 30:194–240, 1980.

American Cancer Society. Mammography guidelines 1983: Background statement and update of cancer-related checkup guidelines for breast cancer detection in asymptomatic women age 40–49. *CA* 33:255, 1983.
Five recent recommendations on periodic health examinations.

132. PROSTATE CANCER SCREENING

J. Pack Hindsley, Jr.

Cancer of the prostate is a disease of older men. The prevalence of this tumor dramatically increases from 9.3 per 100,000 at age 50 to 937 per 100,000 for those 85 and above; it is found in 20 to 40% of autopsy specimens in men in the eighth decade, although many of these tumors were not recognized in life. Only 1% of cases are in patients less than 50 years old. Other characteristics such as race, ethnicity, and socioeconomic status do not affect the incidence of prostate cancer.

Natural History

Cancer of the prostate is thought to occur peripherally, in the outer posterior portion of the gland, and to grow centrally; thus, it is usually readily detectable on rectal examination. Only one extensive study has been done, but this study supports the traditional clinical wisdom. Of 208 patients with prostatic cancer, 94 had peripheral tumor, 109 had both peripheral and central growth, and 1 had a lesion that was entirely central. Only one of the tumors may not have been detectable by rectal examination.

Most, but not all, prostatic cancers progress through orderly steps, from microscopic disease, to nodule, to local extension, to distant metastases. If confined to the prostate gland, prostatic cancer is a curable disease. With all modes of treatment, 5-year survival rates are much better for those with localized disease than those with metastases.

Patient Evaluation

Screening

Since cancer of the prostate is such a common condition and its prognosis is improved by early detection, screening would seem to be important in the management of prostatic cancer. Of all the screening tests, digital examination remains the most efficient and cost-effective. Many other tests, including radioimmunoassay, counterimmunoelectrophoresis, ultrasonography, and cytology have been tried in recent years, but none is better and all are more expensive. Moreover, digital examination has the added advantages of detecting other problems, such as infection or benign prostatic hypertrophy, and of providing stool for Hemoccult testing. Acid phosphatase is ineffective as a screening test because levels rise only after prostatic cancer has spread beyond the prostate.

Unfortunately, screening for prostatic cancer has not yet been studied to delineate the frequency with which a digital exaination of the prostate should be performed or whether mortality is reduced by a rigorous screening program. Data now available suggest that the majority of patients have advanced disease when discovered by an examination, but whether this reflects inadequate examinations or inadequate frequency of examinations is unknown. Because of the wide age-related difference in incidence of prostatic cancer, different screening programs might be designed for each decade of life. Nevertheless, it seems prudent to examine the prostate gland in men over age 50 no less frequently than once every year. The novel suggestion of teaching self-examination has appeared in the literature but has lain unexplored.

Clinical Characteristics
The hallmarks of prostate cancer on digital examinations are irregularity and induration. To differentiate between benign prostatic hypertrophy (BPH) and cancer, imagine a tight fist with the palmar surface to the examiner. The thenar eminence has a consistency similar to BPH, while the first knuckle of the thumb is similar to the induration of cancer.

Diagnosis
Once induration is detected, it must be assumed to be cancer of the prostate until proved otherwise. Several reports have shown that 50% of prostate nodules are cancer. Other conditions causing hard prostatic nodules include granulomatous prostatitis, prostatic infarct, calcific nodules (stones), and senile atrophy. The only reliable way of differentiating among these lesions is by biopsy. When a nodule or induration is discovered, the patient should be referred to a urologist for evaluation. Ordinarily, a needle biopsy is done, either through the rectum or perineum. The procedure can be done without admission to the hospital, but it is more difficult to prevent pain and to get a good specimen with local anesthesia. In the hospital, a brief general anesthesia can be given. Complications, primarily bleeding and prostatitis, are infrequent and usually not severe.

Silberg E. Cancer statistics. *CA* 31:13–28, 1981.
  American Cancer Society statistics.
Higginson J, Muir CS. Epidemiology in Holland. In JF Frei and E Frei, *Cancer Medicine.* Philadelphia: Lea & Febiger,1973. P. 283.
  Epidemiology of prostatic cancer.
Guinan P, et al. What is the best test to detect prostate cancer? *CA* 31:141–145, 1981.
  Cost analysis of various tests for cancer of the prostate.
Byar DP, Mostofi FK. Carcinoma of the prostate. *CA* 30:5–13, 1972.
  Report demonstrating peripheral (capsular) occurrence of prostatic cancer.

133. LIPIDS AND LIPOPROTEIN SCREENING
Bernard Lo and Stephen B. Hulley

Blood tests available for screening asymptomatic adults for abnormal lipid and lipoprotein levels include serum total cholesterol, its fractions, high-density lipoprotein (HDL) cholesterol and low-density lipoprotein (LDL) cholesterol, and triglycerides. Recommendations for screening are controversial; and some recommend that no screening be done, while others suggest measuring only total cholesterol. Complete lipoprotein profiling (as in the Frederickson classification for hyperlipidemia) is no longer recommended for typical outpatients. The occasional patient whose history (e.g., pancreatitis, strong family history of CHD), examination (e.g., xanthomas, xanthelasmas), or serum cholesterol (i.e., above 300 mg/dl) suggests an inherited metabolic disorder is evaluated and treated differently and is not discussed here.

In considering which screening tests to order, the physician should ask three questions: (1) Is the lipid or lipoprotein level a causal risk factor for coronary heart disease (CHD)? (2) Is there an effective and safe intervention to modify the risk factor and reduce the risk of CHD? (3) Will the test results influence the clinical decision to recommend the intervention?

Serum Cholesterol
Many rigorous prospective studies have shown that elevated serum cholesterol is an independent risk factor for CHD. Of the several possible explanations for the association between cholesterol and CHD, the most likely is that cholesterol is a cause of CHD. The risk of CHD for middle-aged men rises sharply only above 220–240 mg/dl. Thus, patients with cholesterol levels above the cut point of 240 mg/dl will probably reduce their risk of CHD by lowering their cholesterol, but the 60% of the population with levels below 220 mg/dl can expect little or no benefit. For women, a similar cut point exists, although the overall risk of CHD is lower. The risk attributable to a high serum cholesterol is greater when other risk factors are present.

Further reservations about lowering serum cholesterol in patients who already have low cholesterol levels are raised by the recent discovery that serum cholesterol is inversely associated with non-CHD mortality, especially cancer deaths. The magnitude of this association is about the same as that between cholesterol and CHD, so that total mortality is increased at both high and low serum cholesterol levels, relative to those in the mid-range. While there is as yet no evidence that low serum cholesterol is a cause of increased cancer, it seems prudent not to recommend lowering serum cholesterol to people whose levels are already low.

Intervention
Conclusive evidence that lowering serum cholesterol reduces the incidence of CHD has been provided by the Lipid Research Clinics Trial. In this randomized, double-blind study of asymptomatic middle-aged men whose total cholesterol was 265 mg/dl or greater, the intervention of cholestyramine and dietary changes reduced serum cholesterol by 8.5% compared to diet alone and, more important, reduced cardiac deaths and nonfatal myocardial infarctions by 19%. Total mortality was slightly but not significantly reduced.

Cholestyramine is the only drug that has been shown to reduce CHD incidence without serious adverse effects. In fact, clofibrate is associated with increased total mortality. Until further information becomes available, drugs other than cholestyramine should not be prescribed for asymptomatic patients, except possibly for patients with familial hypercholesterolemia and other metabolic disorders.

Fat- and calorie-controlled diets that avoid excessive use of polyunsaturated oils can reduce the serum cholesterol by about 10%. Methodological problems have precluded definitive clinical trials on the impact on CHD of dietary changes that lower cholesterol levels. However, given the judgment that elevated serum cholesterol is a cause of CHD and the evidence that lowering serum cholesterol with cholestyramine reduces CHD, such diets can be expected to reduce the incidence of CHD, provided they are begun sufficiently early in the process of atherogenesis. Moreover, the diet appears to be safe, except possibly in individuals whose serum cholesterol levels are already low.

The diet consists of avoiding foods very high in cholesterol and saturated fat (e.g., egg yolk, organ meats); substituting margarine for butter, vegetable oils for lard, and skim milk for whole milk; trimming fat from meat; and reducing meat and cheese consumption to 6 to 8 ounces a day. Obese people should lose weight. The reduction in serum cholesterol may result in a 30% reduction in CHD risk, which is about half the projected benefit of successful smoking cessation or hypertension treatment (see Chap. 128).

Patients with Established CHD
In patients with prior myocardial infarction and high serum cholesterol, the risk of subsequent CHD death is estimated to be only 1.4 times that in the low cholesterol group, whereas the relative risk is 2.3 in healthy men with high cholesterol levels. However, the absolute number of deaths attributed to elevated serum cholesterol (the

attributable risk) is higher in the men with prior myocardial infarction that in healthy men: 11 deaths versus 8 deaths per 1000 patients per year. This apparent paradox results from the much higher incidence of subsequent cardiac events after a first myocardial infarction. Hence, in theory, the reduction in risk from lowering serum cholesterol is greater for people who have had a heart attack. Similarly, elderly men through age 80 also have a smaller relative risk but a greater attributable risk from elevated serum cholesterol levels than younger patients have. However, for those with a previous myocardial infarction and for the elderly, the actual benefits of intervention are uncertain. Dietary interventions may need to be sustained for decades to have a beneficial effect.

The serum cholesterol level is useful in identifying which patients should be advised to adopt a fat-controlled diet. Substantial reduction in CHD risk is most likely in patients with levels above the cut point of 240 mg/dl, especially middle-aged men with other risk factors. We recommend that dietary measures be used first and reserve cholestyramine for those patients whose serum cholesterol cannot be reduced below 240 mg/dl with dietary interventions. If the serum cholesterol is below this cut point, the test need not be repeated for 5 to 10 years, since serum cholesterol levels do not change rapidly. As the likelihood or magnitude of benefit decreases, individual preferences become especially important. With women, older patients, and those with established CHD, screening and dietary modification is justifiable only to those who are eager to adopt preventive measures even though the benefit may be small or uncertain.

Serum HDL Cholesterol
High-density lipoprotein cholesterol may protect against CHD. Levels of HDL cholesterol are inversely associated with risk of CHD in several well-designed prospective studies. However, the interpretation of this association is still unclear: it is possible that both HDL cholesterol and CHD result from a confounding factor that was not measured.

Intervention
Increasing physical activity, losing weight, and quitting smoking may raise HDL cholesterol levels, but the effects are small and not convincingly established. Dietary interventions have not been shown to raise HDL cholesterol, with the exception of alcohol intake, which may affect a fraction of HDL cholesterol that is not related to atherogenesis.

Clinical Usefulness
Levels of HDL cholesterol usually do not influence clinical decisions. There are cogent reasons for recommending physical fitness, weight reduction, and smoking cessation, apart from the serum HDL cholesterol level. Conversely, there are reasons for *not* recommending increased alcohol intake, regardless of the HDL cholesterol level. Elevated HDL cholesterol levels occasionally influence dietary recommendations in patients with total cholesterol levels above 240 mg/dl. The total cholesterol level can be adjusted by subtracting the amount by which the HDL cholesterol exceeds the population mean (45 mg/dl for men and 55 mg/dl for women). For example, if a man has a total cholesterol of 260 mg/dl and HDL cholesterol of 80 mg/dl, the adjusted total cholesterol is [260 − (80 − 45)] or 225 mg/dl. The use of a ratio such as HDL to total cholesterol provides less information for clinical decisions than the two separate test results and is therefore discouraged.

LDL Cholesterol
Since LDL carries the chief atherogenic component of circulating cholesterol, it is potentially a more helpful test than total cholesterol. However, LDL cholesterol is highly correlated with total cholesterol and provides nearly equivalent prognostic information. Interventions that lower LDL cholesterol levels are the same as those that lower total cholesterol levels. Moreover, the tests for LDL are more difficult, less available, and more expensive than those for total cholesterol. Thus screening for LDL cholesterol is not recommended.

Triglyceride

High serum triglyceride levels are not an independent risk factor for CHD, and measurements of triglyceride do not influence treatment decisions, except perhaps in rare patients with specific metabolic disorders. In general, screening for elevated triglyceride levels cannot be recommended.

Practical Matters

All lipid measurements should be repeated at least once because of substantial within-individual variability, and the average of several determinations should be used for making clinical decisions. Fasting is not necessary for total or HDL cholesterol measurements. Plasma levels are 3% lower than serum levels. Some commercial laboratories yield values that differ systematically from research methods; it is wise to ask how the method compares with reference values and to use the same laboratory for serial measurements on a patient.

Hulley SB, et al. Epidemiology as a guide to clinical decisions: II. Dietary fat and CHD. *West J Med* 135:25–35, 1981.
  Review of evidence that dietary fat is a cause of CHD.
Feinleib M. On a possible inverse relationship between serum cholesterol and cancer mortality. *Am J Epidemiol* 114:5–10, 1981.
  Editorial on the association between low serum cholesterol and the incidence of cancer.
Connor WE, Connor SL. The dietary treatment of hyperlipidemia. *Med Clin North Am* 6:485–518, 1982.
  Comprehensive review, including practical suggestions.
Grundy SM, et al. Rationale of the diet-heart statement of the American Heart Association. *Circulation* 65:839A–854A, 1982.
  Policy statement by AHA that recommends a cholesterol-lowering diet for all Americans, with no screening for elevated cholesterol levels.
Oliver MF. Risks of correcting the risks of coronary disease and stroke with drugs. *N Engl J Med* 306:297–298, 1982.
  Brief discussion of the dangers of drug therapies to correct risk factors for CHD.
Eder HA, Gidez LI. The clinical significance of the plasma high density lipoproteins. *Med Clin North Am* 66:431–440, 1982.
  Review of HDL cholesterol and its inverse association with CHD.
Hulley SB, et al. Epidemiology as a guide to clinical decisions: The association between triglyceride and CHD. *N Engl J Med* 302:1383–1389, 1980.
  Argument that triglyceride is not an independent risk factor for CHD.
Hulley SB, Lo B. Choice and use of blood lipid tests: An epidemiologic perspective. *Arch Intern Med* 143:667–673, 1983.
  The material discussed in this chapter is presented here in greater detail.
Lipids Research Clinics Program. The lipid research clinics coronary primary prevention trial results: Reduction in incidence of coronary heart disease. *JAMA* 251:351–363, 1984.
  A randomized double-blind study showing that reducing serum cholesterol with cholestyramine significantly reduces cardiac deaths and nonfatal myocardial infarctions.

XIX. MISCELLANEOUS

134. SYNCOPE
Mac A. Greganti

Syncope is a sudden loss of consciousness that is transient and usually followed within minutes by full recovery. A feeling of detachment precedes the loss of consciousness; however, there is no true prodrome, and the patient can only describe the initial sensation in terms such as "fading" or "blacking out." Syncope usually occurs when the patient is upright, since the most frequent underlying pathophysiology—a fall in cerebral perfusion—is more likely to occur in that position. However, some causes, particularly less common ones, result in syncope in any position.

Usually, syncope is easily recognized, but at times it resembles other syndromes resulting in altered consciousness or dysequilibrium, including seizures, vertigo, and "dizziness" (see Chaps. 1 and 105). Hypoglycemia and hypoxemia cause altered mental status, but rarely so abruptly that they are confused with syncope.

The first task is to distinguish true syncope from other syndromes. Usually a history and physical examination will suffice. When difficulty is encountered, it is usually in separating syncope from seizures. Some observations that are helpful in making this distinction are listed in Table 134-1.

Of these characteristics listed, the presence or absence of postictal confusion discriminates best between the two. Occasionally, syncope is followed by transient tonic-clonic activity as a result of prolonged cerebral ischemia—for example, when a patient is prevented from falling to a horizontal position. Although this raises the question of central nervous system disease, primary neurologic abnormalities are not necessarily present.

The various causes of syncope can result in attacks of greater or lesser severity. At one end of the spectrum is "near-syncope," which presents as light-headedness, dizziness, or faintness that is not followed by loss of consciousness. These attacks are particularly difficult to distinguish from other syndromes resulting in altered consciousness. At the other end of the spectrum is permanent loss of consciousness (sudden death), particularly from cardiac disease, which has been referred to as "irreversible syncope." On occasion, classic syncope can be a harbinger of these more serious attacks.

Frequency
The frequency with which the various causes of syncope are encountered varies with clinical setting and patient age. In the community and in first-contact office practice, vasovagal syncope is by far the most common; many cases are not even brought to a physician's attention. In referral practices, and particularly with older patients, more serious causes are found with greater frequency. In one study of hospital practice, a definite cause of syncope was established, after extensive testing, in only 62 of 150

Table 134-1. Characteristics distinguishing syncope from seizures

Characteristic	Syncope	Seizure
Position	Usually standing	Standing or supine
Onset	Gradual—may be heralded by a "fading" sensation	Abrupt—no prodrome
Skin color	Pale	Normal
Tonic-clonic activity	Occasionally one or two clonic jerks	Frequent
Personal injury	Occasional	Frequent
Incontinence	Occasional	Frequent
Tongue biting	Occasional	Frequent
Postictal phase	Usually return to consciousness is prompt; no post-episode confusion	Return to consciousness is slow; post-episode confusion

patients (41%); cardiovascular causes were responsible for 56% of these. Regardless of frequency, relatively uncommon conditions (e.g., heart block) should always be considered because they are particularly dangerous and treatable.

Causes and Treatment

Since syncope is, by definition, self-limited, the physician is rarely called on to terminate an attack. Rather, the challenge is to find the underlying cause in order to predict future attacks, prevent them, and respond to the infrequent situations in which syncope is a manifestation of serious, life-threatening disease.

Vasodepressor (Vasovagal) Syncope

Vasodepressor (vasovagal) syncope is secondary to a transient decrease in cardiac output because of a combination of peripheral vasodilation and bradycardia. The diagnosis is totally dependent on an accurate history. The episodes typically occur in the setting of physical injury or the threat of physical injury, actual or symbolic, and only in the upright position. Premonitory symptoms include a feeling of warmth, light-headedness, and sweating. Associated physiologic changes include a temporary (1- to 2-minute) increase in heart rate, blood pressure, total systemic resistence, and cardiac output. This is followed by a reversal of these physiologic changes and increased vagal tone. The result is a pallid, unconscious patient who is hypotensive and bradycardic, but who rapidly recovers when placed in the supine position. A history of other episodes under similar circumstances is especially helpful in making the diagnosis.

Postural Hypotension

If reflex vasoconstriction is inadequate, a reduction in systemic blood pressure can occur on assuming the upright position. The classic history is that of a patient who faints on getting out of bed or up from a chair. Diagnosis is dependent on a careful history of the circumstances surrounding an attack and on the measurement of supine and standing blood pressure. Although there is no strict definition of what a clinically meaningful decrease in orthostatic blood pressure is, a drop of 10 to 20 mm in systolic and diastolic pressure increases the likelihood that orthostatic hypotension is the cause of syncope. Any decrease that is associated with symptoms is significant.

When the onset is recent, volume contraction is a common cause, particularly in the elderly. Protracted diarrhea, recurrent emesis, poor oral intake, and excessive use of diuretics are the common precipitating factors. When syncope is more chronic, autonomic nervous system dysfunction is usually the problem. This may result from aging, the sympathetic neuropathy of diabetes mellitus, adrenergic blocking drugs given for hypertension, or less common causes like amyloidosis. Prolonged bed rest predisposes to syncope by deconditioning autonomic reflexes.

Most postural hypotension can be treated by removing the underlying cause(s). When that is not possible (e.g., autonomic neuropathy), relief can often be obtained by having the patient rise more slowly. Alpha-adrenergic agents and 9-alpha fluorohydrocortisone (0.1 mg daily) have been used with success in individual cases.

Cough, Micturition

Syncope can occur during severe paroxysms of coughing. In such cases, a sudden drop in mean systemic blood pressure is probably related to the combination of the standing position plus a depletion of central blood volume secondary to splanchnic pooling. Micturition syncope is less well understood but probably represents the sudden loss of vascular tone related to the emptying of a full bladder in the standing position. Making either of these diagnoses is totally dependent on an accurate history.

Arrhythmia

A precipitous fall in cardiac output secondary to arrhythmia—either tachycardia or bradycardia—results in syncope. The patient may occasionally experience an "odd sensation," a "fluttering" or "jerking" in the chest, but there are often no symptoms referable to the heart. Abrupt loss of consciousness is followed by a similarly abrupt clearing. The routine electrocardiogram (ECG) rarely identifies the problem. Holter monitoring is more effective, particularly when attacks are frequent (and thus likely to be recorded) and in older patients (who are more likely to have arrhythmia as a cause of syncope). Whether the frequency of heart block or tachyarrhythmias is sufficient to support routine 24-hour monitoring in patients with fainting of uncertain etiology can be debated. If a specific abnormality occurs with the patient's symptoms, a specific therapy can be chosen (e.g., an antiarrhythmic agent or pacemaker insertion). In many patients who have chronic, recurrent syncope and who are suspected of having underlying cardiac disease, the syncopal episodes are so infrequent that monitoring is unlikely to be helpful. Cardiology consultation for more invasive diagnostic studies (e.g., intracardiac electrophysiologic techniques) should be considered in these situations.

Other Primary Cardiopulmonary Diseases
Careful cardiac auscultation may provide evidence for entities that commonly produce syncope, which include aortic stenosis, hypertrophic subaortic stenosis, mitral stenosis, mitral valve prolapse, pulmonary hypertension, and atrial myxoma.

Pulmonary Embolus
Massive pulmonary emboli may obstruct the main pulmonary artery and produce a severe drop in cardiac output with hypotension. Most patients with pulmonary emboli causing syncope do not live long enough to obtain medical care. On occasion, central obstruction of blood flow is transient because the clot dislodges and moves to peripheral pulmonary vessels. In such cases, patients present with normal blood pressure and a history of syncope, and pulmonary emboli are not considered unless the clinician maintains a high index of suspicion in any patient presenting with fainting.

Carotid Sinus Syndrome
A hypersensitive carotid sinus can cause transiently depressed cardiac output. Patients should be asked about the relationship of syncope to movement of the neck or to wearing a tight shirt collar. Unfortunately, these questions and physical examination are usually low in yield. This diagnosis should be considered after other cardiac-related problems have been excluded. The diagnostic test is carotid sinus massage during ECG and hemodynamic monitoring in a setting where resuscitative equipment is readily available. Two abnormal responses are observed: asystole with a significant drop in blood pressure (cardioinhibitory and vasodepressor responses) and a significant drop in blood pressure without a significant decrease in cardiac rate (vasodepressor). Treatment of the cardioinhibitory type requires pacemaker insertion.

Cerebrovascular Disease
Transient ischemic attacks resulting in hypoperfusion of the vertebrobasilar system may present with a sudden transient loss of postural muscle tone and consciousness. Often there are other symptoms related to structures in the posterior fossa, for example, visual, auditory, or vestibular symptoms. Ischemia secondary to arteriosclerotic disease of the carotid vessels usually does not produce loss of consciousness.

This diagnosis is suspected by history alone. The physical examination is often of little help, although the suspicion is supported by posterior cervical and infraclavicular bruits or a difference in arm blood pressure (vertebral steal syndrome). Definitive diagnosis depends on aortic arch and cerebral angiography.

Panic Attacks
Syncope can result from panic attacks, particularly if the attacks are accompanied by hyperventilation, which reduces cerebrovascular perfusion by lowering blood P_{CO_2} and, as a result, produces vasoconstriction. It is usually possible, on careful questioning, to elicit one or more of the following, which are characteristic of hyperventilation: stereotyped attacks, onset during times of interpersonal stress or crowding, symptoms of anxiety, heaviness in the chest, paresthesias (hands > perioral > feet), and, in extreme cases, carpopedal spasm and periods of apnea without cyanosis. Having the patient voluntarily hyperventilate during examination may produce the symptoms and provide support for this diagnosis.

Approach to Diagnosis
Successful diagnosis of the cause of syncope, and hence prevention of subsequent attacks, is primarily dependent on taking a methodical history and doing a focused physical examination. A limited number of laboratory tests can be done to substantiate or refute the initial clinical impression. Commonly utilized tests include electroencephalography and 24-hour Holter monitoring. Other tests such as carotid sinus massage,

cerebral angiography, echocardiography, and intracardiac electrophysiologic studies are utilized less often but are worth doing if their indications are considered carefully.

Noble RJ. The patient with syncope. *JAMA* 237:1372, 1977.
An in-depth discussion of differential diagnosis based on pathogenetic mechanisms.

Matthews WB. *Practical Neurology.* Oxford, Engl.: Blackwell, 1975. Chap. 3, pp. 30–47.
A review of the various causes of "blackouts" with a brief discussion of each.

Scherokman B, Massey EW. Evaluating loss of consciousness in the elderly. *J Am Geriatr Soc* 28:504, 1980.
Presents a helpful clinical approach to separating syncope from seizure.

Moss, AJ. Classifying and evaluating syncope. *Geriatrics* 33:103, 1978.
Presents a useful clinical approach to differentiating arrhythmic syncope from other types.

Luxon LM, et al. Controlled study of 24-hour ambulatory electrocardiographic monitoring in patients with transient neurological symptoms. *J Neurol Neurosurg Psychiatry* 43:37, 1980.
Presents data that support the value of 24-hour ECG monitoring as a diagnostic tool.

Dimarus JP, et al. Intracardiac electrophysiologic techniques in recurrent syncope of unknown cause. *Ann Intern Med* 95:542, 1981.
Presents data on 25 patients with recurrent, unexplained episodes of syncope. Full electrophysiologic evaluation with programmed stimulation was useful in diagnosis and therapy.

Thanes MD, Alpert TS, Dalen JE. Syncope in patients with pulmonary embolism. *JAMA* 238:2509, 1977.
Discusses the occurrence of syncope as an initial or predominant clinical feature of pulmonary embolism.

Walter PF, Crauley IS, Dorney ER. Carotid sinus hypersensitivity and syncope. *Am J Cardiol* 42:396, 1978.
An in-depth discussion of hypersensitive carotid sinus syndrome: pathogenesis, clinical presentation, and treatment.

Engel GL. Psychologic stress, vasodepressor (vasovagal) syncope, and sudden death. *Ann Intern Med* 89:403, 1978.
A detailed discussion of the psychosocial factors that predispose to vasodepressor syncope. The associated physiologic changes are correlated with the clinical syndrome.

Kapoor WN, et al. Prospective evaluation and follow-up of patients with syncope. *Clin Research* 30:301A, 1982.
Describes the causes, yield of diagnostic tests, and natural history of patients with syncope seen in office practice.

135. EDEMA
William F. Finn

The amount, composition, and distribution of fluid within the body are exquisitely controlled and under normal conditions remain relatively constant. An abnormal accumulation of fluid in the interstitial space is termed edema.

The hallmark of excessive interstitial fluid is transient pitting of the skin or subcutaneous tissue from the brief application of firm pressure. Nonpitting edema is the peculiar bogginess of the skin that occurs in myxedema and the increased thickness of the subcutaneous tissue that occurs as a result of fibrosis induced by chronic inflammation or venous stasis. The specific cause of edema may be suggested by its distribution. Localized edema suggests damage to tissue or mechanical problems; generalized edema suggests abnormalities in the systemic control of salt and water excretion due to heart, liver, or kidney disease.

Localized Edema
Common causes of localized edema include changes in the permeability of capillary walls, an increase in the protein concentration of the interstitial fluid, and/or an in-

crease in venous hydrostatic pressure. Depending on the specific abnormality, the edema may be unilateral or bilateral and, in either case, more prominent in areas below or above the diaphragm.

Loss of Vascular Integrity
Loss of vascular integrity occurs with urticaria and angioneurotic edema. Release of vasoactive substances (histamine, bradykinin, and other polypeptides) alter the permeability of the capillary wall, resulting in leakage of plasma proteins and fluid movement into the interstitial space. Electrothermal injury, excessive radiation, cold exposure, and severe ischemic injury also cause loss of vascular integrity.

Increase in Tissue Oncotic Pressure
Increase in tissue oncotic pressure may result from reduction in lymph flow, which leads to an increase in interstitial protein concentration. Causes include surgical or traumatic injury, radical mastectomy, radiation therapy, compression or infiltration of the lymphatics with malignant cells, recurrent inflammation (lymphangitis), and Milroy's disease, a form of inherited, congenital lymphedema. The edema associated with lymphatic obstruction often becomes nonpitting and firm because of secondary fibrotic changes in the skin and subcutaneous tissues.

Increase in Hydrostatic Pressure
Increase in hydrostatic pressure, generally due to an increase in venous resistance, favors the movement of fluid into the interstitial space. An increase in the systemic arterial blood pressure does not directly result in edema formation.

Edema above the diaphragm, particularly of the face, is often due to compression of the superior vena cava. The "superior vena cava syndrome" is commonly caused by metastatic carcinoma of the lung, less frequently by tumors or inflammatory lesions of the mediastinum, occasionally by aortic aneurysms or traumtic thrombosis, and rarely by endothoracic goiters, mitral stenosis, pericarditis, and mediastinal emphysema.

Unilateral edema of an upper extremity may be due to thrombosis of a subclavian vein, obstruction from neoplasms, or compression from enlarged lymph nodes.

Unilateral leg edema is most commonly the sequelae of old fractures, phlebitis, or surgery, which has resulted in abnormalities of the veins or lymphatics. Because these conditions are so common, fluid accumulation from systemic causes may also appear unilaterally. Thus, while unilateral leg edema is usually a result of local problems, cardiac, hepatic, or renal disease cannot be excluded on this basis alone.

Unilateral edema of a lower extremity also frequently results from incompetent valves in the superficial venous system (often accompanied by varicosities), venous thrombosis, or external compression from benign or malignant masses located in inguinal or intra-abdominal areas. A less common cause is tight-fitting clothing.

Bilateral edema below the level of the diaphragm may signify an increased resistance to flow in the right side of the heart or pulmonary vasculature or to obstruction of the inferior vena cava. Conditions such as pulmonary hypertension, pulmonic stenosis, tricuspid insufficiency, and constrictive pericarditis are associated with venous congestion and edema formation. The most common causes of bilateral, lower extremity edema, however, are diseases of the kidney, liver, or heart that result in generalized edema.

Generalized Edema

Except when complicated by hypoalbuminemia, generalized edema indicates an increase not only in the interstitial fluid but also in the sodium content of the extracellular compartment and signifies potentially serious renal, cardiac, or liver disease. In general, edema implies an increase in interstitial fluid of at least 3 liters. While this is usually associated with a proportional weight gain, the simultaneous loss of lean body mass may obscure the gradual retention of sodium and water.

Renal Disease
Edema develops as a result of both acute and chronic renal disease. Abnormalities of renal function are usually present, except in the nephrotic syndrome in which edema formation may precede changes in creatinine or urea clearance.

Liver Disease

Liver disease results in ascites when disorganization of the normal architecture of the liver leads to portal venous hypertension. Alone or in combination with other factors, impaired ability to synthesize albumin may result in generalized edema.

Cardiac and Pulmonary Disease

When the classic signs of congestive heart failure are present, the diagnosis is not difficult to establish. However, these abnormalities may be intermittent or associated with other causes of edema. Frequently overlooked is the coexistence of chronic obstructive pulmonary disease.

Nutritional Disease

Kwashiorkor results from a diet high in carbohydrates but insufficient in protein. This condition is frequently associated with hypoalbuminemia, which, along with other factors, results in edema formation. In marasmus due to a low intake of all nutrients, edema is uncommon. When "starvation edema" or "famine edema" occurs, it may be a consequence of the loss of elasticity in tissue structures and the tendency for the extracellular fluid volume to remain at prestarvation levels despite the loss of body weight.

Gastrointestinal Disease

Many diseases are associated with protein-losing enteropathy, including inflammatory diseases, disorders of the mucosal cells, and diseases associated with abnormalities of absorption. In these conditions, edema formation occurs because of an impaired ability to absorb amino acids and subsequent protein depletion and hypoproteinemia.

Other Causes

Idiopathic Edema

Idiopathic edema occurs most commonly in young women in the absence of hepatic, cardiac, or renal disease and without other demonstrable causes. The periodic or cyclical nature of the edema formation and the apparent relation to the menstrual cycle suggest a hormonal basis; however, its pathogenesis remains enigmatic. In overt cases, there is a substantial weight gain during the day, which may range from 1.5 to 2.5 kg. Pitting edema of the lower extremities may occur. The most distressing symptoms include a bloated feeling with abdominal distension, headaches, excessive thirst, and emotional liability. The weight gain occurs over several days or weeks and often remits with a spontaneous diuresis coincident with or soon after the onset of menses. Signs generally attributable to intravascular volume depletion (a rapid, thready pulse with a narrow pulse pressure along with an orthostatic drop in blood pressure and, in severe cases, syncope) may be present during the early phase of edema formation. In addition, evidence of hemoconcentration with an elevation of the hematocrit can be found in some patients. This constellation of signs and symptoms suggests that women with idiopathic cyclical edema alternate between periods of intravascular volume contraction and edema formation.

Orthostatic Sodium Retention

Some patients are thought to have an abnormal capillary leak of protein resulting in a reduction in blood volume, which is most pronounced in an upright posture. Characteristically, these patient may have no evidence of pitting edema in the morning, but by evening, because of the excessive salt and water retention, the edema is present. In some cases, elevated renin and aldosterone and a significant fall in plasma volume have been found after only 1 hour of standing. There is also a tendency in these patients to retain sodium and water when standing and to be unable to excrete a water load in a normal manner when first given a sodium load.

Diuretic and Laxative Abuse

Diuretic and laxative abuse may paradoxically result in edema formation. Prolonged use of either agent may lead to increased renin and aldosterone levels. When the diuretics are precipitously stopped, rapid salt retention occurs, which may last several days. Unfortunately, the response, particularly in people who are overly concerned with their weight and appearance, is to increase the dose and frequency of the diuretic.

It has been claimed that this is the most common cause of idiopathic cyclical edema. If diuretic or laxative abuse is suspected but denied by the patient, the urine can be tested for thiazides or phenolphthalein.

Carbohydrate Loading
Fasting is associated with natriuresis, and conversely, refeeding with antinatriuresis. Patients who alternate between periods of low and high carbohydrate and sodium intake are likely to notice periods of weight gain and even edema formation. Groups of people particularly prone to carbohydrate-induced edema formation include patients who fast during the week but binge on the weekends, travelers forced to alter eating patterns, and some patients with personality traits similar to those with anorexia nervosa. The feeling of bloatedness or the appearance of edema may lead to diuretic use and the possibility of diuretic-induced edema as well.

Heat Edema
Heat exposure is not ordinarily associated with weight gain, but occasionally a transient weight gain of up to 5 kg occurs over several days, accompanied by a decrease in urine volume, edema of the lower extremities, and a feeling of bloatedness. The urine tends to be concentrated with a high sodium content and the serum sodium is depressed, a series of events that resemble inappropriate antidiuretic hormone secretion. After several days, a spontaneous diuresis usually occurs. The frequency of the occurrence of heat edema is unknown, but it is likely to be more common than generally believed.

Altitude Edema
Life-threatening pulmonary and cerebral edema may develop singly or together during the first week of high-altitude exposure, when acute mountain sickness is most common. Peripheral edema also occurs at high altitudes but may occur in low-altitude hill walkers in the absence of the symptoms of acute mountain sickness. It is possible that the effects of altitude and exercise may be additive in producing the altitude edemas. The specific cause is unknown but may result from an increase in venous pressure.

Drugs
Pharmacologic agents other than diuretics can be the proximate cause of edema formation. Drugs that promote salt and water retention include potent vasodilators such as minoxidil, phenothiazine tranquilizers such as thioridazine (Mellaril) and chlorpromazine (Thorazine), and nonsteroidal anti-inflammatory agents.

Approach to Patients with Edema
The primary consideration in patients with edema is to look for systemic disease. This can usually be accomplished by asking about symptoms of cardiac, pulmonary, hepatic, renal, and gastrointestinal disorders and by a physical examination directed toward possible abnormalities of these organs. In patients with generalized edema, posteroanterior and lateral chest films are indicated to look for congestive heart failure. To look for renal disease, a careful analysis of a freshly voided urine specimen and determination of the serum creatinine or blood urea nitrogen (BUN) levels should be performed. Renal insufficiency may be present without striking abnormalities in the microscopic examination of the urine sediment, and conversely, proteinuria and the nephrotic syndrome may occur without a rise in serum creatinine or BUN levels. Liver function studies are useful because generalized edema may be an early manifestation of liver disease and portal hypertension. The serum albumin concentration should be measured when heavy proteinuria is found, when liver disease is suspected, or when protein-depletion malabsorption is suspected. If the patient has ascites, an abdominal paracentesis should be performed. The fluid should be characterized as a transudate or an exudate, examined for abnormal cells, bacteria, and fungi, and cultured for acid-fast bacilli.

If the chest films, urinalysis, serum creatinine and BUN levels, liver function studies, and serum albumin concentration are all normal and there is no evidence of severe pulmonary or gastrointestinal disease, the cause of the generalized edema formation may be assumed to be idiopathic or cyclical in nature, to be related to drug ingestion, or to be due to changes in climate, diet, or altitude or to one of several endocrinopathies. Further diagnostic efforts are warranted because these situations are not uncommon, are often the source of great anxiety, and may be alleviated by relatively simple changes. A detailed history should be taken about those events that are temporarily related to the onset of the edema; specifically, a chart of daily morning and evening weights through several menstrual cycles should be obtained from female patients. All patients should be asked about drugs that can cause edema, diuretic or laxative abuse, patterns of carbohydrate and salt intake, and sudden changes in climate and altitude. If drug abuse is in question, the urine can be tested for thiazides or phenolphthalein.

In patients with localized edema, a search should be made for evidence of allergic reactions as indicated by the presence of wheals or urticaria. These patients frequently complain of intense itching. The edema from burns or cold exposure is accompanied by inflammatory signs or evidence of tissue damage.

With chronic lymphatic obstruction, reduction of edema may minimize secondary fibrotic changes. Frequent elevation of the involved extremity (to a point above the level of the right atrium), use of support hose, dietary sodium restriction, and diuretics may all be helpful.

When edema is associated with varicose veins, there is usually irreversible deep venous obstruction and incompetent valves. Treatment is designed to reduce the hydrostatic pressure when the patient is erect through the use of fitted stockings and periodic elevation of the legs. Occasionally, it may be necessary to recommend ligation of the perforating veins and removal of the superficial veins (see Chap. 45).

Patients who are believed to have cyclical or idiopathic edema should not be given diuretics, which may eventually worsen the edema. Instead they should be put on salt restriction and other dietary or drug manipulations.

Kaloyanoties GJ. Pathogenesis and Treatment of Edema with Special Reference to the Use of Diuretics. In MH Maxwell and CR Kleeman (Eds.), *Clinical Disorders of Fluid and Electrolyte Metabolism.* New York: McGraw-Hill, 1980. P. 647.
  An excellent review with particular emphasis on treatment.
Levy M, Seely JF. Pathophysiology of Edema Formation. In BM Brenner and FC Rector, Jr. (Eds.), *The Kidney.* Philadelphia: Saunders, 1981. P. 723.
  Definitive explanation of mechanisms of edema formation.
Rose BD. *Clinical Physiology of Acid-Base and Electrolyte Disorders.* New York: McGraw-Hill, 1977.
  Extremely well organized summary suited for the general reader.

136. LYMPHADENOPATHY
Robert H. Fletcher

Peripheral lymphadenopathy (enlarged lymph nodes) occurring without other findings that point to the cause presents a difficult dilemma for clinicians. On the one hand, many of the potential causes are both serious and treatable. On the other hand, the only way to make a certain diagnosis is, in nearly all instances, by means of an invasive procedure, usually lymph node biopsy. Therefore, a great deal rests on the clinician's judgment as to whether aggressive evaluation is necessary.

Causes
The list of possible causes for lymphadenopathy is extensive. General categories include malignancies, either intrinsic to the node or metastatic; infections of virtually all kinds; antigenic stimulation (e.g., secondary to local injections or systemic, autoimmune diseases); and drugs (specifically phenytoin, but also others if they cause serum sickness). Sarcoidosis is associated with granulomatous adenopathy. For a large proportion of enlarged lymph nodes, no specific cause is determined.

Initial Evaluation
The likelihood of finding an important and treatable cause of lymphadenopathy can be estimated from information available at the time the patient is first seen. The judg-

ment whether to pursue to diagnostic workup or wait is based, in large measure, on the following observations.

Likely Causes
For nodes that are biopsied, whether at referral centers or community hospitals, a small set of possibilities accounts for nearly all results. Many of the nodes, about 40%, are abnormal but without findings from histologic examination or culture that allow a specific diagnosis. Three conditions account for nearly all of the remaining 60% of nodes that yield a specific diagnosis: metastatic malignancies (25%), intrinsic malignancy (e.g., lymphoma, 20%), and tuberculosis (10%). The remainder (5%) includes a variety of normal and abnormal tissues. Therefore, the probability that a lymph node will be nonspecifically involved, or reflect one of these three conditions, is extremely high even before considering other information.

Age
The likelihood of cancer increases with age. In one series, 25% of biopsied nodes from young people revealed cancer, while 75% of nodes from patients over 75 years old were malignant. Normally, the lymphatic tissue in adolescents and young adults is larger than later in life, so that minor degrees of node "enlargement" may not be abnormal in this age group.

Location
The likelihood of finding a specific diagnosis varies with the location from which a node is taken. Nodes are most often positive in the neck (70%), followed by the axilla (50%) and the groin (40%). This is presumed to be because of minor infections in the extremities, particularly the lower ones, which increase the prevalence of nonspecific, "reactive" nodes in their region. For example, palpable, firm inguinal nodes up to 1 cm in diameter are common in adults. Therefore, one is more inclined to biopsy a neck than a groin node. Similarly, if there is a choice of nodes to biopsy (e.g., with generalized lymphadenopathy), it is best to biopsy one in the neck.

Rate of Change
Nodes that arise rapidly are more often pathologic than those of long duration. Unfortunately, patients often do not notice when the node first appeared, even in prominent places like the neck. Also, fear and wishful thinking may color their reports.

Physical Findings
Examination of involved nodes can yield relatively accurate information about the underlying pathophysiologic process. Five observations are made: size, localization, consistency, inflammation, and fixation. As mentioned, large size (e.g., > 2 cm) weighs in favor of specific pathology. Generalized adenopathy is caused by systemic disease, whereas local or regional adenopathy may represent either local (e.g., infection, tumor) or systemic (e.g., rubella, plague) disease. Hard nodes represent metastatic cancer or fibrosis from previous inflammation (particularly if the nodes are small). Firm or rubbery nodes are associated with lymphomas and leukemias, as well as a variety of infections and antigenic processes. Fluctuant nodes usually represent pyogenic infection, although advanced tuberculosis, and occasionally necrotic tumors, can also result in central liquefication. Signs of inflammation (e.g., heat, redness) suggest infection or antigenic stimulation. Fixation of nodes to adjacent structures—to each other or to the deep fascia or dermis—represents either neoplasm invading outside the node capsule or organizing inflammation.

Diagnostic Tests

Biopsy
Biopsy of abnormal lymph nodes is the most accurate means of diagnosis. Usually a node is excised in its entirety rather than partially removed, because having as much tissue as possible is useful for histologic diagnosis and because the diagnosis and treatment of some conditions (e.g., mycobacterial adenitis) begins with excision. Most pathologic nodes can be removed under local anesthesia, without admission. The morbidity of the procedure is negligible and is mainly related to infection or damage to local neurovascular structures when the procedure is done in the axilla or groin. Usually it

is sufficient to send excised nodes for routine histology and culture. Occasionally, other tests are suggested by the clinical situation, such as cultures for bacteria, mycobacteria, viruses, and fungi. When the official pathology report is equivocal (e.g., "atypical hyperplasia"), it may be helpful to talk to the pathologist; so much rests on their interpretation that they are inclined to be conservative for the record.

Needle Biopsy
Needle biopsy, using a thin-bore needle, can be accomplished with negligible morbidity. In published series, about 85% of attempts yield sufficient tissue for diagnosis. Since only a small number of cells are obtained, and tissue architecture is disrupted, it is sometimes not possible to make a firm diagnosis, particularly for intrinsic malignancies. When the biopsy is positive for cancer, one can have confidence in the result—that is, there are few false positives. However, if the results are negative for malignant cells, one cannot conclude that cancer is ruled out. In one series, 31 of 52 patients (60%) in whom biopsies were read as negative for cancer subsequently proved to have cancer. Therefore, needle biopsy is most useful when metastatic cancer, as opposed to lymphoma, is suspected and when the results are positive rather than negative.

Aspiration
If a node is fluctuant, it is tempting to aspirate it, since that is a relatively noninvasive procedure. Indeed, aspiration might make the diagnosis if the cause is infection, either pyogenic or tuberculous, although it is by no means perfectly sensitive for this purpose. However, most of these nodes require either incision and drainage (for pyogenic infection) or excision for diagnosis (e.g., lymphoma) or for cure (e.g., infection with mycobacteria other than *Mycobacterium tuberculosis*). Therefore, aspiration is not, in itself, a particularly useful diagnostic maneuver.

Lymphangiography
Lymphangiography demonstrates the anatomic distribution of abnormal nodes. But it is not possible to determine, with reasonable certainty, the specific process taking place in the nodes.

Strategy for Evaluation
In most situations, the management of lymphadenopathy involves two options: biopsy or wait. Beyond routine tests such as complete blood count and chest film, efforts to find out the cause of isolated peripheral lymphadenopathy indirectly (e.g., by means of elaborate serologic and skin tests) are usually not helpful. Waiting, at least for a short time, is often the preferred cause of action. There are virtually no situations in which waiting up to 2 weeks will result in a lost opportunity for treatment, particularly if the clinical findings do not change appreciably during that time.

When the decision is made to biopsy, one must expect a certain number of nondiagnostic results (in most series about 40%) in order to safely include nearly all pathologic nodes. At times, biopsy is undertaken because of concern, on the part of the patient or physician, that cannot be relieved in any other way.

Specific Presentations

Hard Cervical Nodes
A hard cervical node, particularly in the elderly, often represents a metastasis from a cancer arising on the mucosal surfaces of the head and neck. The primary cancer often cannot be visualized without using special instruments to examine relatively inaccessible surfaces (e.g., the nasopharynx) and even then may not be found. There is evidence that the likelihood of recurrence is less if definitive surgery (often involving radical neck dissection) is done immediately following biopsy, rather than as a second procedure. For this reason, when head and neck cancer is suspected biopsy should be done by a specialist and in the hospital, so that when surgery is necessary it can be completed at the same time as the biopsy.

Fluctuant Cervical Nodes
Fluctuant cervical nodes, particularly in children and young adults, are usually the result of infection with *Staphylococcus, Streptococcus,* or both. Several features of this

syndrome are counterintuitive. Usually no primary focus of infection is seen in the mouth or pharynx. Also, patients are often not very febrile or "toxic," although they are usually uncomfortable because of local swelling. If the node is just beginning to break down, many clinicians treat first with antibiotics, chosen to cover *Staphylococcus* and *Streptococcus,* and proceed to incision and drainage only if there is no improvement. If the node is frankly fluctuant, it is unlikely that surgery will be avoided.

Tuberculous Adenitis

Tuberculous adenitis presents as an enlarging, mildly symptomatic node of several weeks' to months' duration (occasionally many years). The disease is usually in the neck and rarely in the axilla or groin. About three-fourths of tuberculous nodes are not fluctuant at diagnosis. Tuberculous adenitis is suspected in the presence of a history of tuberculosis, a positive skin test, or abnormal chest film, although only 40 to 90% of cases have these findings. Systemic signs are infrequent, and the disease is usually not active at other sites. The majority of infections in adults are caused by *M. tuberculosis;* in children the majority of cases are caused by atypical mycobacteria. When tuberculous adenitis is suspected, antituberculous drugs are given following node excision until the culture results are available. If cultures grow *M. tuberculosis,* antituberculous drugs are continued for 1 year. If there is evidence of infection elsewhere and the diagnosis can be made without node excision, drugs alone may be curative. For infections with mycobacteria other than *M. tuberculosis,* excision alone is often sufficient.

Greenfield S, Jordan MC. The clinical investigation of lymphadenopathy in primary care practice. *JAMA* 240:1388–1393, 1978.
   An algorithm for evaluating adults whose initial and most prominent problem is peripheral lymphadenopathy.
Lee YTN, Terry R, Lukes RJ. Lymph node biopsy for diagnosis: A statistical study. *J Surg Oncol* 14:53–60, 1980.
   The results of 925 consecutive lymph node biopsies for diagnosis, done at LA County-USC Medical Center between 1973 and 1977.
Harwick RD. Tumors of the Neck. In HF Conn and RB Conn, Jr. (Eds.), *Current Diagnosis (4th ed.).* Phildelphia: Saunders, 1974.
   A discussion of neck masses, with particular attention to the spread of local tumors and of masses that might be confused with tumor. Previous editions of Current Diagnosis *are by different authors and tend to complement each other.*
Schroer KR, Franssila KO. Atypical hyperplasia of lymph nodes: A follow up study. *Cancer* 44:1155–1163, 1979.
   Pathologists were asked to review slides reported as "atypical hyperplasia," a term used to express concern about neoplasia when lymphoma cannot be diagnosed with certainty. The pathologists were able to predict outcome with a high degree of accuracy.
Betsill WL Jr, Hajdu SI. Percutaneous aspiration biopsy of lymph nodes. *Am J Clin Pathol* 73:471–479, 1980.
   The results of 361 cytologic examinations of specimens aspirated by percutaneous needle biopsy from superficial lymph nodes. Adequate material was obtained for 85%, and 81% were positive for malignant cells. There were no false-positive tests, but over half of the negative results were false negatives.
McGuirt WF, McCabe BF. Significance of node biopsy before definitive treatment of cervical metastatic carcinoma. *Laryngoscope* 88:594–597, 1978.
   A survey of 714 radical neck dissections, some of which were preceded by a cervical node biopsy. Complications of wound necrosis, local recurrence, and distant metastases were more common among patients who were biopsied prior to definitive surgery, and the differences persisted after matching for other prognostic factors.
Huhti E, et al. Tuberculosis of the cervical lymph nodes: A clinical, pathological and bacteriological study. *Tubercle* 56:27–36, 1975.
   A review of 59 patients with cervical lymph node tuberculosis.
Lai KK, et al. Mycobacteria cervical lymphadenopathy. Relation of etiologic agents to age. *JAMA* 251:1286–1288, 1984.
   Reports mycobacteria isolated in a reference laboratory for Massachusetts. Mycobacterium tuberculosis was isolated from 147 of 154 adults. Other mycobacteria were isolated from 55 of 60 children.

137. HYPOTHERMIA AND COLD INJURY

Alan K. Halperin

Exposure to cold can cause hypothermia or injury in the form of frostbite, trench or immersion foot, or chilblains.

Hypothermia

Hypothermia is defined as a spontaneous drop in core body temperature below 95°F (35°C). It occurs in two very different populations. One group is composed of the elderly sick and derelicts of any age in whom hypothermia accompanies exposure or medical problems. The other group is composed of young, usually healthy people who by bad luck or ignorance have been caught unprepared in severe, cold weather. Approximately 650 deaths per year are attributed to hypothermia; however, this is probably an underestimate because many cases are unrecognized or unreported. Since 1977, the incidence has been increasing.

Risk Factors

In healthy individuals, hypothermia usually occurs in people exposed to prolonged, cold ambient temperatures. However, it can also occur from exposure at higher temperatures (as high as 70°F or 21°C) if thermoregulatory mechanisms are impaired. Most cases of hypothermia, especially in the elderly or infirm, are a result of exposure to cold plus other factors, such as dampness, alcohol (which causes vasodilation with resultant heat loss and also predisposes to inactivity and trauma), hypoglycemia (which decreases heat production), and infection. Also associated are tranquilizers, sedatives, and hypnotics (which interfere with central hypothalamic regulation); metabolic disturbances (hypoglycemia, hypothyroidism, and hypoadrenalism); miscellaneous diseases, such as sepsis, malnutrition, uremia, and hepatic failure; lesions of the hypothalamus; and spinal cord transection (loss of vasoconstriction). The elderly appear to be particularly susceptible to hypothermia because of an inadequate vasoconstrictive reponse to cold, a decreased ability to generate heat in response to cold, impaired cold perception, decreased muscle mass, and frequent immobility due to disease or trauma. In a cold environment, any disease, particularly in the elderly, can cause hypothermia.

Evaluation

The initial symptoms of hypothermia—fatigue, weakness, slowness of gait, incoordination, apathy, confusion, decreased judgment, and hallucinations—are nonspecific and can easily be confused with other metabolic disorders. Companions of people developing hypothermia may not recognize the early symptoms, and medical personnel may also overlook this possibility unless there is a high index of suspicion.

If hypothermia is suspected, the patient's temperature should be taken with a low-range rectal thermometer or probe. Errors occur when the thermometer is not shaken down properly or when the patient's temperature is actually below 94°F (34.4°C), the lowest point on the usual rectal thermometer.

The physical findings of hypothermia are also nonspecific. These include decreased blood pressure, heart rate, and respiratory rate; generalized edema of the skin; decreased level of consciousness; dilated and poorly reactive pupils; depressed deep tendon reflexes; and increased muscle tone. Shivering is often absent, particularly in severely hypothermic patients. The remainder of the physical examination should include a thorough search for the associated problems, particularly sepsis and myxedema, that increase the risk for hypothermia. Because of the prominent neurologic findings, signs of head trauma can be obscured, making the evaluation of brain injury difficult.

A continual assessment of cardiovascular findings is important because of the effects of the cold on myocardial irritability and conduction. Atrial fibrillation and sinus bradycardia are the most common arrhythmias. The risk of ventricular fibrillation increases as the core temperature drops below 86°F (30°C) and is greatest below 75°F (24°C). Electrocardiographic changes may include prolonged PR interval, prolonged QRS complex, and the J wave (Osborn wave), which is a small upward deflection or hump early in the ST segment of lateral precordial leads.

In addition to cardiac complications, other important potential metabolic complications include aspiration pneumonia (due to increased secretions and decreased level of consciousness and cough reflex), ileus, pancreatitis, decreased renal function (due to hypovolemia, fluid shift to extravascular space), metabolic acidosis (due to poor tissue perfusion), respiratory acidosis (due to hypoventilation), hyperglycemia (due to an inhibition of insulin release), hypoglycemia, electrolyte disturbances, and rarely disseminated intravascular coagulation. Blood gases must be corrected for temperature, or mistakes in evaluation or treatment can occur. For each 1°C decrease in temperature below 98.6°F (37.5°C), the pH is increased by 0.015, the P_{CO_2} is decreased by 4.4%, and the P_{O_2} is decreased by 7.2%.

Treatment
Treatment of hypothermia falls into two categories: first aid in the field and management in a medical facility. In both situations, the approach to rewarming patients is controversial. In mild hypothermia, efforts at rewarming in the field are warranted. But in severe hypothermia, particularly in patients with frozen extremities who have quit shivering and are stuporous, immediate transportation to the nearest hospital is indicated. These patients must be handled gently because jostling may precipitate a cardiac arrhythmia. Wet clothes should be removed and replaced by warm, well-insulated, dry clothing or covering. Both thawing of the extremities and hot liquids taken internally can cause shunting of blood from the extremities into the central circulation, causing a "secondary chill" or "after drop," which can lead to ventricular fibrillation. For patients who are conscious and shivering, tepid sweet drinks are advocated (some recommend warm Jell-O because of the sugar and protein content). In addition to the above, when the patient cannot be removed from the cold environment quickly or when hypothermia is mild, gentle rewarming by direct skin-to-skin contact may be helpful.

Since many patients have hypoglycemia, 50% glucose should be given immediately. If alcoholism is suspected, thiamine should be given with the glucose because a carbohydrate load may precipitate psychosis. Drugs need to be used with extreme caution, as pharmacokinetics are disturbed in hypothermic patients. All drugs are less metabolically active in the hypothermic patient.

All patients with a temperature less than 90°F (32°C) should be admitted to an intensive care unit for continuous monitoring until the temperature is greater than 95° (35°C). Rewarming can be accomplished by external or internal core warming. External warming can be passive (removing the patient from the cold and wrapping with blankets) or active (immersing the patient in a warm-water bath at 105–133°F [40–45°C] or using a heating blanket). Numerous methods for active core rewarming are available, including warmed intravenous (IV) fluids; inhalation of warmed humidified oxygen through an endotracheal tube or mask; peritoneal dialysis; colonic, gastric, or mediastinal irrigation; and hemodialysis. Of the above, rewarming with warmed IV fluids and warmed humidified oxygen is generally the preferred technique. In cases of severe hypothermia (temperatures below 75°F or 24°C) or refractory arrhythmias (ventricular fibrillation or asystole), peritoneal dialysis should be started.

Prognosis
Because of decreased metabolic requirements, patients may appear dead. However, patients have been revived with core temperatures as low as 60.8°F (16°C) and have fully recovered after as long as 6 hours of cardiopulmonary resuscitation or 90 minutes under water. No conclusions about the reversibility should be made until the patient is rewarmed.

Mortality is more related to the presence of associated diseases than to the degree of hypothermia. When a serious underlying disease is present, such as sepsis, mortality approaches 75%, whereas for accidental hypothermia in healthy individuals, mortality is approximately 6%. The death rate is reduced by prompt recognition, awareness of the potential metabolic complications, and prompt treatment.

Cold Injury

Chilblains
Chilblains come from exposure to nonfreezing cold and thus are most often found on cheeks, hands, and shins. The injury results from the vascular response to cold—va-

soconstriction, then vasodilation and edema. After rewarming, the area will appear cyanotic and mildly edematous with burning and pruritus. Re-exposure causes more severe damage in the same areas. These areas may have a heightened response to cold for several years. Treatment is by warming and prevention by wearing protective clothing.

Immersion Foot and Trench Foot
Immersion foot and trench foot are nonfreezing problems caused by exposure to water. In immersion foot, there is direct contact with water; in trench foot, the shod foot is wet. Both are usually associated with more than 12 hours of exposure. The foot appears mottled to waxy, feels cold, and has no pulsations. There is usually no sensation in the foot. On rewarming, there is local swelling, pain, and occasionally blistering. If severe ischemic damage occurs, there may be focal areas of gangrene. This is followed by a phase of recovery that may be associated with weakness, increased sensitivity to cold, and pain with walking. These patients should be evaluated as soon as possible. However, these conditions are often associated with frostbite or hypothermia and frequently should receive inpatient care.

Frostbite
Frostbite is caused by exposure to temperatures below freezing, causing ice crystals to form in tissues. Damage comes from cellular dehydration and ischemia. High-altitude rapid freezing produces less damage than slow freezing. A combination of high winds and cold is much more dangerous than cold alone. People at risk are those who become wet or immobile, who have compromised arterial circulation to the extremities, who are intoxicated from alcohol, or who have had previous frostbite. The parts of the body most likely to develop frostbite are fingers, toes, nose, and earlobes. The frostbitten extremity appears white, feels firm, has lost sensation, and is usually immobile.

The degree of damage is described as follows:

First degree: Hyperemia and edema on rewarming.
Second degree: Blistering following the above.
Third degree: Necrosis leading to hemorrhagic vesicles and edema.
Fourth degree: The same as above, but there is small-vessel obstruction that leads to ischemic demarcation and loss of tissue.

For "frost nip" (blanching of skin), wrapping the affected part in a dry parka or placing it on the abdomen or axilla of a companion can prevent further injury. In frostbite, the frozen part should not be thawed if there is a chance of refreezing, because refreezing may increase tissue damage. Alcohol, despite giving a temporary feeling of warmth, causes further loss of body heat; tobacco is also contraindicated. The extremity should not be rubbed with snow, immersed in hot or cold water, or covered with salves. Restrictive clothing should be removed and the extremity wrapped in a bulky, loose dressing. Activity should be stopped, and patients should not walk on frostbitten feet. Breaks in the skin, particularly in partially thawed tissue, can lead to infection.

If at all possible patients should be hospitalized for treatment. The accepted rewarming technique is to immerse the frozen part in a water bath at 104°F (40–42°C) until a flush has returned to the most distal part (usually 20–30 minutes). The last steps of thawing can be very painful, and analgesics may be required.

After rewarming, extreme care needs to be taken to avoid infection and trauma. The affected parts should be gently cleaned and cotton placed between the digits. Surgical debridement should be delayed until a sharp line of demarcation between viable and nonviable tissue develops. Blisters should not be broken.

Prevention
Cold injuries can best be prevented by wearing warm, loose, dry clothing in multiple layers on the head, body, and extremities to prevent heat loss. One should keep dry at all costs; materials lose insulation properties when wet. People expecting to be outside for a long time should carry spare dry clothing and food for continuous nibbling (a mixture of nuts, raisins, and candy is ideal).

Reuler JB. Hypothermia: Pathophysiology, clinical settings, and management. *Ann Intern Med* 89:519–527, 1978.
Excellent overall review of the literature.
Miller JW, Danzl DF, Thomas DM. Urban accidental hypothermia: 135 cases. *Ann Emerg Med* 9:456–461, 1980.
Comparison of different rewarming methods.
PaVee TS, Reineberd EJ. Extreme hypothermia and ventricular fibrillation. *Ann Emerg Med* 9:100–101, 1980.
Demonstrates value of prolonged cardiopulmonary resuscitation in hypothermia.
Besdine RW. Accidental hypothermia: The body's energy crisis. *Geriatrics* 34(12):51–59, 1979.
Review of hypothermia in the elderly.
Davidson M, Grant E. Accidental hypothermia from a community hosital perspective. *Postgrad Med* 70:42–49, 1981.
Data on 60 patients.
Reuler JB, Parker RA. Peritoneal dialysis in the management of hypothermia. *JAMA* 240:2289–2290, 1978.
Technique is reviewed.
Fitzgerald FT, Jessop C. Accidental hypothermia: A report of 22 cases and review of the literature. *Adv Intern Med* 27:127–143, 1982.
Excellent review of practical considerations.
Mills WJ. Out in the cold. *Emergency Med* 8:134–147, 1976.
Review of hypothermia and frostbite.

138. HEAT INJURY
Alan K. Halperin

The spectrum of local and systemic reactions to excessive ambient temperature includes heat cramps, heat exhaustion, and heat stroke. Heat cramps are painful tonic contractions of muscles occurring in alert individuals with normal temperatures. Heat exhaustion is characterized by fever greater than 102°F (39°C), sweating, headache, nausea or vomiting, chills, and weakness, with central nervous system changes usually limited to lassitude, mild dizziness, or unsteady gait. Heat stroke is associated with high fever (up to 106°F [41°C]); severe central nervous system disturbances such as confusion, delirium, or coma; absent or diminished sweating; and occasionally hypotension and circulatory collapse. There is no sharp distinction among these three syndromes, and they may occur together.

Heat injury arises under two circumstances. One, called exertional heat injury, occurs in athletes or military recruits who overexercise in a hot and humid environment. The other, classic heat injury, is principally a disease of the elderly with chronic diseases who are exposed to an elevated ambient temperature. The presentation, metabolic complications, and treatment are similar, but the means of prevention are different.

Risk Factors

Exertional Heat Injury
Exercising in a hot and humid environment is the most common cause of heat injury. Approximately 1% of runners participating in road races develop heat-related injuries, usually heat cramps and heat exhaustion. Risk factors for heat injury include the following:

1. Weather conditions: The incidence of heat injuries increases with ambient temperature, solar radiation, and humidity. An index called the "wet bulb globe temperature index" (WBGT) is a summary of these three conditions; when the WBGT rises above

84.4°F (28°C), the American College of Sports Medicine recommends not running, including races. Running should be done before 9:00 AM or after 4:00 PM during the summer months.

2. Insufficient acclimatization: Exercising in a hot environment produces higher core temperature, higher heart rate, and a marked reduction in exercise capacity. It takes approximately 5 to 10 running sessions in a hot environment for a conditioned athlete to acclimatize. This can be lost after only 2 to 4 weeks.

3. Lack of conditioning: Less-conditioned athletes are less heat tolerant and take longer to acclimatize. Runners who develop heat injury usually have not run for long and have been running few miles, and their training distances have been shorter than race distances.

4. Dehydration: Progressive dehydration commonly occurs during prolonged exercise, even if fluids are supplied. Extreme fluid losses, especially if exercise is begun in a dehydrated state, predispose to heat injury.

5. Age extremes: Both young children and older adults are more susceptible to heat injury because of lower sweating rates and decreased aerobic capacity.

6. Obesity.

7. Prior heat stroke: Runners with previous history of heat stroke have higher rates of recurrence. It is not known whether these individuals had preexisting defects in thermoregulation or whether defects developed during the heat stroke episode.

Classic Heat Injury

Heat injury is more common in tropical climates. However, yearly epidemics occur during the summer in temperate climates in places such as the United States. For example, in the summer of 1980, approximately 1265 people died of heat injury; many more were less severely affected and survived. Most reported epidemics occur after more than 48 hours of temperature averaging over 90°F and relative humidity over 50%. Classic heat injury is predominantly a disease of the elderly exposed to an elevated ambient temperature without air conditioning or adequate shade and at least one of the following risk factors:

1. Chronic disease, such as cardiovascular disease, is the single most important factor in the development of heat injury. Patients with cardiovascular disease have limited cutaneous vasodilatation, do not increase their tolerance to heat with time, have impaired sweat production, and do not increase their cardiac output or heart rate with increasing temperature. Diabetics have some of these same defects.

2. Drugs that can predispose to heat injury include diuretics, which prevent volume expansion and impair vasodilatation; anticholinergics, which inhibit sweating; phenothiazines, which disrupt the hypothalamic thermoregulatory center; and alcohol, which impairs vasomotor control and judgment.

3. Inability to care for self, such as bedridden or demented patients.

4. Obesity.

5. Acute infections.

Metabolic Complications

The primary defense against hyperthermia is evaporative cooling by sweating. If excessive, this can result in disturbances of body water, electrolytes, and renal function. Either hyponatremia or hypernatremia can occur depending on salt and water intake. Hypokalemia is frequent and may play a role in cardiovascular instability and rhabdomyolysis. It is hypothesized that brief exposure to elevated temperatures causes hyperventilation and respiratory alkalosis. More prolonged exposure results in lactic acidosis from hypovolemia, hypoxemia, hypotension, and increased metabolic requirements. Arterial blood gases in the presence of hyperthermia must be corrected for body temperature. In general, a rise of 1°C above 98.6°F (37.5°C) will increase the P_{CO_2} by 4.4% and the P_{O_2} by 6% and decrease the pH by 0.015. Impaired renal function usually reflects dehydration.

Approximately 10% of patients with severe heat injury develop acute renal failure. Contributing factors include thermal injury, hypotension, dehydration, and rhabdomyolysis. Rhabdomyolysis is associated with dark urine (myoglobinuria), tender muscles, elevated creatine phosphokinase, and commonly hypocalcemia and hypophosphatemia. Abnormalities of liver function, including elevated serum bilirubin and transaminases, are common but rarely serious. Hypoglycemia or hyperglycemia can occur. Minor abnormalities of coagulation such as prolonged prothrombin time and partial thromboplastin time are common, but disseminated intravascular coagulation is a rare complication. Electrocardiographic changes include nonspecific ST and T wave changes and intraventricular conduction abnormalities. Hemodynamic monitoring has demonstrated that exertional heat injury is usually associated with hyperdynamic circulation with increased heart rate and cardiac output and decreased systemic vascular resistance. In contrast, classic heat stroke usually involves decreased cardiac output and increased peripheral resistance. These distinctions are not absolute; the elderly may not have the cardiovascular reserve to compensate with tachycardia and decreased systemic resistance.

Prevention
Prevention of exertional heat injury follows from the risk factors: not running when the weather is hot, humid, and sunny; ensuring adequate training and acclimatization when beginning exercising or changing locations; liberal intake of fluids; and knowledge of the early symptoms of heat injury. Prompt first aid, followed by appropriate care, can reduce morbidity and mortality.

Individuals at risk during heat waves should be encouraged to wear lightweight, light-colored, and wide-pored clothing of cotton, rather than polyester; change wet clothing; decrease activity; take cool showers; and spend as much time as possible in air conditioning. Some cities have established air-conditioning shelters for those at risk.

Treatment
Heat cramps are usually easily treated by giving oral fluids; water is sufficient. Salt tablets and sugar are best avoided because fluid losses are usually hypotonic, and sugar delays gastric emptying. Massaging the affected muscles and rest may also help. Intravenous fluids or muscle relaxants are rarely necessary.

Mild heat exhaustion can be managed where it occurs or in the office. On the other hand, severe heat exhaustion and heat stroke are medical emergencies; usually they require prompt first aid, followed by hospitalization. Treatment is directed toward rapid cooling, support of the cardiovascular system, and increasing renal blood flow. The patient's temperature should be continuously monitored by a rectal probe. Cooling effects should cease when the rectal temperature reaches 102°F, or hypothermia might result. Rapid cooling is best accomplished by spraying the patient with water (maintaining the skin temperature above 86°F, which prevents vasoconstriction), positioning the patient in front of a fan, or placing ice packs to the areas of greatest heat exchange (neck, abdomen, axillae, and groin). Rapid fluid administration at room temperature also promotes cooling. Patients should not be immersed in ice baths, because it promotes vasoconstriction, or given chlorpromazine, because it interferes with central thermoregulation.

Fluids are given to correct dehydration. The amount of dehydration is variable, but patients with exertional heat injury tend to have larger fluid deficits. One liter of hypotonic fluid, such as 0.45% saline and 5% dextrose, should be given rapidly and adjusted as volume and electrolytes dictate.

Acute renal failure should be anticipated if hypotension or rhabdomyolysis has occurred. Mannitol, 12.5 gm, may be used to promote renal blood flow. If rhabdomyolysis occurs, the urine should be alkalinized.

Antipyretics such as aspirin or acetaminophen are ineffective because their action requires the presence of intact heat-losing mechanisms. Oxygen may be helpful.

Prognosis
Exertional heat injury has an excellent prognosis. In a study of 27 military recruits, there were no deaths and only 1 recruit was not able to return to military duty. In these recruits there were no differences in recovery time or disability between patients with exertional heat exhaustion and heat stroke. Studies of classic heat injury report a mortality of 40 to 70%. Most of these patients were elderly and were already compromised by having at least two of the following chronic conditions: diabetes mellitus, cardiovascular disease, or mental illness treated with psychotropic drugs. Approximately 50% of those who presented with hypotension died. All those who died failed to

regain consciousness and had irreversible brain injury and other complications, such as pneumonia. Most who regained consciousness recovered fully.

Knochel JP. Environmental heat illness: An eclectic review. *Arch Intern Med* 133:841–864, 1974.
Excellent review of risk factors, pathophysiology, and treatment.
Sutton JR, Bar-Or O. Thermal illness in fun running. *Am Heart J* 100:778–781, 1980.
Review of risk factors for exertional heat injury.
American College of Sports Medicine. Prevention of heat injuries during distance running. *J Sports Med* 16:345–346, 1976.
Recommendations for preventing exertional heat injury.
Sprung CL. Hemodynamic alterations of heat stroke in the elderly. *Chest* 75:362–366, 1979.
Hemodynamic findings of eight elderly patients.
Sprung CL, et al. The metabolic and respiratory alterations of heat stroke. *Arch Intern Med* 140:655–659, 1980.
Pathophysiology and metabolic complications in exertional and classic heat injury.
Costrini AM, et al. Cardiovascular and metabolic manifestations of heat stroke and severe heat exhaustion. *Am J Med* 66(2):269–302, 1979.
Experience from the Marine Corps at Parris Island, South Carolina.
Weiner JS, Khogali M. A physiological body-cooling unit for treatment of heat stroke. *Lancet* 1:507–509, 1980.
Comparison of various cooling techniques.

139. HICCUPS

Raymond F. Bianchi

Clonic spasm of the diaphragm and the external intercostal muscles results in a singultus, commonly known as a hiccup. The characteristic sound occurs when an inspiratory effort, initiated by the spasm, is aborted by glottic closure.

Causes

Traditionally, a hiccup has been considered an involuntary reflex that produces spasm of a hemidiaphragm, usually the left. The respiratory center was thought to mediate a reflex involving the phrenic nerve, vagus nerve, and sympathetic chain from T6–T12 as the afferent limb and the phrenic nerve as the efferent limb. In 1970, however, Davis demonstrated that hiccup is produced by bilateral diaphragmatic and inspiratory muscle spasms; he suggested that hiccup is mediated by a brain stem center physiologically independent of the respiratory center. He also suggested that hiccup is a primitive response, with no apparent useful function, which is normally inhibited by descending signals from higher centers. Hiccups can therefore develop from either excitation along the reflex arc (particularly phrenic nerve stimulation) or suppression of the higher centers (as seen with central nervous system lesions or metabolic abnormalities). Consequently, treatment can be directed toward either the "hiccup center" in the central nervous center or the limbs of the reflex arc.

Treatment

Transient Hiccups
Transient hiccups are usually the result of gastric distention from overindulgence in food or drink. Because these episodes are brief and self-limited, it is difficult to assess the efficacy of individual treatments. Folk remedies include difficult or distracting tasks like breath-holding, tongue traction, breathing into a paper bag, being frightened, and drinking water from the wrong side of a glass while occluding the ears. Stimulation of the pharyngeal mucosa (e.g., by swallowing 1 teaspoon of either vinegar or dry granulated sugar) is believed to suppress hiccups by competitive inhibition of

Table 139-1. Causes of intractable hiccups

Psychogenic

Anesthesia related

Postoperative

Medical

Central nervous system: trauma, vascular insufficiency, tumor, syphilis, encephalitis, sarcoidosis, temporal arteritis, degenerative diseases, syringomyelia, seizure disorder

Neck: goiter, thoracic outlet syndrome

Thorax: diaphragmatic hernia, diaphragmatic tumor, pleurisy, pneumonia, lung abscess, foreign body, aneurysm, asthma, esophageal dysfunction, esophageal cancer, coronary occlusion, pericarditis

Abdomen: duodenal ulcer, cholelithiasis, pancreatic pseudocyst, pancreatic cancer, stomach cancer, colon cancer, metastatic liver cancer, ulcerative colitis, splenomegaly

Urinary tract: hypernephroma, hydronephrosis, prostatism

Toxin/Drug: uremia, alcoholism, benzodiazepines

---

afferent fibers. The transnasal passage of a small, soft rubber catheter to the C2–3 level of the pharynx, oscillating it rapidly for 30 seconds, also inhibits the pharyngeal afferent fibers and is said to be effective.

Intractable Hiccups

Intractable hiccups are empirically defined as persisting for at least 48 hours. The numerous causes are listed in Table 139-1.

The treatment of intractable hiccups remains controversial. In 1932, Mayo stated, "the amount of knowledge on any subject . . . can be considered as being in inverse proportion to the number of different treatments suggested and tried for it. Perhaps one is justified in saying there is no disease which has had more forms of treatment and fewer results from treatment than has had persistent hiccups." The first step in treating intractable hiccups is to identify one of the potentially reversible metabolic or structural etiologies listed in Table 139-1. If none is found, one suggested approach is to insert a nasogastric tube, both to decompress the stomach and to irritate the pharynx. Lack of response indicates the need for drug therapy using an agent that acts either centrally (affecting the hiccup center) or peripherally.

Chlorpromazine has been the most extensively studied of the centrally-acting drugs. The recommended dose is 50 mg given as an intravenous bolus; systemic blood pressure must be monitored for hypotension. Success with this therapy is followed by oral chlorpromazine for 10 days. A variety of other drugs are reported to be of value: diphenhydantoin, haloperidol (5 mg po tid), orphenadrine (60 mg IM or 100 mg po), ketamine (0.4 mg/kg IV), and carbamazepine (200 mg po qid). Evidence that any of these drugs is effective is either anecdotal or difficult to interpret because of the small study sample. Diazepam paradoxically increased the frequency of hiccups in a study of three patients.

Of the peripherally-acting drugs, metoclopramide (10 mg po qid) appears to be the most efficacious. Quinidine sulfate (200 mg po qid) has been shown effective in a small number of patients. Atropine (1 mg IV), edrophonium chloride (10 mg IV), amphetamine (30 mg qd for 1 week), and amyl nitrite have also been recommended. But again, as for the centrally-acting drugs, the number of patients tested has been too small to judge efficacy from published studies.

In desperation, unilateral phrenic nerve anesthesia, or crush, has been advocated. The number of patients thus treated has been small, however, and there have been failures—not surprising because hiccups probably result from bilateral hemidiaphragm spasm, and unilateral phrenic nerve trauma would therefore be inadequate therapy.

Samuels LS. Hiccup. *Can Med Assoc J* 67:315–322; 1952.
  Classic review of the subject; the major work favoring the unilateral hemidiaphrag
  contraction theory of hiccup. Thirty-three etiologies as well as therapy are discussed.
Davis JN. An experimental study of hiccup. *Brain* 93:851–872, 1970.
  The first study to counter the ideas of Samuels. Evidence for bilateral hemidiaphrag
  and inspiratory muscle involvement is discussed. The author also proposes that hic
  cups are mediated by a brain stem center separate from the respiratory center.
Nathan MD, Leshner RT, Keller AP. Intractable hiccups (singulus). *Laryngoscop*
  90:1612–1618, 1980.
  This work adds credence to Davis' theory of an independent hiccup center.
Williamson BWA, MacInture IMC. Management of intractable hiccup. *Br Med*
  2:501–503, 1977.
  Review of all agents that have been advocated in reports in the English languag
  Protocol for therapy is offered.

140. SERUM DRUG LEVELS
John F. Rogers

For some illnesses, it is helpful to monitor therapy by measuring serum drug concer
trations. These are usually chronic conditions whose manifestations are sporadic, ur
predictable, or difficult to assess during the brief interval of an office visit. For exam
ple, seizure disorders and cardiac arrhythmias are infrequent and so difficult t
monitor in outpatients that it is necessary to determine an indirect end point such a
a serum drug level. In contrast, conditions such as pain and hypertension have obviou
end points (pain relief, lowering of blood pressure) that are easily monitored by physi
cians. For these conditions, serum drug levels are useful only in unusual situation
(e.g., as a test of patient noncompliance in refractory hypertension).

Utility of the Test: The Assay
For a serum drug assay to be useful, the test must fulfill several technical criteria.

1. There must be *an accurate, precise assay.*
2. *Results must be promptly available* if therapeutic decisions are to be based on th
   information.
3. *Quality control of laboratory:* Physicians should be aware of their particular labora
   tory's capabilities: the types of assays that are done and the limitations that suc
   assays may impose. A particular problem is the assay that is done infrequently
   which is generally subject to much greater test variation. Variation of a test is com
   monly described by the term *coefficient of variation,* a measure of how reproducibl
   the test is if multiple measurements were to be done on the same sample. Acceptabl
   coefficients of variation for drug assays are usually less than 10%. The responsibl
   laboratory should periodically make such data available to practicing physicians.

Utility of the Test: The Drug
Serum tests are most useful for drugs with certain characteristics.

Low Toxic-Therapeutic Ratios
Drugs with low toxic-therapeutic ratios, such as digoxin and theophylline, may requir
serum drug levels for therapeutic monitoring. On the other hand, serum levels are no
useful for monitoring drugs such as penicillins and cephalosporins, where adverse ef
fects are commonly allergic in nature and are rarely related to dose or concentration
(e.g., seizures).

Marked Individual Variation
Marked interindividual variation in absorption, distribution, elimination, or effects oc
curs with some drugs. A 300-mg daily dose of phenytoin given to adults results in a

15-fold range in steady-state levels because of marked interindividual differences in rates of elimination. Correction of dosage on a body-weight basis reduces, but does not eliminate, such variation in serum levels.

Utility of the Test: The Clinical Situation

Whenever ordering serum drug levels, there should always be a clinical question associated with the test. If none exists, there is a risk that the test will create more problems than it solves.

Failure to Respond

When the patient fails to respond to a drug, serum drug levels can suggest why this has occurred. A low level suggests several possible problems: patient nonadherence or medication error; failure to absorb drug because of decreased systemic availability of the preparation; malabsorption, vomiting, or drug interaction; enhanced elimination (e.g., because of hepatic enzyme induction); or inadequate dosage. Levels in the therapeutic or toxic range should raise questions about the drug's effectiveness.

Favorable Response

When the patient is responding favorably to a drug, the use of serum drug levels is of questionable value. There is usually no hypothesis being tested, and an "abnormal" serum level is likely to tempt the physician to react where no response is needed. For example, a serum digoxin level in the "toxic" range in an asymptomatic patient with atrial fibrillation, but with adequate control of ventricular rate, may cause the physician to reduce the maintenance dose of digoxin inappropriately.

However, a serum drug level can be used to establish the individual patient's therapeutic concentration as a baseline against which future serum levels can be compared. For example, a serum phenytoin level of 15 mg/L in a well-controlled epileptic can be used as a target for future dosing if the patient's clinical status and/or serum phenytoin concentration changes.

Signs of Drug Toxicity

When the patient experiences signs or symptoms that are compatible with, but not diagnostic of, drug toxicity, elevated serum drug levels may increase the strength of the evidence in favor of toxicity. However, levels in the therapeutic range do not exclude toxicity.

Therapeutic Range

Table 140-1 lists drugs for which serum levels are commonly available. Each laboratory should provide its own normal range for each test. The interpretation of serum drug levels in individual patients depends on many aspects of the clinical situation (see below). Serum concentrations of antimicrobial drugs are not listed because their use is largely restricted to inpatients.

Clinical trials that have established therapeutic ranges often have done so retrospectively by examining the concentrations at which a group of patients on a fixed dose of drug appeared to be adequately controlled. There are few dose-ranging studies that establish an optimal range of concentrations for each patient and then derive a "therapeutic range" for the population. The lack of detail concerning variation in individual response in most studies compromises the physician's ability to apply such information to a specific patient.

In certain clinical situations, interpreting drug levels in relation to a therapeutic range may be misleading:

1. When total (bound and unbound) serum drug levels are measured and the drug is largely protein-bound, the usual assumptions about serum drug levels and effects may not hold in settings where protein-binding may be changing. For example, phenytoin is highly (approximately 90%) bound to serum albumin, and only the unbound or free concentration of phenytoin is available for drug action. In uncomplicated settings where variation in protein-binding is small, the serum phenytoin level, which is a measure of the total (bound plus unbound drug concentration level), is useful as a therapeutic end point; phenytoin serum concentrations appear to be directly related to both seizure control and neurologic toxicity (ataxia, slurred speech, altered mental sta-

Table 140-1. Serum drug concentrations available for therapeutic monitoring

Class/Drug	Usual therapeutic range
Antiarrhythmics	
Disopyramide	3–5 µg/ml
Lidocaine	1.5–5.0 µg/ml
Procainamide	4–10 µg/ml
Quinidine	2–5 µg/ml
Anticonvulsants	
Carbamazepine	8–12 µg/ml
Phenobarbital	15–40 µg/ml
Phenytoin	10–20 µg/ml
Primidone	5–12 µg/ml
Valproate	50–100 µg/ml
Antidepressants	
Amoxapine	30–120 ng/ml
Amitriptyline (+ nortriptyline)	160–240 ng/ml
Desipramine	150–300 ng/ml
Doxepin	75–200 ng/ml
Imipramine (+ desipramine)	150–350 ng/ml
Lithium	0.7–2.0 mEq/L
Nortriptyline	50–150 ng/ml
Cardiac glycosides	
Digitoxin	10–35 ng/ml
Digoxin	0.8–1.8 ng/ml
Salicylate	15–30 mg/dl
Theophylline	10–20 mg/l

tus). On the other hand, in pathologic situations associated with reduced protein-binding and higher fractions of unbound drug (e.g., acute and chronic renal failure, hypoalbuminemia), the serum phenytoin level may be more difficult to interpret. In renal failure, levels of 5 to 10 mg/L may be associated with adequate seizure control due to a higher percentage of free drug (10–30%) in this setting.

2. When the test measures only the parent drug and not active metabolites, the physician's ability to interpret drug levels may be compromised. For example, current assays of serum procainamide concentrations are sensitive and specific but often do not measure the active metabolite, N-acetylprocainamide. In individuals who rapidly acetylate procainamide (about 40–60% of the population), this metabolite achieves high concentrations, especially if renal impairment is also present, and may play a major role in drug effects.

3. The assays themselves may be unreliable in certain settings. Serum phenytoin levels measured by the popular EMIT method (enzyme-mediated-immuno-transfer assay) are unreliable and give spuriously (two- to three-fold) elevated values in renal failure (perhaps due to retention of a cross-reacting but inactive water-soluble metabolite of phenytoin).

Monitoring Drug Levels

Serum drug levels are interpreted in relation to the time since the last dose of drug was administered. As a general rule, the best time to draw a sample is after "steady-state" conditions have been approximated and at the "trough" point in a given drug level cycle. When a drug is administered chronically, either continuously or intermittently, steady-state concentrations will be approximated after treatment has been continued for an interval equal to aproximately 3 to 5 drug half-lives. The trough point is defined as the nadir of drug concentration during a given interval. With recurrent chronic dosing, it is the time just before the next dose. The disadvantage of using trough concentrations is that the physician cannot observe the maximum concentrations achieved. On the other hand, it allows a physician to assume that the level (if the drug continues to be taken as directed) should be no lower than what was obtained at the trough.

When a patient appears toxic, the drug level can be drawn at any time, remembering that levels obtained within 2 to 6 hours after drug administration may be in a very rapidly changing "absorptive phase."

An Example: Serum Digoxin Levels

The serum digoxin level has been the most rigorously studied test and thus illustrates problems in the use of serum drug levels in general. A sensitive, specific radioimmunoassay has been available for over 10 years. Early studies of this test compared two groups of patients taking digoxin: patients without symptoms compatible with digitalis toxicity and patients having symptoms or signs compatible with digitalis toxicity that subsided after drug withdrawal. Mean serum digoxin levels were statistically significantly different in the two groups. However, there was enough overlap between the two to compromise severely the sensitivity and specificity of the test. Approximately 15 to 20% of patients with no signs or symptoms of toxicity exhibit serum levels in the toxic range. The presence of such overlap makes it difficult to base therapeutic decisions on an elevated serum digoxin level without supporting clinical information. Reducing the digoxin dose might be harmful to the patient with atrial fibrillation who has no signs or symptoms of toxicity but is maintaining adequate ventricular rate control at an elevated serum digoxin concentration.

When a physician observes a patient who has signs and symptoms compatible with either digoxin toxicity or with the underlying disease for which the patient is being treated (e.g., congestive heart failure), he or she is almost always compelled to stop the drug as a therapeutic trial to ensure that no further toxicity occurs. A high serum digoxin level does not confirm a suspicion of toxicity but simply makes that diagnosis more likely. As with many tests, the serum digoxin level is most valuable at extreme levels: very low levels suggest inadequate therapy, usually due to noncompliance; very high levels (greater than 3 ng/ml) are usually associated with toxicity. Such levels are relatively unusual, and unfortunately, the more common intermediate values are of limited use to the physician.

General Principles

Sheiner LB, Tozer TN. Clinical Pharmacokinetics: The Use of Plasma Concentrations of Drugs. In KL Melmon and HF Morelli (Eds.), *Clinical Pharmacology: Basic Principles in Therapeutics.* New York: Macmillan, 1981. Pp. 71–109.
  General review of concepts and principles of monitoring drug concentrations.

Koch-Weser J. Serum drug concentrations in clinical perspective. *Ther Drug Monit* 3:3–16, 1981.
  This paper reviews the philosophic principles related to use of this test. It also describes one of the few successful attempts to relate the serum drug concentration to the intensity of its pharmacologic effects (procainamide).

Taylor WG, Finn AL. *Individualizing Drug Therapy: Practical Applications of Drug Monitoring.* New York: Gross, Townsend, Frank, 1981. Vols. 1, 2, and 3.
  A series of critical monographs on the pharmacokinetics, utility of serum levels, and dosing of most of the commonly monitored drugs. Well-referenced. (A pocket-size manual, Individualizing Drug Therapy: Clinical Notes on the Applications of Drug Monitoring, *is also available.)*

Individual Drugs

Ingelfinger JA, Goldman P. The serum digitalis concentration: Does it diagnose digitalis toxicity? *N Engl J Med* 294:867–870, 1976.
  This paper showed that most previous clinical studies separated patients into pure toxic and nontoxic groups without using symptomatic controls.

Aronson JK, Grahame-Smith DG, Wigley FM. Monitoring digoxin therapy. *Q J Med* 186:111–122, 1978.
  Evaluates 83 adults who were referred for serum digoxin concentration measurement and clinically categorized both before and after digoxin withdrawal. The ability of the test to separate patients into toxic and nontoxic categories was poor due to overlap, although mean concentrations were higher in toxic than in nontoxic individuals.

Bernabei R, et al. Digoxin serum concentration measurement in patients with suspected digitalis-induced arrhythmias. *J Cardiovasc Pharmacol* 2:319–329, 1980.

*Examined the value of serum levels in patients with electrocardiographic signs of di
goxin toxicity. The predictive accuracy and specificity of the test were 88 and 89%
respectively, but the sensitivity of the test was only 62% (the number of elevated con
centrations in those ultimately proved toxic divided by the total number of toxic pa
tients).*

Greenspan AM, et al. Large dose procainamide therapy for ventricular tachyarrhyth-
mia. *Am J Cardiol* 46:456–462, 1980.

*This group has successfully employed an individualized target concentration of pro-
cainamide, which is determined by the drug's ability (at that concentration) to suppress ventricular arrhythmias induced by programmed stimulation.*

Hendeles L, Weinberger M, Johnson G. Monitoring serum theophylline levels. *Clin
Pharmacokinet* 3:294–312, 1978.

*This test has not been evaluated as critically as that for digoxin, but its clinical use is
different. There are great ranges in the dose required to achieve concentrations in the
therapeutic range; many conditions (e.g., heart failure, liver disease, drugs) are encountered in asthmatics that can alter the drug's clearance and, thus, its steady-state
concentration.*

Buchthal F, Svensmark O, Schiller PJ. Clinical and electroencephalographic correlations with serum levels of diphenylhydantoin. *Arch Neurol* 2:624–630, 1960.

*A 50% reduction in seizure activity was achieved in patients whose serum phenytoin
levels exceeded 10 µg/ml. This increased to 86% if levels were increased to 15 µg/ml
or more.*

XX. DIETS

C. Stewart Rogers

Strict sodium restriction may be required for patients with advanced congestive heart failure (CHF) or renal failure, severe hypertension, or cirrhosis with ascites. In the much larger group of patients with mild to moderate hypertension or CHF, modest sodium restriction may allow reduction in drug therapy to safer or less expensive levels. Dietary sodium restriction may also avoid the need for potassium supplements because potassium loss on diuretics is directly related to sodium intake. A nonpharmacologic approach to sodium reduction is also favored by recent evidence that diuretics raise serum cholesterol.

Goals

Salt is 40% sodium (MW 23) and 60% chloride (MW 35). Diets may be expressed as milliequivalents of sodium or as milligrams (or grams) of sodium or salt. The usual, unrestricted American diet contains 3 to 5 gm of sodium, or 7 to 12 gm of salt (130–220 mEq of sodium). Some persons take in more than this; it is unusual for a person with ordinary tastes who satisfies a good appetite to consume much less.

A reasonable goal for patients requiring diuretics for hypertension or CHF would be reduction to 2 gm of sodium or 5 gm of salt (80 mEq of sodium). This is the level achieved in many studies of salt restriction for hypertension control and has commonly produced a 6- to 8–mm Hg fall in blood pressure. For severe CHF or cirrhosis with ascites, a 1-gm sodium diet is often used, and for refractory ascites, temporary diets of 500 mg of sodium are customary. These severely restricted diets are too stringent to be followed by most outpatients.

Implementations

The process of implementing a low-sodium diet includes

1. Choosing a diet prescription
2. Attracting the serious attention of the patient and family
3. Communicating principles of diet and providing useful sources of information for shopping, menu planning, and cooking
4. Adapting diet to food customs of the family
5. Obtaining accurate data on the composition of available foods
6. Ensuring access to low-sodium foods (e.g., bread, milk, special preparations)
7. Planning for patients who eat out often
8. Coordinating low-sodium diet with special prescriptions for potassium, calorie, lipid, and protein contents
9. Evaluating adherence

Each of these steps presents obstacles, and rarely are all fulfilled for patients outside of the hospital. It is obvious that ready access to a committed dietitian is essential to full accomplishment of this goal.

The simplest approach, and thus perhaps that most often effective, is to teach the patient/family which foods are to be avoided. Realistically, this method can be expected to reduce grossly excessive sodium intake to 3 gm per day and, if sufficiently inclusive, to as low as 2 gm per day. The prescription is simple: the use of pickles, salted snack foods, cured meats, canned soups, and table salt must become exceptional rather than routine. Other foods to be curtailed include vegetable juices, salty condiments (catsup, salad dressing, soy sauce), most cheeses, pastas with cheese and tomato sauces, cold boxed) cereals, and canned vegetables.

Many widely available foods are very low in sodium: all fresh fruits and fruit juices, alcoholic drinks (including beer and wine), hot cereals, fresh meats, and fresh or frozen vegetables, including potatoes. Acceptable levels are found in bread, milk, most desserts, and most seafoods (except for crabmeat and sardines). If patients eat large amounts of margarine or butter, use of unsalted products can save hundreds of milligrams of sodium per day. If severe salt restriction is desired, special bread and milk are available.

Table 141-1 shows that two representative meal plans, composed of standard and

Table 141-1. Sodium and calorie content comparison of two meal plans

	Na (mg)	Calorie
Plan 1		
Breakfast		
Orange juice, 6 oz	4	84
Oatmeal, 1 oz	1	109
Banana	2	68
Eggs (2)	140	160
	147	421
Lunch		
Hamburger, 4 oz	76	249
Lima beans, fresh, ½ cup	1	95
Margarine, unsalted, 1 tsp	1	30
Apple juice, 8 oz	6	110
Ice cream, 1 cup	112	257
	196	741
Supper		
Pork roast, 4 oz	93	292
Applesauce, ½ cup	3	227
Green beans, fresh, ½ cup	3	16
Potatoes, boiled, 5 oz	5	145
Bread, 1 slice	114	76
Margarine, unsalted, 2 tbs	2	200
Beer, 12 oz	18	151
	238	1107
24-hour total	581 mg	2269
Plan 2		
Breakfast		
Tomato juice, 6 oz	659	36
Rice Krispies, 1 cup	340	110
Sausage, two 2-oz patties	520	260
Toast, 1 slice, margarine	150	110
	1669	516
Lunch		
Vegetable soup, 1 cup	823	78
Macaroni and cheese, 1 cup	1086	430
Lima beans, canned, ½ cup	228	82
Dill pickle	1000	10
Buttermilk, 8 oz	257	99
	3394	699
Supper		
Ham, 4 oz	1494	176
Mashed potatoes	632	137
Green beans, canned, ½ cup	319	16
Biscuits, 2	540	208
Margarine, regular, 1 tbs	133	100
Vanilla pudding, ½ cup	200	321
Milk, 8 oz	120	121
	3438	1079
24-hour total	8501 mg	2294

available food, equal in calories and similar in cost, can differ by a factor of twelvefold in sodium content. Plan 1 would satisfy the strictest inpatient approach to refractory ascites, while plan 2 would likely frustrate any routine drug regimen for essential hypertension.

Further information about the sodium and calorie contents of food can be obtained from listings in cookbooks and in pamphlets from the food industry and the American Heart Association. A useful list for physicians and for many patients has been published in *JAMA* (248:541–543, 1982). If specific adjustments of potassium, lipids, or protein are required, it is necessary to consult a dietitian. Likewise, if cost, religious or ethnic customs, or lack of competence are involved, the diet prescription is unachievable without individualization and instruction by a teaching dietitian.

Adherence

Adherence to a diet can be determined by measuring a 24-hour urine sodium. In the steady state, a person remains in sodium balance, excreting sodium in the urine at approximately the rate of dietary intake. If diuretic therapy has been stable for 2 weeks or more, and if there is no intercurrent illness, a 24-hour urine for sodium (with creatinine to assess completeness of collection) will estimate the sodium intake. Once patients are aware of the purpose of the collection, some may be transiently compliant just before the test, confounding interpretation. In practice, this test is usually reserved for redirecting therapy in refractory hypertension; however, it should be considered before adding a third medication, accepting poor control or adverse drug effects.

The American Dietetic Association. *Handbook of Clinical Dietetics.* New Haven: Yale University Press, 1981. G3–16.
  A concise, practical review of the clinical indications for sodium restriction, including detailed information for menu planning. Includes 62 references to clinical studies, as well as to food lists and cookbooks. The entire handbook would be an excellent resource for a course in clinical nutrition or as an office reference for dietary information.
Hayes A. Sodium and calorie content of common foods (table appended to advances in cardiovascular pharmacology). *JAMA* 248:541–543, 1982.
  A simple list—quick, clean, and current—of the sodium and caloric content of foods.
Northeast Ohio Affiliate's Low Sodium Cookbook Task Force. *Cooking Without Your Salt Shaker.* American Heart Association in cooperation with the Cleveland Dietetic Association. Dallas: National Center of the National Heart Association, 1978.
  This is an attractive, small cookbook with primary emphasis on recipes with moderately low sodium content. Included are low-sodium ingredients and use of often neglected alternative flavor enhancers.
McCarron DA, Kotchen TA. Nutrition and blood pressure control. *Ann Intern Med* 98(5,Part 2):697–890, 1983.
  A small textbook, in effect, of the state of knowledge in this area. Far more sophisticated and more critical than most reviews. Individual sections cover the range of nutrients, including potassium, calcium, fiber, lipids, and alcohol, as well as sodium.

142. HIGH-FIBER DIETS

R. Balfour Sartor

High-fiber diets have assumed a major role in the management of constipation, diverticulosis, irritable bowel syndrome, and hemorrhoids. Preliminary but exciting animal and human studies suggest that fiber may also improve glucose tolerance in diabetes mellitus and prevent atherosclerotic cardiovascular disease as well as colonic carcinoma. These benefits are believed to be related to fiber's effects on stool bulk and transit time.

Fiber is known to decrease colonic transit time and pressures by increasing fecal bulk (both fecal water content and dry weight). Nondegradable polysaccharides (cellu-

Table 142-1. Dietary fiber in some common foods

Food	Amount	Dietary fiber (gm)
Cereals		
All-Bran	1 oz	9.0
Cornflakes	1 oz	3.0
Rice Krispies	1 oz	1.3
Total	1 oz	2.0
Oatmeal (dry)	1 oz	4.5
Bread		
White	1 slice	0.8
Brown	1 slice	2.0
Whole wheat	1 slice	2.4
Meats and milk products		
Beef steak	6 oz	0
Whole milk	1 cup	0
Egg	1 large	0
Raw fruits		
Apple	1 small	3.1
Banana	1 medium	1.8
Grapefruit	½	2.6
Orange	1 small	1.8
Peach	1 medium	1.3
Pear	1 medium	2.8
Raisins	1½ tbs	1.0
Vegetables		
Green beans	½ cup	1.2
Cabbage, cooked	½ cup	1.5
Carrots, raw	1 medium	3.7
Celery, raw	1 stalk	1.2
Corn	½ cup	3.2
Lettuce	1 cup	0.8
Peas, cooked	½ cup	3.8
Potatoes, cooked	½ cup	2.3
Rice, white cooked	1 cup	0.4
Summer squash	½ cup	2.2

Table 142-2. Representative methods for adding supplemental fiber to the diet

Agent	Average dose/day	Dietary fiber (gm)	Cost/Day
Metamucil	2 tbs	?	47¢
Miller's bran	3 tbs	10	2.2¢
Fibermed cookies	2 cookies	10	47¢
All-Bran cereal	1 oz (⅓ cup)	9	8.5¢

lose, gums, and lignins) swell in the presence of water to form a gel, which by its spongelike effect prevents the absorption of water and electrolytes. The water-holding capacity of different types of foods varies widely, depending on their fiber content and individual fiber composition. Wheat bran is the most hydrophilic, holding 4.5 gm of water per gram.

The amount of fiber in the diet may be increased both by dietary manipulation (see Table 142-1) and the addition of supplemental bran or commercial psyllium preparations. The best source of dietary fiber is from the cereal group: whole-grain breads, bran cereals, and rye crackers. Bran, which is the outer coat of grain that is removed by modern milling, contains the highest known concentration of dietary fiber (44%). Brown bread contains twice the fiber content of white bread, while whole-grain bread contains three times as much. Legumes (beans and peas) contain more fiber by weight than root vegetables (carrots and potatoes), and both are higher than leafy green vegetables which, because of their 90% water content, contain surprisingly little fiber. Fruits contain a moderate amount of fiber, with the best sources being blackberries, dried dates, prunes, raisins, peaches, oranges, and apples. Nuts and popcorn are also good sources of fiber.

Many patients with long-standing symptoms complicated by laxative dependence require supplemental bulk agents to provide at least 10 gm of additional fiber per day. This can be accomplished by any of the agents listed in Table 142-2. Of these options, miller's bran is the cheapest ($0.50 per pound); it can be mixed with hot cereals or sprinkled on food and in some studies has been found to decrease the colonic transit time more than bulk laxatives. Bran's beneficial effects are frequently obtained with less supplementation as the colon is gradually "retrained" over a period of months.

Potential side effects of a high-fiber diet include calcium, iron, magnesium, and zinc malabsorption by sequestration within the intestines and poor patient acceptance. Nearly all patients experience temporary sensations of gaseousness, abdominal distention, and cramping during the first few weeks of fiber supplementation. The physician must explain these side effects to patients before initiating therapy, or they will discontinue the diet before beneficial results are obtained.

Connell AM. Dietary Fiber. In LR Johnson (Ed.), *Physiology of the Gastrointestinal Tract.* New York: Raven, 1981. Pp. 1291–1299.
A brief but thorough review of the physiologic and potential therapeutic effects of dietary fiber.
Brody JE. *Jane Brody's Nutrition Book.* New York: Norton, 1981. Pp. 146–147.
Table of dietary fiber in foods by serving size.
Southgate D, et al. A guide to calculating intakes of dietary fibre. *J Hum Nutr* 30:303–313, 1976.
A guide to calculate dietary fiber in a wide variety of foods.

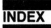

INDEX